FOODS THAT HARM

FOODS THAT HEAL

An A–Z guide to safe and healthy eating

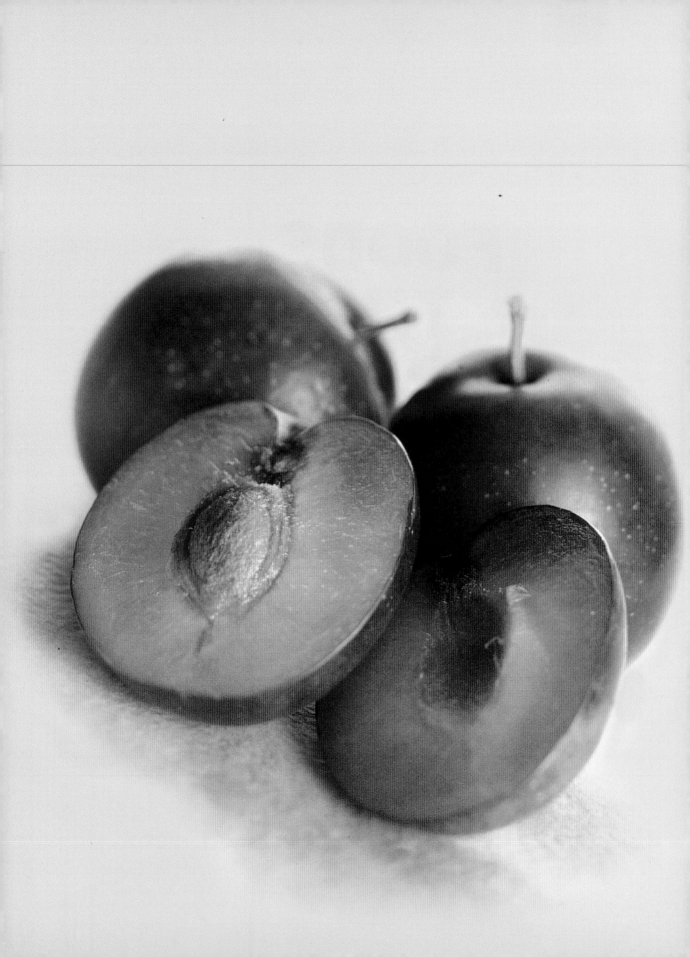

FOODS THAT HARM

FOODS THAT HEAL

*An A–Z guide to safe
and healthy eating*

PUBLISHED BY THE READER'S DIGEST ASSOCIATION LIMITED
LONDON • NEW YORK • SYDNEY • MONTREAL

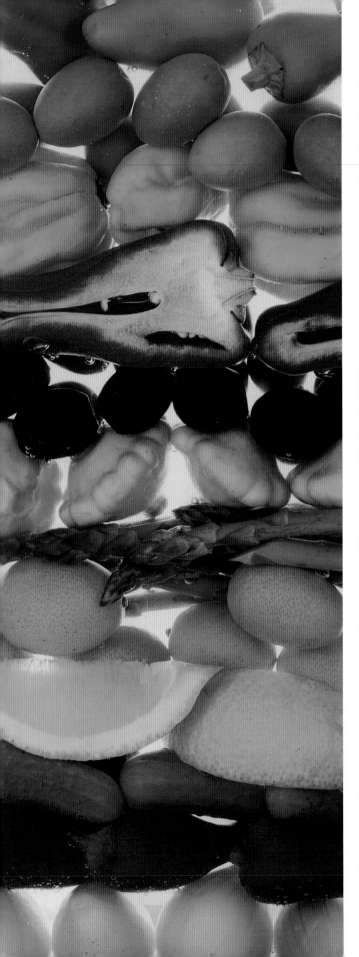

Consultants

Fiona Hunter BSc Hons (Nutrition), Dip Dietetics

Sheena Meredith MB BS

Pamela Mason BSc MSc Phd MRPharmS

Special Features

Contents

Preface **6**

About this book **8**

An A-Z Guide to Safe and Healthy Eating **11**

Glossary **392**

Index **397**

Preface

The quality and variety of food on offer through the UK is greater than ever before. Yet in spite of such abundance (or perhaps because of it) many people make poor nutritional choices. The typical UK diet contains too much fat, salt and sugar and not enough fruit, vegetables or whole-grain cereals. As a result, more than two-thirds of men, just over half of all women and a quarter of our children are overweight, and people of both sexes and all ages continue to grow fatter.

Although rates of coronary heart disease have fallen over the past 50 years, heart disease is still a major cause of premature death. Seventy per cent of UK adults over the age of 40 have high blood cholesterol levels and one in four adults have high blood pressure. A half of all women and one in five men over the age of 50 suffer from osteoporosis (brittle bones). An unhealthy diet increases the risk of many other health problems including Type 2 diabetes, cancer,

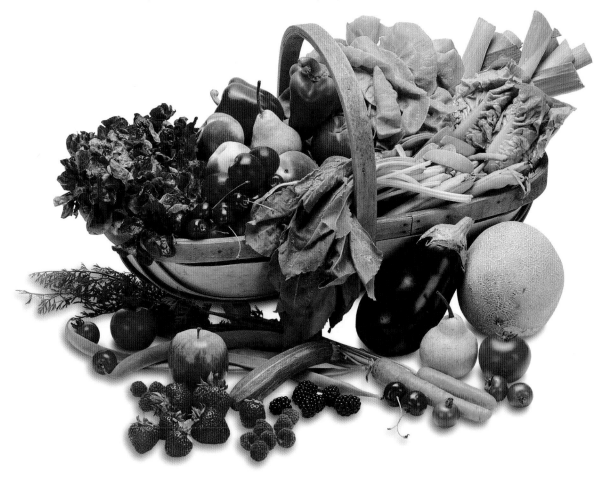

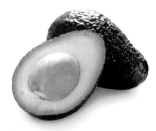

osteoarthritis, and digestive problems. The good news is that it's easy to make changes to reduce the risk of every one of these health problems, once you understand more about food and nutrition.

By altering the balance of foods you eat, you can control your weight (both under and overweight), increase your energy levels to make exercise easier, and help to prevent many health problems. A healthy diet can also reduce the risks associated with high blood fats and it plays an important role in helping to prevent conditions such as Type 2 diabetes, gallstones, high blood pressure, heart disease, certain types of cancer (especially of the bowel, breast and prostate), iron-deficiency anaemia, constipation, joint problems and osteoporosis.

Unfortunately, nutrition is a minefield of misinformation, and confusion is rife. Many people report that they are unsure of what they should be eating, and few know where to go for sound advice that they can easily understand. Facts from genuine experts can make everything clear and provide a simple guide to healthy and enjoyable eating that can make a real difference to your well-being.

Foods that Harm, Foods that Heal was first published in 1996. Since then nutritional and medical research has expanded enormously, allowing us to update and fine tune our original recommendations and offer new advice. In this revised edition we examine new subjects such as 'low-carb' diets and investigate new findings about the Glycaemic Index of foods. We use recent research and clinical trials to investigate certain nutrients and to help to determine which ones fight disease.

Arranged alphabetically, each entry has been written and checked by experts in their field. All facts and figures come from qualified and unbiased sources and reflect the many recent changes to both the food and health industries. This book is refreshingly free of those pushing particular theories through vested interests.

Foods that Harm, Foods that Heal will increase 'food literacy' and as we learn more about food and nutrition, we can free ourselves from conflicting theories and confusion about different diets and understand just how good and easily achievable a healthy diet can be.

Fiona Hunter,
Nutritionist

About this book

Minor changes in your eating habits can lead to major changes in your health: *Foods that Harm, Foods that Heal* explains how. What you eat not only affects your day-to-day health but also helps to determine the quality of your life and even how long you will live. Amid the confusion caused by contradictory claims, scares and reassurances about food and health, this book offers expert, impartial information.

More than 150 food entries, organised from A to Z, give you information on the nutritional value of everything from apples to eggs to yoghurt. Look up 'chocolate' and you'll find out why dark chocolate is probably better for you than milk chocolate. You'll learn that researchers have shown tomatoes could be a powerful weapon in the fight against certain cancers. Elsewhere, read about the potential benefits of alcohol – beer as well as wine.

Food can do more than keep you healthy. Like the best modern medicines, it can also help to heal what ails you. If you have a specific health concern, such as arthritis or diabetes, look it up here to learn what the right diet can do. More than 100 ailment entries reflect the latest, best thinking on foods which can tame inflammation, stop an asthma attack, clean your arteries and even guard against Alzheimer's disease, stroke and cancer. Turn to 'depression' and find some inspiring reasons to eat more fish. And read 'hay fever' to learn which plant foods can actually trigger symptoms.

Beyond the food and ailment entries are special features dedicated to key topics including 'Additives', 'Fast food', 'Genetically modified foods', 'Low-carb diets', 'Pesticides' and 'Probiotics'. Use them to find answers to such questions as: Which fish have the lowest levels of mercury? Is organic produce worth the extra price? Do barbecued foods cause cancer? Turn to 'Glycaemic Index' to find out how to choose foods that will give you more energy and improve your mood. Check 'Dieting' to learn which mineral can help you to lose weight. And in 'Omega-3s and omega-6s', discover how these 'good' fats can benefit people with arthritis, diabetes and heart disease, and where to get them.

Medical and nutritional experts have sifted through the latest scientific studies and reports in order to separate the myths from the facts and help us to create the most authoritative, up-to-date food reference possible. Use it to clear up nagging confusion over carbohydrates, cholesterol, fats and more. Follow its practical advice about the foods you eat every day and how to buy and prepare them. Trust it to help you to make subtle changes to your diet that will pay off in big health benefits over time.

There's no doubt that the right diet is the best prescription for better health. And now we know more than ever before about the power of food to prevent, treat and even cure major ailments and minor annoyances. With *Foods that Harm, Foods that Heal* you can use that information to look better, function better, feel better – and enjoy more years of eating well.

The Editors

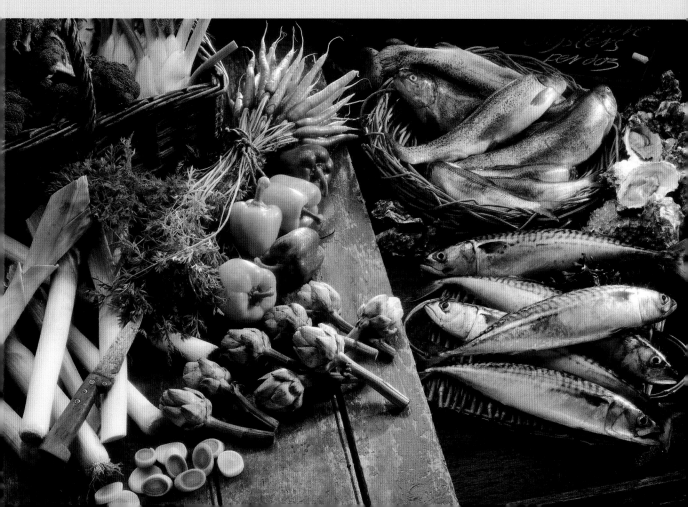

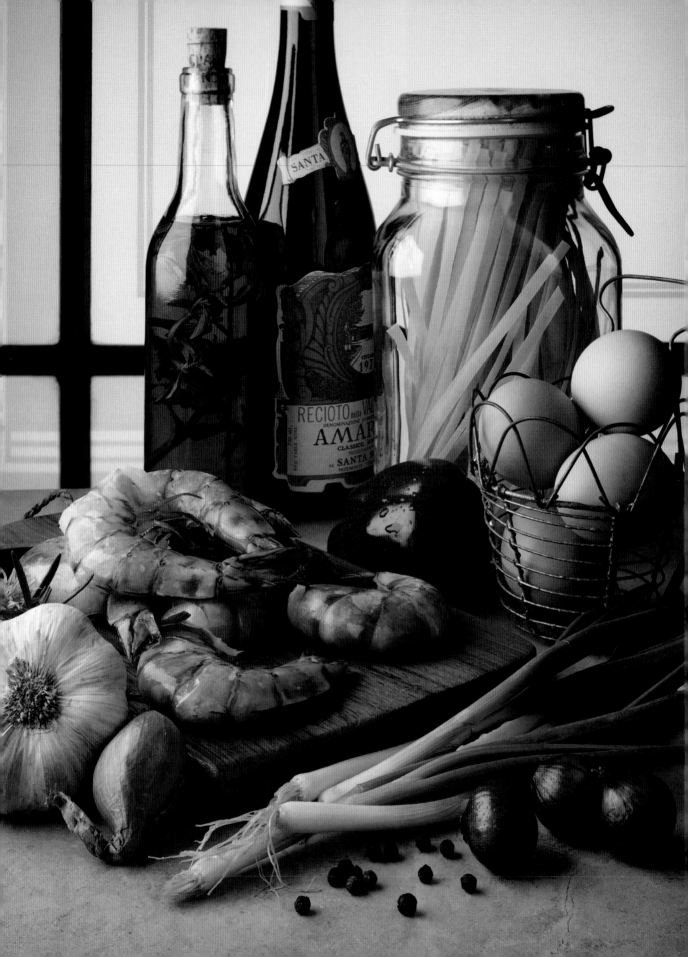

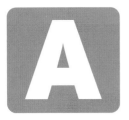

Acne

EAT PLENTY OF

- Fresh fruit and vegetables for beta carotene and vitamin C

- Seafood, lean meat, poultry, yoghurt and whole grains for zinc and vitamin B_6

LIMIT

- Foods high in saturated fat and sugar

- Highly salted snacks and iodised salt

- Kelp supplements

At some time or other during their teens 85 per cent of young Britons suffer from acne – the unsightly spots that are the bane of growing up. Until recently it was a popular belief, though never proven, that it was the high sugar and fat content in 'junk foods' that caused acne.

Although junk food is still thought to be linked to the problem, the fault may lie less with the prime suspects – sugar and saturated fat – than with chemicals that contain iodine. These are often added to the salt that is used liberally on chips, crisps and many other convenience

● **Myth.......**
Some people believe that eating foods like chocolate, French fries, sweets and other high-fat favourites can lead to acne or make it worse.
.......Reality ●
Dermatologists stress that foods do not cause acne, but eating a healthy, balanced diet is vitally important for great-looking skin.

foods. Equally, a bad complexion or dull-looking skin may have more to do with what you do not eat than with what you do. And a diet based on fast foods, sweets, snacks and alcohol is more likely to be low in several vital minerals and vitamins. Either way, youngsters plagued by pimples should cut down on refined carbohydrates found in sugary foods, fatty and fried foods such as burgers and chips, highly salted snacks, soft drinks and sweets, in favour of whole grains, fresh fruit and vegetables, lean meat, a moderate intake of unsaturated fat and plenty of water.

What causes acne

Acne starts when the sebaceous glands overproduce oil, or sebum, secreted through the pores. Sebum carries dead cell debris away with it, but its overproduction blocks pores with a sticky mass of oil and dead cells. When this occurs, the bacteria normally present in skin convert the mass into compounds that irritate and rupture small glands, causing inflammation and pustules.

Some people are genetically predisposed to acne, but the most common triggers are emotional stress and the increased activity of sex hormones, or androgens. These hormones stimulate the oil glands – typically on the face, shoulders, back and chest – and are especially active during puberty. Boys are more prone to acne than girls because they have higher androgen levels, but many girls also suffer, usually in the week before their period.

The zinc link. Research suggests that many acne sufferers are deficient in zinc. Healthy sources include shellfish, nuts, lean meat and skinless poultry. Yoghurt and skimmed milk supply zinc in smaller amounts.

Go for vitamins. Vitamin A, which helps to maintain a healthy skin, is abundant in liver and eggs,

Chemicals and street drugs can also cause acne

The skin disease 'chloracne' is a well recognised clinical sign of exposure to certain chemicals, such as dioxins, which were seen in Vietnam veterans who had been exposed to the defoliant Agent Orange.

Steroids, and the use of the drug Ecstasy, have also been linked with acne-like skin rashes.

while beta carotene, which the body converts to vitamin A, is found in dark green or orange vegetables such as spinach and carrots, and in orange-coloured fruits, such as apricots and mangoes.

An acne-sufferer's diet should contain plenty of unsaturated fats, which have also been claimed to counteract acne. Several of the B vitamins, normally supplied by a well-balanced diet, are believed to prevent blackheads and leave the skin less greasy. A lack of vitamin C is known to make some people more vulnerable to infection, while vitamin E, found in wheatgerm, eggs, and cold-pressed vegetable oils, helps to heal the skin.

Good nutrition is key. Although heredity may be a factor in acne, most persistent mild to moderate acne can be controlled with proper skin care, good nutrition and non-prescription drugs, such as benzoyl peroxide preparations ranging from 2.5 to 10 per cent strength.

A dermatologist may prescribe tretinoin, a topical medication derived from vitamin A, or an antibiotic or, for women, Dianette, a form of the contraceptive pill. Isotretinoin (Roaccutane), a potent oral drug, is reserved for severe cystic acne but can cause severe birth defects. Roaccutane has also been linked with serious psychiatric side effects, but so far clinical trials have not proved these symptoms are caused by the drug.

A

A

Additives
Helpful or harmful?

For centuries, people have enhanced their foods with various flavourings, preservatives and dyes. Many of the 30,000 foods available in our supermarkets contain at least one additive.

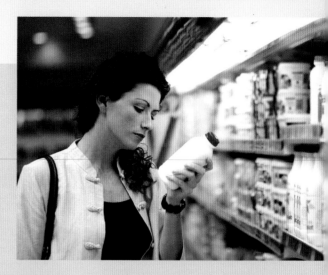

Without additives bread would soon become stale, fatty foods would turn rancid and most tinned fruit and vegetables would lose their firmness and colour. But some additives can trigger allergies and a few may be potentially carcinogenic.

In Britain, some 3,114 substances may be added quite legally to the food you eat. About 2,800 of these are flavourings which need only be described in general terms by the manufacturers who use them. Fewer than 10 per cent of all legal additives are synthetic and they, together with the natural additives that are used, represent less than 0.5 per cent of all the foods we eat. Medical experts place additives a long way down the list of food hazards that face us.

All approved additives must be declared on the food label within the ingredient list, which is arranged in descending order of proportion by weight. Additives can be listed by name or number following the international E numbering system of identification approved by the European Union. The exception is flavourings, where complex mixtures that may include small quantities of many separate substances may simply be listed as 'flavouring'. If an additive or a component of any flavour contains a food product that falls within a list of substances that commonly cause allergies, these must be declared. The products included in this list are cereals containing gluten, as well as eggs, crustaceans, fish, milk, nuts, soya and sesame seed.

ADDITIVES CAN PERFORM USEFUL FUNCTIONS

Additives serve a range of purposes from colouring food, increasing its shelf life or regulating its acidity to making the food more acceptable to the consumer. Some fulfil more than one role.

For example, vitamin C (ascorbic acid) is used to prevent tinned fruit and fruit juice from turning brown, as well as to improve the baking quality of wheat. Citric acid is widely used as both a flavouring agent and as an acidity regulator.

Traditional preservatives, such as wood smoke, salt and vinegar have always been allowed because of their long history of safe use; but approval of new additives is a lengthy procedure involving new tests.

REPLACING LOST COLOURS

Some additives are used to restore colour that has been lost in processing or storage. Without added colour, for example, tinned peas would be an unappetising shade of olive green or grey, and butters and margines would be a pasty white. Some colours, particularly yellow tetrazine, can cause reactions.

Does Chinese Restaurant Syndrome really exist?

Used as a flavour enhancer, monosodium glutamate (MSG) occurs naturally in many foods, contributing to the strong flavours in tomatoes and anchovies. The purified commercial form is made by fermentation and is used like salt in Asian and Oriental cooking. MSG has been blamed for causing Chinese Restaurant Syndrome or CRS. After eating Chinese food, some people experience symptoms of food intolerance, such as swelling of the lips, irritation of the eyes and vomiting.

Studies using capsules containing MSG have failed to prove the existence of CRS. Perhaps the victims of this syndrome are reacting to the high salt content or other components in Chinese food. Histamine, tyramine and phenylethylamine can all cause flushing, palpitations and headaches, and are found in black beans, dried mushrooms and soy sauce, which are all common in Chinese cuisine.

Common food additives

The use of any additive, other than an artificial flavouring is controlled by law. All have to be proved safe, effective and necessary, before they can be used. If an additive has been approved by all the countries in the European Union, it is given an E number, which must appear on the packaging of foods containing it.

TYPE OF ADDITIVE	FOUND IN	FUNCTION
PRESERVATIVES		
Benzoic acid and benzoates (E210-219)	Soft drinks, beer, pickled vegetables, fruit cordials and salad dressings.	Extend shelf life and protect food from bacteria and other micro-organisms.
Nitrites and nitrates (E249-252)	Processed meats, such as sausages, bacon, ham and salami. Smoked fish.	Extend shelf life and protect food from bacteria; preserve colour in meats.
Sulphur dioxide and sulphites (E220-228)	Dried fruit and vegetables, sausage casings, cooked prawns and wines. Desiccated coconut, fruit-based pie-fillings and relishes.	Extend shelf life and protect food from bacteria; preserve colour and moisture in dried fruit.
ANTIOXIDANTS		
Ascorbic acid (vitamin C) and ascorbates (E300-304)	Fruit juices, drinks and cordials, breakfast cereals.	Ascorbates prevent fruit juices from turning brown and improve baking quality in wheat-based cereals.
BHA (butylated hydroxyanisole) and BHT (butylated hydroxytoluene) (E320-321)	Chewing gum, instant potato and fatty foods that can turn rancid, such as baked products, potato crisps and fats and oil.	Extend shelf life and protect food from becoming rancid.
Tocopherols (vitamin E)	Oils and shortenings.	Prevent rancidity in fats and other damage to food due to exposure to oxygen.
COLOURINGS		
Quinoline yellow (E104) Sunset yellow (E110) Beetroot red (E162) Tartrazine (E102) Brilliant blue FCF (E133) Food green (E142)	Many processed foods, especially confectionery and products marketed for children, soft drinks, baked goods, icings, ice cream, jams and margarine. Also used in yoghurts, cheese spreads, pickles, soups, sauces and curry pastes.	Make food look more appealing. Restore colour lost by processing. Provide colour to artificially flavoured foods. Some may cause allergic reactions such as wheeziness or hyperactivity in sensitive people.
FLAVOUR ENHANCERS		
Monopotassium glutamate (622) Sodium inosinate (631) MSG (monosodium glutamate) (621)	Chinese food, gravy powders, stock cubes, packet soups and canned, processed and frozen meats.	Improve the flavour of many canned or processed foods. Studies have failed to prove MSG causes symptoms of food intolerance.
EMULSIFIERS, STABILISERS AND THICKENERS		
Guar gum (E412) Glycerol (E422) Gum arabic (E414) Lecithin (E322) Pectins (E440) Cellulose (E460) Sorbitol (E420)	Sauces, soups, baked goods, frozen desserts, ice cream, fat-reduced cream cheese, jams, jellies, condiments, chocolate, quick-setting desserts, milkshakes and spreads.	Improve texture and consistency of processed foods by increasing smoothness, creaminess and volume. Hold in moisture and prevent separation of oil and water. Excessive sorbitol can result in diarrhoea. Gums may cause flatulence and abdominal pain. Some may trigger adverse reactions.

EXTENDING SHELF-LIFE

Extending the shelf-life of foods is a valuable aspect of additives. Without preservatives, canned and frozen foods deteriorate and become toxic. In addition to salt, vinegar, alcohol and spices, some foods are preserved with artificial forms of naturally occurring benzoates. Some people have adverse reactions to benzoic acid; others are allergic to the sulphites and sulphur dioxides that are used to kill the yeasts that cause sugar fermentation.

The organic acids, such as acetic and propionic acid added to cereal to prevent the formation of mould are harmless. Refrigeration has helped to eliminate the need for some preservatives.

HALTING OXIDATION

To halt oxidisation (which can affect the colour of fruits and cause fats to go rancid) producers use a wide range of antioxidants. In addition to vitamin C (ascorbic acid), butylated hydroxytoluene (BHT) and butylated hydroxanisole (BHA) are also widely used to prevent rancidity in fats and oils. There were some concerns about the safety of BHT and BHA, but these have now been largely resolved. Compounds similar to BHT and BHA occur naturally in rosemary, and some producers now use extracts of the herb instead.

MIXING OIL AND WATER

Emulsifiers are used to enable oils to be mixed with water into an emulsion. They are needed to make foods such as mayonnaise, margarine and low-fat spreads. Two widely used emulsifiers are lecithin and monoglycerides, which are constituents of naturally occurring substances such as egg yolk and soya.

NON-STICK ADDITIVES

Until recently, additives known as mineral hydrocarbons were sprayed on dried fruit to prevent individual pieces from sticking together. This was stopped when the government advised

C A U T I O N

Watch out for yellow colouring tartrazine (E102). It has been linked with adverse reactions in sensitive people who are typically aspirin intolerant, allergic or asthmatic. Symptoms may include hives, itching, runny nose and asthma. Although it does not represent a major health risk to most people, its use in children's medications is clearly inappropriate.

manufacturers that these hydrocarbons could gradually accumulate in the body's lymphatic system. However, minute quantities are still allowed in chewing gum and in the non-edible rinds of some cheeses, such as Edam or Gouda. Because neither chewing gum nor cheese rind are meant to be swallowed, they are not regarded as health hazards. Mineral hydrocarbons are still used, however, to prevent bread sticking to baking trays.

THE QUESTIONABLE FEW

The majority of food additives are safe, but there are exceptions, and every now and then, one is removed from the market as new information is evaluated. The fact that some colourings are banned in some countries but allowed in others demonstrates that, in some cases, 'safety' is open to interpretation. A recent scare about the colouring Sudan red 1, which appeared as a 'contaminant' in some imported products containing Indian chilli powder, resulted in the EU taking precautions against further imports, because of concerns that the red colouring used may have been carcinogenic.

Activist groups have fuelled worries about complete groups of additives in some instances. The case of artificial sweeteners is an example.

◀ **Fresh is best**
Eating fresh foods is one obvious way to avoid additives but always wash fruits and vegetables carefully as some people can suffer unpleasant skin reactions to pesticide residues on the skin or leaves of non-organic produce.

AIDS and HIV infection

CONSUME PLENTY OF

- Meat, poultry, liver, eggs, milk, nuts and other high-calorie, high-protein foods to prevent weight loss

- Pasta, rice and other starchy foods, vegetables, juices and fruit for essential vitamins and minerals

- For small appetites, eat small meals/snacks through the day

LIMIT

- Fatty foods and wholegrain products if they cause diarrhoea, which can reduce absorption of some nutrients

AVOID

- Raw or undercooked foods, especially shellfish, eggs and meats

- Alcohol, which can worsen diarrhoea and can interact with some AIDS medications

There is still no cure for AIDS (acquired immune deficiency syndrome), nor is there a special diet for people infected with HIV, the human immunodeficiency virus that causes the disease. But good nutrition can prevent or delay weight loss and other complications.

Asymptomatic HIV-infected people should follow the same sort of diet recommended for healthy people, but with added precautions. Because the HIV organism attacks the immune system, sufferers are more vulnerable to infections, including food poisoning from salmonella, campylobacter, shigella and other bacteria. Such food-borne infections occur more frequently and are more severe in people with reduced immunity.

Keep up your food intake. AIDS is a wasting disease, and anyone with AIDS should avoid missing meals, should take snacks and, unless markedly obese, not worry about gaining weight. The extra weight can prove to be critical in surviving a crisis when eating is difficult.

Unfortunately, maintaining good nutrition is complicated by the ways in which AIDS affects the digestive system. It reduces the absorption of nutrients, especially folic acid, thiamin, riboflavin and vitamins B_6 and B_{12}; it often causes intractable diarrhoea, which causes further nutritional loss; and it increases the risk of intestinal infections. Many AIDS patients also suffer appetite loss and bouts of nausea, either from the disease or from medications.

If rapid weight loss occurs, artificial feeding may be required; this is generally administered through a gastric feeding tube inserted into the stomach or an intravenous line that pumps predigested nutrients into the bloodstream. Some AIDS specialists advise artificial feeding if nutrients are not being absorbed properly.

Food safety

Anyone who is HIV-positive, or a person who prepares food for an AIDS patient, must pay special attention to food safety. Wash hands before handling food, during its preparation and after. Keep hot foods hot and cold foods cold. Avoid contact between raw and cooked foods. Eggs should be boiled for at least 7 minutes; meat and fish should be well cooked, with an internal temperature of 74°C–100°C. Raw shellfish, sushi, steak tartare, rare hamburgers, as well as homemade mayonnaise and ice cream made with raw eggs are best avoided. Bought mayonnaise and hard ice cream are safe.

Wash fruit and vegetables well. They are not as likely to cause problems as animal products, but

Practical hints and tips for HIV-infected people

When mouth or throat infections, such as thrush or ulcers, make eating uncomfortable: Try soft, moist foods that are easy to swallow, such as mashed potatoes and gravy. Use a straw for liquids. Allow cooked food to cool slightly before eating it as hot foods can add to discomfort. Drink low-acid beverages such as milk or smoothies. Avoid foods and juices with high acid content.

When you suffer from nausea or diarrhoea – common side effects of many HIV medications: Drink plenty of fluids to replace what you've lost. Drink water, broth or flat ginger ale, or eat crushed ice. When you are ready to eat, start out with bland foods such as toast or crackers. Try eating small snacks through the day. Eat slowly and chew food well. If you find the smell of food bothers you, ask someone else to prepare it and keep out of the kitchen. As the diarrhoea improves, try some non-irritating foods such as chicken, eggs, fish and yoghurt.

When you suffer from frequent bouts of diarrhoea: Avoid eating raw fruit and vegetables and high-fibre foods, such as whole-grain breads and cereals. You should also avoid gassy foods, such as cabbage, onions and beans, spicy foods and carbonated beverages. Stay away from rich, fatty foods and alcohol.

should be washed thoroughly. Follow the same precautions that you would when travelling in parts of the world where hygiene standards may be low: eat only cooked vegetables and fruit that is peeled, stewed or canned. Never eat food cooked on the street.

Use of supplements

Nutritionists often recommend that HIV-positive people take a multiple vitamin and mineral supplement to prevent nutritional deficiencies; however, supplements with more than 100 per cent of the RDA (Recommended Dietary Amount) should be used only if prescribed by a doctor or dietitian. Many people self-treat with high-dose supplements, a course that can lead to serious problems. High doses of vitamin C, for example, can worsen diarrhoea.

Fighting the virus. Vitamins B_6, B_{12}, pantothenic acid and folate are vital to immune function, as is vitamin A (plentiful in liver, egg yolk and many dairy products).

The antioxidants beta carotene (in dark green leafy vegetables and orange fruits and vegetables), quercetin (in onions), vitamin C (in citrus fruits and kiwi fruit) and vitamin E (in cold-pressed oils, nuts and avocados) are all important as scavengers of free radicals. The minerals zinc and iron, and trace element selenium are also known to boost immune function. Selenium may play a key role in delaying the progress of HIV infection.

A macrobiotic or other restrictive diet, especially one that is restricted to brown rice and a few vegetables, can actually worsen AIDS, because it fails to provide adequate nutrition; and too much fibre can exacerbate diarrhoea.

Infection-fighting mushrooms could help people with AIDS

Many neuropaths and alternative practitioners consider fungi to be champions in the fight against disease, and shiitake mushrooms in particular are known to stave off infection. Lentinan, a compound found in shiitake mushrooms, is thought to have immune-enhancing properties and so may be beneficial to AIDS sufferers.

Herbal medicine is a popular self-care approach, though there is no evidence of its efficacy. Caution is needed as some herbal preparations contain substances that can cause serious side effects or interact with prescription medications. Check with a doctor before taking any herbal or other preparation or before engaging in self-treatment or complementary medicine.

Alcohol

BENEFITS

■ Moderate consumption cuts the risk of heart attack by raising HDL cholesterol and reducing the risk of blood clot formation

■ May protect the brain against age-related dementia

■ In small amounts, it can aid digestion and improve appetite

■ May foster a happy mood

DRAWBACKS

■ Can provoke mood swings, aggression and hangovers and can be addictive

■ Interacts with many medications

■ Over time, moderate to high intake increases the risk of cancers, as well as heart and liver disease

People have used alcohol in one form or another since prehistoric times. While alcohol is primarily drunk for its mood-altering effects, the results of recent studies suggest that there are actually benefits to moderate drinking. 'Moderate drinking' is defined as 3-4 units a day for men, and 2-3 units a day for women. Pregnant women should have only 1-2 units a week.

A unit is the equivalent of a small glass (125ml) of wine or sherry, half a pint of ordinary strength beer or a single measure (25ml) of spirits.

What does 'proof' mean?

The term 'proof' refers to the alcoholic strength. Proof spirit contains 57 per cent alcohol by volume or 48 per cent alcohol by weight. Brandy and whisky are usually 70-80 per cent proof, which equates to 33-40 per cent alcohol.

What is alcohol?

Ethyl alcohol (ethanol), which is the main active ingredient of alcoholic beverages, is made by the yeast fermentation of starch or sugar. Almost any sweet or starchy food – potatoes, grains, honey, grapes and other fruit – even dandelions – can be turned into alcohol.

Unlike most foods, alcohol does not need to be broken down before it is absorbed; 95 per cent of it is absorbed into the bloodstream from the stomach and small intestine within an hour. (The other 5 per cent is eliminated through the kidneys, lungs or skin.)

The liver breaks down, or metabolises, alcohol; the time this takes depends upon whether the alcohol is ingested with food and upon the person's sex, weight, body type and tolerance level, which increases with time and use. On average, however, it takes the liver 3 to 5 hours to completely metabolise 30ml of alcohol.

Latest medical research on alcohol

Recent medical studies have found that drinking small amounts of alcohol, especially red wine, may lower the risk of a heart attack. This is good news for anyone who enjoys a little red wine with their dinner. But does alcohol provide other protective health benefits? And can protection come with red wine only?

One study revealed that having one drink a day lowered the risk of cardiovascular disease by 5 per cent, but having two drinks a day lowered it by 10 to 13 per cent.

▶ **Good health!**
Moderate drinking has been proven to
improve appetite and aid digestion.

The risk of a heart attack is lower
because alcohol reduces the harmful
effects of elevated blood cholesterol
while also preventing clot formation.
This study showed that levels of bad
cholesterol (low-density lipoprotein,
or LDL) became lower, as did
triglyceride levels: high levels of
either raise the risk of heart disease.
Many studies show that a regular
and moderate intake of alcohol may
increase the levels of protective
(high-density lipoprotein, or HDL)
cholesterol. The results are especially
significant for women over 50 since
a woman's risk of heart disease rises
sharply after menopause.

Just how alcohol protects is still
unclear, but some researchers note
that because red wines especially
contain certain polyphenols, which
can act as antioxidants – resveratrol
being the prime example – they can
be expected to protect cells from
damage that normally occurs when
the body uses oxygen. It's believed
that oxidation of LDLs is what
causes blood vessels to clog. The
polyphenols may also fortify LDL
cholesterol against oxidation and
prevent blood cells sticking together
to form clots.

It's not just red wine that is
protective. Results of several studies
have linked moderate consumption
of alcohol with a 32 per cent lower
risk of heart attack and a decrease in
stroke of 20 to 28 per cent. Results
from other studies also suggest that
people who drink light to moderate
amounts of alcohol daily lower their
risk of diabetes significantly but
heavy intake increases the risk.

Alcohol protects the brain
Several studies report that people
who imbibe moderately every day
are about 70 per cent less likely

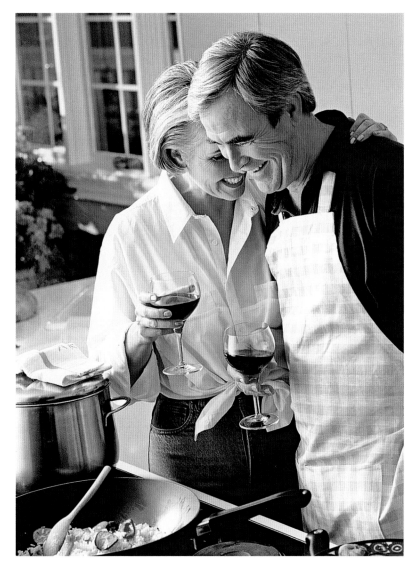

What causes a hangover?

Overconsumption of alcohol invariably results in a hangover; just how much alcohol
is necessary to produce a hangover depends on the biochemical individuality of the
consumer and the type of drink consumed. Spirits, such as whisky and gin, have a
more immediate impact than wines or beers, and all alcohol is absorbed more
quickly when mixed with a carbonated beverage. Once in the bloodstream, alcohol
reaches the brain in minutes. At first it acts as a stimulant, producing euphoria. This
soon gives way to central nervous system depression and feelings of numbness, and
then finally to sleep or unconsciousness. A rapid ingestion of a large amount of
alcohol can be fatal. The severity of a hangover is partially influenced by 'congeners',
which are the by-products of the fermentation process that contribute to the taste
and aroma of an alcoholic beverage. The more congeners in a drink, the more severe
a hangover may be. Brandy has the greatest number of congeners, followed by red
wine, rum, whisky, white wine, gin and vodka.

A

than nondrinkers to develop dementia, an age-related decline in mental ability; they are also more than 30 per cent less likely to develop Alzheimer's disease. Alcohol seems to offer a number of brain-related benefits. It thins the blood and helps to prevent clots from clogging tiny blood vessels in the brain; and it seems to stimulate the release of acetyl-choline, a brain chemical involved in both learning and memory.

However, you should consume no more than the recommended daily limit. Alcohol's protective effects are indeed impressive, but studies show that overconsumption may significantly raise the risk of developing a number of health problems, including high blood pressure, cardiac arrhythmias, liver disease, stroke, dementia and several kinds of cancer, including cancer of the liver, pancreas, oesophagus and mouth. In addition, alcohol is addictive. Over-indulgence quickly

What's in a drink?

Alcohol contains 7kcal per gram, compared with 4kcal per gram of protein or carbohydrate and 9kcal per gram of fat. The British Medical Association has made recommendations for low-risk drinking (designed to minimise harm, rather than for good health). For nonpregnant healthy women, low-risk drinking is defined as an average of 2-3 units per day. Recommended upper limits are 14-21 units over a week. Pregnant women and those hoping to become pregnant should try to avoid alcohol although, after the twelfth week of pregnancy, an occasional drink is not considered harmful. For healthy men, the daily average is set at 3-4 units with never more than 28 units over a week. Saving up the recommended allowance and binge-drinking over a weekend places an extra strain on the liver and can bring on attacks of gout and pancreatitis.

TYPICAL DRINK	ALCOHOL/ VOLUME	NUMBER OF UNITS	KILOCALORIES (KCAL)
SPIRITS			
Standard bottle (750ml)	40%	30	1500
Single pub measure (25ml)	40%	1.5	50
SHERRY OR PORT			
Standard bottle (750ml)	20%	15	1075
Single pub measure (50ml)	20%	1	75
WINE			
Standard bottle (750ml)	8-14%	6-10.5	780
Small pub glass (125ml)	8-14%	1	85
Large pub glass (175ml)	8-14%	1.5	120
ORDINARY BEER, LAGER OR CIDER			
Large can (440ml)	3.5%	1.5	140
Small can (275ml)	3.5%	1	90
1 pint	3.5%	2	180
STRONG BEER OR LAGER			
Large can (440ml)	7%	3	280
Small can (275ml)	7%	2	170
1 pint	7%	4	350

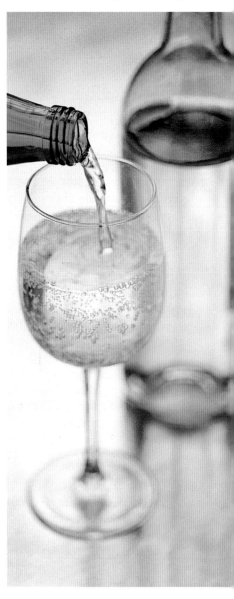

▲ **Wine in moderation**
If you are trying to reduce your alcohol intake, but don't want to forgo the pleasure altogether, try topping up a glass of white wine with soda water. This enjoyable, refreshing drink is known as a wine spritzer.

Facts about alcohol

- The hops that give the distinctive taste and aroma to beer come from a vine that is a relative of cannabis.
- A cold shower, strong coffee and similar remedies are of no value in helping a person to sober up.
- Large amounts of alcohol lower sexual performance in men. Alcohol reduces levels of testosterone, the male sex hormone, while increasing oestrogen levels, which can lead to impotence, shrunken testicles and male breast growth.
- Women absorb alcohol into the bloodstream more quickly than men.

erases any benefits. Even a weekend of heavy drinking causes a build-up of fatty cells in the liver. While this organ has remarkable recuperative powers, continued use of alcohol can lead to liver damage and problems with glucose metabolism and eventually scarring, or cirrhosis. Alcohol also interferes with the body's metabolism of various vitamins and minerals. It has been shown that those women who consume alcohol daily have a higher risk of breast cancer than those who do not. The risk increases with amount of alcohol consumed.

Any heart benefits associated with drinking stop after that second drink. A third drink does more harm than good, actually raising the triglyceride levels without reducing the LDL cholesterol.

The key, with alcohol, as with everything else in life, is moderation. Try to have at least one alcohol-free day a week.

Alcoholism

Alcoholism is as chronic drinking that interferes with one's personal, family or professional life. While an occasional drink is not likely to be

harmful, it is important to recognise that alcohol can be easily abused. Genetic predisposition, learned behaviour and childhood experiences, including abuse, are all thought to foster alcoholism. Progression of the disease varies from one person to another. For some, it develops as soon as they begin to drink; for most people, however, it progresses slowly from periodic social drinking to more frequent indulgence until finally the person is addicted.

Some alcoholics are binge drinkers and can go for weeks or even months without alcohol. But once they have a drink, they are unable to stop until they are incapacitated or pass out. Although these drinkers have difficulty staying sober, they are unlikely to suffer severe withdrawal symptoms when they abstain. In other cases, abstinence of 12 to 24 hours will produce withdrawal symptoms, such as sweating, irritability, nausea, vomiting and weakness. More severe symptoms develop in two to four days and may include delirium tremens (DTs), a condition which is marked by fever and delirium.

The chronic overuse of alcohol takes a heavy toll. Alcoholics often do not appear to be intoxicated, but their ability to work and go about daily activities becomes increasingly impaired. They are very susceptible to depression, mood changes and even violent behaviour. Their suicide rate is higher than that of the general population. On average, alcoholism shortens life expectancy, not only from suicide but also because it raises the risk of life-threatening diseases, including cancer of the pancreas, liver and oesophagus. Women who drink heavily while pregnant may have a baby with foetal alcohol syndrome, a constellation of birth defects, including mental retardation.

Nutritional effects

Alcoholism can lead to malnutrition, not only because chronic drinkers tend to have poor diets, but also because alcohol alters metabolism and digestion of most nutrients. Severe thiamin deficiency (marked by muscle cramps and wasting, nausea, appetite loss, nerve disorders and depression) is very common, as are deficiencies of folate, riboflavin, vitamin B_6 and selenium. Many alcoholics suffer from a deficiency of vitamin D, which helps the body to absorb calcium, so they are at risk of bone fractures and osteoporosis. Impaired pancreatic and liver function may result in poor digestion. As alcohol stimulates insulin production, glucose metabolism speeds up and can result in low blood sugar. Alcoholics are often overweight, as alcohol is high in calories.

Diet and supplements help. Once an alcoholic stops drinking, the nutritional problems are tackled one by one. Supplements are prescribed to treat deficiencies. A diet addresses underlying problems; for example, an overweight person needs a diet that reverses nutritional deficiencies without additional weight gain. If there is liver damage, protein intake must be monitored to prevent any further liver problems.

Danger signs. These are the signs that will tell you your drinking is out of control:
- Needing a drink to feel at ease or forget your worries.
- Forgetting what you have said or done when drunk.
- Surreptitious drinking and preferring to drink alone.
- Drinking and driving.
- Neglecting meals in favour of alcohol.
- Persistent shakes, night sweats and hallucinations.
- Being unable to give up, even though warned by a doctor to do so.

A

Allergies
Reactions to food

The true incidence of adverse reactions to foods is not known, but studies indicate that only a fraction of people who think they have food allergies will test positive to the alleged allergens.

True food allergies involve the body's immune system and can be diagnosed by skin prick or blood tests. Allergies usually begin in infancy and young childhood, and most disappear by school age, although allergic reactions to nuts and seafood may persist throughout life.

An intolerance to various natural or added food chemicals can occur at any age. Food intolerances are less dangerous than allergies, and are more difficult to diagnose as they do not involve the body's immune system and no reliable diagnostic tests are available. Diagnosis involves removing all foods likely to cause a reaction, and if symptoms disappear, specific foods are added in a systematic fashion, preferably by a doctor or dietitian who specialises in this area. It is important to maintain a nutritionally adequate diet during the elimination and the re-introduction phases of diagnosis.

Doctors do not completely understand why the number of people who have adverse reactions to foods is increasing, although heredity is an important consideration. If both parents have allergies, their children are much more likely to have them as well, although the symptoms and allergens may be quite different. There is no doubt that breastfeeding and the delayed introduction of solid foods reduces a child's chances of developing food allergies.

Allergies develop in stages. When the immune system first encounters an allergen (or antigen) – a substance that it mistakenly sees as a harmful foreign invader – it signals specialised cells to make antibodies, or immunoglobulins, against it. There is no allergic reaction in that first exposure; however, if the substance again enters the body, the antibodies programmed to mount an attack against it will go into action. In some cases, the response will not produce symptoms; but the stage will have been set for a future antigen-antibody reaction and an allergic response.

Food intolerances may develop at any age and are related to the quantity of the substance ingested. This makes diagnosis difficult as small quantities of a natural or added chemical may build up and it is only when the total amount consumed goes over one's limit that a reaction will be apparent. One example is when the amines in chocolate or red wine are blamed for causing a headache or skin rash, but the problem may occur only if chocolate or red wine are the 'last straw' to a build-up of related amines from foods such as avocado, cheese, ham, banana, tomato, oranges and mushrooms consumed earlier in the day.

COMMON SYMPTOMS

Common symptoms of food allergies include nausea, vomiting, diarrhoea, skin rashes or hives, itching, shortness of breath (including asthma attacks) and, in severe cases, widespread swelling of the skin and mucous membranes. Swelling in the mouth

The latest on peanut allergy

An allergy to peanuts is one of the most dangerous food allergies, both because peanut products are widely used in processed foods and because even minute amounts of peanut protein, in rare cases, can be enough to trigger fatal anaphylactic shock. Researchers have determined that diagnosis of a peanut allergy is not necessarily a lifelong sentence. A blood test to measure peanut specific antibodies can identify children who may have outgrown their allergies. They can then be tested in a controlled situation with a small amount of peanut protein to see if they are still allergic. Children with a peanut allergy should be retested under strict medical supervision every few years.

A

Common food allergies and intolerances

Almost any food can provoke an allergic reaction. This chart lists the eight most most common culprits and their symptoms. They account for 90 per cent of allergic reactions or intolerances, although no established figures exist for them.

FOOD TYPES	MAIN FOODS	SYMPTOMS
MILK AND MILK PRODUCTS	Dairy products, such as milk, butter, cheeses, yoghurt, ice cream, cream and cream soups.	Constipation, diarrhoea, wind, rhinitis, catarrh, migraine, irritable bowel syndrome. Wind, colic, catarrh and eczema in babies.
EGGS (ESPECIALLY EGG WHITES)	Cakes, ice cream, meringues, mousses and other desserts; mayonnaise, salad dressings, French toast, waffles, pancakes and Caesar salad.	Rashes, swelling and stomach upsets. Can cause asthma as well as eczema.
SOYA AND SOYA PRODUCTS	Soya milk, soya beans, tofu, textured vegetable protein, miso, soy sauce, cake and pancake mixes, tempeh, canned and condensed soups, some gluten-free breads and cereals.	Headaches and indigestion.
WHEAT AND WHEAT PRODUCTS	Flour, bread, biscuits, barley, rye, beer, canned soups, stock cubes, any processed foods containing 'rusk' or hydrolised vegetable protein.	Migraine, coeliac disease (characterised by diarrhoea and weight loss) and irritable bowel syndrome.
NUTS	Peanuts (also called ground nuts) and peanut oil, peanut butter; walnuts, cashews and pecans; baked goods and muesli bars with nuts; nut-flavoured breads, biscuits and ice cream.	Rashes, swelling, asthma and eczema. In severe cases, potentially fatal anaphylactic shock.
ADDITIVES	Packaged, processed and takeaway food and drinks; the colouring agent tartrazine and the preservative benzoic acid.	Hyperactivity and behavioural changes have been attributed to some additives.
FISH	Smoked fish, such as kippers, mackerel, haddock and smoked salmon; fresh fish such as cod and sole.	Migraine, nausea, skin rashes, swelling and stomach upsets.
SHELLFISH	Crustaceans, such as prawns, crab, lobster, langoustine and crayfish; molluscs, such as clams, oysters, mussels and scallops; seafood dishes and fish-flavoured soups.	Prolonged stomach upsets, migraine and nausea.

What is anaphylactic shock?

Severe allergic reactions to foods can result in a life-threatening collapse of the respiratory and circulatory system, known as anaphylactic shock. If you have had, or believe you may be susceptible to, an anaphylactic reaction, you should wear medical identification, and carry emergency medical information in your wallet. Parents should provide a child's school with an EpiPen if a child is known to have a severe nut or seafood allergy.

or throat is rare, but potentially fatal because it can block the airways to the lungs. In the most severe cases, anaphylactic shock (see above) may develop.

Allergens usually provoke the same symptoms each time, but many factors affect intensity, such as how much of the offending food was eaten, and how it was prepared. Some people can tolerate small amounts of an offending food; others are so hypersensitive that they react to even a minute trace.

Symptoms of food intolerance vary but may include hives and eczema, headache, mouth ulcers, nausea, stomach cramps and sinus problems. Feeling generally unwell or becoming moody may also be symptoms, although these are also symptoms of many other problems.

ALLERGENS AND CHILDREN

Some allergens are easily identified because symptoms develop immediately after eating the offending food. The most allergenic foods in infancy are egg, milk, peanuts, wheat and soya (about 85 per cent of children lose their sensitivity within the first three to five years of life), whereas in older children and adults nuts and seafood are the most likely to cause severe reactions. Cooking can often reduce the allergenic potential of foods as the proteins responsible for allergies are degraded by heat. This, however, is not always the case. Roasting peanuts makes them more allergenic.

PINPOINTING ALLERGIES AND INTOLERANCES

Foods that cause allergies and intolerances are not always readily identified. It is useful to keep a documented diary of the time and content of all meals and the appearance and timing of subsequent symptoms. After a week or two, a pattern may emerge. If so, eliminate the suspected food from the diet for at least a week, and then try

it again. If symptoms develop, chances are you have identified the offending food. In cases of a true allergy (as opposed to intolerance), one or more of the following tests may be required.

SKIN TEST: The most common test, where food extracts are placed on the skin, which is then pricked or scratched, allowing the penetration of a small amount of the extract. Development of a hive or itchy swelling usually indicates an allergic response.

RAST (radioallergosorbent test) blood study: Small amounts of the patient's blood are mixed with food extracts and then analysed for signs of antibody action. This may be safer for hypersensitive people, who may have a severe reaction to the skin test.

LIVING WITH FOOD ALLERGIES AND INTOLERANCES

Once problem foods or ingredients have been identified, eliminating those foods from the diet should solve the problem. But this can be more complicated than it sounds. Some of the most common food allergens are hidden ingredients in many processed foods. Also it would be impossible to guess the sources of problem chemicals that are widely distributed in natural foods. Dietitians can provide lists of food to avoid and alternative ingredients. In some cases of food intolerance, people may be able to build up their tolerance to problem food chemicals by starting with a low intake of carefully selected foods and gradually increasing the intake.

When an allergic reaction is too weak or elusive to identify, a diet rich in antioxidants (from fruit and vegetables) and omega-3 fatty acids (from oily fish) has an anti-inflammatory effect and will reduce the body's inflammatory reaction.

ALLERGIES AND MEDICATIONS

Certain medications can predispose some people to food intolerances: teenagers may develop digestive disorders after long-term use of tetracycline antibiotics for acne.

Some people develop irritable bowel syndrome after treatment with antibiotics; others experience allergic reactions after taking steroids or oral contraceptives. To make diagnosis even more difficult, it is possible for several mechanisms to produce the same result.

Almonds

See Nuts and seeds

Alzheimer's disease

CONSUME PLENTY OF

- Fruit and vegetable juices

- Leafy green vegetables, orange juice, liver, cooked beans and lentils, peas, sweetcorn, asparagus, nuts, breads and cereals with added folate

- Lean meat, fish, poultry or dairy products for vitamin B_{12}

- Meat, fish, poultry, whole grains, lentils, beans, avocados, bananas, potatoes, nuts and leafy greens for vitamin B_6

- All types of seafood, especially salmon, swordfish, mackerel, herring, trout and sardines for omega-3 fatty acids

- Eggs, liver, soya products, whole grains, brewer's yeast and wheatgerm – all reasonably good sources of lecithin and choline

AVOID

- Antacids with aluminium

- Obesity

Alzheimer's disease is a brain disease that affects memory, language and reasoning. It is the most common form of dementia in people over the age of 65, accounting for up to 70 per cent of cases of dementia.

There are more than 400,000 Alzheimer's sufferers in Britain, and the number is rising. The disease usually begins after 60, afflicting more women than men. It is characterised by abnormal deposits of a protein called beta-amyloid (plaque) in the brain as well as by twisted fibres caused by changes in a protein called 'tau' (tangles). Before arriving at a diagnosis, tests are needed to rule out other conditions which present with similar symptoms, such as stroke, a brain tumour and other possible causes of senile dementia.

Blood tests can uncover genetic markers. The cause of Alzheimer's disease is unknown, but researchers believe that chromosomal and genetic factors are responsible for some cases. The increased incidence of Alzheimer's among those with Downs syndrome, which is caused by a chromosomal abnormality, seems to support this theory. Researchers have discovered a genetic marker, called apolipo-protein E, which can be detected by blood tests, that identifies those people likely to develop the disease. About 40 per cent of sufferers have the gene that produces this protein.

Thyroid disorders have also been linked to the disease, while the long-term use of nonsteroidal anti-inflammatory drugs (NSAIDs) has been associated with a reduced Alzheimer's risk. These drugs may reduce inflammation in the brain linked with the disease. There is insufficient evidence, however, for physicians to recommend taking NSAIDs in the hope of warding off Alzheimer's disease.

Foods that fight Alzheimer's

Researchers are finding some links between diet and dementia, and there is evidence that some foods may help in the battle against Alzheimer's.

SEAFOOD, especially fish like salmon, mackerel, herring, trout, tuna and sardines are rich in omega-3 fatty acids and should be eaten at least three times a week.

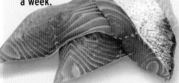

EGGS are a good dietary source of choline – a component of lecithin. They are also a good source of vitamin B_{12} and other B vitamins, an excellent source of protein and very easy to eat and digest.

WHEAT GERM AND WHOLE GRAINS high in lecithin and choline, carbohydrate, vitamin E, B vitamins and numerous minerals may help to forestall Alzheimer's.

SOYA products are rich in choline and provide protein, calcium and fibre. They are a good source of folic acid and are known to lower blood levels of homocysteine.

A

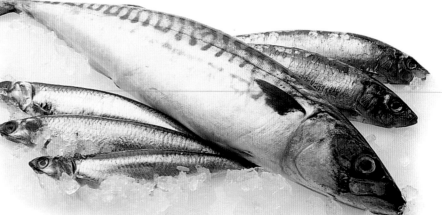

▶ **Feed on fish**
Increase the amount of cold-water, deep-sea fish in your diet and you'll be increasing your chances of avoiding Alzheimer's disease. The anti-inflammatory properties of the omega-3 fatty acids present in these fish may help to prevent the formation of plaques in the brain.

Predicting Alzheimer's

Exciting studies have shown that brain scans (PET scans) of regions connected with memory may help to predict Alzheimer's. Another means of prediction is a urine test which detect damage associated with mild cognitive impairment, such as memory loss, which is a precursor to Alzheimer's There is also a new formula to help doctors predict the likelihood of a patient developing Alzheimer's. It is based on age, sex, level of education, body mass index, blood pressure level, physical activity and genetic factors. Each is given a risk score and by combining these an overall score is reached. If this is done early enough, therapeutic action can be taken to help the person to avoid or at least delay, the development of dementia.

Diet and Alzheimer's

Researchers are studying the role of the B-vitamin folic acid in reducing the risk of Alzheimer's. This vitamin helps to regulate blood levels of homocysteine, an amino acid, high levels of which may play a part in the development of the disease. Studies have shown that

Medical proof that risk can be cut by diet
Researchers at Chicago's St. Luke's Medical Center found that people aged 65 and older who had fish once a week had a 60 per cent lower risk of developing Alzheimer's disease than those who did not eat fish.

people with Alzheimer's have high homocysteine levels and there is evidence that high concentrations of homocysteine in healthy adults may lead to Alzheimer's.

Vitamins B_6 and B_{12} also help to regulate homocysteine levels. People with high blood cholesterol and high blood pressure are also at greater risk and taking cholesterol-lowering drugs, particularly 'statins', has been shown to reduce the risk. Blood-pressure-lowering drugs and diuretics are also helpful. It appears that what is good for the heart is also good for the brain – which is rich in DHA (docosahexaenoic acid), an omega-3 fatty acid plentiful in seafood, especially salmon, mackerel, trout, herring and sardines. Low levels of this essential fat have been linked with Alzheimer's disease and other age-related forms of dementia.

Antioxidants may prevent it. A recent study suggests that the risk of developing Alzheimer's may be cut by by 76 per cent by drinking fruit and vegetable juices. They mop up free radicals and have been touted as possible preventives for Alzheimer's since the body's ability to neutralise these rogue substances declines with age. Fruit and vegetables may also lower the risk by helping to lower blood pressure and keeping the blood vessels in good order.

People with Alzheimer's disease have abnormally low levels of choline acetyltransferase, an enzyme necessary to make acetylcholine, a brain chemical believed to be instrumental in learning and memory. Also, the brain cells most affected by Alzheimer's are those that normally respond to acetyl-choline. Some nutrition researchers theorise that supplements or foods high in lecithin or choline (the major component of acetylcholine) can also slow the progression of Alzheimer's by raising acetylcholine production. So far, studies have failed to document its value, but some nutritionists feel that foods high in lecithin and choline may help forestall symptoms and will certainly do no harm; these foods include egg yolks, offal, soya products, peanuts, wheatgerm and whole grains.

Monitor nutrition carefully. As the disease progresses, its victims may forget to eat or eat only sweets or foods with low nutritional value. Nutritionally balanced meals are important, even if spoon-feeding is required for those who cannot feed themselves. Taking a multivitamin may also be advisable; high-dose supplements should not be given unless specifically recommended by a doctor. In large amounts, alcohol destroys brain cells. A healthy person can tolerate this loss, but it can accelerate the progression of Alzheimer's disease. Small amounts of wine, however, are associated with a lower incidence of Alzheimer's. Alcohol may interact with antidepressants, sedatives and other medications prescribed for Alzheimer's patients.

Evidence is accumulating for the 'use it or lose it' theory of reducing Alzheimer's risk. People who exercise their brains with puzzles, games, and education seem to be less sensitive to brain damage.

Danger: aluminium?

There have been other intriguing theories, but researchers have been unable to pinpoint any specific dietary factors that increase the risk of Alzheimer's disease. Some research appeared initially to implicate aluminium, which has been found in the abnormal tangles of brain cells in some Alzheimer's patients. However, extensive studies since have failed to prove that aluminium actually causes the disease, and it now seems more likely that aluminium is found in Alzheimer's brains simply because the diseased brain retains it.

Avoid taking antacids with aluminium. Although most researchers discount the aluminium factor, some argue that while the metal may not cause the disease, its increased concentration in the Alzheimer's brain worsens the condition. They suggest that patients avoid taking antacids with large amounts of aluminium or using aluminium cookware that could allow the metal to leach into food if the food is acidic (such as tomatoes, rhubarb and fruit).

Concern has also been raised about the aluminium content of drinking water in areas where aluminium compounds are used as flocculating agents in city water treatment.

Anaemia

EAT PLENTY OF

- Red meats, especially beef, poultry and seafood, especially oysters and mussels for iron and vitamin B_{12}
- Beans and peas, dried apricots, nuts, seeds and green vegetables which are all useful sources of iron
- Iron-enriched breakfast cereals
- Fresh fruit or vegetables at each meal – their vitamin C increases the body's iron absorption
- Green leafy vegetables, lentils, beans, asparagus, sweetcorn and enriched cereals for folic acid

LIMIT

- Strong tea, which hinders iron absorption

AVOID

- Iron supplements, unless prescribed by a doctor

Anaemia is the umbrella term for a variety of disorders characterised by the inability of red blood cells to carry sufficient oxygen. This may be due to an abnormally low level of haemoglobin, the iron and protein-based red pigment in blood that carries oxygen from the lungs to all body cells. Symptoms of anaemia, therefore, reflect those of oxygen starvation. In mild anaemia, this may include general weakness, pallor and fatigue. The more severe cases of anaemia are marked by shortness of breath, fainting and cardiac arrhythmias.

Iron-deficiency anaemia

The most common type of anaemia is due to iron deficiency, usually caused by blood loss of some type. Women with heavy menstrual periods, especially adolescents, are at risk. Young children, chronic dieters, female athletes, distance runners or people on restricted vegetarian diets may also develop low iron levels. Pregnant women are predisposed to anaemia because of the demands of the growing baby and placenta. People with a bleeding ulcer or those with chronic or repeated bleeding such as nosebleeds may also have iron-deficiency anaemia. In men, a blood test that shows iron deficiency often prompts a doctor to investigate the possibility of colon cancer.

Other types of anaemia

Haemolytic anaemia occurs when red blood cells are destroyed more rapidly than normal. The cause may be hereditary or the result of one of various diseases, including leukaemia, other cancers, abnormal spleen function, auto-immune disorders or severe hypertension.

Pernicious, or megaloblastic, anaemia is caused by a deficiency of vitamin B_{12}, which is necessary to make red blood cells. Stomach acid releases B_{12} from protein in food. The vitamin then binds to a substance called intrinsic factor that enables B_{12} to be absorbed in the bloodstream. This means that you can develop a B_{12} deficiency if your stomach produces insufficient acid.

Supplements for older adults. Up to a third of elderly people produce inadequate amounts of stomach acid and can no longer properly absorb B_{12} from food. Elderly people may have to meet

Do one simple thing

Cook in iron pots

Cooking tomatoes and other acidic foods in iron pots can add significant amounts of iron to food. Half a cup of tomato sauce cooked in a regular pot provides 0.7mg of iron; cooking it in an iron pot adds 5mg. This may be desirable for iron deficiency, but would create problems for those predisposed to iron overload (or haemochromatosis).

A

C A U T I O N

Do not take iron supplements unless
you have had a blood test to confirm
an iron deficiency. Excess iron can
be dangerous for anyone with
undiagnosed haemochromatosis,
or 'iron overload' disease. For these
people, taking iron supplements can
have catastrophic results.

their B₁₂ need by eating food that
has been fortified with B₁₂ or by
taking B₁₂ supplements. Because the
vitamin is found only in animal
products, vegetarians are potentially
at risk of B₁₂ deficiency and should
eat fortified foods and/or take a
B₁₂ supplement.

Deficiency of another B vitamin,
folic acid, which is not found in
foods of plant origin, can cause a
type of anaemia in pregnant women
(who need extra folate for the
developing foetus), alcoholics, the
elderly, vegetarians and vegans.

Relatively rare types of anaemia
include thalassaemia, an inherited
disorder and aplastic anaemia,
which may be caused by infection,
exposure to toxic chemicals or
radiation or a genetic disorder.

How much iron do you need?

The human body recycles iron to
make new red blood cells. Even so,
the body loses an average of 1mg for
men and 1.5mg for women during
reproductive years. The body takes
in only a 10 per cent of dietary iron,
(pregnant women absorb more) so
the Reference Nutrient Intake (RNI)
calls for more than the amount lost:
8.7mg a day for men and post-
menopausal women; 14.8mg for
women aged 19-50.

Those who have nutrition-related
anaemias can benefit from a session
with an accredited dietitian or a
qualified nutritionist in order to
help to structure a healthier diet.

There are two main types of iron
found in the body: haem iron and
non-haem iron. The best sources of
haem iron are found in animal
products such as meat, fish and
poultry. The body absorbs 20 to 30
per cent of the haem iron found in
these foods compared with the 5 to
10 per cent of non-haem iron from
plant sources, such as green
vegetables, dried fruit, soya and
other pulses, nuts, seeds, iron-
enriched breads and cereals, whole
grains, tofu and eggs.

Strict vegetarians, or those people
who rely heavily on plant food to
get iron, need to ensure an adequate
intake of foods such as pulses, green
vegetables, whole grains and tofu.
Adding a vitamin C-rich food to a
plant-based meal can enhance the
body's absorption of non-haem iron.
Haem iron also promotes the
absorption of non-haem iron from
other foods when eaten at the
same meal. The amount of non-
haem iron absorbed increases when
the body's iron reserves are low.

**Watch out for natural
compounds in tea, called tannins.**
They can bind with iron and make
it unavailable for absorption. It is
best to drink your tea between

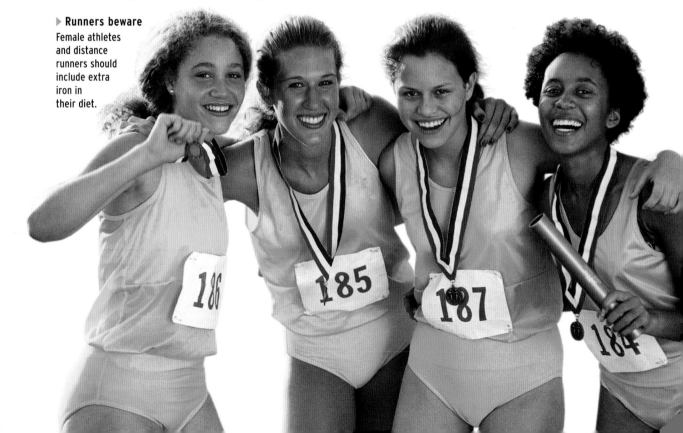

▶ **Runners beware**
Female athletes
and distance
runners should
include extra
iron in
their diet.

meals rather than during. Oxalates found in spinach, rhubarb and chocolate as well as phytates found in nuts and bran cereal also can bind with iron and prevent the body from using it.

It is possible to be genetically predisposed to iron 'overload' – a condition called haemochromatosis – which can damage heart and liver.

Anorexia nervosa

CONSUME

- A variety of nutritious foods in small amounts
- High-protein liquid supplements and multivitamin supplements, if approved by a doctor or dietitian

AVOID

- Diet soft drinks and low-calorie or low-fat diet foods
- Appetite suppressants, diuretics and laxatives

The self-starvation that is a hallmark of anorexia nervosa is caused by a complex psychiatric disorder. It is estimated to occur in approximately 90,000 Britons, mostly adolescent girls or young women. (Only about 10 per cent of people with anorexia are males; they are often weight-conscious adolescent boys who are dancers or athletes.)

The cause of anorexia nervosa – a medical term for a relentless pursuit of extreme thinness and refusal to eat to maintain normal weight – is unknown. Researchers believe that a combination of hormonal, social and psychological factors are responsible. The disease often begins in adolescence, a time of hormonal and psychological change. Convinced of being too fat, often regardless of actual weight,

the individual begins to diet obsessively. Some adopt a very restricted diet while others become overly preoccupied with food, often planning and preparing elaborate meals that they then refuse to eat. When they do eat, they may resort afterwards to self-induced vomiting or laxative abuse to avoid gaining weight. Many exercise obsessively.

Take note of telltale signs. As the disease progresses in girls, menstruation ceases and nutritional deficiencies develop. Many girls with anorexia try to hide their thinness by wearing oversized clothes. Physical signs of anorexia include nervousness, fatigue, hyperactivity, dry skin, hair loss and intolerance to cold. More serious consequences include cardiac arrhythmias, loss of bone mass, kidney failure and in about 6 per cent of cases, death.

Treatment strategies

Anorexia often requires intensive long-term treatment, preferably by a team experienced with eating disorders: a psychiatrist, a doctor to treat starvation-induced medical problems and a dietitian. Family members will often benefit from counselling, too.

Sufferers tend to defend their eating habits and resist treatment. Most are treated as outpatients; in severe cases, hospitalisation and nutritional therapy are necessary.

The biggest hurdle is to help toovercome the abnormal fear of food and distorted self-image of being fat. Counselling tries to uncover the source of these fears.

In the beginning, the patient is offered small portions of nutritious and easily digestible foods, perhaps eggs, custard, soups or milk shakes. Portion sizes and the variety of foods are increased gradually to achieve a steady weight gain. This does not require huge amounts of

> ## CAUTION
>
> Younger women are particularly vulnerable to eating disorders like anorexia nervosa, a serious, often chronic and life-threatening condition. Although the word 'anorexia' means loss of appetite, people with anorexia nervosa ignore hunger and deliberately control their desire to eat.
>
> Constant obsessive dieting may result in severe anorexia and sufferers may be at risk of death from starvation.
>
> Should someone you know exhibit the following warning signs, contact a doctor knowledgeable about eating disorders immediately.
>
> - Preoccupation with food
> - Distorted body image, thinking they are fat when they are actually bone-thin
> - Intense fear of gaining weight
> - Refusal to eat
> - Deliberate self-starvation
> - Denial of hunger
> - Obsessive exercise
> - Loss of scalp hair
> - Brittle nails and hair
> - Constant complaining about feeling cold (due to low body temperature)
> - A fine layer of hair on the body or face (like on a newborn baby)
> - Depression
> - Irregular or absent periods

food; instead, doctors strive for a varied diet that provides adequate protein for rebuilding lost lean tissue, carbohydrate for energy and a moderate amount of fat for extra calories. Extra calcium and multivitamins may also be given.

Monitor food intake closely. People with anorexia are skilled at deceiving others about their eating. Relapses are common and close monitoring may be necessary to ensure that the person is really eating. But avoid making food a constant source of attention and conflict; group therapy can be more helpful than parental nagging.

A

Anti-ageing diet
Eat wisely to age well

As you get older, your body's energy needs drop; at the same time, demands for some nutrients increase. New studies indicate that paying more attention to the foods you eat and making good nutritional choices may slow the ageing process.

Ageing is inevitable, but some degenerative changes that manifest themselves after middle age are not, if preventive steps are taken. Good nutrition can prevent, or at least slow, such debilitating conditions as osteoporosis, diabetes and heart disease. In fact, one report estimates that a third to a half of the health problems of people over the age of 65 are related to their diet.

Proper nutrition is an important part of any 'ageing-well' strategy. Yet, some people fail to eat well. There are many reasons for this: a person's appetite and the senses of taste and smell decline with age, making food considerably less appealing. Many older people experience difficulty chewing; in addition, heartburn, constipation and digestive problems increase with age and contribute to poor nutrition. Stomach acidity also declines with age, and this impairs the absorption of nutrients. The loss of a partner, or difficulty in shopping or preparing meals, may result in a person subsisting on tea, toast, sweets, canned soups and other foods that provide little nutrition.

Interesting facts about longevity

◼ A few years ago, gerontologists revealed that residents of the Okinawan Islands in southern Japan lived longer than anyone else in the world. Their diet secret? Lots of grains, vegetables, soya and fish; less meat and poultry, and fewer dairy products. Now Okinawan life expectancy is falling, say the team who first drew attention to the phenomenon, as younger Okinawans succumb to a fast-food diet that is causing rising obesity levels.

◼ Various studies of Mormons, Seventh-Day Adventists and Trappist monks – all people who follow a vegetarian diet and engage in a prudent lifestyle – also show that they enjoy increased life expectancy.

◼ A recent Spanish study of people aged between 65 and 80 showed that those who ate a Mediterranean diet were 31 per cent less likely to die in the next nine years than those who didn't. The diet includes bread, fish, fruit and olive oil, but very little red meat, ice cream or processed foods.

▶ **A healthy diet**
Choose foods that are low in saturated fat and rich in whole grains, fruit and vegetables.

A

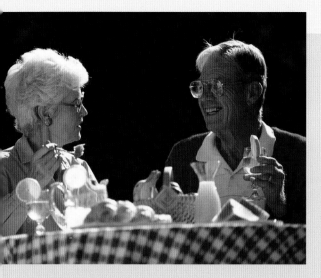

◀ **Eating a healthy, nutritional diet**
As you age, make sure you still enjoy a wide variety of nutritious foods. Remember, the more diversity in your diet, the better the quality, in terms of vitamins, minerals, trace elements and fibre.

CHANGING NEEDS

A person's body composition changes with age, as muscle mass decreases, often due to disuse, and fatty tissue increases. Because metabolism slows down, fewer calories are required; experts estimate that the average person should consume 10 per cent fewer calories for every decade after the age of 50. Therefore, a 50-year-old who needs 1,500kcal a day may require only 1,225kcal at the age of 70.

People who fail to cut back on their food intake are likely to gain weight, thus increasing the risk of heart disease, diabetes and osteoarthritis.

With increasing age, the body is less efficient in absorbing and using some nutrients; osteoporosis and other medical conditions common among older people also change nutritional needs. Consequently, an older person may need extra amounts of the following essential nutrients:

- Calcium for healthy bones and to prevent osteoporosis.
- Vitamin D, which the body needs in order to absorb the calcium.
- Vitamin B_{12} to build red blood cells and maintain healthy nerves.
- Zinc to counter lowered immunity due to ageing.
- Potassium, especially in the presence of high blood pressure or the use of diuretic drugs.

Medical proof that food is a powerful medicine

According to a 2003 medical study there's nothing fishy about fish oil's ability to protect your heart. Omega-3 fatty acids from fish oils can prevent sudden cardiac death by blocking fatal heart rhythms, researchers say. Sudden cardiac death accounts for at least half of heart-related deaths. Eating seafood, particularly fish such as salmon, trout, mackerel, herring and sardines, has long been associated with a reduced risk of heart disease. Omega-3 fats are credited with keeping arteries healthy and reducing the stickiness of platelets in the blood.

Elsewhere, researchers found that, in older people, eating fish more than once a week was associated with a 50 per cent reduced risk of macular degeneration, the chronic eye disease which accounts for a third of all cases of vision loss that gradually destroys central vision.

Studies also indicate that fish oils may protect against Alzheimer's disease.

If you don't like fish, consider omega-3 supplements; these are made from fish liver oils that contain vitamins A and D as well as omega-3 fats. Because of the vitamin A, they are not recommended for pregnant women, and no one should exceed the recommended dose. Some people choose a supplement made from fish body oils, instead, which have a lower level of vitamins A and D and as seen as a safer option.

- Folic acid, a B vitamin, which the body uses to make DNA and red blood cells, may also help to lower blood levels of homocysteine, a compound in the blood that has been associated with an increased risk of heart disease.
- Fibre to prevent diverticular disease and constipation.

SUPPLEMENTS MAY BE NEEDED

A lack of attention to diet may mean that older people face the risk of developing vitamin deficiencies. Some doctors recommend a daily vitamin and mineral supplement to ensure that an older person takes in 100 per cent of the recommended daily amount. However, a multivitamin cannot take the place of healthy food because foods contain additional important components such as fibre, plant chemicals and essential fatty acids. Also, high-dose supplements should be avoided unless prescribed by a doctor

A

or dietitian, as they can lead to nutritional imbalances. For example, zinc supplements can interfere with the body's use of folic acid, and iron can inhibit proper calcium and zinc absorption.

MAKE THE MOST OF MEALTIMES

Although nutrition is all important for ageing well, healthy eating isn't just about the nutrients. Sharing a meal with family and friends provides many more benefits than just the food on your plate. Sharing your food and your life enables you to build up a support system to help you to weather physical ailments, stress and emotional problems, and derive more pleasure from life. If the thought of cooking and eating meals holds little pleasure, for whatever reason, try some of these practical tips to make dining an enjoyable occasion.

Do one simple thing

Drink lots of water every day

Water is essential to health. It helps to regulate body temperature, transports nutrients to your body's cells and helps to remove waste. Because sensitivity to thirst diminishes with age, older adults are susceptible to dehydration, which can cause confusion, fatigue, headache and more. The exact amount a person requires varies with body size and the climate. Most people need six to eight glasses each day, and tea and coffee count towards the total.

■ Try to make your meals pleasurable, even if you're eating alone. Set the table or prepare an attractive tray for yourself. Play your favourite music.

■ If you dislike eating alone, why not organise regular 'bring and share' meals with friends and neighbours. Or perhaps you could consider joining a dining club which provides an opportunity to eat with other members.

■ Select those foods that supply contrasts in colour, texture and flavour. Avoid adding salt in order to improve the flavour; instead, use herbs and spices. Remember that a sprinkling of nutmeg or cinnamon can compensate to a large degree for a diminished sense of taste. Using garlic to flavour your food not only makes it more delicious, but it may help to lower high cholesterol.

■ Eat at least five servings a day of fruit and vegetables, which are rich in fibre, potassium, folic acid and antioxidants. Include a serving each time you eat. Many of these contain compounds that protect against diseases of ageing such as heart disease and cancer. Choose brightly coloured fruit and vegetables such as carrots, broccoli, peppers, pumpkin, melons and oranges. The more colourful your diet, the more antioxidants you are getting – and that cuts down the effects of free radicals in your body.

■ A small glass of wine or beer with a meal aids digestion and adds to eating pleasure. But don't substitute alcohol for food, and check with your doctor to make sure that it does not interact with any medications you might be taking.

■ Make sure you drink six to eight glasses of water, juice, or other non-alcoholic fluids every day. Older people often experience decreased thirst or they reduce fluid intake because of bladder-control problems. This can contribute to constipation and kidney problems and increase the risk of dehydration in hot weather. Water also helps to regulate your body temperature.

■ If you have trouble chewing, see a doctor or dentist first, in case your problem is treatable. If it's not, prepare fish or minced meat and puréed vegetables, soups and other nutritious foods. A purely liquid diet can lead to digestive problems.

■ Take daily walks or engage in other exercise, but first consult your doctor for an appropriate routine. Exercise not only preserves muscle strength but also improves your appetite and your general mood.

C A U T I O N

If you do not regularly expose at least some portion of your skin to the sun, your body may be seriously lacking in vitamin D, which is essential for the absorption of calcium. The majority of this vitamin is made in our skin when it is exposed to sunlight. Our desire to protect our skin against the sun's harmful rays lead many people to shun it altogether. Vitamin D is important in helping calcium to shore up bones to protect older people against fractures. An average 20 minute, daily exposure of some part of the skin (for example, the forearms) to the sun is all that is required. If that isn't possible, older people might consider taking 10mcg of vitamin D a day.

A

- If you're on a tight budget, why not organise a co-operative shopping arrangement with others in a similar situation. Buying larger quantities is more economical. You can share with others, or divide the food into smaller portions and freeze them for future use.
- Be informed and read the labels. Even if you have to take along a magnifying glass to see the small print, reading the breakdown of the nutrients on a food package's label will help you to make healthier food choices.

EAT LESS TO LIVE LONGER?

Since the 1930s, scientists have known that restricting calories not only delays ageing but even reverses some of its consequences in laboratory rats and mice. By feeding these animals a very low-calorie diet, a mere 30 to 50 per cent of what they normally eat, scientists have been able to extend the lives of both mice and fruit flies.

One study was designed to see whether monkeys, fed a diet that included all the required nutrients but two-thirds the usual calories, would live longer than normal. Data suggests that the primates who ingested a lean meal, as compared with their peers who ate all the food they wanted, had a lower incidence of heart disease, diabetes and cancer.

▶ **Fresh vegetables**
New US research has shown that eating a wide variety of vegetables actually helps people to consume fewer calories overall. They play a key role in weight management.

One theory as to why there's a link between eating less and living longer, is that the metabolism of food leads to the production of free radicals; and the less food consumed, the fewer damaging free radicals are produced.

Energy restriction is risky to try on your own. While it's generally known that older people require fewer calories, it is important to remember that the ageing body is also less efficient in absorbing and using some nutrients.

Knowing how to cut your calories without compromising the essential nutrients can be tricky. Becoming undernourished would erase any benefits that there might be in such a diet. Low-calorie diets are likely to be deficient in some nutrients.

Far more effective, in the long run, is to avoid becoming obese in the first place. Obesity can reduce your lifespan by an average of nine years.

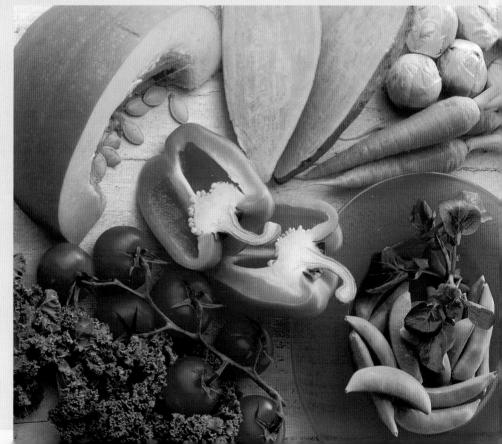

A

Antioxidants
Sorting facts from hype

Recent research on antioxidant supplementation in the form of pills has yielded conflicting results. But there is no doubt about one thing – eating a diet high in foods that are rich in antioxidants, such as brightly coloured fruit and vegetables, is a wise choice. And studies show that the reasons for this seem to mount as you get older.

There are hundreds of studies linking fruit and vegetables that are rich in antioxidants to a lower risk of heart disease, cancer and many other illnesses. But why is eating fruit and vegetables so healthy? Is it due to some specific compounds found in plant products or is it some special combination of nutrients? Or is it that people who eat lots of fruit and vegetables eat less meat, or that in general they consume fewer calories? Whatever the case, the antioxidant theory merits investigation.

Top 10 antioxidant fruits and vegetables

The Oxygen Radical Absorbance Capacity score (or ORAC score) is an analysis that is used to measure the total antioxidant power of foods and other chemical substances. The higher the ORAC score, the greater its antioxidant capacity. This is a laboratory measurement and its relevance to the diet is, as yet, unclear.

ORAC scores per 100g

Fruit		Vegetables	
Prunes	5770	Kale	1770
Raisins	2830	Spinach	1260
Blueberries	2400	Brussels sprouts	980
Strawberries	1540	Broccoli florets	890
Raspberries	1220	Beetroot	840
Plums	949	Red peppers	710
Oranges	750	Onions	450
Grapes	739	Sweetcorn	400
Cherries	670	Aubergine	390
Kiwi fruit	602	Carrots	210

Just as a burning fire needs oxygen, every cell in our body needs a steady supply of oxygen to derive energy from digested food. But consuming oxygen comes with a price; it also generates free radicals, unstable molecules that can damage healthy cells. Free radicals are highly reactive because they contain an unpaired electron, and electrons prefer to pair up. So these free radicals search for a molecule from which they can steal an electron. The molecular victim then goes in search of an electron to satisfy its deficiency and sets off a chain reaction in the body that results in the creation of more free radicals. A molecule that has lost electrons in this manner is said to have been 'oxidised'.

Although all healthy cells produce small amounts of free radicals, a variety of other factors can promote free-radical formation in the human body, such as radiation (including X-rays), cigarette smoke, alcohol and environmental pollutants. Excessive free radicals can damage DNA and other genetic material. The body's immune system seeks out and destroys these mutated cells in much the same way as it eliminates invading bacteria and other foreign organisms. This mechanism declines with age, however, and the body becomes more vulnerable to free-radical damage.

Antioxidants are molecules that interact with and stabilise free radicals, preventing the damage they might cause. Researchers have identified hundreds of antioxidants in our foods, including vitamins C and E, selenium and carotenoids such as beta carotene and lycopene. There are many other phytochemicals (chemicals derived from plants), such as the polyphenols in tea and wine that have antioxidant properties. Coffee and chocolate are also high in antioxidants.

Over time, without the neutralising action of antioxidants, the damage that free radicals cause to cells can become irreversible. Antioxidants also help to prevent heart disease by hindering oxidation of LDL (low-density lipoprotein), the harmful cholesterol. It is actually oxidised cholesterol that damages arteries. There are hundreds of studies linking diets rich in antioxidants to a lower risk of both cancer and heart disease, as well as other degenerative diseases.

POSSIBLE DETRIMENTAL EFFECTS

Less clear is the effect of antioxidant supplementation on health. Although the research is ongoing, recent large-scale, randomised clinical trials have reached inconsistent conclusions. In five separate clinical trials that studied the effects of antioxidant supplements on cancer in the last decade, results ranged from a reduced incidence of gastric cancer, to a possible increase in lung cancer rate.

A survey of more than two dozen of the latest studies on the use of antioxidants to reduce the risk of cancer and heart disease concluded that people taking antioxidant supplements for the sole purpose of preventing heart disease or cancer 'are basically creating expensive urine'. Results from studies that have examined the relationship between cardiovascular disease and antioxidant vitamins found that vitamin E provides no benefits to people suffering from cardiovascular disease and that beta carotene supplements actually increase the risk slightly.

RESEARCH IS ONGOING

Although results to date have been disappointing, research continues. It may be that the benefits of supplements show up only after many years. It is possible that while vitamin E is of no help once cardiovascular disease exists, it could help to prevent the condition in the first place.

There are many current clinical trials investigating the effect of antioxidant supplementation on degenerative disease. Results are expected in the next few years.

A

It is possible that antioxidants may have more effects on other diseases. One study reported modest benefits with supplements of vitamin C (500mg), vitamin E (400 IU) and beta carotene (15mg), along with 80mg of zinc and 2mg of copper a day for macular degeneration, a common cause of blindness in the elderly.

If you are taking supplements with amounts of nutrients higher than the RNIs, talk to your doctor, particularly if you are on any prescription drugs.

CAUTION

Smokers who take high-dose beta carotene supplements actually increase their chances of developing lung cancer, say the results of two large medical trials. Ongoing studies continue to stress that everyone should get beneficial antioxidants the natural way – by eating their fruit and vegetables.

High doses of vitamin E, for example, can interfere with blood clotting and can increase the risk of a haemorrhage. Some antioxidants may also reduce the effectiveness of the statin drugs, which are taken to reduce cholesterol levels. The antioxidant level in tea is so good that experts recently said that it is a healthier drink than water. Pomegranate juice has even more antioxidants than green tea or red wine and is the latest weapon against heart disease, high cholesterol and prostate cancer.

Antioxidant power

Researchers have investigated and identified literally hundreds of antioxidant phytochemicals in our food, from vitamins to pigments, that protect against disease, and the list continues to grow. Here are the main ones:

ANTIOXIDANT	FUNCTION	FOOD SOURCES
VITAMIN C	Protects against heart disease, cataracts and possibly macular degeneration.	Citrus fruit, tomatoes, melon, strawberries, kiwi fruit, peppers, broccoli.
VITAMIN E	May help to prevent heart disease and prostate cancer, and slow progression of Alzheimer's.	Nuts and seeds, oils, fruits and vegetables.
CAROTENOIDS		
Beta carotene	Protective against some cancers and heart disease.	Orange and dark green vegetables, including carrots, sweet potatoes, pumpkin, broccoli, kale, spinach, apricots, peaches and melon.
Lutein, zeaxathin	Protects against macular degeneration.	Dark green leafy vegetables, sweetcorn, peppers, spinach, cabbage, oranges.
LYCOPENE	May protect against prostate cancer, lung cancer and heart disease.	Tomatoes, pink grapefruit, watermelon.
FLAVONOIDS		
Anthocyanidins	Protective against cancer.	Blueberries, cranberries, blackberries, plums, blackcurrants, cherries, black grapes.
Hesperidin	Protective against heart disease and cancer.	Citrus fruit and juices.
Isoflavones	Protective against heart disease and cancer.	Soya, pulses, peanuts.
Quercetin	Protective against heart disease and cancer.	Onions, apples, berries, black grapes, kale, broccoli, red wine.
SELENIUM	May help to prevent prostate cancer, colon cancer and lung cancer.	Whole grains, nuts, onions, garlic, poultry, seafood, meat.
CO-ENZYME Q_{10}	May help to reduce the risk of heart disease. Works together with vitamin E.	All plants and animal foods.

A

Appetite loss

EAT PLENTY OF

- Fresh fruit and vegetables for vitamin C

- Lean meats, seafood, nuts, seeds and whole grains for zinc and B vitamins

- Foods containing healthy fats, such as avocados, nuts and olive oil

AVOID

- Smoking and excessive alcohol, which dull the appetite

- Liquids before meals

- Bran and other high-fibre foods

The pleasant anticipation of eating, that we call appetite, is controlled by two centres in the brain: one is the hypothalamus, which stimulates the release of hunger-producing hormones until hunger is satisfied; the other is the cerebral cortex, the centre of intellectual and sensory function. Thus, a healthy appetite reflects both an unconscious response and learned behaviour.

Many disorders and conditions cause loss of appetite; most are temporary, such as a cold, an upset stomach, dental problems or stress. However, a persistent loss of appetite can reflect a more serious illness; for example, clinical depression, anaemia, kidney disease, AIDS or cancer.

In unusual cases, appetite loss stems from nutritional deficiencies, usually of vitamin C, thiamin, niacin, biotin and zinc.

Excessive drinking of alcohol not only reduces appetite but may also cause nutritional deficiencies. Smoking is another activity that blunts appetite. Food loses its appeal when smoking is excessive.

Eating large amounts of bran can interfere with the absorption of zinc and other minerals. High-fibre foods may also lessen appetite because they are filling.

Try to avoid drinking large quantities of liquid before a meal, because that reduces appetite too. Loss of appetite related to illness usually corrects itself with recovery. But there are several strategies, that may help to trigger an appetite when it is lost inexplicably.

Eat small snacks throughout the day rather than three large meals. Keep snacks available to eat whenever you feel the urge.

Have a lemon drop. Before a meal, have a lemon drop; sucking something sour increases saliva flow, which in turn stimulates appetite.

Create a pleasant eating atmosphere. Put flowers on the table, play quiet music, use soft light – whatever makes you feel good. Surround yourself with appetising odours, spices like cinnamon or a favourite food.

Try a little exercise. Take a walk before meals; some people find that activity increases their appetite.

A little alcohol may help. Try drinking a glass of sherry, wine or beer – it may increase your appetite.

Apples

BENEFITS

- High in fibre, including soluble fibre that helps to lower cholesterol

- Good source of bioflavonoids. May help in the treatment of asthma and other lung diseases

- Packed with numerous protective phytochemicals, such as quercetin

A fresh apple is an ideal snack. It's easy to carry, tastes good and is filling and low in caloriees; a 150g apple contains only 70kcal. Apples can be eaten fresh or cooked in myriad ways. When cut, the surface of an apple will go brown as oxygen from the air reacts with an enzyme

in the apple flesh. The reaction can be halted by cooking the apple or by brushing with lemon juice. Drying also kills the enzyme, so the dried apple stays a pleasant cream colour. Apple cider vinegar is a popular folk remedy for many health problems, but claims that its value is due to high levels of nutrients are not supported. It contains only insignificant quantities of nutrients, but its acidity may be helpful in reducing the rate at which carbohydrates in a meal are converted to blood glucose. Apple juice and cider are popular drinks.

Apples should always be washed before eating; some experts even suggest peeling them, especially if they have been waxed. The wax itself is not a problem but it may prevent pesticide residues from being rinsed off.

Nutritional value

'An apple a day keeps the doctor away' is an old adage, and no-one quite knows why it came into use. The average apple provides 10mg of vitamin C, so its value probably involves other components. It contains a good dose of pectin, the soluble fibre that thickens jams and helps to lower artery-damaging LDL blood cholesterol levels.

However, the most positive nutritional aspect is the mix of antioxidants apples contain. Flavonoids, such as quercetin, prevent LDL cholesterol from being oxidised to a more dangerous form.

Researchers have shown that as little as one and a half glasses of apple juice a day can significantly reduce the oxidation of LDL. Another study found that eating five or more apples a week was linked to slightly better lung function.

It's a myth that all the goodness of an apple is just under the skin, because the skin is an important source of antioxidants, and also prevents loss of nutrients that occur when the flesh is exposed to air.

Because stewed apple is pleasant-tasting and easily digested, doctors recommend it as an early baby food. Apples have long been called nature's toothbrush; while they don't actually cleanse the teeth, they still enhance dental hygiene. Biting and chewing an apple stimulates the gums and the sweetness of the apple prompts an increased flow of saliva, which reduces tooth decay by lowering the levels of bacteria in the mouth.

Dried apples

Usually served as a snack, dried apples are a more concentrated source of energy than the fresh form. It takes about 2.5kg of apples to make 500g of dried apple slices, which provide about 72kcal per 30g.

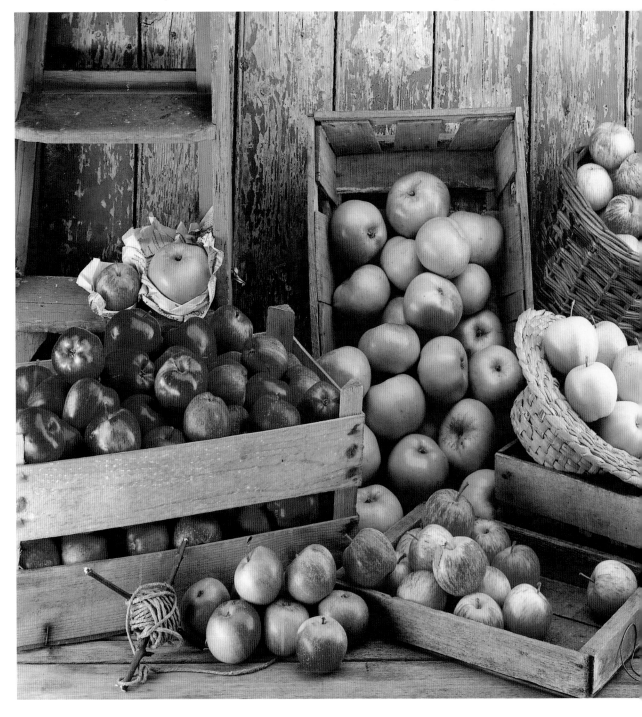

Except for fibre and a small amount of iron, most nutrients are lost in the drying process.

Sulphur dioxide is often added to dried apples to preserve their moistness and colour, however, it can provoke an allergic reaction in a susceptible person.

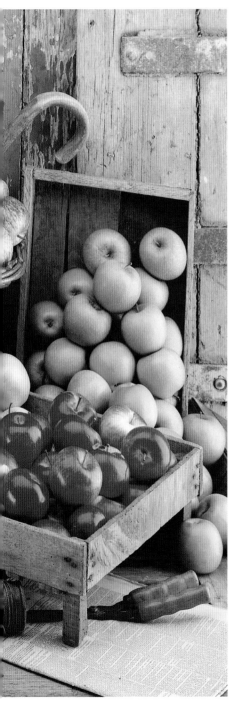

◀ **Apple harvest**
Apples that are widely available in the UK include (from left to right): Red Delicious, Cox, Bramley, Royal Gala, Golden Delicious, Granny Smith and Empire.

Apricots

BENEFITS

■ A good source of beta carotene, potassium and vitamin C

■ High in fibre, low in calories

■ Dried apricots are nutritious, fat-free foods, and a source of iron

DRAWBACKS

■ Sulphite preservatives in some dried apricots can trigger an allergic reaction or asthma attack in people susceptible to sulphites

■ Dried apricots leave a sticky residue on teeth that can lead to cavities

Apricots are ideal for both snacks and desserts. They are tasty, easy to digest, high in fibre, low in calories (about 40kcal in three fresh apricots and 75kcal in ten dried apricots), virtually fat-free and highly nutritious.

Apricots' deep colour indicates the presence of carotenoids, more specifically beta carotene, which is an important antioxidant, linked with prevention of some cancers. Apricots are also a source of the soluble fibre pectin, which helps to lower LDL cholesterol.

Although eating fresh apricots is a way to get vitamin C (which is depleted by heat and exposure to air when apricots are dried), other substances such as beta carotene and pectin are actually made more available to the body when apricots are cooked. However eaten, apricots provide iron and potassium, a mineral essential for proper nerve and muscle function that also helps to maintain normal blood pressure

Is laetrile an effective cancer treatment?

Laetrile is a controversial substance derived from apricot kernels. Legally, it cannot be sold as a medical treatment, but it is available, often called vitamin B_{17}, through the Internet. It is promoted as an alternative treatment for cancer, heart disease and other ailments. However, there is no scientific evidence of any benefit from laetrile and clinical trials are needed. Indeed, laetrile from apricot kernels carries a risk of cyanide poisoning. Apricot kernels in any form should not be ingested.

and the balance of body fluids. It is interesting that dried apricots are a regular item in the diet of the inhabitants of the Hunza Valley in Pakistan who profess to have legendary longevity (although they have no proof of it).

Apricots also contain a natural salicylate, a compound similar to the active ingredient in aspirin. People who are sensitive to aspirin may experience allergic responses after eating apricots.

Dried apricots

Apricots are more nutritious when they are dried. This is because dried apricots are only 32 per cent water, compared with 85 per cent water content in the fresh fruit. They are a more concentrated source of calories – 31kcal in 100g of fresh apricots versus 188kcal in 100g (about 25 halves) of the dried form. When eaten in moderation, dried apricots are a compact and convenient source of nutrition.

People who suffer from asthma should buy the natural fruit, which does not contain sulphur. Apricots are often treated with sulphur dioxide before they are dried in order to preserve their colour and certain nutrients. Sulphites may trigger an asthma attack or allergic reaction in susceptible people.

A

Top foods that fight arthritis

- **FISH** Eat a portion of salmon, sardines and other ocean fish, which are rich in omega-3 fatty acids, two to three times a week.

- **VEGETABLES** Eat at least five servings every day of dark green or bright orange vegetables to provide beta carotene; broccoli, peppers, cabbage and Brussels sprouts for vitamin C; and avocados for vitamin E.

- **FRUIT** Eat daily: any yellow or orange-coloured fruit for its beta carotene content; citrus fruit, berries, melons and kiwi fruit for extra vitamin C.

- **NUTS AND WHOLE GRAINS** Eat nuts, seeds and whole grains regularly, because vitamin E, which is a potent antioxidant, is believed to help to relieve inflammation.

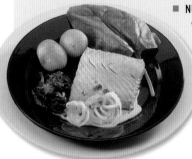

Arthritis

EAT PLENTY OF

- Salmon, sardines and other seafood to counter inflammation

- High-fibre, low-calorie foods to help to control weight

AVOID

- Any foods that provoke symptoms

More than eight million people in the UK suffer from one type of arthritis or another – there are more than 100 disorders characterised by joint inflammation, stiffness, swelling and pain. The most common types are: osteoarthritis, a painful condition in which joint cartilage gradually breaks down; gout, where uric acid crystals are deposited in the joints; and rheumatoid arthritis, a systemic disease that can cause severe pain and eventual crippling.

Doctors do not understand why some people develop arthritis and others don't, but a combination of factors plays a role. People with

osteoarthritis may have inherently defective cartilage that makes it vulnerable to normal wear and tear. Rheumatoid arthritis (RA) develops when an overactive immune system attacks connective tissue in the joints, causing inflammation and pain. It is much less common but may occur in young adults.

Arthritis and fish

New research shows that for some patients, diet can make a difference. Studies have found that some people with rheumatoid arthritis who add omega-3 fatty acids to their diets experience a marked reduction in swelling, pain and redness of joints. The fats are found in salmon, mackerel and sardines, as well as in other seafood. Omega-3 fats have

Foods may be the culprits

For some people who develop rheumatoid arthritis, an allergy to or intolerance of particular foods may be a contributing factor. Pinpointing the culprit food can be difficult, especially if there is more than one. Common suspects include dairy products, eggs and cereals. One of the best ways to identify problem foods is to follow an exclusion diet – which involves cutting one suspect food at a time from the diet and then reinstating it to see if there is a reaction. But this should only be done under medical supervision.

anti-inflammatory properties, whereas the more common omega-6 fats found in soya, corn, safflower and sunflower oils can increase inflammation. The best results with fish oils are seen when the omega-6 fats in the diet are reduced, and the omega-3 fats increased so they are consumed in roughly equal amounts.

Gamma linolenic acid (GLA) is another type of fat that has anti-inflammatory properties. The best sources are borage oil (it contains up to 24 per cent GLA), evening primrose oil (8 to 10 per cent) and blackcurrant oil (15 to 17 per cent). Benefits in rheumatoid arthritis can occur, with recent studies indicating that 1 to 1.5g a day may be needed. Fish oils and GLA should be taken together as GLA on its own can increase the risk of blood clots. But it may be months before any improvement occurs. Excessive fish oil consumption can also increase the risk of bleeding problems.

Eat more vitamin C-rich foods. Since vitamin C is important for the manufacture of collagen, eating vitamin C-rich foods may help to slow the progression of osteoarthritis. The best food sources are citrus fruit, berries, kiwi fruit, melons, broccoli, peppers, potatoes and cabbage. It is also possible that antioxidants such as vitamin C, beta carotene and vitamin E will fight the effects of free radicals, which are generated by inflammatory compounds and which are thought to cause tissue damage in people with rheumatoid arthritis.

Other food theories

Studies now show that the anti-inflammatory properties of ginger may be useful for both osteoarthritis and rheumatoid arthritis. Before you take ginger in large doses, however, check with your doctor, as it may interfere with some or any other medications you are taking.

Green tea contains compounds called polyphenols, which may help to relieve inflammation. It's available in capsules and tea bags – but don't take it with milk, which may block the effect of the polyphenols.

Acidic foods such as oranges, lemons, tomatoes and pineapple are often avoided by people with arthritis. In fact, the level of acid in these foods is very low compared with normal stomach acidity, and they need not be avoided unless you have a specific intolerance for other reasons.

Cider vinegar is often used by those with arthritis but there is no scientific evidence that it helps with the prevention or the relief of symptoms. However, as it also does no harm, its use on salads or in drinks is not a problem.

The weight factor

Obesity greatly increases the risk and severity of osteoarthritis. Even a little bit of extra weight strains the knees and hips. Losing weight and gradually increasing exercise is often found to improve symptoms.

Patients with rheumatoid arthritis often have the opposite problem; they may be too thin due to a lack of appetite, depression or chronic pain. A doctor may recommend high-calorie and nutrient-enriched liquid supplements.

Vegetarian diet

Researchers have found that fasting followed by a strict vegetarian diet for at least three months can bring about significant symptom relief for a small number of people. They theorise that one benefit of this strict diet comes from fruit, grains and vegetables, which contribute important antioxidants that, in turn, can help to counter some of the inflammation. The diet is also very low in – or free of – animal fats, which may promote the

● Myth.......
Wearing a copper or magnetic bracelet reduces arthritis pain

.......Reality ●
No scientific studies support this belief, although traces of copper may be absorbed through the skin. It is more likely the strength of the wearer's belief that triggers some relief.

production of inflammatory immune compounds. A strict vegetarian diet requires professional supervision to ensure proper nutrition.

Other treatments

One promising approach entails rubbing painful joints with a cream containing capsaicin, a derivative of chillies. Capsaicin produces a stinging or burning feeling, but it appears to reduce inflammation.

Studies have been conducted that show a marked improvement to osteoarthritis when patients take glucosamine sulphate in dosages of 500mg three times a day. It is a natural compound extracted from the shells of crabs, oysters and prawns, which is helpful in building and maintaining cartilage.

Beware unproven remedies. Because arthritis has no cure, sufferers often turn for help to alternative therapies. Some may help, but others are worthless, often costly and sometimes dangerous. Treatments such as bee venom injections do nothing for arthritis. The treatment process called chelation, which is used to remove toxic metals from the body, has been touted in a series of 20 to 30 intravenous treatments as a remedy, especially for reactive arthritis, but to date there has been no scientific evidence that it is effective. When in doubt about any treatment, talk to your GP or specialist.

Artichokes

BENEFITS

- A good source of folate, vitamin C and potassium
- Low in calories, high in fibre
- May improve liver function

Served either hot or cold, the globe artichoke is both a delicacy and a low-calorie, nutritious vegetable. A globe artichoke is actually the flower bud of a large, thistle-like plant, with only a few edible portions – the heart and the tender, fleshy part at the base of the tough outer leaves. While both the heart and the meaty leaves of the artichoke are edible, it's the leaves that contain many of the vegetable's phytochemicals.

To prepare a fresh artichoke, the thorny top and leaf tips are trimmed away and the vegetable is boiled, steamed or baked. It can be served in many ways, but one of the most popular is to dip the edible portion of the leaves in a sauce. Try to use a light sauce, as it's this sauce that dictates whether an artichoke is a healthy treat or an indulgence.

High-fat sauces, such as Hollandaise and melted butter are traditional favourites, but a much healthier choice is lemon juice with just a dash of a good olive oil. Artichokes contain cynarin, an organic acid that stimulates the sweetness receptors in the taste buds of some people, causing the

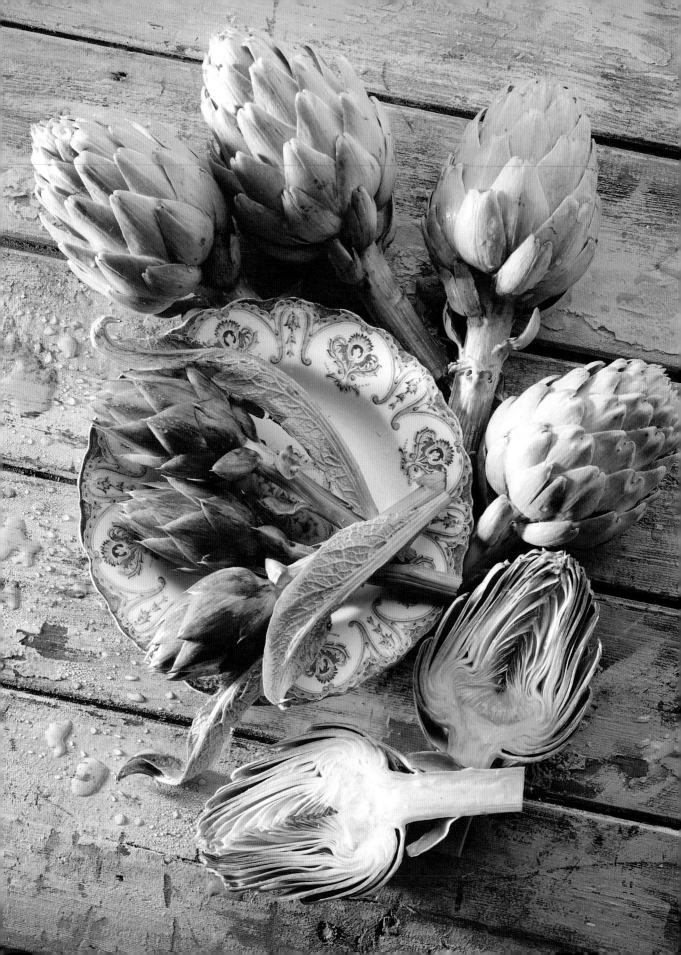

foods eaten afterwards to taste sweeter. This chemical is thought to improve liver function and possibly also to lower blood cholesterol, making it potentially useful for protecting against artery and heart disease. German researchers have shown that artichoke extract has a cholesterol-lowering effect. But claims that artichokes lower blood sugar and stimulate bile flow are unproven.

Artichokes are members of the sunflower, or composite, plant family. People allergic to ragwort pollen may react to artichokes because of cross-reacting antigens that respond to both allergens.

Artificial sweeteners

BENEFITS

■ Provide a sweet taste with virtually no calories

■ Can be used as a sugar replacement for people with diabetes

■ They do not promote tooth decay

DRAWBACKS

■ Pregnant or lactating women should discuss the use of sweeteners with their doctor

■ Aspartame should not be used by people with phenylketonuria (PKU)

Artificial sweeteners are popularly used to reduce both the total calorie intake and the amount of sugar consumed. They are many times sweeter than table sugar but, in measured amounts, add a taste to foods that is similar to that provided by regular sweeteners such as sugar or honey. Because they do not contain any calories, or cause an increase in blood sugar levels, they are useful for people with diabetes and those trying to lose weight.

Check your daily intake. Before any sweetener is approved for sale, it must have been tested extensively. The Acceptable Daily Intake (ADI) is an average daily amount that can be used over a lifetime without causing harm. It is based on body weight and includes a very large safety margin (see *Acceptable Daily Intake* chart below). While sweeteners on the market are safe for consumption and do play a role, especially for people with diabetes, it is prudent to be moderate in your use of them. Here is a rundown of some of the most popular artificial sweeteners:

• Saccharin, sold as Sweet 'n Low, Hermesetas and Natrena, is the oldest of the sweeteners on the market. It is calorie-free, about 300 times sweeter than sugar, but has a slightly bitter aftertaste. Several studies suggested that large quantities of saccharin can cause bladder cancer in rats, no similar effects have been shown in humans. The FDA in the United States has now dropped saccharin from its list of cancer-causing chemicals. It is heat stable and suitable for use in cooking and baking and as an addition to beverages and foods.

• Aspartame, marketed as Flix, NutraSweet and Canderel, is made from two amino acids, phenylalanine and aspartic acid. It contains the same calories, weight for weight, as sugar, but since it is nearly 200 times sweeter, it can be used in minute quantities. Aspartame loses its sweetness when exposed to high temperaures so is not ideal for baking. You'll find it in soft drinks, confectionery, sports drinks and desserts. Some studies suggest that in isolated cases aspartame can trigger seizures, blurred vision or headaches, but most people use it without obvious problems. Because it contains phenylalanine, it should be strictly avoided by people with phenylketonuria (PKU).

• Acesulphame potassium (acesulphame K) is 200 times sweeter than sugar and calorie-free. Marketed under the names Sunett and Diamin, it is highly stable, is able to withstand heat and consequently can be used for baking. It is not broken down by the body and is eliminated without providing any calories. It is found in beverages, confectionery chewing gum and some baked products. However, people on a potassium-restricted diet should discuss the use of Ace-K with their doctor before using it.

Acceptable Daily Intake (ADI) of artificial sweeteners

Here's how to calculate your ADI. If, for example, you weigh 60kg, multiply your weight by the ADI figure of your sweetener in the chart. For Acesulphame K you would be allowed 900mg per day (60kg x 15mg). One packet contains approximately 50mg, so you could use up to 18 packets a day.

NAME	NUMBER	ADI mg/kg body weight
Acesulphame K	E950	0–15
Aspartame	E951	0–40
Saccharin	E954	0–5
Sucralose	E955	0–15
Cyclamate	E952	0–11

A

• Sucralose, made from sucrose, is about 600 times sweeter than sugar. Marketed as Splenda, it is highly stable and can be used in foods and beverages, cooking and baking. It is used as an additive in beverages and processed foods and as a tabletop sweetener. It is not broken down by the body and is eliminated without providing any kilojoules.

• Cyclamates were banned in the UK until 1995, because of the increased cancer risk scare in US laboratory rats, but after lengthy discussion it was accepted that cyclamates were used in such small quantities in the UK that they did not pose a threat. Cyclamates are sold in liquid, tablet and powder forms, marketed under the brand name Sucaryl. You can cook and bake with this sweetener without it losing its sweet taste.

• Sugar alcohols are another category of sweetener, sometimes called bulk sweeteners as they are added to foods as part of the manufacturing process. They are derived from plant products such as fruit and are referred to as nutritive sweeteners because they provide calories and may affect blood sugar. They contain fewer calories than table sugar because they are not well absorbed. The most common include sorbitol, mannitol, xylitol, maltitol and lactitol. One strong benefit of these sweeteners is their role in preventing dental cavities. You will find them in confectionery, chewing gum, jams and jellies and some cough syrups.

In excess, they can cause abdominal discomfort and bloating and have a laxative effect. They can also exacerbate the symptoms of irritable bowel syndrome (IBS) in some people.

Asparagus

BENEFITS

■ A good source of vitamin C and folate; useful source of potassium and vitamin E

■ Contains prebiotic fibre that encourages 'friendly' gut bacteria

DRAWBACKS

■ Contains purines, which may precipitate an attack of gout if eaten to excess

Prized as a springtime delicacy for centuries, this edible member of the lily family is now so widely cultivated that it is available in supermarkets for most of the year; homegrown asparagus appears in May and June.

The ancient Greeks and Romans believed that asparagus possessed medicinal qualities, curing everything from rheumatism to toothache. However, asparagus does provide many essential nutrients such as folate and potassium, the antioxidant glutathione and fibre. Asparagus is low in calories, too – there are only 17kcal in 100g.

Did you know?

Asparagus can cause painful gout attacks

Asparagus contains purines, substances that promote the over-production of uric acid that precipitates attacks of gout. Asparagus should be consumed in moderation by gout sufferers.

Always keep asparagus in the refrigerator or it will lose half its vitamin C and much of its flavour in just two or three days. Canning destroys some flavour while adding large amounts of salt.

Some people find that asparagus gives their urine a pungent odour – a harmless reaction that occurs when the body metabolises the sulphur compounds in the food.

Asthma

EAT PLENTY OF

■ Fruit and vegetables (aim for at least seven servings per day)

■ Foods high in omega-3 fatty acids such as salmon, mackerel, herring and sardines to counter inflammation

AVOID

■ Any foods, including additives, that seem to bring on attacks

■ Mushrooms, cheese, soy sauce and yeasty breads if moulds trigger attacks

■ Foods containing tartrazine, or additive E102

■ Salicylates, an ingredient in aspirin, tea, vinegar, salad dressings and many fruit and vegetables, if sensitive to aspirin or salicylates

■ Any food preserved with sulphites

Asthma is a chronic lung condition estimated to affect about 20 million people in the UK. The rising toll of asthma has puzzled doctors, but many attribute it to a combination of factors, such as family history of asthma or other allergies, parental smoking, major respiratory infection during infancy and exposure to environmental pollutants.

Wheezing, chest tightness, laboured breathing and other asthma symptoms occur when the tiny muscles that control the airways to the lungs constrict, causing a bronchospasm. Normally, the airways narrow somewhat when exposed to smoke, pollutants, very cold air or substances that are harmful if inhaled. In asthmatic people, however, the response is exaggerated and often triggered by otherwise harmless substances or activities, such as pollen and other allergens, and exercise.

Heredity is a factor. The reason why some people have hyper-reactive airways is unknown; but heredity plays a definite role, because the disease runs in families. Heritary factors are thought to account for some 30 to 50 per cent of the risk. Many people with asthma also have hay fever and eczema. Although stress and emotional upsets can trigger or worsen an attack, experts emphasise that asthma is a lung disease, not a psychological disorder; as such, it should be treated as a serious and even debilitating physical condition.

Some asthma attacks are rapidly reversed by taking a broncho-dilator medication. These ease symptoms by opening the constricted airways. Other episodes may be more prolonged and, as the airways become more inflamed and clogged with mucus, breathing becomes increasingly difficult. In such cases, an injection of adrenaline and perhaps a corticosteroid drug may be needed to stop the attack.

Although asthma is a chronic disease, the changes that occur during an attack are temporary, and the lungs generally function normally at other times. When asthma starts during childhood, the frequency and severity of the attacks tend to lessen as the youngster grows, and may disappear by adulthood. Some adults, however, suffer a recurrence, often occurring as an aftermath of a viral infection. In such cases, the asthma may be even more severe than it was in childhood.

Eliminating triggers

Doctors agree that the best treatment for asthma entails identifying and then avoiding its triggers. In some instances these are obvious – for example, exposure to tobacco smoke and other noxious fumes, cold air, exercise or an allergy to animal dander. Seasonal asthma is usually due to pollens, moulds and other environmental factors. Suspected allergens can usually be identified by blood and skin tests.

Food allergies can cause attacks. In a small percentage of asthma sufferers, food allergies are a trigger; in these cases, identifying the culprits may require some detective work, especially in the case of children. Because food allergies vary from person to person, there is no handy list of offenders. Occasionally, foods that trigger asthma can be identified by keeping a careful record of the time and ingestion of all foods and drinks, as well as any asthma symptoms. After a few weeks, a pattern of offending foods may emerge. A doctor can then do skin or other allergy tests to confirm the findings.

For some people, inadvertently ingested environmental allergens are the problem rather than the foods. People allergic to ragwort, for example, may also react to pyrethrum, a natural pesticide made from chrysanthemums, or to other allergens related to plants. Similarly, a few people allergic to mildew and other environmental moulds may react to moulds in foods; common offenders include mushrooms, cheese and many processed meats, as well as anything that is fermented, including soy sauce, beer, wine and vinegar.

Salicylates – compounds in the same family as the active ingredient in aspirin and found naturally in many fruits – may trigger asthma in a few people. Additive E102 (tartrazine) is chemically similar to salicylate, although it is less potent.

Helpful foods

There are no specific foods that prevent asthma, but some may lessen its complications. Omega-3 fatty acids, found in salmon, mackerel, sardines and other seafood, have an anti-inflammatory effect and may counter bronchial inflammation, too.

Eat at least seven servings of fruit and vegetables daily. Evidence continues to grow on the protective effects of fruit and vegetables on

Do one simple thing

Drink one or two cups of coffee to abort a mild asthma attack

Coffee and tea are sources of theophylline, a bronchial muscle relaxant used to treat asthma in people who are not sensitive to salicylates. Anyone taking a theophylline drug, however, should avoid large amounts of tea to prevent an overdose.

lung function. All these foods provide a variety of vitamins, minerals and antioxidants important for healthy lung function. Vitamin C helps to promote a healthy immune system and may be helpful in reducing wheezing in children with asthma. This vitamin is also said to be a natural antihistamine, which helps asthma sufferers. Some studies have linked weight gain with adult-onset asthma. In addition, when obese people with asthma lose weight, there can be a marked improvement in asthma symptoms.

Potential problems

Like everyone else, people who suffer from asthma need a healthy, balanced diet. Contrary to some theories, there is no evidence that omitting dairy products will prevent an asthma attack. However, if you are concerned about dietary interactions, a dietitian can ensure that you maintain good nutrition.

Sometimes asthma drugs can create nutritional problems. Long-term steroid use, for example, causes bone loss; supplements of vitamin D and calcium may be needed to strengthen bones.

Another potential problem, potassium deficiency can be cut by eating plenty of citrus fruit, bananas, dried fruit, berries, beetroot, tomatoes and green leafy vegetables.

Adrenaline and bronchodilator drugs can cause nervousness, which may be exacerbated by caffeine. It may be advisable to switch to decaffeinated coffee or tea.

Atherosclerosis

EAT PLENTY OF

■ Fresh fruit and vegetables for vitamin C, beta carotene and folate

■ Wheatgerm, nuts, seeds and vegetable oils for vitamin E

■ Salmon, sardines and other oil-rich fish for omega-3 fatty acids

■ Apples, rolled oats, lentils and pulses for soluble fibre

■ Soya proteins in foods such as soya beverages, tofu or tempeh

CUT DOWN ON

■ Fats, especially saturated ones

■ Biscuits, cakes and snack foods rich in trans fatty acids

■ High-cholesterol foods

AVOID

■ Smoking, obesity, high alcohol intake and physical inactivity

As we become older, our arteries lose some of their elasticity and begin to stiffen. This can lead to a progressive condition referred to as atherosclerosis, the medical term for hardening (sclerosis) of the arteries. These stiffened blood vessels usually become clogged with fatty plaque, the hallmark of atherosclerosis (*athero* is the Greek term for porridge, which describes the thick, cheesy appearance of the deposits).

Some degree of atherosclerosis is a natural part of ageing. It usually progresses slowly over years without producing noticeable symptoms. But serious problems develop when these stiffened blood vessels become severely narrowed with plaque.

Complications include circulatory disorders, especially reduced blood flow to the lower legs and other extremities; angina, the chest pains caused by inadequate oxygen to the heart; and heart disease and stroke.

By the time Western men have reached their late forties, most have some degree of atherosclerosis. In women the process is somewhat delayed, presumably due to the protective effects of oestrogen during the reproductive years. After

◀ **Fruit rich in vitamin C**
Foods that are rich in vitamin C are believed to be particularly helpful in helping asthma sufferers. Citrus fruit and berries are excellent sources of ascorbic acid, the form of vitamin C found in plants.

A

Do one simple thing

Eat more soya

Add 25g of soya protein to your daily diet. Try tofu or soya beverages. A variety of studies have shown that eating this amount daily should lower cholesterol in people with elevated levels by about 9 per cent, and LDL cholesterol, by as much as 15 per cent.

menopause, women quickly catch up with their male counterparts, however, and once in their sixties they are just as likely to develop severely clogged arteries as men are.

Underlying causes

Just what initiates atherosclerosis is unknown, but most experts agree that a genetic susceptibility and a combination of lifestyle factors accelerate the process; these include a diet high in saturated fats, smoking, excessive stress and lack of exercise. Poorly controlled diabetes and high blood pressure also contribute to atherosclerosis.

Arteries can be narrowed by 85 per cent (or more) without producing symptoms. Nevertheless, there is still a high risk of a heart attack or stroke because clots tend to form at the site of fatty deposits. Most heart attacks are caused by a clot blocking a coronary artery (a coronary thrombosis); similarly, a cerebral thrombosis, or a clot that blocks blood flow to the brain, is the most common type of stroke.

Dietary approaches

Researchers agree that diet plays a critical role in both the development and treatment of atherosclerosis. Cholesterol is the major component of atherosclerotic plaque, and numerous studies correlate high levels of blood cholesterol with atherosclerosis. Research indicates that atherosclerosis can be slowed and even reversed by lowering

cholesterol in the blood – in particular the levels of low-density lipoproteins (LDLs), which is the bad type of cholesterol.

Elevated triglycerides, another type of lipid that circulates in the blood, may also contribute to atherosclerosis. People who have diabetes also tend to have high triglyceride and cholesterol levels, which may explain why they are so vulnerable to heart disease.

Limit 'bad' fat intake. The most important dietary treatment for atherosclerosis involves reducing saturated fats to comprise no more than 10 per cent of calories. For most people, this means keeping these fats to no more than 20g a day for women and 30g a day for men. Saturated fats are found in animal fats (meat and dairy products) and also in some processed vegetable fats used in biscuits, cakes, crackers, crisps, confectionery, fried foods (especially fast foods) and some margarines. Trans fats produced when vegetable fats are hydrogenated can also raise your LDL cholesterol. Many brands of margarine no longer contain trans fats, but check the label on generic brands before buying. Trans fats are widely used in frying fats, baked goods, crisps and French fries.

People who are overweight need to reduce total calories and one of the simplest ways to do this is to replace 'bad' fats with 'good' ones, as well as reducing alcohol and refined sugar. Very strict low-fat diets, along with exercise and methods for dealing with stress have also been proved effective in reversing atherosclerosis. These diets limit fats to 10 per cent of the calorie intake, which translates to a diet with no obvious sources of fat.

Eating a high-fibre diet can reduce the amount of cholesterol absorbed from the diet, although this is a neglible source of blood

cholesterol, most of which is made from saturated fats in the diet. Some experts recommend limiting dietary cholesterol to 300mg a day – about the amount in 1½ egg yolks.

The omega-3 fatty acids in salmon, sardines and other seafood lower blood levels of triglycerides;

Ten ways to cut down on saturated fat

1 Choose skimmed or semi-skimmed milk and low-fat yoghurt. Limit cheese and ice cream intake to twice a week. Avoid butter.

2 Choose lean meat and skinless chicken and remove visible fat. Avoid sausages and delicatessen meats such as salami.

3 Include fish, especially ocean fish, three times a week.

4 Include pulses (dried or canned beans) in two meals a week.

5 Cook with olive oil (or rapeseed, peanut, sesame, sunflower or soya bean oil) instead of butter or margarine.

6 Snack on fresh fruit or nuts, especially almonds or walnuts.

7 Make vegetables and grain-based foods (bread, cereals, rice, pasta) the major part of every meal.

8 Make your own salad dressings using extra virgin olive oil, wine or cider vinegar or lemon juice, pepper and mustard.

9 Limit takeaway foods to no more than once a week. Where possible, select those with less fat such as sushi or sashimi, or fresh salads or sandwiches.

10 Limit cakes, pastries, biscuits, chocolate and crisps to no more than once a week.

A

they also reduce the tendency to form blood clots. Oats, lentils and pulses, as well as fruit containing pectin such as pears, apples and citrus fruit, barley, guar gum and psyllium all contain soluble fibre that lowers blood cholesterol, probably by interfering with the intestinal absorption of bile acids, which forces the liver to use circulating cholesterol to make bile.

A group of compounds known as phytosterols are available in various food forms, and will help to lower the cholesterol in your body. They are available in margarines and low-fat spreads, yoghurts and yoghurt drinks under brand names such as Benecol.

Antioxidants may help. Theoretically, beta carotene and vitamins C and E may protect against atherosclerosis by preventing LDL cholesterol from collecting within atherosclerotic plaque. In practice, current studies show that there are greater benefits for foods rich in antioxidants than for supplements. Regular intake of soya protein may raise HDL cholesterol (the 'good' cholesterol) as well as provide antioxidant protection.

Many studies are looking at homocysteine, an amino acid, which is one of the building blocks of protein, that some scientists say is as risky or may be even riskier than cholesterol. High levels of homocysteine have been shown to damage the lining of the artery walls, potentially leading to a build-up of plaque. Folate, as well as vitamins B_{12} and B_6, appear to help to lower homocysteine levels.

Diet is not the only factor. Keep to an ideal weight, abstain from smoking, increase exercise, develop effective methods of coping with stress and keep blood pressure and blood sugar levels within normal limits – these are all important in the fight against atherosclerosis.

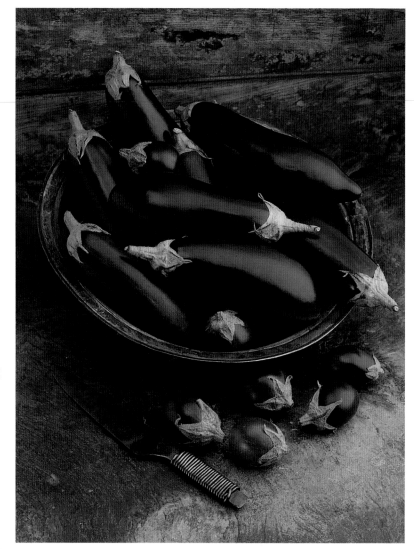

Aubergines

BENEFITS

■ Low in calories (unless cooked in fat)

■ Satisfying flavour and texture lend themselves to vegetarian dishes.

DRAWBACKS

■ Soak up fat during cooking.

Aubergines provide fibre; they are among our most versatile vegetables and a component of many popular ethnic dishes, including Indian curries, Greek moussakas, Middle Eastern baba ghanoush and French ratatouille. Aubergine are filling, yet

Did you know?

Oriental origins

The aubergine is native to India, but was also a common food in China as long ago as 600 BC, when it was called the Malayan purple melon. Chinese ladies of the time used it as a beauty aid, staining their teeth black with a dye made from its skin. The first varieties that English-speakers came across probably bore egg-shaped fruits, hence its other name – eggplant.

low in calories – 100g has only 15kcal. An aubergine's spongy texture, however, soaks up fat. Deep-fried aubergines soak up four times as much fat as French fried potatoes, so they should be eaten only as a treat.

The tastiest aubergines are firm, with thin skins. Larger ones are more likely to be seedy, tough and bitter. Their skins range in colour from deep purple to light violet and white.

Aubergines are members of the nightshade family, which also includes tomatoes, potatoes and peppers. Some have a bitter flavour, which can easily be eliminated with salt before cooking. Slice or cube the aubergine, then sprinkle it with salt. Let it stand for half an hour, then rinse and drain it and blot it dry. The salt draws out the excess moisture and reduces bitterness. Small and freshly harvested aubergines do not need salting. Aubergines can be stuffed and baked or barbecued, roasted or stewed. If sautéeing, use a nonstick pan and minimal oil.

Avocados

BENEFITS

■ A good source of vitamins C, E and B_6, potassium, lutein and dietary fibre

■ Useful amounts of iron, magnesium and folate

DRAWBACKS

■ High in calories, with 85 per cent coming from fat

Although it is often mistaken for a vegetable, the avocado is actually a fruit – the reproductive part of the plant. The rich, buttery flavour and smooth texture of an avocado make it a complementary addition to salads and sandwiches.

When mashed and seasoned with spicy chilli, it can also be served as a dip (as in guacamole) or a spread. It should always be mixed with a little lemon or vinegar to prevent the flesh from discolouring as it is oxidised by exposure to the air.

Half a medium avocado contains about 143kcal, and it has more calories and fat than any other fruit. A whole avocado may contain up to 371kcal and 37g fat. However, because most of the fat in avocados is monounsaturated, it does not raise blood cholesterol levels, unlike the saturated oil that comes from palms and a number of other tropical plants.

When served as part of an otherwise low-fat meal or snack, an avocado contributes a number of important nutrients. One tablespoon of avocado has about 40kcal compared with 143kcal in a tablespoon of butter or margarine. To make a delicious difference to sandwiches that are to be eaten immediately, try mashing avocado and spreading it on the bread in place of butter.

Avocados are also rich in two phytochemicals: beta-sitosterol, an important phytochemical linked with lower cholesterol levels; and glutathione, an antioxidant that may offer protection against several cancers. Vitamins C and E, also found in good quantities in avocado, are antioxidants that help to prevent free radical damage. Vitamin B_6 is important for the proper functioning of the nervous

helps to prevent cataracts and macular degeneration. Potassium helps to control blood pressure and maintain a regular heartbeat and healthy nervous system.

Avocados should always be served raw; they have a bitter taste when cooked. But they can be added to hot dishes that have already been cooked – for example, tossed with a spicy pasta sauce, or sliced on top of a grilled chicken breast.

An avocado primer

■ Avocados are rich in mono-unsaturated oil, the same heart-friendly fat found in olive oil, and have more soluble fibre than most other fruit.

■ Avocados are full of a plant sterol called beta-sitosterol, which can help to prevent cholesterol from being absorbed through the intestine.

■ The avocado is popularly known as the alligator pear because of the shape and rough skin of its most common variety.

■ Avocados start to ripen only after being cut from the tree. Mature fruit can be left on the tree for six months without spoiling. Once picked, it will ripen in a few days.

■ Avocado is suitable for infants from six months of age.

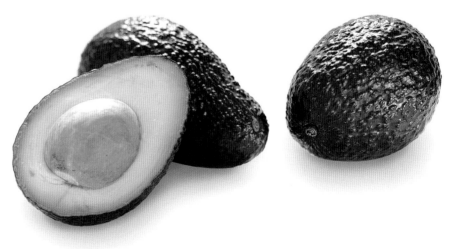

B

Baby food
Healthy choices for toddlers

Proper early nutrition is important, even vital. The eating patterns that parents help their baby to establish in infancy determine how well a baby grows. Establishing and encouraging a healthy approach to food influences lifelong food habits and attitudes.

New parents probably worry more about feeding their baby than any other aspect of early child care. Much of the advice they receive from well-meaning friends and family is often conflicting and adds to a parent's feelings of confusion. So here are a few tips and truths to help you to stay calm:

- Get to know your baby. No two are alike. Some enter the world ravenously hungry and demand to be fed every hour or two. Others seem to prefer sleeping, and may even need to be awakened to eat.
- Try to relax. It's natural for new parents to feel nervous and apprehensive, but this should be a happy time.
- Trust your own judgment and common sense. A baby who is developing and growing at a normal pace is getting enough to eat.
- Keep food in its proper perspective. It provides the essential energy and nourishment infants need to grow and develop. But an infant quickly learns how to use food as a manipulative tool, which can set the stage for later eating problems.

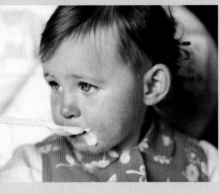

IN THE BEGINNING, THEY ARE WHAT *YOU* EAT
Good nutrition starts during pregnancy. A mother who is well nourished herself provides plenty of nutrients that her baby can use for proper development in the uterus, as well as to store for later use. If a woman skimps on food to avoid gaining excessive weight while she is pregnant, she can produce a low-birth-weight baby who has serious medical problems. A woman who is anaemic may have a baby with low iron reserves. A woman who does not consume adequate folate may have a baby with serious neurological problems. High doses of vitamin A before and during early pregnancy can cause birth defects.

BREAST MILK – BABY'S FIRST FOOD
Doctors agree that breast milk provides the most complete food to achieve optimal health, growth and development for full-term infants. The World Health Organisation says that a full-term, healthy infant should be exclusively breastfed up to six months of age (premature and low-birth-weight babies may need specialised formula in addition to breast milk). As an alternative to breast milk, a commercial infant formula provides similar nutrition but lacks many of the unique benefits of breast milk.

Although breastfeeding for six months may not be possible for every mother, a baby can benefit from any amount of breast milk – even a few feedings. Colostrum, the breast fluid that is secreted for the first

> ● Myth.......
> One glass of beer a day increases a mother's supply of breast milk.
>
> ....Reality ●
> There is no scientific evidence to support the claim that drinking beer boosts milk production or improves mother's milk, researchers say. However, studies have shown that beer can increase levels of a hormone necessary for milk production. In the late 1800s an American brewery marketed a new beer blend that was touted as a 'tonic' for breastfeeding women.

Introducing new foods in the first year

During the first six months of life, breast milk or formula provides all the nutrients a newborn baby needs. The following chart summarises the generally accepted guidelines for introducing new foods to babies under one year of age. It should be noted, however, that all babies are different; consequently, the timing varies considerably from one baby to another.

UP TO 6 MONTHS
If giving breast milk, allow the baby to feed until satisfied. Generally you can be sure the baby is taking enough milk if he or she is growing, passing regular, soft stools and has six or more wet nappies a day. If giving formula, start with 60-120ml per feeding (every 2 to 4 hours), but be guided by your baby's needs and the advice from your GP or post-natal clinic.

MILK AND DAIRY	CEREALS AND STARCHY FOODS	VEGETABLES AND FRUIT	MEAT AND MEAT ALTERNATIVES	OCCASIONAL FOODS AND FOODS TO AVOID
6 TO 7 MONTHS Total intake: breast milk or formula as demanded by the baby.				
Breast milk or formula feeding five or six times a day.	Iron-fortified cereals—rice first, then barley and oats.	Plain, cooked puréed vegetables; plain, soft puréed or mashed fruit.		Avoid honey in the first year due to its link to botulism in infants, and egg white to reduce risk of egg allergy.
8 TO 12 MONTHS Continue breastfeeding if possible. Give four to six feedings per day. For formula, give 180-240ml per feeding four or five times each day. Yoghurt; cheese; cottage cheese; cow's milk*.	Toast, soft breads, dry unsweetened cereals; plain muffins; other grains, such as pasta and rice Daily intake: ¼ to ¾ cup starchy food over three meals.	Plain, cooked mashed vegetables; soft bite-sized pieces of vegetables; plain, soft, ripe fruit. Daily intake: four to six ¼ to ½-cup servings of fruit and vegetables.	Plain, puréed, minced or finely chopped meat, poultry, fish or strips of lean tender meats; cooked egg yolk; mashed or whole, well-cooked pulses, lentils and tofu.	Limited amount of unsweetened, diluted fruit juice in child-size cup. May use moderate amounts of butter (unsalted) and a small scrape of yeast extract on bread or toast. Do not give peanut butter or peanuts, which can cause choking.

*Whole cow's milk can be offered at around 12 months of age and continued until the age of two.

few days after birth, is higher in protein and lower in sugar and fat than later breast milk. It has a laxative effect that activates the baby's bowels. Colostrum is also rich in antibodies, which increase the baby's resistance to infection. Hormones released in response to the baby's sucking increase the flow of breast milk, and within a few days women produce mature milk which is easy to digest and provides just about all the nutrients a baby normally needs for the first six months. A breastfed baby should remain on breast milk exclusively until about four to six months old.

THE ADVANTAGES OF BREASTFEEDING
Breast milk is convenient economical, sterile, portable and always the right temperature. It may protect infants with a strong family history of allergy from developing one themselves. Breastfed babies appear to have fewer infctions. The benefits extend beyond childhood: studies show that adults who were breast-fed have a reduced incidence of obesity, asthma, diabetes heart disease and some kinds of cancer. Mothers who breastfeed have a reduced risk of post menopausal breast cancer and osteoporosis.

HOW TO TELL IF YOUR BABY IS GETTING ENOUGH

Many new nursing mothers worry that their babies are not getting enough to eat. A baby who has regular stools and produces six or more wet nappies a day is most likely getting plenty of food. Although this varies, breastfed babies generally feed every 2 to 4 hours for the first month or so. Growth is an important indicator of whether or not a baby is getting enough to eat. Remember, however, that babies tend to grow in spurts. During a growth spurt, an infant will want to feed more often and longer than usual, but the mother should not be concerned if, a week or two later, her baby is less interested in eating.

Finally, hungry babies send out plenty of signals that they are hungry. Common cues are crying, irritability and a variety of lip and tongue movements – such as lip smacking and fists in mouths.

BOTTLE-FEEDING

Many mothers elect to bottle-feed and commercial formulas can provide all the essential nutrients to help babies thrive. Choosing an iron-fortified formula is recommended. Babies under one year of age should not be given regular cow's milk because it does not contain the appropriate concentrations of protein, fat

Commercial baby food

Most babies' introduction to solid food comes in the form of small jars of puréed vegetables, fruit and meats. For a young baby, the commercial foods offer some advantages – they are safe and most are free from salt and sugar. For the mother, they offer convenience. If you use commercial baby foods, follow these precautions:

- Never feed the baby straight from the jar and then save the remaining food; saliva on the spoon can transmit bacteria to the food and result in spoilage.

- Commercial baby food typically tastes bland; resist the temptation to season it with salt. Excessive salt can cause future health problems.

- Commercial baby foods have little texture. As a baby's teeth come through, remember to give home-cooked foods with more texture. Finger foods are excellent.

Do one simple thing

Try, try and try again when introducing new foods to baby

Refusal to eat new foods is common and may not reflect an actual dislike of the food. Offer the rejcted food from time to time. Persistence will help a child to develop a varied diet in the long term.

and carbohydrate. The cow's milk in most infant formulas is modified. Some babies who have an allergic reaction to cow's milk protein may require a special formula. Generally, bottle-fed babies consume more than breastfed infants do; they may gain weight more rapidly, although the breastfed babies will eventually catch up with them.

On average, most babies double their birth weight in four to five months, and triple it by the time of their first birthday. Formula mixed in advance should be refrigerated, but not longer than 24 hours; after that, it should be discarded. Discard any formula that is left in the baby's bottle after a feeding; if not, there is a possibility of its being contaminated by micro-organisms entering through the teat opening.

INTRODUCING FOODS

Babies should be introduced to solid foods at six months. Starting solids early can be harmful because the digestive system may not be ready to handle solid foods; also, the early introduction of solid foods may increase the risk of a baby developing food allergies. The first solid food must be easy to digest and unlikely to provoke an allergic reaction – infant rice cereal is a good choice. For the first few feedings, put a small amount on the spoon, gently touch the baby's lips - this action will encourages babies to open their mouths - and place the cereal at the back of the tongue. Don't expect all feedings to go smoothly; babies often spit and protest. The baby should be hungry, but not ravenous. Some experts suggest starting the feeding with a few minutes of breastfeeding or bottle-feeding, then offer a small amount of the moistened cereal – no more than a teaspoon or two – then finish with the milk. After a few sessions, you can start with the cereal, then gradually increase the amount of solid foods. Ideally, continue breastfeeding as well as giving solids until the baby is at least 12 months old. Begin slowly, introducing only one or two new items a week. If you use home-cooked foods, purée them or put them through a blender. In addition to rice cereal, try oat and barley cereals; vegetables and fruit; and puréed chicken and beef.

Do not introduce fruit juice before six months, and preferably not until the infant can manage a cup. If there is a family history of allergies, potentially allergenic foods, such as cheese, yoghurt, ice cream, fish and wheat cereals, should be delayed until the baby is nine months old, or even later. Withdraw any food that provokes a rash, runny nose, unusual fussiness, diarrhoea or any other sign of a possible allergic reaction or food intolerance.

Dental hygiene

Many parents mistakenly assume that baby teeth are not important because they are eventually replaced by the permanent teeth. In fact, early dental decay not only threatens the underlying secondary teeth, it can cause severe toothaches. As soon as the first tooth comes in, parents should begin practising preventive dental hygiene. Babies should not be allowed to fall asleep while breastfeeding or sucking a bottle; this allows milk to pool in the mouth, and the sugar (lactose) in it can cause extensive tooth decay. Offering a little water at the end of a feeding rinses any remaining milk from the baby's mouth. The gums and emerging teeth can be wiped gently with a gauze-wrapped finger.

Sugar is the major cause of childhood tooth decay; avoid offering sugary soft drinks and sweet snacks. A chunk of cheese, a piece of fruit, a rusk or other hard biscuit are better alternatives that provide important nutrients without harming the teeth.

SELF-FEEDING

When they are about seven or eight months old, most babies have developed enough eye-hand co-ordination to pick up finger food and manoeuvre it into their mouth. The teeth are usually beginning to come in at this age; giving a baby a finger of toast or a rusk to chew on can ease gum soreness as well as provide practice in self-feeding. Other good starters are finger foods, which could include banana, slices of apples and pears, peas and cooked carrots and small pieces of soft-cooked boiled or roasted chicken. The pieces should be large enough to hold but small enough so that they don't lodge in the throat and cause choking.

As soon as the baby can sit in a high chair, he or she should be included at family meals and start eating many of the same foods, even though they may need mashing or cutting into small pieces. Offer a spoon, but don't be disappointed if a child prefers to use hands. At this stage it's more important for the baby to become integrated into family activities and master self-feeding than to learn proper table manners. These will come eventually, especially if the parents and older siblings set a good example.

● **Myth.......**

Vegetables should be introduced to baby's diet before fruit in order to increase the acceptance of vegetables.

.......Reality ●

This is not the case and fruit and vegetables should be introduced to baby's diet in an alternating manner.

WEANING

Giving up the breast or bottle is a major milestone in a baby's development, but not one that should be rushed. When a woman stops breastfeeding it is largely a matter of personal preference, but ideally, breastfeeding should continue for 12 months. Some babies decide to give up their bottles themselves at nine or ten months; yet others will still want it – especially at nap or bedtime. If a baby under a year old drinks milk from a cup, it should still be expressed breast milk or a formula.

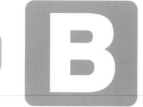

Backache

EAT PLENTY OF

- Oily fish
- Citrus fruit, papaya, kiwi fruit and peppers for their vitamin C

CUT DOWN ON

- Coffee, tea and other drinks containing caffeine
- Fat and sugar if you are overweight

Damage to spinal discs, pressure on nerves, damaged ligaments, misalignment or inflammation of joints, or diseased vertebrae can all lead to backache. Other common causes include pregnancy, poor posture, a bed that does not support your body correctly, lifting heavy objects or suddenly taking up a new sporting activity. A chiropractor or osteopath should be able to relieve most forms of backache, but in the long term, a healthy diet may prevent it in the first place.

There are no nutritional 'cures' for backache but a sensible programme of diet and exercise to lose weight may help to ease the pain in those who are overweight; the increased strain extra weight puts on the spine can contribute to the problem.

By ensuring that your diet contains all the nutrients needed for healthy bones and muscles you can also reduce the risks of developing back problems. You need protein to build up the strong muscle tissue that your back needs. B vitamins, particularly niacin, strengthen and nourish nerve tissues. Liver and oily fish, such as sardines, mackerel and salmon, are good sources of niacin and vitamin D, which aids the body's absorption of calcium and is important in developing and maintaining healthy bones and nerves. A twice weekly 100g helping of any oily fish will provide you with the equivalent of the recommended weekly intake of both these vitamins, while the fatty acids that the fish contain can help to suppress inflammation, and so reduce pains in the joints.

Citrus, cabbage, guavas, papaya, kiwi fruit and peppers are all excellent sources of vitamin C, which is needed for the development and maintenance of strong bones and a healthy nervous system. It is generally recommended that a healthy adult should take about 40g of vitamin C every day – this is about as much as you would get from eating two portions of cabbage, a mango, a small papaya or half a guava. However, smokers need twice this amount.

If you are suffering from backache it is wise to cut down on coffee and tea and any other drink containing caffeine as this relatively mild stimulant narrows the smallest blood vessels at the tip of the arteries. This reduces the flow of blood and nutrients carried in the blood to the spinal tendons, which may slow the healing process.

Joints need to keep moving in order to stay healthy. So whether you want to relieve back pain now or help to prevent it in the future, one of the best things you can do is to keep active.

Persistent backache is a common problem, especially with increasing age. But it is important to consult your doctor for a proper diagnosis, as the pain could be the symptom of a more serious disorder, such as osteoporosis or, in rare cases, cancer.

Bad breath

TAKE PLENTY OF

- Raw vegetables and apples to help to protect the gums
- Ginger, cinnamon, mustard and horse-radish for the sinuses
- Whole-grain cereals and water to avoid constipation
- Carrots, broccoli, spinach and citrus fruit for beta carotene and vitamin C
- Probiotic supplements and water

CUT DOWN ON

- Sugar, sweets, sweet drinks, cakes and biscuits to protect the teeth and gums and reduce plaque

AVOID

- Garlic, onions and curry
- Alcohol and all tobacco products

Unless it is caused by illness, bad breath can usually be cured by sensible eating habits and thorough oral hygiene. It is often caused by curry, garlic, alcohol or cigarettes.

Digestive disorders and ongoing constipation can also cause bad breath, and here again a healthy, sensible diet can often help.

Food odours can be avoided by chewing a few dill seeds or a couple of coffee beans after a meal. Caraway and cardamom seeds are

Did you know?

Sometimes breath odour can be a key to medical diagnosis – the acetone smell of a diabetic coma, the ammonia smell of uraemia or the fishy smell of liver failure.

But the most common cause of bad breath can usually be found in the mouth – a bad tooth or abscess, a build up of tartar, inflamed and infected gums or rotting food in crevices or mouth ulcers. Take action straight away in all these cases, to prevent problems.

also effective, while chewing a sprig of fresh parsley will rid the breath of garlic and alcohol odours. Eating plenty of fibre-rich foods such as raw vegetables, apples and pears help to massage the gums and keep them healthy. Reduce plaque formation by cutting down on sugary drinks and foods, and brush and floss your teeth regularly.

A gargle and mouthwash made by adding 30 drops of tincture of myrrh (available from most chemists) to a glass of warm water will help to keep your breath sweet. It is important to remember that patent antiseptic mouthwashes can kill good as well as harmful bacteria.

Problems in the mouth, the nose and sinuses, the lungs or the stomach and digestive tract can all lead to bad breath; so can use of the prescribed sedative paraldehyde. To relieve sinus problems and catarrh, try reducing your intake of dairy products and eat decongestant spices such as ginger, cinnamon, mustard and horseradish. It may also help to add 5 or 6 drops of eucalyptus oil to a bowl of hot water then inhale the pungent steam.

Chronic chest infections require medical attention, but you may avoid them by not smoking and by eating plenty of carrots, broccoli, spinach and citrus fruits for their beta carotene and vitamin C, which help to protect lung tissue.

Constipation, ulcers and indigestion can provoke bad breath. Sucking peppermints or chewing gum may hide it, but it is best to deal with the cause by increasing your fibre and fluid intake. Try eating wholemeal bread instead of white, and drinking a couple of extra glasses of water a day.

If the cause of your bad breath is not easily identified or remedied, it is important to seek professional dental or medical advice. Do not leave it, in case the cause is serious.

Bacon

See Pork

Bananas

BENEFITS

- An excellent source of potassium and vitamin B$_6$, as well as a source of folate and fibre

Healthy, filling and tasty, bananas are one of nature's ideal snacks. The fruit is harvested while still green. When stored at room temperature, most bananas ripen in a few days; the ripening process can be hastened by placing them in a plastic or paper bag along with an apple. Banana skins have a naturally high serotonin content.

Try bananas for your baby's first food. Because bananas are easy to digest and unlikely to produce allergies, they are an ideal early food for babies. Some ulcer patients report that green bananas and plantains alleviate some pain. While an intolerance to bananas is rare, it is more common in people who are allergic to rubber products. It is thought that bananas may contain proteins that resemble latex.

Nutritional value

A medium banana contains 400mg of potassium, a mineral that plays a role in lowering blood pressure – higher potassium levels are linked with lower blood pressure. Bananas also contain the amino acid tryptophan, which stimulates the production of serotonin, a neurotransmitter that has a calming effect on the body.

Bananas are an excellent source of vitamin B$_6$; a medium 100g banana supplies 40 per cent of the amount we need daily. Some of the dietary fibre in bananas is soluble fibre, which is helpful in lowering blood cholesterol levels. Bananas contain about 95kcal each, mostly in the form of fruit sugar and starch. The riper the banana, the more its starch is converted to sugar.

Plantains. These resemble large green bananas, but they are not as sweet. Plantains can be baked or fried and are usually served as a starchy side dish. They can also be a delicious addition to soups, stews and meat dishes. Nutritionally, plantains are comparable with bananas, except that they contain about ten times more beta carotene than an ordinary banana.

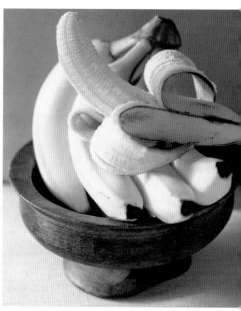

Did you know?

Bananas can be served just like ice cream

Frozen bananas – with nothing added – will whip into a frothy substitute for soft-serve ice cream. Peel and freeze four or five bananas, then place chunks of the frozen fruit into a food processor. The yellow lumps will gradually turn into a deliciously healthy dessert. The foam can be kept in the freezer for about 24 hours.

B

Barbecued foods
Examining the risks

Barbecuing has been a popular method of cooking for thousands of years. Barbecued foods retain a lot of flavour and cooking them doesn't require added fats. Fish and vegetables cook quickly on the barbecue with little loss of moisture or vitamins. In short, barbecuing is a truly healthy cooking method – with one potentially major caveat.

CAVEMAN COOKING

Involving direct exposure of food to the source of heat, barbecuing is the modern and controlled version of man's oldest culinary technique – namely, roasting over an open fire. The intense flavour of barbecued food results from the numerous chemical reactions that take place when a food surface is subjected to very high temperatures. Barbecuing – whether by gas flame, wood fire, electric element or charcoal – demands temperatures four to six times higher than can be reached in an oven; an electric barbecue heats to about 1000°C and a gas flame to about 1650°C, compared with a maximum of 260°C for domestic ovens.

Unfortunately, the high heat that causes the appealing caramelisation of browning has a less desirable aspect: the outside of the food may become unpalatably charred before the inside is cooked through. Barbecuing is best reserved for quick-cooking foods, such as fish and thinner cuts of meat and poultry. It is an excellent method of cooking such vegetables as aubergines, courgettes, peppers and mushrooms. Apples, peaches and other fruit are also delicious when barbecued. Preparation requires little more than a light brushing with oil to prevent food from sticking to the barbecue or drying out.

THE DOWNSIDE OF GRILLING

At high temperatures, the surface fat on meat quickly burns away, releasing acrid fumes and creating a risk of fire. There's a further hazard to barbecuing. Cancer-causing substances called polycyclic aromatic hydrocarbons form when the fat from meat drips onto hot coals, and are deposited onto the food through smoke. You can minimise exposure to the fumes by partly baking or parboiling the food, then finishing it off with a few minutes on the barbecue to achieve a crusty exterior and succulent interior. Choose lean cuts, and trim all visible fat from meat. Whether you're using an oven griller or an outdoor barbecue, place a pan to catch melted fat under a spatterproof metal shield.

Heating meat, poultry and fish to a high temperature also creates substances called heterocyclic amines (HCAs), which have been linked to cancer in animals. HCAs can also form in foods – especially red meat – that are fried or barbecued. This may be one reason that frequent consumption of red meat has been linked in some studies with an increased risk for cancers such as colon cancer.

B

Other potentially toxic compounds are generated by chemical reactions that take place when foods are cooked at high temperatures. Carcinogenic nitrosamines, for example, form when foods that contain nitrite as a preservative, such as bacon or smoked sausages, are heated.

There's no direct evidence that substances causing cancer in animals necessarily cause the disease in humans, but there is enough epidemiological evidence to suggest that foods cooked at a high temperature should be consumed only in moderation.

COMBINE PROTECTIVE FOODS AND NUTRIENTS AS A PRECAUTION

The risks of eating barbecued meats can be modulated by combining them with certain protective nutrients. Vitamins C and E, for example, block the chemical reaction that generates nitrosamines. As antioxidants, these vitamins, as well as beta carotene, can neutralise some carcinogens. Wheatbran binds with nitrite and makes it unavailable for nitrosamine formation. So, you can balance your barbecued breakfast bacon with a glass of vitamin C-rich citrus juice and whole-grain cereal or a bran muffin for essential vitamin E.

Substances found in vegetables and fruit bind directly to carcinogens, such as the polycyclic hydro-carbons, and prevent them from reacting with DNA. Bioflavonoids, the pigments in many fruits and vegetables, appear to block many carcinogens. Fibre may bind with or dilute carcinogens and speed their elimination from the digestive tract. When you barbecue, serve lots of leafy greens and whole grains with the meat or fish to ensure a healthy mixture of fibre and vitamins. Make a vegetarian barbecue; add low-fat cheese to satisfy a desire for protein. Grilled fruit ends a meal with a colourful cocktail of vitamins, fibre and flavour.

A WARNING ABOUT MARINADES

Marinades can add exotic flavours. A small amount of honey or other sugar in the marinade will hasten the caramelisation process because simple sugars brown at lower temperatures than proteins and starchy foods do. Some studies show lower levels of HCAs in meats that have been in a sweet marinade. But don't make the mistake of assuming that a marinated meat is cooked just because the outside is browned. And despite the instructions in many recipes to marinate for hours, there's nothing to be gained from prolonged marination. The marinade cannot penetrate past the surface of the meat, no matter how long the meat is soaked. In addition, the acid of the marinade will eventually tenderise the surface of the meat by denaturing the surface proteins.

Minimising your cancer risk

Charcoal-grilling foods, especially fatty meats, can create compounds that are potentially carcinogenic. The factors involved are the charring of the food and the smoke produced when fat drips on the coals, which is then carried back up to the meat. To minimise the risks, do this:

1 Avoid flare-ups, since burning juice or fat can produce harmful smoke. If smoke from dripping fat is too heavy, move the food to another section, or reduce the heat.

2 Cook meat until it is done without charring it. Remove any charred pieces – don't eat them.

3 Don't place the heat source directly under the meat. For example, place coals slightly to the side so the fat doesn't drip on them. Keep a water bottle handy for coals that become hot or flare up.

4 Cover the barbecue bars with punctured aluminium foil before you cook. The foil protects the food from the smoke and fire.

5 Keep meat portions small so they don't have to spend as long on the barbecue.

6 Defrost frozen meats thoroughly before grilling. In trying to get the frozen meat cooked, there is a tendency to cook it for too long and burn the surface.

Beans and pulses

B

BENEFITS

- Contain more protein than any other plant-derived food

- A good source of B-complex vitamins, iron, potassium, zinc and other essential minerals

- Most are high in soluble fibre

DRAWBACKS

- May cause bloating and intestinal gas

- Can trigger allergies in some people

- Must be cooked to destroy numerous toxic substances.

Beans and pulses belong to a food group called legumes. The 13,000 varieties of legume that are grown worldwide share two major characteristics – they all produce seed-bearing pods, and have nodules on their roots, which harbour bacteria that can convert nitrogen to nitrate, a form that the plant uses for nutrition.

Otherwise, these members of the *Leguminosae* plant family differ greatly: some are low-growing plants (bush beans, lentils and soya beans) or vines (many peas and beans); others are trees (carob) or shrubs (mesquite). Peanuts are not nuts, they are actually legumes.

Did you know?

Losing weight is easier when you eat legumes

If you are trying to lose weight, a serving of beans or pulses will help you to feel full more quickly. The rich fibre content fills your stomach and causes a slower rise in blood sugar, staving off hunger for longer and giving you a steady supply of energy.

Because beans and pulses may lack certain amino acids (the building blocks of protein), it was thought that vegetarians should eat these foods with other foods which contain the missing amino acids to provide a 'complete' protein. As a result, most legumes are served with plant foods and whole grains such as rice or bread. These combinations are referred to as complementary proteins and have been used by vegetarians the world over. However, it is now known that if there is a mix of amino acids throughout the day, then having complementary proteins at the same meal isn't necessary. Soya beans contain almost all of the essential amino acids that make complete protein; they are also high in other nutrients.

Thus, strict vegetarians whose diets exclude all animal foods can rely on tofu and other soya products for protein as well as iron, calcium and other nutrients.

Nutritional winners

Legumes are among our most nutritious plant foods – high in protein, B-complex vitamins, iron, potassium and other minerals. They provide large amounts of fibre, both soluble and insoluble. The soluble type is important in controlling and lowering blood cholesterol levels, reducing the risk of heart disease and stroke. Insoluble fibre aids digestion by helping to cut down constipation and thereby reduce the risk of cancers of the colon and rectum.

Legumes contain a range of important phytochemicals that have a number of disease-fighting properties. Some of the important ones include: isoflavones, which are protective against heart disease and cancer; saponins, which help to lower cholesterol; and phytosterols, which have anticancer and cholesterol-lowering properties.

Sound effects

The gas-causing culprits in beans are carbohydrates called oligosaccharides. Rinsing canned beans and presoaking dried beans should help.

Legumes are also a good food for a diabetic diet because they have a low glycaemic index (GI), which provides a slow, steady source of glucose instead of the sudden surge that can occur after eating carbo-hydrates that are converted to glucose more rapidly.

Most legumes are low in fat, but soya beans and peanuts are high in mostly unsaturated fats.

The downside

Despite their many advantages to the human diet, legumes harbour a number of toxic substances that can interfere with the absorption of vitamins. Soya beans, for example, contain substances that interfere with the absorption of beta carotene and vitamins B_{12} and D. Beans and peas have an anti-vitamin E compound. Although heating and cooking can inactivate most of these substances, legumes should be eaten with lots of fresh fruit and yellow or dark green vegetables (for beta carotene), lean meat or dairy products (for vitamin B_{12}) and nuts, wheat germ fortified cereals, seeds and poultry (for vitamin E).

People with gout are sometimes advised to avoid dried peas and beans, lentils and other pulses because of their high purine content. In susceptible people, purines increase levels of uric acid and can precipitate a gout attack.

Some people of Mediterranean or Asian descent carry a gene that makes them susceptible to favism, a severe type of anaemia contracted from eating fava beans. Others can develop an allergic reaction and migraine headaches from peanuts.

Beans, more beans and other legumes

There are hundreds of different varieties of beans and other legumes; the following are among the more popular.

ADUKI These small red beans are lower in B vitamins but higher in minerals than their larger red cousins, the kidney beans. Sweet flavoured, they are used in Oriental cuisine.

BLACK BEANS A staple in Latin American, Chinese and Japanese dishes, these earthy-flavoured beans are somewhat lower in folate than kidney beans but otherwise comparable in nutritional value.

BLACK-EYED PEAS A creamy, kidney-shaped bean with the chacteristic black spot. It is an excellent source of folate, supplies useful amounts of phosphorus and manganese, and contains zince, iron, magnesium and thiamin.

BORLOTTI BEANS A speckled, light brown bean that is popular in Italy.

BROAD BEANS Strongly flavoured beans that can be eaten raw. A useful source of phosphorus and manganese, they also contain iron, zinc, folate, niacin, magnesium and vitamin E. They are high in soluble fibre.

CANNELLINI These large white kidney beans are used in minestrone and other Italian dishes; they are available canned.

CHICKPEAS Round, with a nutty flavour, they are used in central Asian and Middle eastern cuisines; also available as a flour. A good source of manganese, iron, folate and vitamin E. Chickpeas form the basis of hummous.

FLAGEOLET BEANS Pale green, immature kidney beans. Popular in France.

HARICOT BEANS Small, white bean, these have a milder flavour and slightly more folate and iron than most types of bean. They are used for baked beans.

KIDNEY BEANS These large, red beans derive their name from their shape and are among the most nutritious of the dried types. Meaty-flavoured, they are a favourite for chilli con carne, stews and soups.

LENTILS A staple of south Asian cuisine, they are available in various colours. Green and brown varieties are a good source of selenium, offer useful amounts of iron and manganese, and also contain phosphorus, zinc, thiamine, vitamin B_6 and folate.

LIMA BEANS Also called the butter bean. Used fresh or dried, lima beans are highly nutritious. They contain phosphorus and iron.

PINTO BEANS This mottled, long, multi-coloured bean is one of the most nutritious types and is very high in fibre. Popular in the USA and latin America.

RED BEANS Often combined with rice or used in chilli dishes, red beans are similar to kidney beans.

SOYA BEANS Among the most nutritious of all the legumes, soya beans give rise to many widely consumed products, including bean curd, soya milk, soya flour and soy sauce. They are rich in potassium, and are a useful souce of magnesium, phosphorus, iron, folate and vitamin E. They also contain manganese, vitamin B_6 and thiamin.

SPLIT PEAS Yellow or green dried peas; excellent in soups and purées.

▲ **The power of beans**
Beans are a source of non-animal protein and may help to reduce LDL cholesterol, stabilise blood sugar and even control weight.

Pulses such as dried beans, lentils and peas are notorious for causing intestinal wind or flatulence. Some herbs, in particular thyme, rosemary, sage, summer savory, lemon balm, fennel and caraway, can help to prevent flatulence.

Fresh broad beans

Pale green or creamy white broad beans are at their best in late spring and early summer. Their pods should be crisp and bright green when you buy them; brown patches indicate rot.

Young beans, no thicker than a finger, with pods around 7.5cm long, are the most delicious and can be cooked and eaten in their entirety. Mature broad beans should be shelled before cooking. The pods are high in tyramine, which can cause migraine and trigger an adverse reaction with the class of antidepressants called MOIs.

Freezing does not greatly affect the nutrients in broad beans, but the canning process destroys some of their vitamin C.

Beef

BENEFITS

- Major source of high-quality protein

- Contain a wide range of nutrients, especially vitamin B_{12}, iron, niacin and zinc

DRAWBACKS

- Fatty cuts contain saturated fat, which can increase blood cholesterol levels and the risk of cardiovascular disease

- A high-meat diet may raise the risk of colon cancer and other cancers

- Rare beef may be a source of *E. coli*

Although its consumption has decreased in recent decades, beef is still a popular red meat. One of the most versatile meats, beef may be prepared by roasting, stewing, barbecuing, frying and grilling.

There is no question that beef is a highly nutritious food source; not only is it a leading source of high-quality protein, but a 120g serving provides more than 100 per cent of the RNI of vitamin B_{12}, an essential nutrient found only in animal products. Beef is also an excellent source of vitamin B_6, niacin and riboflavin, as well as such essential minerals as iron and zinc.

A case of less is best

Although beef contains immune-boosting nutrients, its major drawback is the large amount of saturated fat in some cuts, especially in hamburgers and marbled steaks. Medical studies have linked the consumption of large amounts of meat to an increased risk of heart attacks and colorectal cancers.

The key factors concerning fat are the cut, portion size and cooking method. Choose the leanest cuts – fillet, rump or round are good. Then, trim all visible fat from your meat. Reduce fat further by grilling, barbecuing or roasting on a rack (so fat can drip away).

Another approach is to cook casseroles, curries and soups in advance, chill them so that the congealed fat can be removed easily and then reheat the dishes before serving. Instead of gravy or sauce, serve your meat 'au jus', after skimming off all the fat.

> ### Beef facts
> - The fat content of today's beef is lower than in the past, in response to popular demand and as a result of modern breeding techniques and feeding methods.
> - Lean beef contains less than 5 per cent fat; less than half of this is saturated fat.

Offal

The liver, kidneys and other types of offal are the most concentrated source of iron and vitamins A and B_{12} in beef. At one time, women were urged to eat an occasional serving of liver in order to prevent iron-deficiency anaemia. Now, pregnant women are advised to avoid liver or liver products, such as paté, because of the high level of vitamin A, which can adversely affect the foetus when taken in large amounts.

Kidneys are also an extremely rich source of vitamin B_{12}; a typical serving can provide about 20 times the adult daily requirement.

Veal

Very young calves produce the delicate light-coloured, low-fat veal that has always been considered a luxury meat. It is an excellent source of high-quality protein and a source of iron, zinc and vitamin B_{12}. On average, a trimmed, cooked 85g serving of veal contains about 190kcal and less than 8g of fat. The leanest cuts include the cutlet, veal roast and the loin chop.

Scares and chemicals

The scare involving BSE (bovine spongiform encephalopathy), or 'mad cow disease', which happened in the late 1980s changed public perceptions about eating beef, but since stringent steps were taken to change the manner in which cattle were fed, and the acceptance of

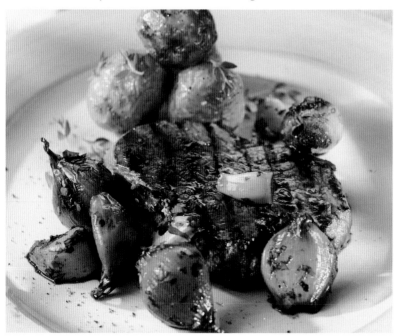

British beef back into the European market, beef has regained much of its former popularity.

BSE is not contagious, but the disease can be transmitted when rendered materials from an infected animal are fed to another animal. By banning the feeding of rendered materials, the major transmission method of BSE between animals has largely been eliminated.

After a similar disease, Creutzfeldt-Jacob Disease (CJD), was found in humans, potentially infectious material was removed from the human food chain, but because the incubation period of CJD may be as long as 20 years, it is hard to predict how many people will develop the disease.

Another major concern is about the illegal use of chemicals in beef farming. Antibiotics have long been banned as additives to animal feed and, in 1988, the European Union banned the use of growth-promoting hormones aimed at increasing the amounts of lean meat each animal produced. The ban was introduced because of the unknown consequences of such eating beef treated in this manner. However, researchers have found signs that hormones are still being used illegally in Europe.

Beer

BENEFITS

- Is lower in alcohol concentrations than wine and spirits

DRAWBACKS

- Overconsumption can cause unwanted weight gain and obesity

- Heavy drinking can lead to inebriation and alcoholism

- Causes feelings of aggression in some people

Historians believe that humans began to brew beer some time around 5000 BC in the areas that are now called Iraq and Egypt. Barley, which is the grain that still dominates beer brewing, was abundant in those regions at that time. Over the centuries, almost every society worldwide has, independently, developed ways of making beer from local cereal grains: African tribes use sprouted corn, millet and sorghum; Russians turn rye bread into a low-alcohol beer, which they call *kvass*; the Chinese and Japanese use rice; and the Native Americans from South and Central America rely on corn to make their respective beers.

The brewing process

Although many societies around the world continue to use their traditional methods to make beer, modern brewing is a scientific process that begins with malting to convert grain starch into sugar that will ferment. To do this, the grain is sprouted in order to activate enzymes that will eventually turn the starch into sugar. The precise methods vary according to the type of beer being produced, but at some point the germination is stopped, the sprouts are removed and the malted grain is then prepared for mashing. The malt is

heated slowly to allow the enzymes to continue converting starch into a sugary broth called wort. The grain is allowed to settle, and the wort is heated and filtered through it into the brewing kettles. (The grains are then rinsed and salvaged for livestock feed.)

Hops, which are dried flowers from the hop vine, are added to the wort, and the mixture is boiled and

Beer for the ages

A long-term study found that having 1.5 alcoholic drinks a day offered some protection against heart failure in 20-50 per cent of men and women with an average age of 74. Too much alcohol, however, has the opposite effect.

then strained. (The used hops are added to livestock feed.) The wort is allowed to settle so that the protein can be removed; the clear liquid is then fermented with yeast and aged. Eventually, yeast residue is skimmed off and used as a nutritional supplement (brewer's yeast) or added to livestock feed. The process may be varied and other ingredients added to give beer a distinctive flavour, colour or aroma. Adding extra hops produces the British draft beer known as bitter; ale, a more concentrated beer, uses a type of yeast that rises to the top; stout is a bitter ale brewed from a dark malt.

The specific brewing method influences the nutritional quality of beer. The cloudy German *weisse bier*, for example, retains many of the B vitamins found in brewer's yeast, but these are strained away to make clear beer.

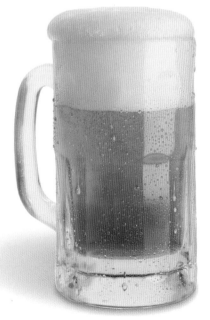

Native African beers remain unfiltered; as a result, they retain many of the nutrients found in the grains, roots and tubers that are their main ingredients.

Nutritional value of beer

Beer's nutritional value is often overstated because most of the nutrients in the grain are lost in the brewing process. About three-quarters of the 113kcal in 375ml of ordinary beer come from the alcohol itself, with the rest coming from sugars; in contrast, only a trace of protein remains after brewing and straining. A 375ml can of ordinary beer provides 5 to 10 per cent of the RNIs of folate, niacin and vitamin B_6.

How much is enough?

Typically, the alcohol content of beer ranges from 3 to 8 per cent, compared with an average of 12 per cent in wine, and about 40 per cent in spirits. Some people who are very sensitive to alcohol will react almost immediately to even this modest amount, often with feelings of aggression. Many people, however, can consume a couple of beers without any obvious mental or physical effects.

Beer drinking can, however, add a significant number of calories, which may result in weight gain. The excessive urination resulting from the diuretic effect of the alcohol may also wash away important vitamins and minerals before the body can absorb them. Chronic over-consumption of beer can lead to problem drinking and alcoholism.

Watch what you eat with it

Beer is frequently served with nuts, potato crisps, pretzels and other salty foods. Because these increase feelings of thirst, they actually promote the consumption of excessive amounts of beer.

Beetroot

BENEFITS

■ A source of folate, fibre and potassium

■ The greens are a rich source of potassium, calcium, iron, beta carotene and vitamin C

■ Low in calories

■ Rich in phytochemicals such as anthocyanins and saponins, which may bind cholesterol in the digestive tract, lowering the risk for heart disease

DRAWBACKS

■ Turns urine and stools red, a harmless condition that nonetheless alarms people who mistake it for blood

Beetroot is a versatile vegetable. It can be baked, steamed or barbecued and served as a side dish; pickled and eaten as a salad or condiment; or used as the main ingredient in borscht, a popular Eastern European soup. The most nutritious part of the vegetable, the grens, can be cooked and served like spinach.

According to folklore, beetroot was believed to possess curative powers for headaches and other painful conditions. Even today, some naturopaths recommend beetroot to bolster immunity; they also suggest using the juice of raw beetroot to speed convalescence. Although beetroot is a reasonably nutritious food source, to date there is no scientific proof that it confers any special medicinal benefits.

Don't forget the tops

An 80g serving of cooked beetroot provides 85mcg of folate, about 40 per cent of the adult RNI. However, the tops, if eaten while young and green, are also nutritious. They provide vitamin C, beta carotene, as well as some calcium, iron and potassium.

The most tasty beetroot is small, with greens still attached. The best way to cook beetroot is to boil it unpeeled, or bake it wrapped in foil, which retains most of the nutrients, as well as the deep red colour. After the beetroot has cooled, the skin slips off easily; the root can be sliced, chopped or puréed. Beetroot may also be canned and pickled with vinegar; some nutrients are lost in the processing, but the sweet flavour remains.

Effects on body wastes

Many people notice that their urine and stools have turned pink or even red after eating beetroot. This is harmless and occurs in about 15 per cent of people who lack the gut bacteria that normally degrade the bright red pigment present in beetroot. Known as betacyanine, this pigment is totally harmless and passes straight through the digestive system. The urine and stools will usually return to their normal colours after a day or two.

Facts about beetroot

- Beetroot has one of the highest sugar content of any vegetable, yet is relatively low in calories – about 37kcal in an 80g serving.
- Beetroot contains betacyanin, a type of plant pigment, which some preliminary research indicates might be helpful in defending cells against harmful carcinogens. It is also being studied for its potential as a tumour-fighting compound.
- Many cooks today discard the beetroot tops and use only the roots. In ancient times, however, only the tops were eaten as a vegetable; the roots were used as a medicine to treat painful disorders such as headaches and toothaches.
- Betalains, which are the bright red pigments in beetroot, are extracted and can be used as a natural food colouring or a dye.

Bioflavonoids

BENEFITS

- Thought to function as antioxidants and also to enhance the antioxidant effects of vitamin C

- Believed to be instrumental in proper capillary function

- Some appear to be natural antibiotics and anticancer agents

Bioflavonoids are naturally occurring phytochemicals that act primarily as plant pigments and flavouring. Numerous compounds fall into this family of substances, which are linked by some common features in their molecular structure. Some of the sub-categories of bioflavonoids include isoflavones, anthocyanidins, flavans, flavonols, flavones and flavanones.

Where are they?

Bioflavonoids are found in a wide range of foods, but particularly in fruit and vegetables. For example, flavanones are found in citrus fruit, isoflavones in soya products, anthocyanidins in wine, flavans in apples and tea, and rutin in the buckwheat plant. Other foods that are high in bioflavonoids include apricots, blackberries, bilberries, blackcurrants, broccoli, cherries, grapefruit, grapes, lemons, papayas, peppers, plums, melons and tomatoes, as well as in coffee and cocoa.

Potential health-boosting effects include the following:

- Capillaries are highly permeable blood vessels that allow oxygen, hormones, nutrients and antibodies to pass from the bloodstream to the cells. If the capillary walls are fragile, blood will seep out into the cells. This can result in brain and retinal haemorrhages, bruising, bleeding gums and other problems. Bioflavonoids improve capillary strength by helping to maintain the proper degree of permeability in the capillary wall.
- Recent research indicates that some bioflavonoids are inhibitors that prevent blood clot formation. These bioflavonoids may be useful in treating phlebitis and other clotting disorders.
- Bioflavonoids are also believed to protect against heart disease. Resveretrol and quercetin, the bioflavonoids in grape skins, are thought to reduce the risk of heart disease among moderate wine drinkers.
- Many bioflavonoids prevent cellular damage caused by free radicals – unstable molecules that are formed when the body uses oxygen. Some bioflavonoids are used as food preservatives to prevent oxidation of fats. Others enhance the antioxidant action of nutrients.

- Bioflavonoids enhance the action of vitamin C. Bioflavonoids and vitamin C are present in the same foods, and the body metabolises both in a similar way. This has led researchers to theorise that some of the functions attributed to vitamin C are actually due to bioflavonoids instead; others feel that the two work together in a synergistic manner.
- Cancer-causing substances may be hampered by bioflavonoids. Recent laboratory studies indicate that some bioflavonoids stop or slow the growth of malignant cells and may also help to protect against cancer-causing substances.
- Some bioflavonoids destroy certain bacteria, retarding food spoilage and protecting humans from food-borne infections.

Potential therapeutic uses

A number of bioflavonoids are currently being studied for potential therapeutic uses:

- **Hesperidin**, a bioflavonoid in the blossoms and peels of oranges, lemons and other citrus fruit, is being considered for treating easy bruising and other types of bleeding problems.
- **Rutin**, found in buckwheat leaves and some other plants, is being studied for treating glaucoma and the retinal bleeding that may occur in diabetes, as well as for reducing tissue damage from the effects of frostbite, radiation exposure and haemophilia.
- **Quercetin**, found in apples, onions, tea, red wine and grapes, raspberries, citrus fruit, cherries and other foods, is being investigated to improve lung function and lower the risk of certain respiratory diseases, such as asthma, bronchitis and emphysema. It may also help to treat or even prevent prostate cancer by blocking male hormones that encourage the growth of prostate cancer cells.

Dietary requirements

No Reference Nutrient Intake (RNI) has been established for bioflavonoids, but studies show that if a diet contains enough fruit and vegetables to supply 60mg of vitamin C, it will provide adequate bioflavonoids.

Good sources of vitamin C include oranges, lemons, grapefruit, nectarines, strawberries, kiwi fruit, mangoes, tomatoes, blackberries, broccoli and peppers.

Should you take bioflavonoid supplements?

There is no justification at this time for taking individual bioflavonoids in supplement form. These substances almost certainly act synergistically with other vitamins, minerals and phytochemicals found in foods. The optimal doses, long-term adverse effects of high doses and possible interactions with medicines are unknown.

Scientists at the University of Chicago Medical Center have expressed concern that certain bioflavonoids in supplement form, if taken during pregnancy, may result in childhood leukaemias. They found that 10 out of 20 bioflavonoids tested caused DNA breaks in a gene known to be involved in infant leukaemias. An earlier study had found that these rare leukaemias were twice as common in large Asian cities where soya intake (soya contains a number of bioflavonoids) is two to five times as high as in North America.

The benefits of foods high in flavonoids is unquestioned but the benefits of supplements are not convincing. Pregnant women especially should be careful about taking bioflavonoid supplements. The best way of ensuring an adequate intake of bioflavonoids is to eat a variety of plant foods daily, especially fruit and vegetables.

◀ **Beneficial pigments**
These and many other brightly coloured fresh fruit and vegetables are rich in bioflavonoids.

Blackberries

BENEFITS

- Low in calories and high in fibre

- A good source of vitamin C, useful source of vitamin E; also contain folate

- Contain anthocyanins, bioflavonoids with health benefits including lowering risk of cancer and heart disease Also contain ellagic acid, which has anticancer properties

DRAWBACKS

- Contain salicylates, which can cause a reaction in aspirin-sensitive people

When fully ripe, blackberries are sweet and juicy. Wild berries have a much more concentrated flavour than commercially grown berries.

Their many seeds make blackberries high in fibre. An 80g serving supplies 20kcal and 12mg of vitamin C – 30 per cent of the Reference Nutrient Intake (RNI) – as well as 27mcg of folic acid (15 per cent of RNI) and small amounts of iron and calcium.

Blackberries contain anthocyanins, which have numerous possible health benefits, such as inhibiting cholesterol, preventing cancer and heart disease and even combating some of the effects of ageing.

They also contain ellagic acid, a substance that is believed to help to prevent cancer. Cooking does not appear to destroy ellagic acid, so even blackberry jam may confer this health benefit.

People allergic to aspirin may find that they experience a similar reaction from eating blackberries. The reason for this is that blackberries are a natural source of salicylates, which are substances related to the active compound in aspirin. For this reason, people susceptible to asthma and hyperactivity should avoid them.

Bleeding problems

EAT PLENTY OF

- Spinach, broccoli and other leafy greens and offal

- Lean meat, poultry, seafood and other foods high in iron and vitamin B_{12}

- Citrus and other fresh fruit and vegetables for vitamin C

LIMIT

- Fish oil supplements

AVOID

- Alcohol, aspirin and other drugs that suppress blood platelets and clotting

Some bleeding disorders, such as haemophilia, are hereditary; others develop as a result of nutritional deficiencies, or taking aspirin and other medications that suppress clotting, or as the consequence of certain diseases, including some cancers. Most of these bleeding disorders stem from some type of thrombocytopenia, which is the medical term for a reduced number of platelets, the blood cells vital to clotting. Symptoms vary, but they typically include easy bruising, frequent nosebleeds and excessive bleeding from even minor cuts. Bleeding gums unrelated to dental problems are common. Affected women may experience very heavy menstrual periods. In some cases, there are no obvious symptoms, but blood tests reveal a low platelet count and reduced clotting time.

The blacker the berry, the sweeter the fruit
Delicious plump blackberries are an excellent source of vitamin C, and have more fibre than a serving of some bran cereals. Eat them when freshly picked, and remember to lightly rinse them just before serving.

Check all medications. The overuse of aspirin or other drugs that suppress normal platelet function or production is the most common cause of platelet abnormalities; stopping the offending medication usually solves the problem. In other cases, transfusions of platelets and blood cells may be necessary.

Nutritional influences

Bleeding disorders due to nutritional deficiencies are uncommon, but they do occur. For example, vitamin K – necessary for the blood to clot normally – is made by bacteria in the human intestinal tract; it is also found in green peas, broccoli, spinach and other green leafy vegetables, Brussels sprouts and offal. Sometimes prolonged antibiotic therapy destroys the bacteria that make vitamin K, resulting in bleeding. Increasing your intake of foods that are high in vitamin K may help, but often supplements of the vitamin are given.

Limit foods high in vitamin K if you are taking anti-coagulants, such as warfarin. This vitamin can counteract the desired effect of the drug. Omega-3 fatty acids, found in salmon and other seafood, suppress platelet function, but are unlikely to cause problems if consumed, say, once a week. People taking high doses of fish oil supplements have an increased risk of developing bleeding problems; the risk is compounded if they are also taking aspirin.

Vitamin C deficiency can cause bleeding gums. This deficiency may occur in alcoholics or people who eat little fruit and vegetables.

Chronic blood loss can lead to anaemia, a blood disorder that is characterised by inadequate levels of red blood cells. Dietary sources should supply extra iron, folate and vitamins B_{12} and C, but supplements may be needed in some cases.

Blood pressure

EAT PLENTY OF

- Fresh vegetables, fresh and dried fruit, beans, pulses for potassium
- Oily fish for omega-3 fatty acids
- Low-fat dairy products

LIMIT

- Canned and other processed foods with added salt
- Fatty foods, especially saturated fats

AVOID

- Pickled and very salty foods
- Excessive alcohol and caffein

As blood circulates through the body, it exerts varying degrees of force on artery walls; this is known as blood pressure. According to the World Health Organization, between 10 and 30 per cent of people throughout the world have blood pressure that is too high – or hypertension. In its early stages, high blood pressure is symptomless, so many people do not realise they have a potentially life-threatening disease. If the condition goes unchecked, it will damage the heart and blood vessels and can lead to a stroke, heart attack and other serious consequences.

In about 5 per cent of cases, there's an underlying cause for high blood pressure; for example, a narrowed kidney artery, pregnancy, an adrenal gland disorder or a drug side effect. Most often, however, there is no identifiable cause, and this is referred to as primary, or essential, hypertension.

Blood pressure rises when the body's smallest arteries, narrow or constrict, requiring the heart to beat more forcefully in order to pump blood through them. Increased blood volume, often caused by the body's tendency to retain excessive salt and fluids, raises blood pressure; so do high levels of adrenaline and other hormones that constrict blood vessels.

Monitor underlying factors. With age, blood pressure rises somewhat; no one fully understands precisely what leads to hypertension, although a combination of factors, especially salt intake, seems to be involved. It tends to run in families, so inherited susceptibility is suspected. Diabetes, obesity and certain other disorders increase risk. Stress prompts a surge in adrenal hormones and a temporary rise in blood pressure; some researchers believe that constant stress may play a role in developing hypertension. Other contributors include smoking, excessive alcohol and a generally sedentary lifestyle.

Proper control of high blood pressure and cholesterol can halve the risk of heart attacks. It seems that the death rates from different forms of cardiovascular disease, have been steadily declining since the 1960s, thanks largely to lifestyle changes and improvements in hypertension treatment.

Diet and hypertension

Diet plays a role in both prevention and treatment of high blood pressure. Simple things can help to keep your blood pressure in check.

Limit your salt intake. A high-salt diet also contributes to the condition in people who have a genetic tendency to retain sodium. In these individuals, restriction of salt, from an early age, reduces the risk of developing hypertension. A portion of the population, including older people and people with diabetes, appears to be particularly sensitive to sodium and may benefit significantly from eating low-salt foods. Experts agree that most people should aim to consume no more than 6g of salt each day. The

best way to reduce intake is to avoid adding salt, and to avoid processed foods, which are usually loaded with sodium. Check labels carefully – look for the term 'sodium' to find hidden salt. It may be a good idea to switch to a potassium-based salt substitute, as potassium lowers blood pressure.

Keep your weight down. Being even slightly overweight contributes to hypertension; losing excess weight is often all that is needed to return blood pressure to normal. Even a modest weight loss will cause a drop in blood pressure.

Eat less fat. A high-fat diet not only leads to weight gain but may also contribute to high blood pressure. Limit fat intake to 30 per cent or less of total calories, with 10 per cent or less coming from saturated fats. This means cutting back on butter and margarine; reading food labels to check the saturated fat content; switching to skimmed milk and other low-fat dairy products; choosing lean cuts of meat and grilling instead of frying.

Reduce alcohol and caffeine consumption. Although a glass of wine or other alcoholic drink daily seems to reduce the chance of a heart attack, consuming more than this will negate any benefit and may increase the risk of hypertension. Too much caffeine can also raise blood pressure. Older adults with hypertension may be more sensitive to the effects of caffeine and should limit their intake.

Boost your mineral intake. Some nutrients may protect against high blood pressure. Potassium, an electrolyte that helps to maintain the body's balance of salt and fluids, helps to ensure normal blood pressure. Potassium is found in fruit (especially bananas) and vegetables, dairy products, beans and pulses.

A few US studies have linked calcium deficiency to hypertension, and have suggested that increased intake of low-fat dairy products may be beneficial.

Get more garlic. Other research appears to suggest that garlic can help to lower blood pressure. The amount of garlic necessary to lower blood pressure, however, can cause other problems, especially unpleasant breath and body odour. Although garlic is available in odourless pills, it is not known if these pills produce the same benefits as eating real garlic.

Other lifestyle changes

While a proper diet is instrumental in maintaining normal blood pressure, it should be combined with other lifestyle changes. One of the most important is regular aerobic exercise, which lowers blood pressure by conditioning the heart to work more efficiently. If you smoke, you should give up, because nicotine raises blood pressure.

Did you know?

Limiting sodium and salt content in your diet

Current guidelines suggest you should keep your salt intake below 6g per day. Expressed as sodium (the way salt content is often listed on food labels) that means no more than 2.4g a day. To convert sodium to salt, multiply by 2.5.

Control blood pressure with the DASH diet

The most compelling evidence in support of diet as a means of controlling blood pressure comes from two trials sponsored by the US National Institutes of Health. Together the studies are known as the DASH diet.

The first study, carried out in 1997, was called 'DASH', for Dietary Approaches to Stop Hypertension. It found that blood pressure levels could fall significantly with an eating plan low in total fat, saturated fat and cholesterol, and rich in fruit, vegetables and low-fat dairy products. The diet was shown to prevent hypertension and in some cases reduce blood pressure as much as an antihypertensive drug. Results were seen within two weeks, and benefits remained eight weeks later regardless of a person's gender, ethnicity or initial blood pressure level.

The DASH diet provides foods that are high in fibre, calcium, magnesium and potassium, all of which have been associated with lower blood pressure. It is also low in saturated fat. The diet calls for eating eight to ten servings of fruit and vegetables and two to three helpings of low-fat dairy foods daily. Here are the broad DASH guidelines you can follow in menu planning:

- Grains and grain products: 7 to 8 servings daily
- Fruit and vegetables: 4 to 5 servings of each daily
- Low-fat or nonfat dairy foods: 2 to 3 servings daily
- Meats, poultry and fish: 2 or fewer 85g servings daily
- Nuts, seeds or legumes: 4 to 5 servings per week
- Fats: 2 to 3 servings daily; avoid saturated fat
- Sweets: no more than 5 per week

A follow-up trial, held in 2000, examined whether reducing salt could enhance results even more. Sodium in table salt and in other foods can raise blood pressure by causing the body to retain water, thereby increasing blood volume and thus blood pressure. Sodium also causes small blood vessels to constrict. This study showed that the DASH diet combined with salt reduction was superior to either strategy alone. All the participants benefited from limiting their salt intake.

Giving up smoking can reduce blood pressure markedly – apart from the other health benefits.

Use medications with caution. Non-prescription cold, allergy and diet pills can raise blood pressure. In some women, birth control pills, or hormone replacement therapy, can cause high blood pressure.

Reduce stress. Experts continue to debate the role of stress in hypertension. There is no doubt that stress temporarily raises blood pressure, and some experts think that it may have a long-term effect. Meditation, yoga, biofeedback training, self-hypnosis and other relaxation techniques may help to lower blood pressure. Studies have found that people with pets have lower blood pressure than people who don't own pets.

Drug therapy

Doctors usually recommend about six months of lifestyle changes to see if mild to moderate hypertension returns to normal levels. If not, drug therapy is often instituted. There are dozens of antihypertensive drugs and doctors can usually find one or a combination that lowers blood

B

Understanding blood pressure measurements

Blood does not flow through the body in a steady stream; instead, it courses in spurts. Thus, blood pressure is expressed in two numbers, such as 120/80. The higher number indicates the systolic pressure, the peak force when the heart contracts and pumps a small amount of blood into the circulation. The lower number, the diastolic reading, measures pressure exerted when the heart is resting momentarily between beats. The units of blood pressure measurement are millimetres of mercury; basically this measures how high the pressure of the blood can push a column of mercury in an evacuated tube.

Doctors usually use a stethoscope and a sphygmomanometer to measure blood pressure. The cuff is tightened to stop blood flow, and as pressure is released, they listen for the sounds that indicate systolic and diastolic pressures. If your resting blood pressure is consistently 140/90 or higher, you have high blood pressure. Normal adult blood pressure is defined as below 120/80; hypertension is classified as follows:

	Systolic/Diastolic		Systolic/Diastolic
Optimal:	Less than 120/80	Mild hypertension:	140/90 to 159/99
Normal:	130/85	Moderate hypertension:	160/100 to 179/109
High normal:	130/85 to 139/89	Severe hypertension:	More than 180/110

Note: Some people have a normal systolic reading but a high diastolic pressure; they are classified as hypertensive. Other people have isolated systolic hypertension.

pressure with minimal adverse side effects. The most widely used drugs are diuretics, which reduce salt and fluid volume by increasing the flow of urine. Some classes of drugs reduce the heart's workload by helping to widen the arterioles to increase blood flow; other drugs can slow the pulse.

It is also important to treat disorders that add to high blood pressure, such as diabetes and high blood cholesterol which increase the risk of developing heart problems.

Did you know?

Dry-roasted soya nuts may reduce blood pressure

Can a snack be this potent? According to research that was presented to the American Heart Association in November 2003, eating a half-cup a day of dry-roasted soya nuts may reduce blood pressure readings as much as some prescription blood pressure medications.

Blueberries

BENEFITS

- A good source of dietary fibre

- An excellent source of antioxidants

- Provide vitamin C

- May protect against some intestinal upsets

- May help to prevent urinary tract infections

- Anthocyanins may help to prevent heart disease and cancer and may help with memory loss

DRAWBACKS

- Can make stools dark and tarry, which may be mistaken for intestinal bleeding

- May cause allergic reactions in some people

Blueberries are naturally sweet and, as cooking destroys vitamin C, should be eaten raw to preserve this antioxidant nutrient.

Natural healers also advocate eating one cup of raw berries or drinking one to two cups of unsweetened blueberry juice a day to treat and prevent urinary tract infections. Research appears to support this advice. Blueberries are in the same plant family as cranberries, and both contain a substance that prevents bacteria from adhering to the bladder walls, where they can multiply. These berries also make urine more acidic, which helps to destroy bacteria that invade the bladder and urethra.

Blueberries are particularly effective against the *E.coli* bacterium, which explains their traditional use as a cure for diarrhoea and food-poisoning.

Eating large amounts of blueberries, however, can make stools appear dark and tarry; this is a harmless situation but can be alarming when first noticed, because it resembles intestinal bleeding.

Blueberries provide antioxidant power. They contain anthocyanins, which are flavonoids that give the fruit their distinctive blue colour. These compounds are associated with numerous health benefits such as the prevention of heart disease and cancer and may even combat ageing. Studies on animals have shown that blueberries help to prevent and may even reverse age-related memory loss. The specific substance has not been identified, but scientists speculate that the antioxidant power of blueberries protects brain cells from free-radical harm. More work is needed to see if this extends to humans as well.

Like many fruits, blueberries are potential allergens in susceptible people. Common symptoms are swollen lips and eyelids.

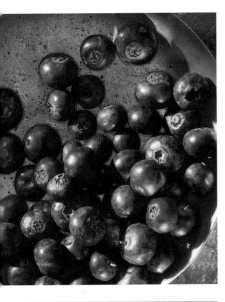

Blueberries: antioxidant superstars

Blueberries are rated third in the ORAC (oxygen radical absorbance capacity) scores, which rates the antioxidant capacity of foods. Fresh blueberries have a high level of ORAC, 2,400 per 100g. (This is almost equal to five servings of some fruit and vegetables.)

Nutritional value

Although they are sweet and tasty, blueberries are not especially high in nutrients other than vitamin C; 50g of raw berries or two 200ml glasses of juice provides 12mg of vitamin C. The same amount of raw raw blueberries has 5mg of fibre and only 28kcal but only very small amounts of other nutrients. However, they do contain some important disease-fighting anthocyanins, so they're an ideal low-calorie fruit treat.

Bran

BENEFITS

■ Helps to prevent constipation

■ Oat and rice brans help to lower blood cholesterol levels

■ Promotes a feeling of fullness, which can help to control appetite

■ May reduce the risk of some cancers

DRAWBACKS

■ Excessive consumption of unprocessed wheat bran reduces the absorption of calcium, iron and zinc

■ Can cause intestinal irritation, bloating and flatulence

Bran, one of the richest sources of dietary fibre, is the indigestible outer husk of wheat, rice, oats and other cereal grains. At one time most bran was discarded when grains were milled. Then in the 1960s Dr Dennis P Burkitt, a British medical officer in Africa, published several scientific reports in which he theorised that bran and other types of fibre could prevent heart attacks, diverticulitis and other intestinal disorders, and cancers of the breast, colon, prostate and uterus.

Burkitt developed this theory after observing that these diseases are rare among rural Africans, who consume large amounts of whole grains. Prompted by the resulting number of best-selling books, bran became the fad food of the 1970s, and unprocessed bran was added to everything from bread to such unlikely dishes as meat loaf and baked apples.

Since then, much of the enthusiasm for using raw bran has dissipated as researchers have learned more about its health benefits and possible hazards. We also know now that various types of bran have different properties and functions. Wheat bran, for example, is mostly insoluble fibre; although it absorbs large amounts of water, it makes its way through the intestinal tract intact. If used in moderation, insoluble fibre helps to prevent constipation by producing a soft, bulky stool that moves quickly and easily through the colon. Excessive amounts, however, should not be taken as they can cause bloating and intestinal gas.

Does bran prevent colon cancer?

Dr Burkitt had theorised that bran prevented colon cancer by reducing the amount of time required for the stool to travel through the bowel. But studies to document this protective effect have produced mixed results. An Australian study found that women taking large amounts of wheat bran actually had a slightly increased incidence of colon cancer. In contrast, a four-year study involving 58 high-risk adults with precancerous colon polyps found that those taking wheat bran achieved a reduction in the size and number of these growths.

Two 2003 medical studies – one on Americans and one on Europeans – showed that high intake of dietary fibre is associated with a lower risk of colorectal cancer. In the American study, investigators compared the daily fibre intake of more than 3,500 people who had precancerous colon polyps to the fibre intake of about 34,000 people who did not have these growths. They found that the people who ate the most fibre, about 35g daily, had a 27 per cent lower risk of precancerous growths than those who ate the least, about 12g per day. The association was strongest for fibres from grains, cereals and fruit. In the European study, researchers examined the link in more than 500,000 people in ten countries. Those who ate the most fibre, about 35g daily, had about a 40 per cent lower risk of colorectal cancer compared to those who ate the least, about 15g a day.

An editorial accompanying the publication of the studies concludes that 'Eating a diet rich in plant

B

foods, in the form of fruit, vegetables and whole-grain cereals probably remains the best option for reducing the risk of colon cancer and for general health protection'.

It also appears that including wheat bran in a high-fibre diet can help to prevent diverticulitis, an intestinal disorder in which small pockets bulging outwards from the colon wall become impacted and inflamed. And because it helps to prevent constipation, bran may also be beneficial for people suffering from haemorrhoids.

People with diabetes may benefit from oat bran. Oat bran is high in soluble fibre, which is sticky and combines with water to form a thick gel. Some researchers have reported that this type of fibre reduces blood cholesterol levels. It also appears to improve glucose metabolism in people with diabetes, which reduces their need for insulin and other diabetes medications.

More recently, there have been reports that rice bran also reduces cholesterol levels. Researchers are not sure, however, whether this benefit comes from the insoluble fibre found in the bran or from the highly unsaturated oil in the rice germ – which is not separated from the grain husks during the milling process.

All types of bran, as well as other high-fibre foods, play an important role in weight control by promoting a feeling of fullness without overeating. This may provide an explanation for the lowered incidence of some obesity-related cancers and heart attacks among populations whose diets are high in fibre – such as Dr Dennis Burkitt's African patients.

Possible hazards

When the benefits of bran were first announced, many people started adding three, four or even more

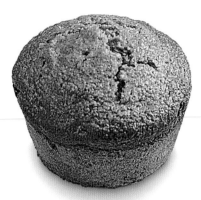

◄ **Fibre food**
If you get your bran in a muffin, make sure it's of the low-fat variety.

- good source of niacin, riboflavin and other B complex vitamins
- Whole-grain breads are high in fibre
- White bread contains calcium

DRAWBACKS

- People with coeliac disease cannot tolerate the gluten found in breads
- May trigger an adverse reaction in people allergic to moulds
- Major contributor of hidden salt
- Some breads made from refined flour and may have a high glycaemic index

tablespoons of unprocessed bran to their daily diet. It soon became apparent that this practice could cause bloating and discomfort, and also aggravate irritable bowel syndrome. In addition, the phytic acid in raw bran inhibits the body's absorption of calcium, iron, zinc, magnesium and other important minerals. During bread baking, the enzymes in yeast destroy much of the phytic acid. The heat that is present during processing also destroys most of the phytic acid in high-bran cereals. Thus, these processed products are safer than unprocessed bran.

There have been several reports of severe bowel obstruction in people who consumed large amounts of bran; it is especially dangerous if a person doesn't drink enough water.

Many nutritionists now advise people to eat whole-grain bread, cereals and other products that contain bran rather than straight bran. For instance, try rolled oats and cereals made with whole oats; substitute brown rice for the white. These foods are more palatable than unprocessed bran, which tastes like sawdust, and more beneficial.

Bread

BENEFITS

- A good source of complex carbohydrates

Since prehistoric times, bread has been a staple food in virtually every society. As early hunter-gatherers settled into agricultural societies, they learned how to transform various grains into bread. This simple food required only stones to grind grain into flour or meal, water or another liquid to mix it into dough, and a means of baking or cooking it.

Over the centuries, each society developed its own unique types of bread. The huge variety of baked goods that are available to us at our supermarkets and bakeries today – different-shaped loaves of white, wholemeal, rye, pumpernickel, sourdough and multigrain breads, croissants, bagels and muffins, tortillas, pita, wraps and chapattis, among many others – represent a dietary melding of dozens of diverse cultures.

Giving dough a lift

The simplest and oldest breads are flat, or unleavened; they are made by mixing flour or meal with water and then baking, frying or steaming it. Examples include matzo, tortillas, chapattis and some types of crackers. The addition of yeast, baking

The language of bread

Descriptions and definitions of breads vary widely. The following are some general guidelines for interpreting the labels:

- White bread is made from refined wheat flour, to which thiamin has been restored.
- Multigrain bread is usually made from white flour with varying quantities of added whole grains.
- Wholemeal bread will contain mostly whole-grain wheat flour, but unless it specifically states on the label '100 per cent whole wheat', it may also contain some refined white flour.
- High-fibre bread is usually made from white wheat flour with varying amounts of added bran or the ground husks of legumes.

There is a difference between wholemeal and whole-grain bread. Wholemeal is usually smooth-textured whereas whole-grain breads usually contain 'bits' of various grains.

soda or other leavening agent to the flour-and-water mixture allows the dough to expand, or rise, and gives the bread a lighter, finer texture than unleavened types.

The type of flour used and the manner in which it and the other ingredients interact give the various kinds of breads their unique textures and flavours. In many industrialised countries, the most popular breads are made from wheat flour, which produces a product with a light texture. When wheat flour is kneaded with liquid, the gluten proteins absorb water to form an elastic dough that traps gas from the fermenting yeast; bubbles of carbon dioxide are formed, resulting in the light texture.

Rye and some other flours contain varying amounts of gluten, but none comes close to that of wheat which is why breads made from other grains tend to be heavy and coarse. To make a lighter-textured bread from rye, barley or other grains, some wheat flour is usually added to the dough.

Flavour and texture are also influenced by the type of liquid mixed into the dough – plain water, milk, beer and fruit juice are common choices. Sugar or honey may be added to 'feed' the yeast and make the bread rise at a faster rate; it also results in a moister product. A small amount of salt is needed to strengthen the gluten and to temper the rate at which the yeast multiplies. Vegetable fats are often added to flavour commercial breads; butter also makes pastry-like breads, such as croissants, so rich and flaky.

Check the ingredients. Breads may contain various preservatives and emulsifiers to extend their shelf life and improve their appearance. These additives do not alter nutritional value, but most commercial bread may be too high in salt for people on low-sodium diets. Also, people who have coeliac disease cannot tolerate the gluten in bread. People with food allergies may react to specific ingredients; for example, those people allergic to moulds may react to sourdough or very yeasty breads. Some supermarkets and many health-food and specialty shops offer breads that are gluten-free; people with food allergies should always check the labels for any offending ingredients.

Nutritional value

Traditionally, bread has been called the staff of life, implying that it alone is all that is required for total nutrition. This is inaccurate.

Bread provides starch, protein and some vitamins and minerals, but it is far from being nutritionally complete. It lacks such essentials as vitamins A, B_{12}, C and D. Many of the nutrients in the grain are destroyed by milling and processing, although thiamin is added to flour to restore this nutrient to its original level. In general, wholemeal and whole-grain flours are held to be more nutritious than their highly processed counterparts; and they also provide more dietary fibre.

Look for added nutrients. The addition of other ingredients also increases the nutritional value of bread. Depending upon the type, these may include soya, linseeds, raisins and other dried fruit, whole grains, nuts, olives, seeds and various types of cheese.

▶ **Rye bread**
Bread made from rye flour is usually quite dense and heavy. It has a coarse texture. To make it softer and lighter, some wheat flour can be added to the dough.

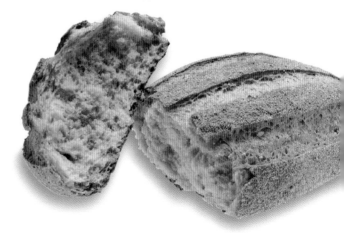

B

Do one simple thing

For good health, buy bread which has 'whole' goodness.

Twenty grams of additional dietary fibre per day, as found in wholemeal or whole-grain breads, is associated with an approximate 26 per cent reduction in the risk of coronary heart disease.

Contrary to popular belief, bread is not especially fattening; a medium slice of white or wholemeal bread contains only about 70kcal. But smothering bread with butter, margarine or other fatty spreads does make the snack considerably more calorific; low-fat mayonnaise, low-sugar jam or an all-fruit preserve are much healthier.

The world's breadbasket

The ever-growing popularity of international breads is reflected in the many types sold in delis, supermarkets and bakeries. Here are some common breads :

Bagel. This doughnut-shaped roll, identified with many Eastern European and Jewish communities, is boiled and then baked.

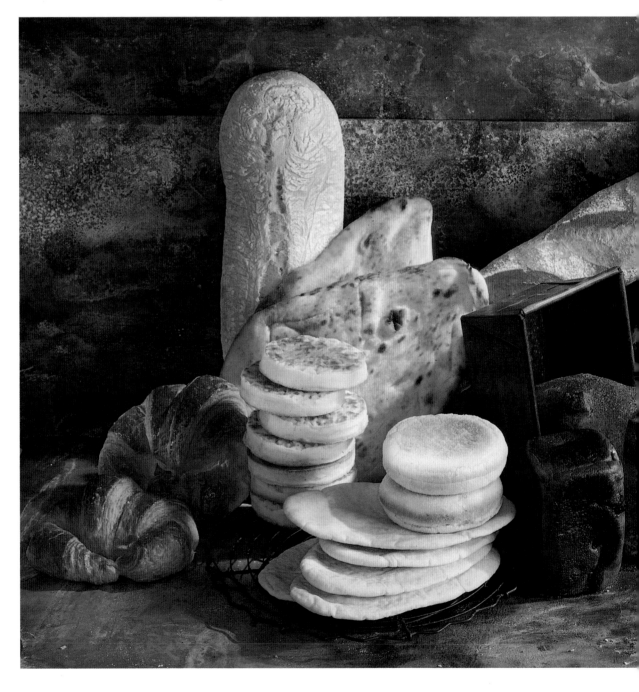

Traditionally, bagels are made from a high-gluten white flour, but whole wheat, rye, linseed, pumpernickel, sourdough and other versions are also commonly available. Bagels may be topped with caraway, sesame seeds, poppy seeds, chopped onions or coarse salt. Cinnamon and raisin bagels are also popular and low-fat versions are sometimes seen.

Brioche. A light yeast roll that originated in France, brioche is half bread and half cake in texture and taste. Made with white flour, it is enriched with butter and eggs.

Chapatti. A flat Indian bread that is made with whole wheat or white flour and may be leavened or unleavened. Some chapattis are brushed with butter or oil.

Ciabatta. Olive oil is added to this Italian raised bread, making it moist and chewy; oregano, basil and various other herbs may also be added.

Croissant. A rich, flaky breakfast roll, shaped as a crescent. It is high in fat, as it is made with butter.

Crumpet. A circular, yeasted bread, baked on one side, with a honeycomb texture on the other.

English muffin. High-protein white flour is used to make this flat, round roll; it is usually split and toasted before eating.

Focaccia. An Italian yeast bread that is made from a dough similar to that of pizza, it is usually baked in a large disc and flavoured with olive oil, onions, garlic and herbs. The added oil in this recipe contributes extra calories.

Fruit breads. Usually made from malted or white bread dough with sugar and dried fruits added.

Matzo. Made from wheat flour, water and salt, this crisp unleavened Jewish bread is traditionally served at Passover meals.

Multigrain or granary. Often promoted as a health food, this bread is usually made with a

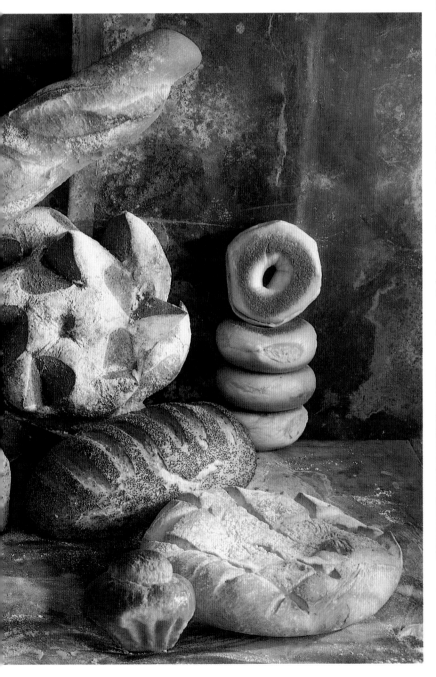

B

> ## Did you know?
> ### Coeliac disease is much more common than previously thought
> As many as one in every 1,500 people in the UK may have coeliac disease, an auto-immune disease in which a protein found in many grains causes problems such as diarrhoea, anaemia, constipation and abdominal pain.

◀ **Choosing your loaf**
Breads from around the world include: croissant, pitta, muffin, crumpet, Italian, naan, raisin, whole wheat, baguette, crusty whole wheat, bagel, poppy seed, pain de campagne and brioche.

combination of flours, whole grains and various seeds. Some multigrain breads are more nutritious than others, but a close check of their labels will often show that many are comparable to ordinary breads.

Naan. Baked on the hot side of a tandoori oven, this flat yeast bread originated in India. It is a source of thiamin and niacin.

Pitta. This flat, leavened Middle Eastern bread puffs up during baking and can be split to form a pocket, that can take a variety of fillings. White and wholemeal versions are available.

Pumpernickel. This heavy rye German bread derives its dark colour from molasses or caramel. One dense type of pumpernickel is steamed and baked for hours, then cut into thin slices.

Quick bread. Made from a variety of flours, it is leavened with baking powder or baking soda and rises as it bakes. Scones, cake-style muffins, coffee cakes and loaf breads are all quick breads.

Rye. All-rye bread is heavy and dense; most of the softer rye breads are made mostly of wheat flour. The low gluten in rye flour makes the breads heavier and denser.

Soda bread. This bread is made with buttermilk, bicarbonate of soda and cream of tartar.

What's in a slice of bread?

- One medium slice of white or whole-meal bread contains about 70kcal.
- The fat content in different breads will vary but is generally low. Breads with more nuts and seeds will be higher in fat.
- Bread flour contains thiamin.
- Wholemeal and whole-grain breads contain more fibre.
- All breads contain small amounts of zinc, potassium and magnesium. Some can be quite high in sodium.

Tortillas. This unleavened Mexican bread is made of corn or wheat flour, salt and water. Finely ground limestone is often added.

Broccoli

BENEFITS

- An excellent source of vitamin C
- A good source of beta carotene and folate
- Significant amounts of iron, potassium and other minerals
- Rich in glucosinolates, effective natural cancer fighters
- Low in calories and high in fibre.

DRAWBACKS

- Overcooking releases unpleasant-smelling sulphur compounds and may cause flatulence

A very nutritious vegetable, broccoli's powerful disease-fighting properties give it the ability to protect against many common cancers. Over the past 20 years, numerous studies have found that people who eat an abundance of broccoli have a significantly reduced incidence of numerous cancers, including cancers of the colon, breast, cervix, lungs, prostate, oesophagus, larynx and bladder.

While other cruciferous vegetables (members of the cabbage family, whose flowers resemble crosses) are recognised as protective foods, broccoli seems to have even more cancer-fighting compounds. Some of these block the action of hormones that stimulate tumours; others work by inhibiting tumour growth or by boosting the action of protective enzymes.

Broccoli contains glucosinolates, which, once ingested, break down into healthy compounds, including indoles, sulforaphane and

---

Mum was right: you should eat your broccoli

Researchers at the Johns Hopkins University School of Medicine have discovered that sulforaphane, a chemical contained in broccoli and broccoli sprouts, has been found to kill *Helicobacter pylori*, a bacterium that causes stomach ulcers and often fatal stomach cancers.

---

isothiocyanates, all of which may be cancer fighters. The most interesting compound is sulforaphane, which shows decided anti-cancer activity in both cultured rat and human cells. Broccoli sprouts are roughly 50 times richer in sulforaphane than mature broccoli. Broccoli is high in bioflavonoids, including quercetin and other phytochemicals that protect cells against mutation and damage from unstable molecules.

Broccoli has an abundance of essential vitamins and minerals. An 80g serving of broccoli contains 19kcal, yet it provides more than 100 per cent of the Reference Nutrient Intake (RNI) of vitamin C, almost half the RNI for folate and a healthy amount of beta carotene. The same sized helping also provides 1.5mg of iron and 5g of protein, and because the same amount of cooked broccoli has 6g of fibre, it is often suggested as a preventive measure for constipation.

Fresh broccoli is available year-round; frozen broccoli is just as nutritious. When shopping for broccoli, avoid florets that are turning yellow – they are past their prime and less nutritious.

Broccoli can be eaten raw, but most people prefer it cooked. Steaming or stir-frying it until crispy tender retains the most nutrients; and boiling it in a large amount of water destroys many of the cancer-fighting compounds, vitamin C and other nutrients.

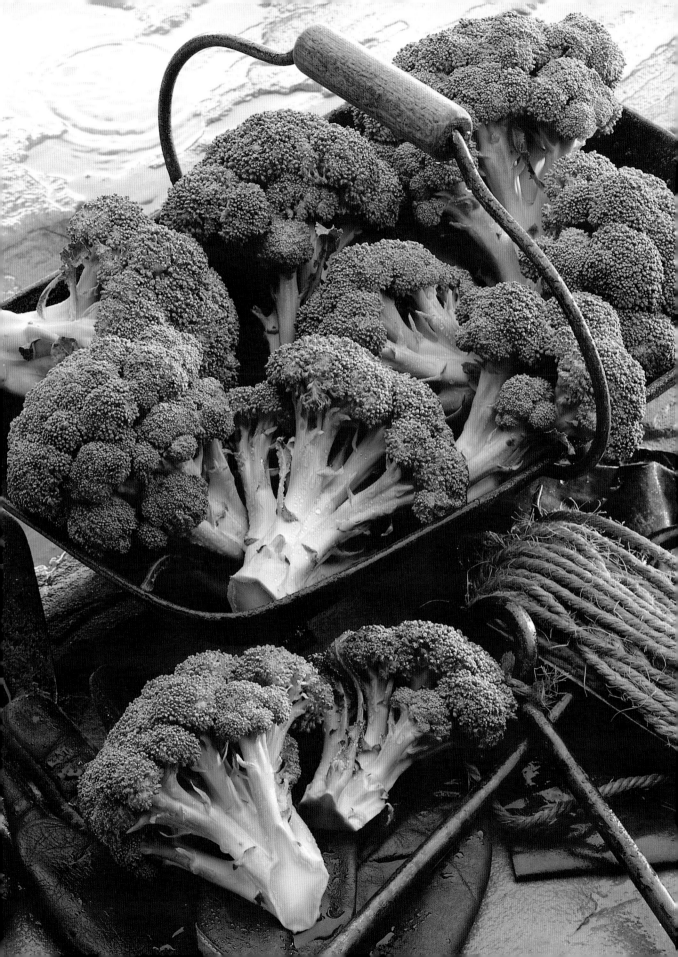

Brussels sprouts

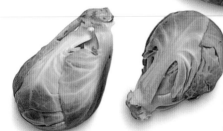

BENEFITS

■ An excellent source of vitamin C

■ A good source of folate, beta carotene and potassium

■ Contain bioflavonoids and other substances that protect against cancer

■ Low in calories and high in fibre

DRAWBACKS

■ Can cause bloating and flatulence

Brussels sprouts resemble small cabbages and share many of the same health benefits as broccoli, cabbage and other cruciferous vegetables: they contain chemicals that appear to protect against cancer. They are also very high in vitamin C; a cup of cooked Brussels sprouts provides more than 100 per cent of the Reference Nutrient Intake (RNI); it also provides 70 per cent or more of the folate and a healthy amount of beta carotene that our bodies need. An 80g serving has about 20kcal. Serving Brussels sprouts with a small amount of cheese, rice or another grain adds complementary amino acids to make a complete protein.

The cancer factor

Brussels sprouts have high amounts of bioflavonoids and indoles, plant chemicals that protect against cancer. Bioflavonoids have an antioxidant effect that helps to prevent cellular damage and mutation caused by the unstable molecules released when the body uses oxygen. Bioflavonoids, along with indoles and perhaps other plant chemicals, inhibit hormones that promote tumour growth. Indoles are particularly active against oestrogen, the hormone that stimulates the growth of some breast cancers.

Other studies indicate that bioflavonoids and indoles may protect against cancers of the prostate and uterus. These plant chemicals may also slow tumour growth and spread of the disease.

Low blood levels of folate may predispose some people to lung cancer. Brussels sprouts are a good source of folates and so eating them may offer some protection against this condition.

Sprouts at their best

When buying fresh Brussels sprouts, select small, bright green ones with tightly packed leaves. Those past their prime will have patches of yellow, and when cooked will be spongy and have an unpleasant sulphurous smell and a bitter taste. Frozen Brussels sprouts retain most of their nutrients and flavour.

Sprouts can be boiled or steamed. To ensure that they are evenly cooked, cut a small cross into their base before cooking. When boiling, allow a cup of water for each cup of sprouts. Bring it to a rapid boil, add the sprouts, and cook uncovered until they are crisply tender.

Overcooking Brussels sprouts destroys their vitamin C and also gives them a bitter taste. When steaming sprouts, uncover the steamer for a few seconds every 2 or 3 minutes to prevent a build-up of the sulphurous gases.

Buckwheat

BENEFITS

■ A good source of iron and magnesium

■ High in starches, protein and fibre

DRAWBACKS

■ Strong flavour and the dark colour of the flour does not appeal to some people

Although it's not a grain and is unrelated to wheat, buckwheat is generally used as if it were. In North America buckwheat is commonly used in pancakes, which are made from the flour of the plant's seeds. The hulled roasted seeds, commonly called groats or kasha, can be boiled to make cereal, pudding or a side dish similar to bulghur wheat.

Sprouted buckwheat seeds are a nutritious and tasty addition to salads, stir-fried foods and other dishes. Fresh unhulled seeds suitable for sprouting are available from health-food shops.

▶ **Gluten-free** Buckwheat flour is used to make a number of tasty gluten-free products, including pasta, bread, muffins, pancakes and breakfast cereals.

Did you know?

Rutin, found in buckwheat, is a known cancer fighter

It also helps to lower cholesterol levels, strengthen blood vessels and lower blood pressure.

Bulghur wheat

BENEFITS

■ A useful source of dietary fibre and B complex vitamins

The basis of many Lebanese dishes, such as tabbouleh, bulghur wheat is sometimes called cracked wheat, but it is actually a more refined version. It is produced by cooking grains of wheat which contain everything but the bran, until they crack. They are then dried and ground between rollers to fine, medium or coarse consistency. Being precooked, bulghur wheat needs only a little cooking or it can be soaked in boiling water for about 30 minutes to achieve its attractive golden colour and nutty texture.

Bulimia

EAT PLENTY OF

■ Fresh vegetables, fruit and high-fibre foods to promote a feeling of fullness

■ Bananas, dried fruit and a variety of fresh vegetables and fruit for potassium

AVOID

■ 'Trigger' foods that are associated with binges

Bulimia is an eating disorder in which secretive bouts of over-eating are interspersed with unhealthy attempts to curb weight gain through self-induced vomiting, laxative or diuretic abuse, fasting or fanatical exercising.

Although bulimia literally means 'the hunger of an ox', the majority of people with bulimia do not have excessive appetites. Instead, their tendency to overeat compulsively seems to arise from psychological problems. These are possibly complicated by abnormal brain chemistry or perhaps a hormonal imbalance.

Far more women than men are affected by bulimia. Despite their overeating, most people with bulimia are of normal weight, although many have a frequent gain or loss of 5kg or more. Their ability to maintain normal weight is attributed to their compensating behaviour of purging, exercise and strict dieting. Those affected typically have a distorted body image and feelings of low self-worth and helplessness.

Some purge after eating any food. About half of people with anorexia suffer from bulimia, and both disorders are characterised by a perfectionist focus on dieting and weight and a fear of being unable to control their eating behaviour. These disorders sometimes begin with a strict weight-loss diet. After a time, the dieter may succumb to gorging, usually on sweet food that is high in calories, such as cake and ice cream. Then, feeling guilty and ashamed, the dieter may purge to compensate for the indiscretion. Before long, the dieter may be caught in a cycle of binging and purging. Episodes are characteried by a loss of control and a need to numb uncomfortable feelings such as sadness or anger. A binge may be brief, or it may last for several hours.

Nutritional deficiencies

Repeated purging can have serious consequences, including nutritional deficiencies and an imbalance of sodium and potassium, leading to fatigue, fainting and palpitations. Acids in vomit can damage tooth enamel and the lining of the oesophagus. Laxative abuse can irritate the large intestine and produce rectal bleeding. Overuse of laxatives disrupts normal bowel function, leading to chronic constipation when they are discontinued. Perhaps one of the most severe consequences, however, is depression and the high suicide rate that is common among those with bulimia, either as a result of the condition, or as part of its symptoms.

Treatment

Like all eating disorders, bulimia can be difficult to treat and usually requires a team approach involving nutrition education and some psychotherapy. If the sufferer appears to be suicidal or the intractable binge-purge behaviour does not respond to outpatient therapy, hospitalisation may be necessary. Don't expect instant success, however; treatment often takes three years or more, and even then, relapses are common. Many sufferers resist treatment, and then some degree of compulsion is used.

Treat nutritional deficiencies early. This is especially important if the body's potassium reserves have been depleted by vomiting or laxative abuse. Eating foods high in potassium, such as dried fruit, bananas, and fresh fruit and vegetables, usually restores the mineral; if not, a supplement may be needed.

Keep a diary. Nutrition education typically begins with asking the person with bulimia to keep a diary

Bulimia warning signs

A complete medical check-up is the only way to be absolutely certain of a diagnosis of bulimia. There are, however, some warning signs that are obvious and should warrant concern. Stomach acids from repeated self-induced vomiting causes damage to teeth and gums, and one or more fingers may be scarred as a result of pushing them down the throat to induce vomiting.

to help to pinpoint circumstances that contribute to binging. A nutrition counsellor may also give the patient an eating plan that minimises the number of decisions that must be made about what and when to eat. This diet should emphasise foods high in protein and starches while excluding favourite binge foods until the bulimia is under control; they can then be reintroduced in small quantities.

At this stage of treatment, people with bulimia learns how to give themselves permission to eat desirable foods in reasonable quantities, in order to reduce the feelings of deprivation and intense hunger that often lead to loss of control in eating.

Those who abuse laxatives may need a high-fibre diet to overcome constipation. Whole-grain cereals and breads, fresh fruit and vegetables and adequate fluids should help to restore normal bowel function.

Drug therapy

Because chronic clinical depression often accompanies bulimia, treatment may include giving selective antidepressant drugs that restore normal levels of serotonin, a brain chemical instrumental in mood control and appetite. Among the drugs prescribed for bulimia are the serotonin-reuptake inhibitors like fluoxetine (Prozac), which is specifically licensed for bulimia in the UK and which suppresses appetite, and sertraline (Lustral). As patients recover from their depression, they are better able to control their compulsive eating.

Psychotherapy may be an option. It can take several forms, including family and group therapy, and cognitive behavioural therapy to help sufferers to shift the central focus of their lives away from food.

People with bulimia also learn to recognise the warning signs of a binge and how to deal with stress or situations that make them vulnerable to binges.

Some people with bulimia find that participation in self-help groups can be useful. Alternative therapies, such as meditation, guided imagery and progressive relaxation routines, can also help to reduce obsession about weight and eating habits.

Burns

CONSUME PLENTY OF

- Foods high in protein and zinc, such as lean meat, poultry, fish and shellfish, eggs and legumes, to promote healing and tissue repair

- Water, broth, fruit juices and other nonalcoholic beverages to replace fluid loss

- Fresh fruit and vegetables rich in vitamin C to foster healing

AVOID

- Alcohol

To promote healing and tissue repair, victims of extensive burns should have a well-balanced diet that provides extra calories, protein, vitamins and minerals. They also require extra fluids, sodium and potassium to replace the substances that seep out through damaged skin. If this isn't done, there is a danger of dehydration and an imbalanced body chemistry.

Second and third-degree burns are very serious and there is a high risk of infection. Those hospitalised with extensive burns are usually given intravenous fluids and antibiotics. If they are unable to eat, they will also be fed intravenously. A diet that provides extra calories, protein and zinc is needed for tissue repair. Zinc, found in seafood, meat,

poultry and in slightly lesser amounts in eggs, milk, beans, nuts and whole grains is essential for wound healing; it also helps the immune defences to fight infection.

Include vitamin C in the diet to build and maintain healthy skin and ward off infection. Liquid supplements are necessary to maintain a high-calorie intake during the day, but alcohol should be avoided.

Butter and margarine

BENEFITS

- Improve flavour, moistness and texture of baked goods

- Good sources of vitamins A and D

- Margarine made with polyunsaturated oil contains essential fatty acids and vitamin E

- Some margarines contain plant sterol and stanol additives, which can reduce cholesterol

DRAWBACKS

- High in calories, all of which come from fats, which increase the risk of obesity, cancers and other diseases

- Butter is high in saturated fats, which increase the risk of heart disease

- Cooking margarine or margarines that are made from hydrogenated oils may contain trans fatty acids, which lower good cholesterol and raise bad cholesterol levels

- Polyunsaturates in margarine have been linked with increased asthma risk in children

Eating habits have changed over the last few decades, and nowhere is this more obvious than in the supermarket dairy cabinets. Where butter once reigned supreme, there

B

is now a bewildering array of margarines and other types of spread, making great health claims, from which to choose.

More people than ever now use margarine instead of butter because they believe it is the healthier of the two spreads. Although most people agree that butter tastes better than margarine, they also know the fat in butter is mostly saturated, and it is these fats that raise cholesterol levels more than most others.

So is margarine healthier than butter?

Yet, many nutritionists now say that butter is better – as long as it is eaten in moderation. Butter is certainly a more natural product than margarine, which relies heavily on colourings and other additives.

Butter and margarine usually have the same total fat content and provide the same amount of energy (typically 81 per cent fat and 740 kcal per 100g), but some makers of margarine have lowered the fat in their product to 71 per cent and 635kcal per 100g.

By law, margarine has to be fortified with vitamins A and D – which are found naturally in butter.

▶ **Fat statistics**
Butter and margarine contain, on average, 143kcal per tablespoon and 16g of total fat (10g saturated fat in butter compared with 2.5g to 4.5g saturated fat in margarine).

Choosing a margarine

In the making of margarine, liquid oils are converted into a solid spread by a process called hydrogenation. As well as hardening the oils, the process changes their chemical structure, turning some of the unsaturated fatty acids into trans fatty acids – a far less healthy form. They raise the level of cholesterol and research indicates that they increase the risk of heart disease.

Choose mono or polyunsaturated margarines made from rape seed, safflower, sunflower, olive and corn oils. Avoid products that list hydrogenated or trans fats.

Margarines that have added plant sterols that reduce blood cholesterol are now widely available. Scientists theorise that due to their chemical similarity to cholesterol, these compounds compete with cholesterol for absorption into the bloodstream from the intestine. This interferes with the uptake of cholesterol from the diet, and also lowers the amount of cholesterol that gets into the blood from cholesterol synthesis in the liver.

Cholesterol is made in the liver from saturated fats. You need a certain amount of it in your bloodstream to stay alive and well. It is only when you have too much of it that cholesterol becomes a problem. Most cholesterol arrives in the bloodstream in an indirect fashion.

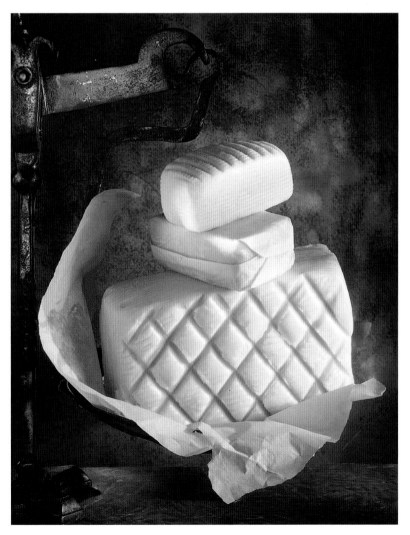

Comparisons of various spreads (values per 100g)

CALORIES	FATS	VITAMINS	DID YOU KNOW?
BUTTER			
740	Total 81g of which saturated 54g, monosaturated 20g, polyunsaturated 3g, trans fat 4-8g	A 887mcg D .76mcg E 2mg	'Spreadable' butters contain less salt than standard butters. The natural trans fats in butter do not raise blood cholesterol in the same way as artificial trans fats in margarine.
MARGARINE, HARD			
740	Total 81g of which saturated 36g, monounsaturated 33g, polyunsaturated 9.8g trans fats 9-14g	A 790mcg D 7.94mcg E 8mg	Margarine is fortified with vitamins A and D; the vitamin E content varies according to the oil used and whether it has been added as an ingredient.Beta carotene is added to give a golden colour. Like butter, margarine is 16 per cent water.
MARGARINE, POLYUNSATURATED			
740	Total 81g of which saturated 16g monounsaturated 21g, poly-unsaturated 41g, trans fats 0.7-6g	A 900mcg D 7.94mcg E 8mg	Similar in nutrition to hard margarine. Sunflower and safflower types are highest in vitamin E, but are also high in omega-6 fatty acids that promote inflammatory conditions.
LOW-FAT SPREAD			
390	Total 40g of which saturated 11g, monounsaturated 18g, poly-unsaturated 10g, trans fats 0.4-7g	A 1084mcg D 8mcg E 6.33mg	Low-fat spreads are 50 per cent water. They contain 6 per cent protein (compared with 4 per cent in butter and margarines) which produces a 'creamy' feeling in the mouth.
VERY LOW-FAT SPREAD			
270	Total 25g of which saturated 7g, monounsaturated 11g, poly-unsaturated 4g, trans fats 0.2-3.5g	A 820mcg D 8mcg E6.7mg	These spreads have a higher salt content than butter, margarine and low-fat spreads. Very low-fat spreads are more than 60 per cent water and about 6 per cent protein.
LOW-FAT SPREADS WITH PLANT STANOLS – Flora pro.activ (A) and Benecol Light Spread (B)			
A) 331	Total 35g of which saturated 8.1g, monounsaturated 9g, poly unsaturated 17,5, trans fats 0.4	A 800mcg, D 7.5mcg, E 20mg B_6 5mg	For optimal cholesterol-lowering benefits, three portions of Flora pro.activ foods daily are recommended. One portion of spread is 10g.
B) 329	Total 35g of which saturated 6.9, monounsaturated 19.1, poly-unsaturated 9.0, trans fats 0.1	A 750mcg D 7.2mcg	For optimal cholesterol-lowering benefits, Benecol recommends 2-3 servings of its products daily. One serving of Benecol spread is equivalent to 12g or 2½ teaspoons.

It is first secreted into the intestine via the bile, where it plays a role in fat absorption, then absorbed into the blood. Plant sterols have been found to block this absorption. One to two tablespoons of margarine that contains plant sterols are needed daily to benefit from the cholesterol-lowering effect.

A matter of calories

Butter and margarine are both highly calorific. Regular varieties of both have about the same number of calories. Both also contain about 16-20 per cent water. Their calorie content can be reduced by adding extra water and/or air, so anyone who aims to cut fat intake should select the reduced-fat varieties.

A question of flavour

It's no secret that butter tastes better than margarine. Mixing a little butter with margarine gives it a more satisfying taste. Salt is used in both butter and margarine; anyone on a low-sodium diet should look for unsalted varieties.

Used sparingly, both butter and margarine can be part of a healthy diet. You can further reduce your use of butter or margarine by combining it with herbs, spices or low-fat ingredients. It will make the dish more interesting, and you'll find you won't notice the absence of the exra fat. You could also try using half or two-thirds of the amount of butter or margarine suggested in recipes.

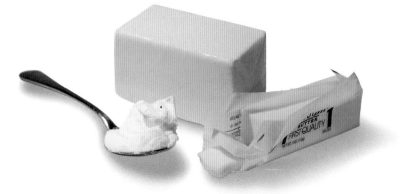

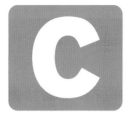

Cabbage

BENEFITS

- An excellent source of vitamin C
- Low in calories and high in fibre
- May help to prevent colon cancer and malignancies stimulated by oestrogen

DRAWBACKS

- Can cause bloating and flatulence
- Gives off strong, somewhat unpleasant sulphurous odour when cooked
- Coleslaw can be high in calories; sauerkraut is loaded with salt

Although cabbage is not quite as nutritious as broccoli, Brussels sprouts and cauliflower, it does outrank these plant relatives in

Types of cabbage

There are hundreds of different kinds of cabbage; the following are the most popular varieties:

- Green, the most common cabbage, has a mild flavour that can be enjoyed raw or cooked.

- Red cabbage is similar to the green varieties, but it is much higher in vitamin C than other types.

- Savoy cabbage has ruffled green outer leaves and is higher in beta carotene than other varieties.

- Bok choy, or Chinese cabbage, forms a celery-like stalk of white leaves; it is higher in calcium.

consumption. In fact, in some parts of the world, cabbage consumption is on a par with that of potatoes. Very high in fibre and very low in calories (80g of cooked cabbage contains a meagre 14kcal), the lowly cabbage is a rich source of vitamin C (with over 15mg in 80g). Red cabbage contains even more vitamin C than the green cabbage, but the green variety contains twice as much folate as the red; both red and green cabbages contribute potassium and fibre. Savoy cabbage is a good source of beta carotene.

Cabbage is rich in cancer-fighting compounds

Cabbages are members of the cruciferous family of vegetables, associated with numerous health benefits. It has long been known that people who eat large amounts of cabbage enjoy a low rate of colon cancer. This protective effect is assumed to come from indoles, bioflavonoids, monoterpenes and other plant chemicals that inhibit tumour growth and protect cells against damage from free radicals, those unstable molecules released when the body uses oxygen. Some of these chemicals also speed up the body's metabolism of oestrogen, which may explain why women whose diets provide ample amounts of cabbage and related vegetables have a reduced incidence of breast cancer. This chemical action may also protect against cancers of the uterus and ovaries. Of particular interest is indole-3-carbinol, a cabbage component that in animal studies had reduced the risk of cancer. However, advice to take this compound in pill form, as advocated by some supplement manufacturers, would appear to be premature.

● **Myth.......**
Prevailing folk wisdom states that cabbage juice is a miracle cure for ulcers.

.......Reality ●
There is little scientific evidence to prove that cabbage juice works. But there is probably no harm in trying cabbage juice along with conventional medical treatment for ulcers.

Preparation methods

Cabbage can be served raw as coleslaw, pickled into sauerkraut or cooked. Commercial coleslaw is high in calories (about 200kcal in an 80g portion) because it has large amounts of mayonnaise. You can reduce the calories by making your own and using low-fat yoghurt, vinegar and oil. Sauerkraut is soaked in salt brine and then fermented; to lower the sodium content, you should rinse it before heating. Use your blender to make cabbage juice, which can effectively relieve heartburn.

Steaming and stir-frying preserves most nutrients. You should avoid using aluminium cookware, which causes a chemical reaction that discolours the vegetable and alters its flavour.

Caffeine

BENEFITS

- Temporarily enhances mental alertness and concentration

- Can improve athletic performance by temporarily increasing endurance

- May abort an asthma attack by relaxing constricted bronchial muscles

DRAWBACKS

- Is mildly addictive and can result in withdrawal symptoms

- Can cause insomnia

- Excessive amounts can produce tremors, palpitations and feelings of anxiety

- In large quantities, lowers the body's absorption of calcium by increasing the amount lost in urine and stools

- Can increase blood pressure

By far our most popular (and least harmful) addictive drug, caffeine is the stimulant in coffee, chocolate, tea and cola soft drinks; it is also added to some painkillers, cold medications, weight-loss supplements and drugs used to promote mental alertness. Within a few minutes after caffeine is ingested, it is absorbed from the small intestine into the bloodstream and carried to all the body's organs. It speeds the heart rate, stimulates the central nervous system, increases the flow of urine and the production of digestive acids and relaxes smooth

Did you know?

Coffee may keep Alzheimer's at bay

It is possible that drinking coffee could help to stave off Alzheimer's disease. In one small study, drinking three cups a day reduced the risk of developing Alzheimer's by as much as 60 per cent.

▶ **Coffee beans for caffeine boost**
The caffeine in coffee inhibits one of the brain's calming transmitters, making you alert. But don't overdo it, or you may end up jittery and unable to concentrate.

muscles, such as those that control the blood vessels and the airways.

Although caffeine in moderation is generally harmless, sudden withdrawal can often cause headaches, irritability and other symptoms that vary in severity from one person to another. For example, in some people who are sensitive to caffeine, the substance can trigger migraine headaches, while in others it might actually abort a migraine by relaxing the constricted blood vessels that are causing the head pain. People with some types of heart-valve disease may be advised to avoid caffeine altogether because it can provoke heart palpitations or other cardiac arrhythmias. Research also suggests that people with Type 2 diabetes should avoid coffee at mealtimes as it may interfere with their ability to control blood sugar.

Boosting performance

The stimulant in caffeine enhances mental performance by increasing alertness and concentration. Coffee helps many people 'get going' in the morning; coffee or tea breaks give a boost when energy lags.

Athletes have observed that one or two caffeine drinks an hour before competition can improve their performance, especially in endurance sports like distance running. Studies confirm that 250mg of caffeine – which is the amount in two cups of strong coffee – increases endurance, presumably because caffeine increases the body's ability to burn fat for fuel. However, while high doses may improve

performance, they can also cause side effects and athletes must be aware of their individual tolerance.

Potential side effects

Ingestion of caffeine late in the day can result in a sleepless night, and excessive intake can lead to caffeinism, a syndrome marked by insomnia, feelings of irritability and anxiety, a rapid heartbeat, tremors and excessive urination. These symptoms abate with the gradual withdrawal of caffeine. Otherwise, caffeine is relatively nontoxic; a fatal adult dose would require the rapid consumption of the caffeine in 80 to 100 cups of coffee.

Because caffeine, and other compounds in coffee, increase the production of stomach acid, those who suffer from indigestion are often advised to limit coffee consumption (including decaffeinated) to one cup after a meal. Many of these patients can tolerate tea, however. Caffeine can prompt a modest temporary rise in blood pressure; it also speeds up the heart rate. Most heart patients need not eliminate coffee or tea from their diets, but cardiologists generally advise no more than two cups of coffee a day. Older people with hypertension may be more sensitive to caffeine and should limit their intake to a cup per day.

Controversy over the safety of caffeine consumption during pregnancy. Drinking more than 300mg of caffeine a day (equal to four cups of instant coffee or six cups of tea) increases the risk of low-birth-weight babies and even miscarriage. (300g of caffeine is also the eqivalent of three cups of brewed coffee, eight cans of cola drinks, four cans of 'energy drinks' and 400g of normal chocolate. Some experts suggest that pregnant women should avoid coffee altogether during pregnancy, while others recommend that pregnant women should limit their daily caffeine consumption to about 150mg, which is the amount found in one-and-a-half mugs of coffee, spread over the entire day. Because caffeine enters breast milk, nursing mothers are advised to either skip caffeinated beverages altogether or to drink them at least 3 hours before they commence breastfeeding.

Large quantities of caffeine reduce calcium absorption, which in turn can increase the risk of osteoporosis, especially in older women. Those people who are heavy coffee drinkers should either consume more milk, low-fat yoghurt and other high-calcium foods, or consider taking calcium supplements.

Some people worry that the decaffeination process used in teas and coffees introduces some undesirable substances into the drink. While the process may be harmful to the flavour of the coffee, it is not harmful to its drinker. Look for those products whose labels say that only water extraction is used in decaffeination. If the method is not stated, a solvent was probably used – it's unlikely to be harmful but you may find that it affects the flavour.

Sources of caffeine

Coffee is our most prevalent caffeinated drink; however, many other products also contain caffeine. The following chart shows how much caffeine can be found in some of the most common sources.

AVERAGE CAFFEINE CONTENT	milligrams
COFFEE (150ml)	
Cappuccino	90–100
Decaffeinated	2–4
Espresso, short black (60ml)	90–100
Ground:	
Drip method	100–180
Percolated	75–170
Instant	60–100
TEA (250ml)	
Brewed, 1 minute	10–20
Brewed, 3 minutes	30–40
Brewed, 5 minutes	50–80
Decaffeinated	1–5
Green tea	25–35
SOFT DRINKS (375ml)	
Cola, regular or diet	35–55
Red Bull (250mg can)	80
CHOCOLATE	
Cold chocolate milk (250ml)	2–7
Hot cocoa (250ml)	10–70
Chocolate bar (60g)	10–20
Dark chocolate (60g)	40

▶ **Potent soft drinks**
One source of caffeine is the kola nut, from which cola is made.

Cakes, biscuits and pastries

BENEFITS

■ Delicious occasional snacks or treats

DRAWBACKS

■ Most are high in fat and calories

■ Generally contain low amounts of most vitamins and minerals

■ Can contain trans fatty acids

Although high on most people's list of favourite foods, cakes, biscuits, pies and other pastries are low on the scale of nutritious choices. Most are high in fats, sugar and other sweeteners, and calories – but relatively low in vitamins, minerals, protein and dietary fibre. Worst of all, most packaged biscuits and baked goods are loaded with saturated and trans fats, introduced fats that contribute to heart disease (see *atherosclerosis*). The word 'hydrogenated' on the nutrition label means the food contains trans fats. Anyone who wants to avoid gaining weight should cut consumption of these foods. Many people can't resist overindulging in them, at the expense of healthier items.

Flour, sugar, fat, eggs and milk are the basic ingredients in most cakes, biscuits and pastries. Solid and highly saturated fats, such as vegetable shortening, butter and palm and coconut oils, are generally more suitable for baking than liquid vegetable oils and reduced-fat margarines. So the fats found in most baked goods are the types that are most likely to raise the blood levels of the detrimental LDL cholesterol.

The high sugar content can hasten tooth decay and may pose a problem for some people with diabetes. Recent studies show,

C

Eight tips for healthier baking

Commercial and home bakers have now developed low-fat versions of many cakes, biscuits and pies. Some lack the flavour and texture of their traditional counterparts, but others are quite acceptable alternatives. Experiment with favourite recipes; fat can often be cut by a third or more and sugar by up to a half without jeopardising texture and flavour. Here are a few tips for cutting fat and sugar.

1 Try using puréed apples or prunes, mashed bananas and other puréed fruit as substitutes for at least some of the fat in biscuit and cake recipes. The fruit adds the moisture and texture generally contributed by fat; it also imparts sweetness and extra flavour.

2 Reduce or even eliminate sugar in fruit pies; use extra cinnamon and other spices to perk up the flavour. Offset a sour fruit without using sugar by combining it with a much sweeter fruit.

3 Cut the fat content in pies by using pastry on the top, only (not at the bottom, too); reduce it even more by making a deep-dish crustless pie or cobbler.

4 Discard half the egg yolks and increase the number of whites when baking a cake; this increases the protein and at the same time cuts down on the amount of both fat and cholesterol.

5 Substitute evaporated skimmed milk for cream in pie fillings. Similarly, try strained fromage frais instead of high-fat cream cheese for toppings and fillings. Fruit and fruit sauces are other options for low-calorie toppings.

6 Increase the nutritional content and cut the fat calories in biscuits by sticking with old favourites such as oat cookies or fruit bars. These can be made even healthier by substituting puréed apples or prunes for part of the fat. Try using wholemeal flour and raisins and other dried fruit instead of nuts.

7 For a festive occasion, serve an angel food cake with fresh berries and strawberry or raspberry sauce; it has virtually no fat and a fraction of the calories contained in a comparable piece of rich chocolate cake with chocolate icing.

8 Make a light lemon cheesecake by using a combination of nonfat cottage and ricotta cheeses and evaporated skimmed milk, lemon zest and egg whites. Top the cake with natural yoghurt instead of cream.

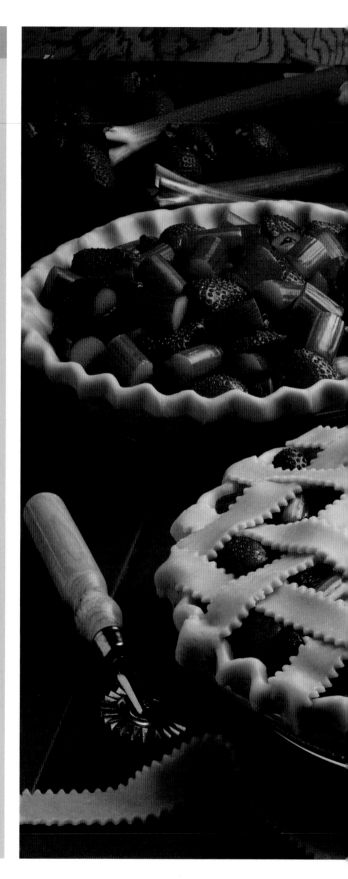

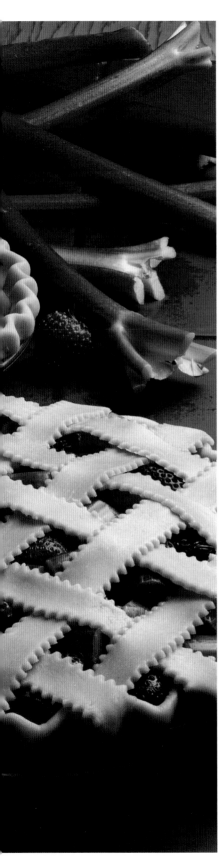

▶ **Sweet and sour**
To reduce the amount of sugar needed to sweeten rhubarb pie, combine the rhubarb with a sweet fruit, such as strawberries.

● **Myth.......**
Low-fat biscuits are better for you than regular biscuits.
.......Reality ●
According to the latest thinking, it doesn't do any good to replace the fat in your diet with sugar. And low-fat biscuits often contain more sugar.

however, that most people with diabetes can tolerate small amounts of sweet foods, especially if they are low in saturated fat.

Carrot cakes, courgette and banana breads and other such baked goods are often promoted as healthy alternatives. But most of these contain only negligible amounts of the fruit or vegetable, are still high in fat and sugar and are often topped with rich icing. However, these can be made healthier by using low-fat substitutes for some ingredients. Try to incorporate some of the baking ideas shown in the panel on the left.

Cancer

EAT PLENTY OF

■ Citrus and other fruit and dark green or yellow vegetables for vitamin C, beta carotene, bioflavonoids and the plant chemicals that protect against cancer

■ Wholegrain breads and cereals and other high-fibre foods to promote smooth colon function

LIMIT

■ Fatty foods, especially those high in saturated fats

■ Alcoholic beverages

■ Salt-cured, smoked, fermented and charcoal-grilled foods

AVOID

■ Foods that may contain pesticide residues and environmental pollutants

Recent research has dramatically changed our thinking about the role of diet in both the prevention and the treatment of cancer. It is increasingly clear that some dietary elements may help to promote the development and spread of malignancies, while others slow or block tumour growth. It's estimated that at least 35 per cent of all cancers may be related to diet, especially one high in saturated fat and processed foods; it is also believed that many cancers could be prevented by dietary changes. There is strong evidence that more vitamin D in the diet (whether from sunlight, eating oily fish or taking supplements) can help greatly in reducing the risk of cancer of the breast, colon and prostate.

The anti-cancer diet

Eat more fruit and vegetables.
Compelling data associate a diet that provides ample fruit and vegetables with a reduced risk of many of our most deadly cancers. These foods are rich in bioflavonoids and other plant chemicals; dietary fibre; folate and antioxidants from the carotenoid family and vitamin C. All of these substances may slow, stop or reverse the processes that can lead to cancer through several protective mechanisms such as by neutralising or detoxifying cancer-causing agents (carcinogens); by preventing precancerous changes in cellular genetic material due to carcinogens, radiation and other environmental factors; by inducing the formation of protective enzymes; and by reducing the hormonal action that can stimulate tumour

growth. Folate is crucial for normal DNA synthesis and repair and low levels are thought to make cells vulnerable to carcinogenesis.

Reduce saturated fat intake. Numerous studies link a high-fat diet and obesity with an increased risk of cancers of the colon, uterus, prostate and the skin (including melanoma, the most deadly form of skin cancer). The link between fat consumption and breast cancer is more controversial. Experts stress that no more than 30 per cent of total calories should come from fats, and many advocate a 20 per cent limit on fat calories. Often, it takes only a few simple dietary changes to lower fat intake; for example, choosing lean cuts of meat; trimming away all visible fat; eating vegetarian dishes several times a week; adopting low-fat cooking methods, such as baking and steaming; and limiting the use of added fats such as butter, margarine, mayonnaise, shortening and oils.

Eat more fibre. Increased intake of fibre may protect against cancer. It speeds the transit of waste through the colon, which some researchers think cuts the risk of bowel cancer. A high-fibre, low-calorie diet also protects against obesity and the increased risk of cancers linked to excessive body fat.

Break high-risk habits

Limit your alcohol intake. Heavy use of alcohol is associated with an increased risk of cancers of the mouth, larynx, oesophagus and liver. Excessive alcohol consumption hinders the body's ability to use carotenoids, which appear to protect against these cancers. Alcohol can deplete reserves of folate, thiamin and other B vitamins, as well as selenium. Folate is known to reduce the proliferation of cancer cells; low levels of folate are also associated with an increased risk of cervical cancer. Researchers have found that giving folate supplements slows the spread of other precancerous cells.

Stop smoking. Smoking, more than any other lifestyle factor, increases the risk of cancer; stopping the habit is the most important step that a smoker can take to avoid cancer. In addition to lung cancer, smoking is strongly associated with cancers of the oesophagus, mouth, larynx, pancreas and bladder; recent studies also link it to an increased risk of breast cancer. For people who can't stop smoking, there are some dietary measures that can somewhat lower their cancer risk. One is to eat broccoli or other cruciferous vegetables several times a week. These members of the cabbage family are known to be appreciably high in some cancer-fighting compounds, including bioflavonoids, monoterpenes, indoles, phenolic acids and plant sterols, the precursors to vitamin D. Sulforaphane, a chemical that is abundant in broccoli, is one of the most potent anti-cancer compounds identified to date; various studies show that eating broccoli several times a week lowers the incidence of lung cancer among smokers compared with those whose diet does not include the vegetable.

Low levels of vitamin C are linked to an increased risk of many of the cancers related to smoking. Because smoking depletes the body's reserves of vitamin C, it's a good idea for smokers to eat more citrus fruit and other good sources of this nutrient. Similarly, smoking can deplete the body's stores of folate and other B-complex vitamins. Eating more lean meat, grains, fortified cereals, legumes and green leafy vegetables may help to counter this effect.

Top cancer-fighting foods

APPLES, BERRIES, BROCCOLI AND OTHER CRUCIFEROUS VEGETABLES AND CITRUS FRUIT contain flavonoids, which act as antioxidants. Flavonoids are also thought to prevent DNA damage to cells.

TOMATOES AND TOMATO PRODUCTS contain lycopene, which has been found to have protective effects against prostate cancer. Eat plenty of tomato sauce and tomato paste.

ONIONS AND GARLIC contain sulphur compounds that may stimulate the immune system's natural defences against cancer, and they may have the potential to reduce tumour growth. Some studies suggest that garlic can reduce the incidence of stomach cancer by a factor of 12.

GREEN TEA contains EGCG, a catechin that may help fight cancer in three ways: it may reduce the formation of carcinogens in the body, increase the body's natural defences and suppress cancer promotion. Some scientists believe that EGCG may be one of the most powerful anti-cancer compounds ever discovered.

BRAZIL NUTS, SEAFOOD, SOME MEATS AND FISH, BREAD, WHEATBRAN, WHEATGERM, OATS AND BROWN RICE are the best sources of selenium, a trace mineral that is another powerful cancer-fighter. In one major study, selenium significantly reduced the incidence of lung, prostate and colorectal cancers in participants who received 200mcg selenium for 4½ years. This has led to follow-up studies investigating whether selenium in combination with vitamin E has a protective effect against prostate cancer. Other studies show that selenium in a test tube works relatively quickly, protecting cells from becoming cancerous. Researchers believe that these cancer-fighting properties will work fast in the body, too.

Limit your consumption of processed foods. People who eat large amounts of smoked, pickled, cured, fried, charcoal-grilled and processed meats have a higher incidence of stomach and oesophageal tumours. Smoked foods contain polyaromatic hydrocarbons that are known carcinogens. The salt in pickled foods can injure the stomach wall and aid the formation of tumours. Nitrites, commonly found in bacon and hot dogs, as well as in processed meats, can form nitrosamines, known carcinogens. However, eating these foods along with good sources of vitamins C and E reduces nitrosamine formation.

When cancer strikes

A qualified dietitian should be part of any cancer treatment team, because both the disease and its treatment demand good nutrition as an aid to recovery. Surgery, which is still the major treatment for cancer, also requires a highly nutritious diet for healing and recuperation. The cancer itself can cause nutritional problems that will require treatment along with the underlying disease; colon cancer, for instance, will often cause iron-deficiency anaemia because of chronic intestinal bleeding. Weight loss is common among many cancer patients, too. Most experience a loss of appetite as a result of the cancer itself; depression brought on by a diagnosis of a potentially fatal disease, as well as pain, will quite understandably lessen any desire to eat. Cancer treatments, especially radiation and chemotherapy, curb appetite and may produce nausea and other side effects. Surgery, too, can affect appetite and make eating unappealing, especially if it involves the digestive system. A qualified dietitian can devise a diet or suggest supplements to provide the calories,

Eat your vegetables and fruit!

The pigments and other chemicals that give plant foods their bright colours also seem to contribute to their cancer-fighting properties. Nutritionists now agree with the age-old urging of mothers, and advise people to eat at least three different coloured vegetables and two different types of fruit daily. Choose from among the dark green leafy vegetables and the dark yellow, orange and red fruit and vegetables. Include one serving of citrus a day, and try to have at least one cruciferous vegetable such as bok choy (or pak choi), broccoli, Brussels sprouts, cabbage, cauliflower, kale, kohlrabi, mustard greens and turnips.

Most fruit and vegetables have more than one cancer-fighting benefit. Broccoli, for example, contains beta carotene, vitamin C, fibre, as well as the phytochemicals found in the vegetables of the cruciferous family. This is why nutritionists recommend a variety of foods instead of supplements as your first line of defence. Here are some of the fruit and vegetable superstars:

BEST VITAMIN C: citrus fruit, strawberries, melon, kiwi fruit, mango, broccoli, Brussels sprouts, cauliflower, peppers and potatoes.

BEST CAROTENOIDS: sweet potatoes, carrots, squash, pumpkin, broccoli, red peppers, apricots, melon, mangoes and some papaya.

BEST FIBRE: sweetcorn, pears, broccoli, Brussels sprouts, potatoes (with skin on), carrots, apples, berries, figs, prunes, peas and spinach.

BEST FOLATE: green leafy vegetables, spinach, orange juice, broccoli, avocado, asparagus and Brussels sprouts.

◀ **Cancer-fighting foods**
A variety of fresh fruit and vegetables, high-fibre legumes and wholegrain breads are not only high in vitamins and minerals, but may also protect against cancer.

Did you know?

Diet can help to keep breast cancer in remission

Evidence suggests that a wholegrain, fish, vegetable and fruit-based diet that is low in fat may be the best regimen for a patient in remission, post chemotherapy. Some data suggests that recurrence rates are lower in those who decrease their total calorie intake by 10 to 15 per cent. This should not be practised by those with active disease, undergoing treatment or without medical supervision.

Eating when you have cancer

In many instances, loss of appetite, nausea and other eating problems of cancer patients can be dealt with by changing daily habits and routines. The following tips have worked for many people.

- Plan your major meal for the time of day when you are least likely to experience nausea and vomiting. For many cancer patients, this is in the early morning. Otherwise, eat small, frequent meals and snacks throughout the day.

- Let someone else prepare the food; cooking odours often provoke nausea. You'll find that food that is served cold or at room temperature gives off less odour than hot food.

- If mouth sores are a problem, eat bland, puréed foods – for example, custards, rice and other puddings made with milk; and eggs, porridge and blended soups. Avoid salty, spicy or acidic foods. Sucking on zinc lozenges may speed the healing of mouth sores.

- Try to eat with others in a pleasant social atmosphere. Ask family members to bring home-cooked food to the hospital (but make sure they check with the dietitian first). Once you are home, try to make meals fun and relaxed.

- Get dressed to eat, if possible, and strive to make meals visually attractive. A few slices of a colourful fruit give visual appeal to a bowl of rolled oats; a colourful napkin and small vase of flowers perk up a tray of food.

- To overcome nausea, try chewing on ice chips, eating a little ginger or a sour lemon drop before meals. Sipping flat ginger ale or cola may also help.

- Rest for half an hour after eating, preferably in a sitting or upright position; reclining may trigger reflux, nausea and vomiting.

- Pay extra attention to dental hygiene. If mouth sores hinder tooth brushing, make a baking soda paste and use your finger and a soft cloth to gently cleanse the teeth. Then rinse the mouth with a weak solution of hydrogen peroxide and baking soda. Diluted commercial mouthwashes freshen the breath, but avoid full-strength products that can further irritate sores.

- If a dry mouth makes swallowing difficult, liquefy foods in a blender or moisten them with low-fat milk, sauces or gravies.

- If diarrhoea is a problem (as is often the case during chemotherapy), avoid fatty foods, raw fruit, wholegrain products and other foods that can make it worse. Instead, eat binding foods, such as rice, bananas, cooked apples and dry toast.

protein and other nutrients that are needed to maintain weight and promote healing. Extra vitamin D is recommended as an accompaniment to treatment to enhance the effects of surgery or radiotherapy.

Dietary guidelines for cancer patients must take into account the stage and type of malignancy. In most cases of early or localised cancer, patients are generally advised to follow a diet that is low in saturated fat; high in wholegrain products and other starches; and high in fruit and vegetables. Saturated fats are discouraged because they may support tumour growth. In contrast, fruit and vegetables contain a variety of natural plant chemicals that are thought to retard the growth and spread of cancers.

Protein is essential because it helps the body to repair tissue that has been damaged during treatment of the disease. Protein is also important to counteract muscle wastage and for wound healing. So patients should eat at least two – more, if possible – daily servings of lean meat, low-fat dairy products, eggs, fish and shellfish or meat alternatives such as tofu and other soya products. Many cancer patients find it difficult to tolerate red meat, because for some it takes on an unpleasant metallic taste; in such instances, substitute egg whites, poultry and a combination of grains, beans and pulses. They will provide the much-needed protein and zinc. In some cases, a prescription for supplements may be required.

Wisdom of the body

Flying in the face of conventional wisdom, however, are recent recommendations from a growing number of cancer specialists who discourage urging some cancer patients to eat when they don't feel like it. In the past, forced feeding in the form of enriched dietary supplements, intravenous nutrition or a gastric feeding tube was recommended to maintain nutrition, but these approaches usually did not result in weight gain or prolonged survival. Instead, many who were force-fed actually died sooner; experts now believe this may be because the feeding actually spurs tumour growth. Consequently, many medical

C

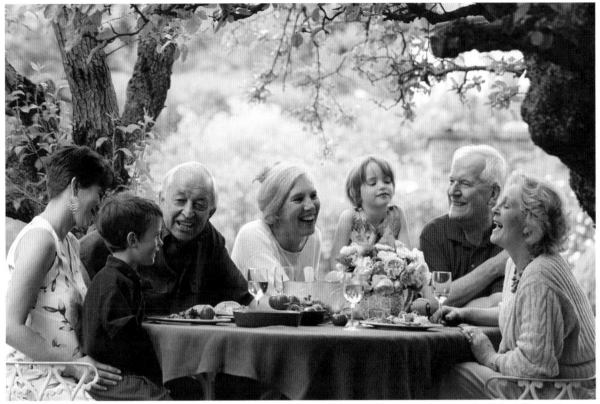

▲ **Delicious, fresh food and a happy atmosphere can make meals pleasurable, even when you don't feel like eating.**

scientists now believe that the anorexia and cachexia (a severe form of malnutrition and body wasting) that occurs in advanced cancer may be an example of the 'wisdom of the body' as it attempts to starve the tumour. Although it may be difficult for family members and friends to watch loved ones stop eating and progressively lose weight, informed doctors now urge that, in some situations, cachectic patients be allowed to limit food intake while doctors undertake aggressive therapy to destroy the tumour. Once this is accomplished, appetite returns, and the lost weight is regained as recovery takes place.

The lure of supplements

Many people take vitamin and mineral supplements, often in high doses. Most do so without consulting a doctor. Recent reports detailing the anti-cancer effects of antioxidants have resulted in greatly increased sales of high-dose supplements of beta carotene and vitamins A, C and E. In theory, it is reasonable to assume that if a small amount of a nutrient protects against cancer, then a high dose should be even more protective. Unfortunately, this does not seem to be true. When consumed in the amounts that are generally found in foods, these nutrients do have an antioxidant effect, which prevents the potentially cancer-causing damage that occurs when the body uses oxygen. But when taken in the form of high-dose supplements, these substances may have an opposite effect; recent research indicates they may become pro-oxidants and may actually increase damage caused by free radicals, the unstable molecules released when the body uses oxygen. In addition, high doses of vitamin A can lead to toxicity. (It is best to consult with qualified professionals, including your doctor and pharmacist, before deciding to pursue high-dose supplement therapy.)

The situation may be quite different, however, for patients who are undergoing cancer treatment. Some may need high-dose supplements, while others may be advised to avoid certain nutrients. As some forms of cancer treatment rely on the generation of free radicals to destroy cancer cells, the use of antioxidant supplements may be counterproductive. This is why it's important to consult an accredited dietitian or nutritionist about any dietary change and supplementation. There is no scientific evidence to suggest that alternative therapies, which include Chinese herbs, blue-green algae or shark cartilage extracts, have any added value in treating cancer.

C

Carbohydrates

A reassessment

There has recently been considerable debate over the role of carbohydrates in our diets. Low-carbohydrate diets such as the Atkins diet captured much greater public attention than most other weight-loss plans.

As a result, more and more people have come to believe that carbohydrates are inherently bad. But that's not the case. Starches and sugars are our major source of energy. Fibre, another form of carbohydrate, also has significant health benefits.

Almost all of the starches and sugars that humans burn for energy come from plants; the only major exception is lactose, the sugar in milk. In effect, each plant is a complex food factory that takes water from the soil, carbon dioxide from the air and energy from the sun to make glucose, a simple sugar that is later converted into starch. As the plant develops and grows, it also makes various vitamins, minerals and other phytochemicals, as well as some fat and protein. Consequently, we can get our carbohydrates and most of the other nutrients needed to sustain us from the thousands of different grains, seeds, fruit and vegetables that can be grown.

Carbohydrates are often classified according to their digestibility and chemical structure; they are divided into two groups: simple and complex.

Simple carbohydrates, or sugars, can generally form crystals that dissolve in water and are easily digested. Naturally occurring sugars are found in a variety of fruit, some vegetables and honey. Processed sugars include table sugar, brown sugar and molasses.

Complex carbohydrates have a range of textures, flavours, colours and molecular structures. Composed of complex chains of sugars, these carbohydrates are further classified as starches or fibre. Our digestive system can break down and metabolise most starches, which are found in an array of grains, vegetables and some fruit.

Our digestive system, however, lacks the enzymes that are needed to break down dietary fibre, including cellulose and other woody parts of the plant skeleton, and pectin and other gums that hold plant cells together. But dietary fibre is still important because it promotes smooth colon function and may help to prevent some types of cancer, heart attacks and other diseases.

ENERGY FOOD

Our body metabolises all carbohydrates into glucose, or blood sugar, the body's primary source of fuel. Carbohydrates are high-quality fuels because – compared to proteins or fats – little is required of the body to break them down to release their energy.

Glucose, the only form of carbohydrate that the body can use immediately, is essential for the functioning of the brain, nervous system, muscles and various organs. At any given time, the blood can carry about an hour's supply of glucose. Any glucose that is not needed for immediate energy is converted into glycogen, a large molecule composed of a chain of glucose units, which is stored in the liver and muscles;

when necessary, the liver turns its glycogen back into glucose. The muscles can store enough glycogen to last for several hours of moderate activity.

Medical researchers have become increasingly aware that the rate at which carbohydrate-rich foods are digested and absorbed into the bloodstream also affects health. The rate at which a food causes blood sugar to rise can be measured and is assigned a numerical value. This measure is referred to as the food's glycaemic index (GI). Foods with a low GI, such as pumpernickel bread, wholegrain bread, brown rice, bulghur wheat, oats, lentils, yams, apples, pears and yoghurt take longer to digest and cause a slower, more gradual rise in blood sugar. This means that energy is released more slowly, leading to more consistent energy levels. Low-GI foods are better for blood sugar control in those with diabetes and may help with weight loss. The carbohydrates in high-GI foods such as white bread, white rice, mashed potato, corn flakes and watermelon are more quickly absorbed and so provide a quicker source of energy. For active people high-GI foods can be a source of quick energy to aid short-duration sports performance and recovery. On the other hand, lower-GI foods are better for endurance.

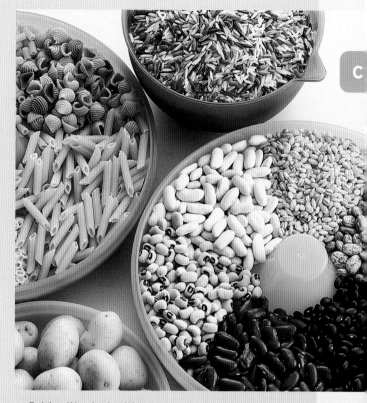

▲ **Eat healthy, be healthy**
Carbohydrates, especially complex ones found in foods such as whole grains, legumes, pasta and potatoes, are the building blocks of a healthy diet. Dietary fibre, especially cereal fibre, is associated with a lower risk of coronary heart disease.

Carbohydrates: myth and reality

Some people feel that the lower their carbohydrate intake is, the healthier they will be. A great deal of research shows that this is not the case. Choosing the healthiest carbohydrates, especially whole grains, fruit and vegetables is important for your well-being. It is well known that all three are important sources of fibre but newer research shows that health benefits can also be attributed to the vitamins, minerals, antioxidants and other plant chemicals found in them. Many people – particularly slimmers – avoid cereals but research shows that whole grains protect against diabetes, cancer and heart disease. In a long-term study of nearly 90,000 women, and in a similar study of about 44,000 men, those who consumed the most cereal fibre had about a 30 per cent lower risk of developing Type 2 diabetes. The UK Nurses' Health Study, an ongoing survey monitored by the Harvard School of Public Health, suggests a lower risk of heart disease and stroke among whole-grain eaters.

When glucose reserves run low, the body turns first to protein for conversion into glucose and then to fat. Burning protein, however, robs the body of lean muscle tissue. In addition, if the body has to burn fat in the absence of carbohydrates, toxic by-products called ketones are released; these can lead to a potentially dangerous biochemical imbalance.

COMPLEX CARBOHYDRATES

The human diet worldwide is based on complex carbohydrates. Populations that eat a higher-carbohydrate, low-fat diet generally enjoy good health. Vegetarian, Mediterranean and Asian diets typically provide a high percentage of calories from complex carbohydrates in foods such as whole grains, lentils, beans, fruit and potatoes. In some countries, too much of the carbohydrate intake is in the form of sugar due to the high consumption of refined and

C

processed foods. Another factor has been the proliferation of low-fat foods. Consumers often assume that these are also low-calorie foods. In many cases, fats have been replaced by carbohydrates with no great saving in calories. The many low-fat, high-carbohydrate foods available, including low-fat biscuits, cakes, muffins and baked chips are all adding to expanding waistlines.

HOW MUCH DO YOU NEED?

There is no Reference Nutrient Intake (RNI) for carbohydrate, but government guidelines suggest that the present level of about 45 per cent of total calories consumed is rather low; recommendations have been made that it should rise to about 50 per cent. Both children and adults should consume at least 130g of carbohydrates a day. This is based on the minimum amount needed to produce enough glucose in order for the brain to function. This amount is easily exceeded in the average diet. The problem is that the excess usually comes from refined carbohydrates.

Although refined carbohydrates, such as white flour and white rice, are just as good energy sources as wholemeal flour and brown rice, processing removes some essential nutrients, including the B vitamins, iron and other minerals, as well as dietary fibre. The best approach is to build a diet around whole or lightly processed grains, legumes, beans and raw or slightly cooked vegetables and fruit, and to avoid a high sugar intake.

Carbohydrate facts

- Legumes, such as dried beans and peas, provide the best food value for your money.

- Just because you don't see 'sugar' listed as an ingredient on a food label doesn't mean it's not there. Look for words ending in 'ose' (sucrose, lactose, maltose, fructose, glucose and dextrose) and anything described as 'syrup' (such as corn or malt syrup), as well as honey and molasses.

- Both carbohydrates and proteins provide 4kcal per gram, while fat supplies 9kcal. Sugar and starches can become fattening if they are consumed with fatty additions such as butter or spreads, or when they are eaten in quantities much larger than the body can readily use, in which case they are converted and stored as body fat.

CARBOHYDRATE LOADING

Nutrition can have a significant impact on athletic performance and vice versa. Regular exercise increases the body's ability to utilise glucose efficiently and to store glycogen in muscle tissue. So the fitter you are, the greater your ability to store the extra glycogen that is needed for endurance events, such as running a marathon or cross-country skiing. That's why carbohydrates are the preferred fuel for most sports.

SPECIAL CONCERNS

Carbohydrates can be worked into almost any diet, but people with certain diseases may need to make special adjustments. Those with diabetes must manage the total amount and type eaten at each meal and snack. Contrary to popular belief, sugar does not cause diabetes, nor do those with diabetes have to avoid sugar completely.

Those with heart disease need to emphasise high-fibre complex carbohydrates in their diet. Soluble fibre, found in rolled oats, legumes and fruit pectin, helps to lower cholesterol and plays an important role in preventing atherosclerosis, the build-up of fatty deposits in coronary arteries and other blood vessels.

Cancer patients are often advised to increase their carbohydrate intake and decrease fat intake, especially if they have cancers of the breast, colon, uterus, prostate or skin. Evidence suggests certain fats may encourage tumour growth.

Cardiovascular disease

EAT PLENTY OF

- Fresh fruit and vegetables, foods rich in vitamin C, carotenoids and other antioxidant nutrients
- Fish
- Soya protein
- Apples, rolled oats and other soluble fibre foods
- Wholegrain breads and cereals
- Nuts

LIMIT

- Saturated fats in fatty meats, chicken skin, full-fat dairy products, coconut oil and solid frying fats
- Eggs, whole milk, offal and other high-cholesterol foods
- Fats, especially those that are saturated
- Trans fatty acids in partially hydrogenated margarine and shortenings, processed foods made with partially hydrogenated fats, and baked goods

AVOID

- Excessive alcohol
- Tobacco use in any form
- Salty foods (especially if you have hypertension)

Heart and blood vessel disease affects 900,000 people in the UK and kills more than 110,000 people every year. As well as the risk for premature death, cardiovascular disease represents a heavy financial burden to the health care system.

There have been numerous population studies since the early 1950s that have confirmed that diet is a major force in both the cause and the prevention of heart disease. One of the most extensive research projects is the US Framingham Heart Study, which has followed more than 5,000 men and women in Boston, Massachusetts, for more than 40 years. Another large-scale study, the 'Seven Countries Study', compared the incidence of heart disease among men in seven countries and correlated these statistics with diet, smoking habits, physical activity and other lifestyle factors. By carefully analysing the results, researchers have identified risk factors that predispose people to heart disease: heredity, advancing age and gender (pre-menopausal women have a lower risk than men and older women) are among those over which people have no control. Tobacco use heads the list of controllable risk factors.

Poor diet is instrumental in most other factors: these include high blood cholesterol, which promotes the build-up of fatty deposits in the coronary arteries and leads to angina and heart attacks; obesity, which increases the risk of heart attack and contributes to other cardiovascular risk factors; high blood pressure, which can lead to a stroke and heart attack; diabetes, a disease that affects the heart, blood vessels, and other vital organs; and excessive alcohol use, which harms the heart and blood vessels.

A heart-healthy diet

If the wrong diet can promote heart disease, the right one can reduce the risk. This is true, even in the face of such unalterable risk factors as advancing age and a family history of heart attacks.

There is nothing radical about a heart-healthy diet; in fact, it's the same commonsense balanced diet that protects against cancer, Type 2 diabetes and obesity. Carbohydrates, especially wholegrain breads and cereals, beans and other legumes, along with ample fresh fruit and vegetables form the foundation. About 15 per cent of daily calories should come from protein foods – lean meat, fish, poultry (without the skin), egg whites and a combination of grains and legumes (beans and rice, for instance, together make up a complete source of protein). Saturated and trans fats, sugars and salt should be used sparingly.

Ideally, sensible eating should be instilled during childhood, which is when atherosclerosis – the clogging of arteries with fatty deposits – begins. It takes 20 to 30 years, or even longer, for the vessels to become clogged enough to produce symptoms. By that time, however, it may be too late; in a number of cases, the first indication of heart disease is a fatal heart attack.

In addition to encouraging a low-fat diet, it's also a good idea to accustom children to the natural flavour of foods, rather than adding lots of salt or strongly flavoured sauces. While there are some conflicting reports, numerous studies show that populations with a high intake of salty foods have an increased incidence of hypertension. A group of researchers in Finland identified excessive iron as another

Wine as medicine?

For years, researchers have tried to determine why the French have fewer heart attacks than their counterparts in other industrialised countries. It would seem that the high-fat diet and pervasive tobacco use for which the French are famous would make them prone to more, not less, heart disease. Increasingly, researchers have settled on wine as the protective factor, although there is uncertainty over exactly what it is in wine that benefits the heart.

The French lifestyle may also play a part. The French are less obese, eat more olive oil, fish, vegetables and fresh fruit. They consume far fewer calories than British or American people and eat much less refined sugar.

C

dietary factor that may well damage the heart and blood vessels. Their research found that men with high levels of iron in their blood also had an increased incidence of heart attacks. While it was already well known that excessive iron damages the heart, liver and other vital organs, this was the first time that iron levels in the high-to-normal range had been linked to a serious health risk. It also reinforces the long-standing advice from doctors and nutritionists not to take any supplements without first consulting a doctor. Athletes in particular should take note of these findings.

▲ **You are what you eat**
Vegetables, beans, whole grains and lean protein make up a heart-healthy diet.

The cholesterol factor

Excessive cholesterol circulating in the blood is the major precipitating factor in atherosclerosis. In rare cases, an inherited disorder, familial hypercholesterolaemia, causes high blood cholesterol. Without a strict low-fat diet and cholesterol-lowering drugs, people with this disorder have a greatly increased risk of an early heart attack – sometimes during childhood. Far more often, high cholesterol is caused by a diet high in saturated fat, lack of exercise and other lifestyle habits.

For most people, moderately elevated cholesterol levels can be lowered by adopting a diet with less than 30 per cent (preferably 20 per cent) of its calories coming from fats, mostly the mono-unsaturated and polyunsaturated types found in plant oils, fish, nuts and seeds. Doctors advise using olive oil and margarine, especially the kinds that are made with corn, safflower and other unsaturated fats, instead of butter.

Superstar foods and nutrients

Fruit and vegetables. Numerous studies correlate a diet rich in fresh fruit and vegetables with a 25 per cent or better reduction in heart attacks and strokes. Researchers believe that it's the ample vitamin C, carotenoids and other antioxidants in fruit and vegetables that account for the difference. Antioxidants protect cells against damage from the unstable molecules that are released when the body uses oxygen. Oxidation of LDL cholesterol – the type that forms fatty plaque – is thought to be instrumental in initiating atherosclerosis. Fruit and vegetables are also quite high in bioflavonoids and other plant chemicals that act as antioxidants.

Fish. Salmon, sardines, herring, tuna, trout and most oily fish are high in omega-3 fatty acids, which reduce the tendency of blood to clot. This benefit can be had from eating two servings of fish a week. Although fish oil supplements are high in omega-3 fatty acids, they should not be taken without approval by a doctor, because they may increase the risk of a stroke. Omega-3 fats are also found in plant sources such as rape seed and soya oils, linseeds, walnuts and unsaturated margarines, but may not offer the same health benefits.

Soluble fibre. Pectin, rolled oats and other types of soluble fibre help to lower cholesterol and improve glucose metabolism in people predisposed to develop diabetes. Rolled oats, oat bran, psyllium, linseeds, lentils, legumes, apples, pears, grapes and other fruit are high in soluble fibre. A combination of legumes and grains is a prudent low-fat meat alternative.

Whole-grain foods. Several studies have found that diets high in wholegrain foods such as wholemeal bread and wholegrain cereals reduce the risk of coronary heart disease. They contain a variety of important vitamins and minerals, as well as phytochemicals, which have antioxidant properties.

Soya. A large body of evidence has shown that adding soya protein to a low-fat diet lowers the risk of heart disease. Soya contains plant compounds called isoflavones that appear to benefit the heart. Together they help to lower cholesterol levels. Soya protein is found in soya beans and a wide range of products made from these beans, including tofu and soya beverages.

Special margarines. Plant sterols and stanols have been shown to help to lower cholesterol levels when consumed as part of a heart-healthy diet. They are found in plant-sterol enriched margarines, such as Benecol, and are also present, in smaller amounts, in vegetable oils, nuts, sesame and sunflower seeds and legumes.

Olive and rape seed oil. Mono-unsaturated fats tend to lower total and LDL cholesterol levels when they replace saturated fats in the diet. They are found in oils such as olive and rape seed.

The omega-6 polyunsaturated fats found in safflower, sunflower, corn, cottonseed and soya bean oils reduce cholesterol levels when they replace saturated fats in the diet.

Folate. Green leafy vegetables, orange juice, lentils, enriched cereals and asparagus are good sources of folate, which can lower heart disease risk by helping to regulate homo-cysteine levels. Homocysteine forms in the body from methionine, a common amino acid, and high levels are considered to be as much a risk factor for heart disease as high levels of cholesterol. Folate works together with vitamins B_6 and B_{12} to keep homocysteine levels from increasing. B_6 is found in meat, poultry, fish, legumes, nuts, seeds, leafy greens, bananas and whole grains. B_{12} is found in animal foods such as meat, fish and poultry.

Nuts. Nuts and seeds, used moderately, are rich sources of fibre, vitamin E, essential fatty acids and minerals all linked to heart health. Recent studies have shown that adding nuts to the diet lowers the risk of heart disease.

Do supplements help?
Although studies suggest that antioxidants from food play a protective role against cardiovascular disease, studies using supplements have proved disappointing. One trial found no significant benefits from taking daily supplements of vitamin E, beta carotene and vitamin C in people at high risk. And, the relationship between vitamin E and prevention of heart disease is still being debated. Some research has even shown that antioxidant supplements may reduce the efficacy of the 'statin' type cholesterol-lowering drugs.

Food as medicine
One study suggests that a low-fat vegetarian diet may be just as good as the 'statin' drugs at lowering high cholesterol levels. Forty-six adults with high cholesterol levels were put on one of three diets: a low saturated fat diet, the same diet plus medication or a strict vegetarian diet that included soya proteins, high-fibre foods and a margarine containing plant sterols. The researchers found that those on the vegetarian diet lowered their cholesterol levels by almost 29 per cent compared with a decrease of 30 per cent in those who followed the low-fat diet with medication during that same time. Those on the low-fat only diet had just an 8 per cent drop in cholesterol.

Although more research is needed, these positive results underline the great importance of diet as an option for those people who are working to lower their cholesterol levels. There are a number of dietary factors in this vegetarian diet that

Did you know?

High homocysteine levels can be just as dangerous to your heart as smoking or high cholesterol

A significant number of people dying from cardiovascular diseases don't have high blood pressure or high LDL cholesterol, don't smoke and aren't overweight. The culprit may be high levels of homocysteines in the blood. This is an amino acid that damages the walls of an artery when it reaches high concentrations in the blood.

C

help to lower cholesterol: the soya protein, the plant sterols and the soluble fibre found in fruit, grains and vegetables.

Carrots

BENEFITS

- An excellent source of beta carotene, the precursor of vitamin A
- A good source of dietary fibre and potassium
- Help to prevent night blindness
- May help to lower blood cholesterol levels and protect against cancer

DRAWBACKS

- Excessive intake can give skin a yellowish tinge

Native to Afghanistan, carrots are our most abundant source of beta carotene, a compound that can function as an antioxidant and can also be converted by the body into vitamin A. The more vivid the colour of the carrot, the higher the levels of this important carotenoid. An 80g portion of cooked carrots contains only 19kcal, 2g of fibre and about 15mg of beta carotene. This provides more than 75 per cent of the Reference Nutrient Intake (RNI) of vitamin A – nutrient that is essential for healthy hair, skin, eyes, bones and mucous membranes. Vitamin A also helps to prevent infections.

A US government study found that volunteers who ate about one cup of carrots a day had an average 11 per cent reduction in their blood cholesterol levels after only three weeks. Lowered cholesterol levels, in turn, decrease the risk of heart disease. The cholesterol-lowering effect is likely to be due to the high soluble-fibre content of carrots, mostly in the form of pectin.

Take carrots to heart

Studies show that high doses of beta carotene may help reduce the risk of cardiovascular disease by about 45 per cent. Carrots are one of the richest sources of this important carotenoid. Studies also indicate that high doses of beta carotene in pill form will not help to prevent heart disease.

Seeing in the dark

Carrots will not prevent or correct our most common vision problems, such as shortsightedness or long-sightedness. But too little vitamin A does cause night blindness, an inability of the eyes to adjust to dim lighting or darkness. Vitamin A combines with the protein opsin in the retina's rod cells to form rhodopsin, which is needed for night vision. Eating one carrot every few days provides enough vitamin A to prevent or overcome night blindness, if this condition is caused by vitamin A deficiency.

Cooked or raw?

Naturally sweet, carrots make an ideal high-fibre, low-calorie snack food. Interestingly, cooking actually increases carrots' nutritional value, because it breaks down the tough cellular walls that encase the beta carotene. To properly absorb beta carotene, the body needs a small amount of fat, because carotenoids are fat, not water-soluble. Adding a pat of butter or margarine to cooked carrots ensures that the body will fully use this nutrient. Cooked and puréed carrots are an ideal beginner food for babies, as they are naturally sweet and high in nutrients.

Carrots also contain other carotenoids, including alpha carotene, as well as bioflavonoids. The beneficial effects of carrots may not be reproduced by taking isolated supplements. Indeed, a number of studies have shown that beta carotene supplements may

actually be harmful, particularly to smokers. This is not a problem with an excessive intake of carrots, but it can result in the skin taking on a yellow-orange tinge. This harmless condition, called carotanaemia, disappears in a few weeks of reducing carrot intake. If the yellow skin colour persists, or if the white portions of the eyes are also discoloured, the problem may be jaundice, a symptom of a liver disorder.

Cauliflower

BENEFITS

- An excellent source of vitamin C
- A good source of folate and potassium
- Low in calories and high in fibre
- An anti-cancer food

DRAWBACKS

- May cause flatulence

Cauliflower is rich in vitamin C, folate and other phytochemicals linked with good health. An 80g portion of raw cauliflower florets has 75 per cent of the Reference Nutrient Intake (RNI) of vitamin C, 25 per cent of the RNI for folate and reasonable amounts of potassium and vitamin B_6. It also has indoles, bioflavonoids and other chemicals that protect against cancer.

Filling, high in fibre and low in calories (80g of cooked cauliflower has 22kcal), this is an ideal food for weight watchers. Raw cauliflower has more folate (20 per cent is lost in cooking).

To retain flavour and reduce nutrient loss, cook cauliflower rapidly by steaming or boiling in a minimum amount of water. Too much cooking turns cauliflower mushy and releases sulphurous compounds, resulting in an

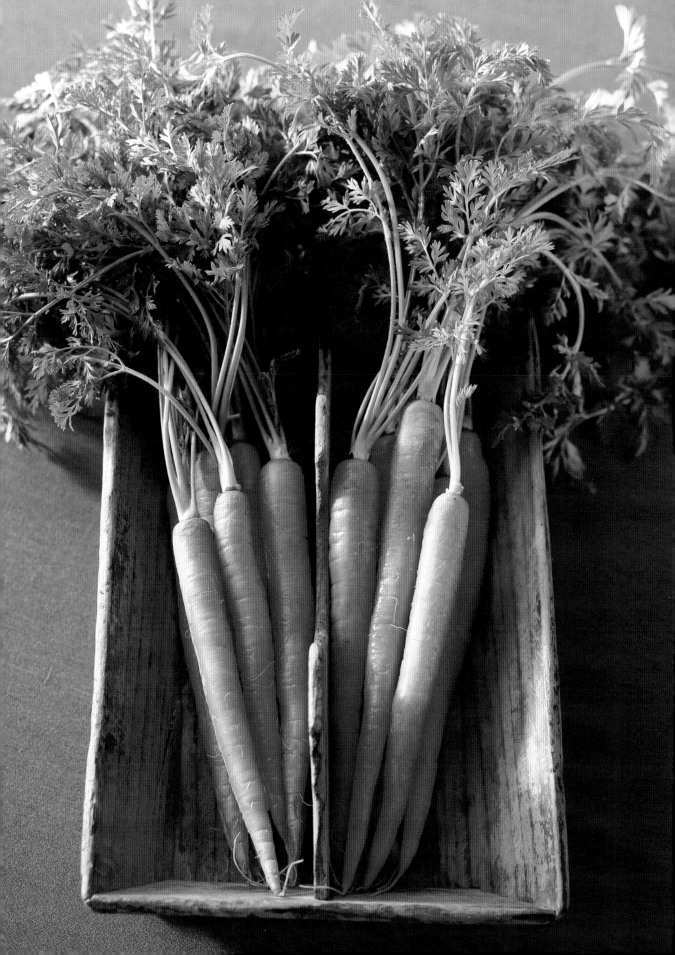

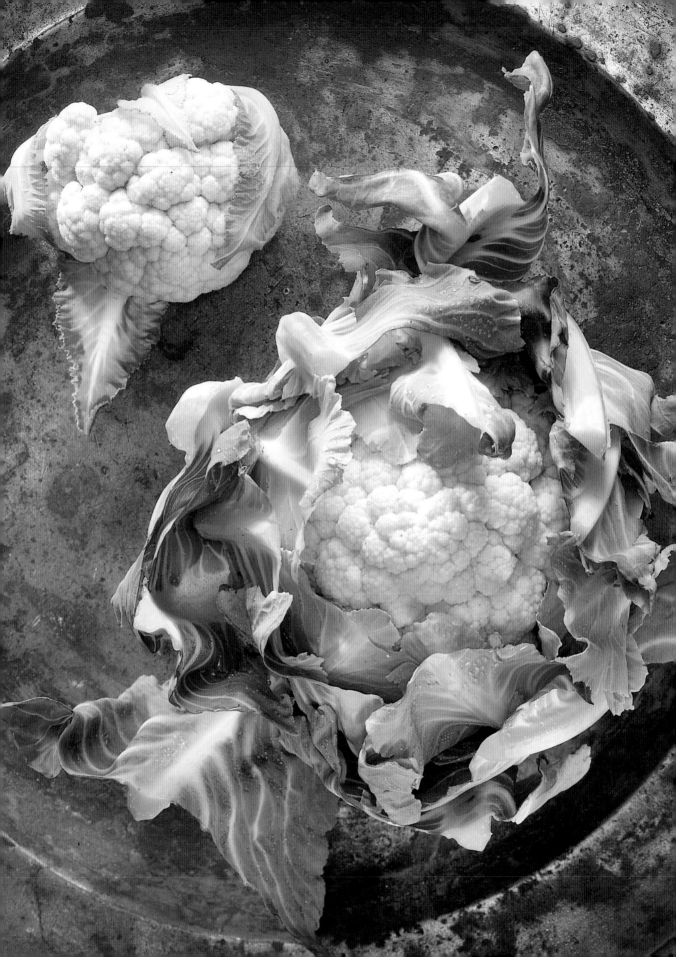

unpleasant odour and bitter taste. Boiling the vegetable in an open pot helps to disperse these compounds. To avoid discolouring cauliflower, don't use aluminium or iron pots.

When buying cauliflower, look for a head with firm, compact florets. If it is fresh, the leaves will be crisp and green, and the head, or curd, snowy white.

Cauliflower may cause flatulence as the gut breaks down the fibrous cell walls. Eating it with spices such as garlic, caraway, ground coriander and cumin will help to ease digestive discomfort. Herbs that can help the digestion are tarragon, bay and fennel.

Celeriac

BENEFITS

- Low in calories and a source of vitamin C and folate
- Good source of potassium

A winter root vegetable, celeriac is a member of the parsley family and is closely related to celery; in fact, its other names include celery root, knob celery and German celery. Fresh celeriac resembles a large, round, knobby turnip, but when the tough outer skin is peeled away, the flesh is white, with a flavour and odour similar to celery.

Celeriac is a good source of potassium and, when eaten raw, 80g of the vegetable contains 14kcal, 3g of fibre, 11mg of vitamin C as well as some folate. It is nutritionally similar to celery, although celeriac offers slightly more folate and iron than the same amount of celery does.

Celeriac lends itself to a variety of dishes. For example, it is often grated raw into salads; boiled and puréed to add body and flavour to soups and stews; chopped into poultry stuffing; or sliced, dipped in an egg batter, and sautéed to serve as a meat substitute.

It is also delicious served as an accompaniment to salmon or spicy pork. The French cut celeriac into thin strips, then blanch them in boiling water and toss them with a mustard-mayonnaise dressing to make an alternative to celery salad.

Celery

BENEFITS

- Low in calories and a source of fibre
- Provides some potassium, vitamin C and folic acid
- In significant amounts may reduce inflammation and protect against cancer

Dieters tend to eat lots of celery because it is so low in calories, but, it is a myth that chewing the stalks consumes more calories than the vegetable provides. Two stalks – about 60g – of celery contain only 4kcal (celery is about 95 per cent water by weight), yet their fibre content makes them filling. It is a good source of potassium; it also contributes small amounts of vitamin C and some folic acid.

Although it is not very nutritious, it adds a unique flavour soups, salads and stuffing.

Celery leaves are the most nutritious part of the plant, containing more calcium, iron, potassium, vitamin C and beta carotene than the stalks. The leaves should be salvaged for soups, salads and other dishes enhanced by the flavour of celery, and even used as a garnish.

Medicinal properties

Herbalists have advocated fresh celery and celery seed tea to treat gout and other forms of inflammatory arthritis, as well as high blood pressure and oedema. Studies indicate that phthalides in celery may reduce the body's levels of certain hormones that constrict blood vessels and raise blood pressure. Polyacetylenes, also found in celery, are said to reduce production of some prostaglandins, which are body chemicals that cause inflammation. There is no scientific proof, however, that celery can ease arthritis pain or lower blood pressure and increase urine output.

In theory, celery may help to reduce the risk of certain cancers. The polyacetylenes destroy benzopyrene, a carcinogen that occurs in foods cooked at a high temperature. This benefit may be offset by celery's high levels of plant nitrates, substances that the body converts into nitrosamines, which have been linked to an increased risk of cancer. However, many researchers believe that this is a minor risk because most plants high in nitrates and other potentially cancer-causing substances also contain chemicals that neutralise any harmful effects. Cooking celery by boiling, braising or steaming lowers its nitrate levels.

Cereals

BENEFITS

- High in complex carbohydrates
- Many are high in fibre
- Enriched cereals are high in iron, niacin, thiamin and riboflavin, along with other B vitamins
- Iron-fortified infant cereals are ideal introductory solid foods

DRAWBACKS

- Many commercial varieties are high in salt, sugar and fat
- High-bran products may cause bloating and flatulence

Served hot or cold, cereals can be a healthy, low-calorie breakfast main dish. Many also make popular snacks and can be used in meat loaves, muffins and biscuits. Since ancient times, rolled oats and other cooked cereal porridges have been valued as much for their economy and ease of preparation as for their nutrition and flavour.

The first ready-to-eat cold cereals were developed by the Western Health Reform Institute in Battle Creek, Michigan, founded by the Seventh-Day Adventists in 1866. The Adventists wanted a vegetarian, libido-suppressing alternative to the traditional cooked breakfast of ham or bacon and eggs. It took another 30 years, however, for cold cereals to gain much of a following. In 1899 Dr John Harvey Kellogg, the medical director of the Battle Creek Sanitarium (a health institute that

Did you know?

Eating breakfast might help you to lose weight

People who eat breakfast instead of skipping this meal have more success in losing weight.

specialised in the treatment of digestive diseases), and his brother Will, invented a wheat-flake cereal to improve bowel function. A few years later they developed another cereal made of corn flakes. Adding to these developments, one of Dr Kellogg's patients, CW Post, came up with a wheat and barley mixture that he called Grape Nut Flakes. Food companies founded by the Kellogg brothers and Post remain North America's leading producers of cold cereals, with dozens of different brands.

Prepared cereals are popular in Europe and other parts of the world, they are generally considered a North American product, with one notable exception – the muesli mixture of oats, wheat flakes, nuts and dried fruit invented by Dr Max Bircher-Benner, a Swiss pioneer of the natural health-food movement in Europe. Variations of his muesli, which is served either hot or cold, are now international favourites.

Wheat, corn, rice, oats and barley are the most familiar grains used to make cereals. Most flaked cereals are varying combinations of flour, water, sugar and salt that are mixed into a dough, rolled thin and then toasted. Some cereal preparations are spun into different shapes, such as tiny doughnuts or cartoon characters; in others, the grains are shredded or exploded.

Nutritional value

Cereals are one of the most popular members of the carbohydrate, or starch, food group. Most packet cereals are enriched or fortified with various vitamins and minerals, especially iron, niacin and thiamin. Unfortunately, many of the cereals that hype their vitamin and mineral content are so loaded with sugar

that eating an unprocessed cereal and taking vitamins could arguably be a healthier option.

Some cereals have added dried fruit and nuts. An economical and healthy approach is to buy plain cereal and then add your own fresh fruit, sultanas, seeds, nuts or other ingredients. Some muesli is high in fat from added oils.

Many commercial cereals are also high in salt. If possible, it's best to make your own. If you do use bought muesli cereal, look for a low-fat brand.

Rolled oats are high in soluble fibre that helps to lower blood cholesterol levels, thereby reducing the risk of heart disease. Some cereals, especially those made from whole grains or those with added bran, are high in insoluble fibre as well. These help to prevent constipation and may also reduce

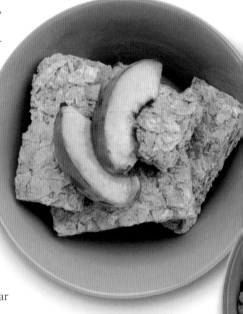

▶ **Something for every taste**
Cold cereal, such as wheat biscuits or muesli, with low-fat milk provides a tasty low-calorie breakfast; for an even heartier start, try hot rolled oats or another cooked cereal. A serving of fruit adds flavour and extra vitamins and minerals.

Do one simple thing

Make your own delicious and nutritious cereal

For a healthy muesli, mix uncooked rolled oats with an assortment of dried fruit and seeds, sweeten with a small amount of brown sugar and toast for a few minutes in a warm oven.

the risk of some cancers, including colon cancer. Wholegrain cereals that are rich in fibre are a very convenient way to add more fibre to your diet. You should look for a cereal that contains at least 3g of fibre per serving.

Be careful not to add too much bran to your diet all at once; it can cause bloating, with abdominal discomfort and intestinal gas and flatulence.

The calories in most cereals can vary considerably, depending on the ingredients and how they are served. If you serve them with whole milk you will more than double the calorie content of many cereals. But if you use skimmed milk or semi-skimmed milk you will save calories and, for children over the age of two and adults, it is much healthier than whole milk.

When you are comparing the calorie content of cereals, pay attention to the serving sizes given on the package's nutrition label; some cereals are low in calories only when consumed in unreasonably small amounts.

Children's cereals, in particular, are often extremely high in sugar. In fact, sugar may top the list of ingredients on the nutrition table, which means that the product actually has more sugar than anything else. Compare the nutrition table of your chosen cereal with the nutrition tables on other cereals to find a product that offers more fibre and less sugar.

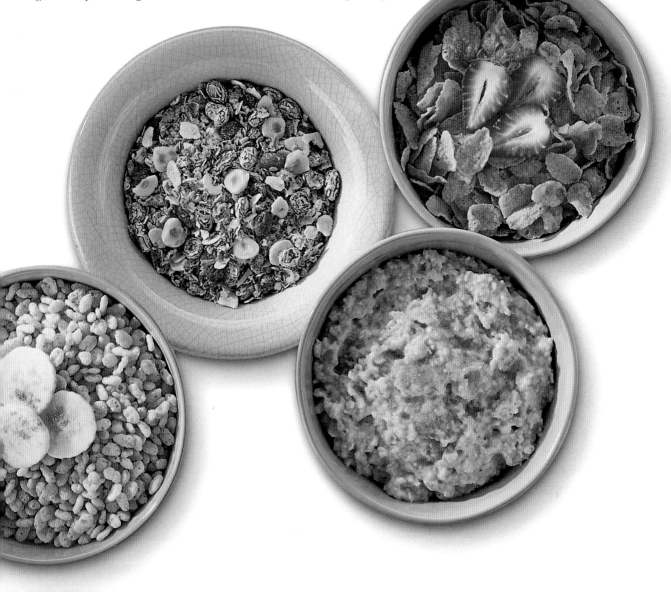

Cheese

BENEFITS

- High in protein and calcium
- A good source of vitamin B$_{12}$
- Cheddar and other cheeses may fight tooth decay

DRAWBACKS

- Most are high in saturated fat and sodium
- Some may trigger migraines or allergic reactions in susceptible people

One of our most versatile and well loved foods, cheese is used for snacks, appetisers, main courses and desserts. It's an ancient food that can be made from the milk of almost any animal – cows, sheep, goats, yaks, camels and buffaloes.

Most cheeses are made by adding a mixture of enzymes, known as rennet, to milk to curdle it. The main enzyme in rennet, which traditionally has been isolated from the stomach lining of calves, is chymosin. Today, it can also be produced by inserting the gene that codes for its production into bacteria. This allows for a more ready production of chymosin and can also cater for the needs of vegetarians. The liquid that remains after the curds have formed is known as whey. When it is drained away, we are left with what's called cottage or farmer's cheese. Or the curds may be mixed with other ingredients such as wines or herbs, injected with special moulds or bacteria, pressed or moulded, smoked or aged to make any of hundreds of different cheeses.

On average, it takes about 4 litres of milk to make 500g of cheddar, Swiss or other firm cheese. A 30g serving of Cheddar cheese contains about 120kcal, about 220mg of calcium and 10g of fat. Cottage cheese has the fewest calories – about 110kcal in a 100g serving, but it has less than half the calcium of milk. Cream cheese is comparable to hard cheeses in calories and fat, but has less calcium.

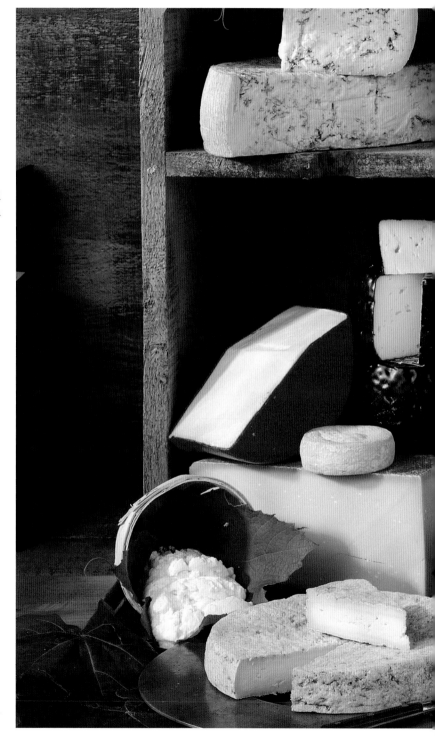

▶ **A rich variety of cheeses**
There's a different kind of cheese to suit almost any palate, from firm to soft cheeses, and from mild to strong-flavoured cheeses.

Eat in moderation

Cheese is rich in both calcium and protein, making it a staple for vegetarians. But it's also high in fat, cholesterol and sodium. Most people – especially those with a weight or cholesterol problem – should use it moderately. Exceptions include adolescents going through a growth spurt, vegetarians and thin older women with osteoporosis, a weakening of the bones. Many people who cannot digest more than small quantities of milk because of lactose intolerance can eat cheese, as the bacteria and enzymes used to make cheese also break down some of the lactose (milk sugar).

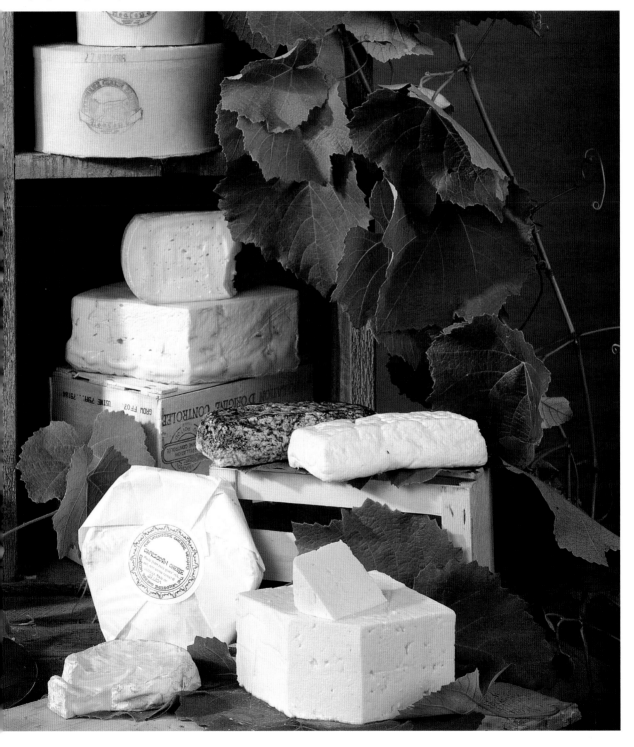

Do one simple thing

Go for flavour, not fat

Use small amounts of a highly flavour-some hard cheese, such as mature Cheddar or Parmesan, to add taste without adding a lot of fat. You need less of a strong-flavoured cheese than you would with a milder cheese.

Health hazards

Doctors often advise patients with heart disease, high blood cholesterol or high blood pressure to reduce the amount of cheese they consume. Because most cheese is high in saturated fat, it may increase the risk of atherosclerosis, the clogging of arteries with fatty deposits. And the sodium it contains can be a hazard for people with high blood pressure.

Matured cheese can also trigger a migraine headache in susceptible people. The likely culprit is tyramine, a naturally occurring chemical in Cheddar, blue cheese, Camembert and certain other ripe cheeses. Tyramine also interacts with monoamine oxidase (MAO) inhibitors, drugs sometimes used to treat depression, and can cause a life-threatening rise in blood pressure. People taking MAO inhibitors should get a list of foods to avoid from their doctor, as they fall into many categories.

People who are allergic to penicillin may react to blue cheese and other soft cheeses that are made with penicillin moulds. Also young children who are allergic to cow's milk will react to cheese. Many cheeses are made from pasteurised milk. The process does not kill all the micro-organisms, although it does destroy the harmful ones. Milk used for cheese cannot be boiled in order to sterilise it as this makes the calcium salts within the milk insoluble and they need to be soluble for rennet to solidify the cheese. Cheeses made from unpasteurised milk may contain micro-organisms such as listeria. Listeria poisoning resembles flu and is particularly hazardous to babies, pregnant women and the elderly, as well as to anyone who is already ill.

Low-fat cheeses

Fat gives cheese its rich texture and delicious taste, but it also adds calories and cholesterol. About 70 to 80 per cent of the calories in cheese comes from fat. Even reduced-fat or part-skimmed milk cheeses can be high in fat; more than 50 per cent of the calories in part-skim milk mozzarella come from fat. Historically, low-fat cheeses often lacked flavour, and tended to be high in salt to improve flavour; sodium phosphate may be used to create a smoother texture. Today, there is a broader range of tasty fat-reduced cheeses on the market. Cholesterol-free imitation cheeses are often made of soya, or tofu; these cheeses, however, can still be high in fat and sodium.

Fresh cheeses made from skimmed milk, such as reduced-fat ricotta and cottage cheese, are lower in fat and calories. Reduced and low-fat soft cheeses have much less fat and can be substituted for regular cream cheese, which gets 85 per cent of its calories from fat.

Did you know?

Cheese fights cavities

Studies have shown that cheese can help you to reduce tooth decay. The fat naturally contained in cheese coats your teeth and acts as a natural barrier against bacteria. All cheese contains casein, which provides a natural tooth protectant. And the calcium and phosphorus found in cheese help to remineralise tooth enamel.

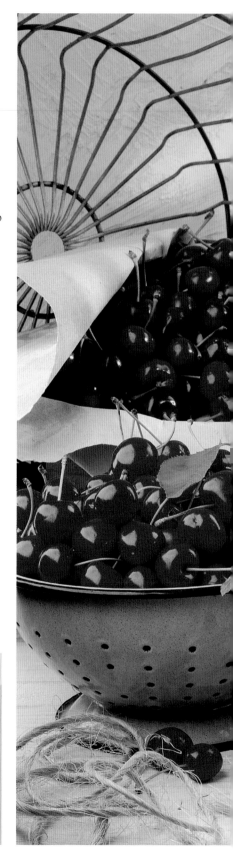

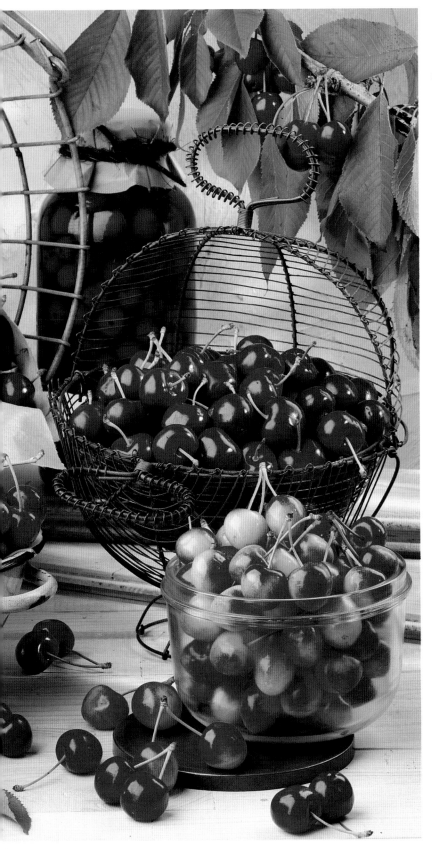

Cherries

BENEFITS

- Low-calorie snack or dessert

- High in pectin, a soluble fibre that may lower cholesterol

- Good source of potassium

- May help to prevent gout and reduce arthritis pain

DRAWBACKS

- Can provoke allergic reactions in susceptible people

- They spoil quickly and are usually only available for a limited season

A member of the plant family that includes plums, apricots, peaches and nectarines, cherries are generally lower in vitamins and minerals than their larger cousins. Still, the flavour and low calorie content of the various sweet varieties make cherries an ideal snack or dessert. Sour cherries are more nutritious than the sweet types, and are used for making jams, or are often bottled or canned.

Facts about cherries

- Maraschino cherries are made by bleaching the fruit in a sulphur dioxide brine, then toughening it with lime or calcium salt. The cherries are then dyed bright red, sweetened, flavoured and packed in jars.

- Cherry seeds contain cyanide. As a result, kirsch, a fruit brandy made from cherries, also contains a very small amount of cyanide.

- Cherries were named after the Turkish town of Cerasus where cherries were grown at least as far back as 300 BC.

◀ **Sweet and sour treats**
Yellowish Queen Anne cherries (right) are sweet, scarlet Morellos are tart but make delicious pies. Deep red Bing cherries (background) are delicious raw or preserved.

C

Nutritional value

There are about 38kcal in 80g of cherries, as well as vitamin C and potassium. They are a good source of pectin, a soluble fibre that helps to control blood cholesterol levels. Cherries are also a wealthy source of quercetin, a flavonoid with anticarcinogenic and antioxidant activities. They are valued in natural medicine for their cleansing properties; the fruit is believed to remove toxins and fluids and cleanse the kidneys. Their mild laxative affect can help to relieve constipation.

A substance in cherries called cyanidin has anti-inflammatory properties and helps to reduce the swelling and pain of gout and alleviate the symptoms of arthritis. In theory, 20 cherries have the same effect as an aspirin. A recent study showed that eating 45 Bing cherries a day for a month reduced inflammation linked with arthritis, heart disease and cancer.

People who are allergic to apricots and other members of the plum family may also suffer a reaction to cherries with symptoms such as hives and a tingling or itching sensation in or around the mouth.

Some studies also link the flavonoid quercetin with a reduced risk of coronary artery disease, in addition to its other activities.

Varieties of cherry

There are more than 1,000 varieties of cherry worldwide. The most popular sweet cherries in the UK are Napoleon and Bing and other dark coloured varieties (ranging from deep maroon to almost black), such as Dukes. Queen Annes are yellow with tinges of red, large and very sweet. Sour varieties, such as Morellos, are smaller than the sweet types and are best for bottling or being made into pies. When buying fresh cherries, you should look for plump, firm fruit with green stems. Both sweet and sour cherries will spoil quickly and have a relatively short season. Imported cherries are not usually as tasty as the local fruit that is picked and marketed at the height of its ripeness.

Chestnuts

BENEFITS

- Source of folate, fibre, riboflavin and thiamin
- Low in fat and with fewer calories than other nuts

DRAWBACKS

- Tend to be expensive

Unlike most other nuts, chestnuts are made up almost completely of carbohydrates and are low in fat and calories. They are also high in a number of important nutrients: a 100g serving of chestnuts provides more than 50 per cent of the adult Reference Nutrient Intake (RNI) of vitamin B_6, and 12 per cent of the RNI of magnesium. The same sized serving contains 170kcal, 2g of protein and 2.7g of fat.

High in natural sugar

After chestnuts are picked, their starch begins to turn to sugar, giving the nuts their mild, sweet flavour. Chestnuts are almost always cooked, either by roasting or boiling, before they are eaten.

When they are heated, the nuts swell and their thin, soft shells crack, which makes them very easy to peel and eat as they are or use in cooking. They are often used in baked desserts.

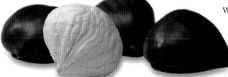

Water chestnuts

These crunchy vegetables, which are served in many Asian dishes, salads and soups, are unrelated to chestnuts; in fact, they are not nuts, nor do they grow on trees. Instead, they are tubers that grow wild in marshes or the shallow water along lake banks in China and Japan and other areas in Asia. The Chinese also cultivate water chestnuts as a second crop in their rice paddies.

Most of the water chestnuts sold in the UK are imported from China. They do contain moderate amounts of protein and vitamin C, however, they are not as nutritious as potatoes and other tuberous vegetables.

Roasted chestnuts can be dried and ground into a flour that makes a rich, tasty crust for tarts or pies. Boiled chestnuts, which have a consistency similar to that of potatoes, can be mashed or puréed to add to cake batter or used as a pastry filling. Marrons glacés, a French delicacy, are peeled whole chestnuts preserved in a sweet syrup. Chestnuts may also be used in soups, salads and pasta dishes, as well as in some liqueur desserts.

They also make an appearance at Christmas – often served with the traditional Brussels sprouts or mixed into turkey stuffing.

The chestnut develops inside a prickly burr that is gathered after it falls from the tree in early autumn. It should not be confused with the horse chestnut, which is inedible. They are best stored in an airtight container or a perforated plastic bag in the crisper section of the refrigerator. Use them within three weeks of purchase. They can be roasted, boiled, baked or microwaved (remember to split the skins first).

Childhood nutrition

Food for the growing years

During the first few years of life, it's vital to meet a child's nutritional needs in order to ensure proper growth and also to establish a lifelong habit of healthy eating.

Eating a meal should be both a healthy and an enjoyable occasion – something that many parents may overlook when they are planning a meal for their growing children. Instead of a fast meal (especially one low in nutritional value) that family members eat at different hours, mealtimes should involve good food and conversation (that doesn't involve criticising table manners or begging children to eat). A calm atmosphere helps to foster family relationships, as well as good digestion. You can also involve children in family meals by having them help out with simple mealtime tasks, such as peeling potatoes, preparing salads or setting the table. If mealtime is a pleasant event, children may practise healthy eating habits later on in life.

THE GROWING YEARS

Between the ages of 2 and 20, the human body changes continuously and dramatically. In general, muscles grow stronger, bones grow longer, height may more than double and weight can increase as much as fivefold. The most striking physiological changes take place during puberty, which usually occurs between the ages of 10 and 15 years in girls and slightly later – between the ages of 12 and 19 years – in boys. Sexual development and maturity take place at this time.

Children need energy for their growing years: varying from 1,230kcal a day for one to three year old boys, 1,165 for girls; 1,715kcal for four to six year old boys and 1,545kcal for girls; up to 2,755kcal for 16 year old boys and 2,110kcal for girls.

Did you know?

The incidence of childhood obesity has almost doubled over the last 10 years

Currently more than 27 per cent of children under 10 in the UK are overweight, according to surveys. This epidemic is occurring in every age group, and in boys as well as girls.

The amount of food that a child needs varies according to height, build and activity level. Left to themselves, most children will usually eat the amount of food that's right for them; however, it is up to the parents to make sure that their children have the right foods available to choose from. Avoid the old trap of making them eat more food than they want or need. Yesterday's notion of 'cleaning your plate' can lead to overeating and weight problems or to a lifelong dislike of particular foods. Parents may find it better to serve smaller portions in the first place or to allow children to serve themselves.

CHANGES IN APPETITE

In most children, appetite slackens as the growth rate slows after the first year; it will then vary throughout childhood, depending on whether the child is going through a period of slow or rapid growth. It is perfectly normal for a young child to eat ravenously one day and then show little interest in food the following day. Eating patterns change markedly with the onset of the adolescent growth spurt.

C

FOODS FOR TODDLERS

After six months when children begin to eat 'solid' foods, they can eat most of the dishes prepared for the rest of the family, suitably chopped or mashed where necessary. Toddlers, however, have high energy requirements and small stomachs, so they may need five or six small meals or snacks a day. Schedule a toddler's snacks so they don't interfere with food intake during meals. An interval of about an hour and a half is usually enough.

Toddlers may develop strange habits – such as eliminating everything that's white or green. Such food rituals are often short-lived, although they can be annoying or worrying if they get out of hand. Respect the child's preferences without giving in to every whim; offer a reasonable alternative.

BALANCE AND VARIETY

Children need a wide and balanced variety of foods. Carbohydrates (breads and cereals), fruit and vegetables should make up the major part of their diet. Protein foods can include meat, fish, chicken, eggs, milk, soya products (such as tofu) and mixes of grains and legumes. Milk is an important source of calories, protein, minerals and vitamins. Children four to nine years old should have 2 to 3 servings of dairy foods every day (some of the milk may be in the form of cheese or yoghurt). Grilled and baked foods are preferable to fried and fatty ones for children of all ages.

THE VALUE OF DIETARY FATS

Fats are probably the most misunderstood nutrients. Although everyone should avoid excess fat, we all need a certain amount of essential fatty acids for important body functions. Several vitamins (A, D, E and K) can be absorbed only in the presence of fat,

Do one simple thing

Ensure they eat a good lunch

Recent attention to school meals means that many schools now provide more nutritious meals for pupils and school vending machines have either been banned or now stock healthier options, too. But if your child refuses to eat a school meal or you don't like what's on offer, pack a healthy lunch, such as wholemeal bread sandwiches with a protein-rich meat or poultry filling, a little salad and some fruit.

and fats are necessary for the production of other body chemicals, including the hormones required in adolescence. Despite the benefits of fat intake, excessive fat intake in childhood may easily lead to obesity and many adult diseases. The current recommendation for fat intake is to limit saturated fat and to moderate total fat intake. The general recommendation is that children older than two years of age consume a diet containing no more than 30 per cent of energy as fat and no more than 10 per cent of energy as saturated fat. The transition to this diet should begin at two years of age with a gradual reduction in fat intake over time.

Encouraging good eating habits

- Do set a good example for your child to copy. Share mealtimes and eat the same healthy foods.
- Do discourage snacking on sweets and fatty foods. Keep plenty of healthy foods, such as fruit, raw vegetables, low-fat crackers and yoghurt, around for children to eat between meals.
- Don't buy junk food when you do your grocery shopping; no matter how well you hide it, children will find it. If it's not there, they can't eat it.
- Do insist a child takes a good mouthful of a new food, to taste it, but don't force him to eat it if he dislikes it.
- Do encourage children to enjoy fruit and vegetables by giving them a variety from an early age.
- Don't give skimmed or semi-skimmed milk to children under the age of two unless your doctor prescribes it; at this stage, children need the extra calories and vitamin A in whole milk.
- Do ask children to help to prepare meals. If parents rely mostly on convenience foods, children may not learn to cook or enjoy cooking.
- Don't add unnecessary sugar to drinks and foods.
- Don't accustom children to extra salt by adding it to food or placing the shaker on the table.
- Don't give whole nuts to children under the age of five, who may choke on them. Peanut butter and chopped nuts are fine as long as the child is not allergic to them.
- Don't force children to eat more than they want.
- Don't use food as a bribe.
- Don't make children feel guilty about eating or not eating any type of food.

EATING THEIR VEGETABLES

It may not be easy to get children to eat vegetables, but you can win them over with bright colours and interesting textures. Choose crisp, raw carrot sticks and other attractive, crunchy vegetables. Add minced vegetables (courgette, aubergine, mushrooms) to minced meat in spaghetti sauce, or chop chickpeas with grains and other vegetables into 'veggie burgers'.

BUILDING BONE

Calcium is important for forming strong, healthy bones during adolescence and preventing osteoporosis later in life. Youths 12 to 18 years old need three milk-product servings a day – such as a 200ml of milk or 40g (two slices) of cheese or 200g of yoghurt. If teens don't like milk, they can try a smoothie, fortified soya or rice drinks, cheese sandwiches or even fat-reduced custard.

A GROWING EPIDEMIC: OBESITY

In the Western world, children are becoming obese or overweight in growing numbers and at earlier ages. The consequence is high blood pressure, high cholesterol, Type 2 diabetes, sleeping disorders and orthopaedic complications. One study found that the arteries of many teenagers are so clogged that the children are at increased risk for a heart attack. Guidelines suggest limiting foods high in saturated fat for children over two; encouraging children to eat more fruit, vegetables and whole grains; and to eat only moderate amounts of sugars and foods containing added sugars. Daily physical activity is also important – but it is rarer, since computers and computer games increased in popularity.

Overweight children tend to become overweight adults. Parents should foster healthy eating, positive body image and active lifestyle early in a child's life. The best approach to controlling weight in obese children is to serve smaller portions and encourage regular, vigorous exercise. Parents should lead by example in this area.

Food for growing up

As children grow, their nutritional needs change; some needs vary between the sexes. The chart below gives an overview of the Reference Nutrition Intake (RNIs) of certain nutrients for children from the ages of 1 to 18.

AGES		1-3	4-7	8-11	12-15	16-18
VITAMIN A (mcg)		300	350	500	725	750
VITAMIN D (mcg)*		10				
VITAMIN E (mg)	Boys	5	6	8	10.5	11
	Girls	5	6	8	9	8
VITAMIN C (mg)	Boys	30	30	30	30	40
	Girls	30	30	30	30	30
NIACIN (mg)	Boys	9-10	11-13	14-16	19-21	20-22
	Girls	9-10	11-13	14-16	17-19	15-17
THIAMIN (mg)	Boys	0.5	0.7	0.9	1.2	1.2
	Girls	0.5	0.7	0.8	1.0	0.9
RIBOFLAVIN (mg)	Boys	0.8	1.1	1.4	1.8	1.9
	Girls	0.8	1.1	1.3	1.6	1.4
FOLATE (mcg)		100	100	150	200	200
VITAMIN B$_6$ (mg)	Boys	0.6-0.9	0.8-1.3	1.1-1.6	1.4-2.1	1.5-2.2
	Girls	0.6-0.9	0.8-1.3	1.0-1.5	1.2-1.8	1.1-1.6
VITAMIN B$_{12}$ (mcg)		1.0	1.5	1.5	2.0	2.0
CALCIUM (mg)	Boys	700	800	800	1200	1000
	Girls	700	800	900	1000	800
IRON (mg)		6-8	6-8	6-8	10-13	10-13
ZINC (mg)		4.5	6	9	12	12

* No RNI has been set for children over three years of age as it is assumed they will receive vitamin D from the action of sunlight on their skin

C

FOODS FOR TEENAGERS

Teenagers usually develop voracious appetites to match their need for additional energy: calories and protein for growth and to build muscles; and protein, phosphorus, calcium and vitamin D for bone formation. At the same time, many develop erratic eating habits – for example, skipping breakfast, lunching at school or at a fast-food restaurant then snacking almost non-stop until bedtime. Although snacking is not the ideal way to eat, a 'food on the run' lifestyle won't necessarily cause nutritional problems as long as the basic daily requirements for protein, carbohydrates, fats, dietary fibre and various vitamins and minerals are met. You can generally keep your teenager out of nutritional danger by providing snacks that are high in vitamins, minerals and protein but low in sugar, fat and salt. This means buying healthy snack foods, such as fresh and dried fruit, raw vegetables, nuts, cheese and yoghurt – not high-fat, high-sugar, high-salt options.

Many teenagers become vegetarians out of a genuine concern for animal welfare or because they do not like the taste or texture of meat. They can thrive on a well-balanced vegetarian diet based around wholemeal bread, pasta, rice and potatoes, eaten with a variety of vegetables, fruits, nuts and seeds. Don't let your children substitute large quantities of dairy products for meat and fish, or their diet will be too high in saturated fats. Children who decide to become vegan and cut out dairy products will need to take supplements of vitamin B_{12}, (found naturally in animal products) or eat fortified cereals served with soya milk or fruit juice. A sensible approach is vital for parent and child.

Easy, healthy snacks

Stock up on healthy snacks that children and teenagers can nibble on throughout the day.
- Fresh and dried fruit.
- Breads and crackers with spreads such as peanut butter, low-fat cheese, canned tuna or sardines and lean cold meats.
- Rice cakes and whole-grain crackers or breadsticks.
- Low-fat yoghurt.
- Sticks of carrot, celery or other raw vegetables and cherry tomatoes with nutritious dips.
- Plain popcorn.
- Water, milk or fruit juice.

IRON DEFICIENCY

Iron is an essential mineral for normal growth and development for a child. Unfortunately, many children have inadequate stores of iron due to insufficient intake of iron-rich foods. There are two types of iron: haem, which is easily absorbed by humans, and non-haem iron, which is poorly absorbed. Foods that contain haem iron include meat, fish, poultry and seafood while breakfast cereals, legumes, eggs, grains, breads, seeds, nuts, dried fruit and dark green, leafy vegetables contain the non-haem variety. Children should have a variety of iron-containing foods in their diet. In addition, the consumption of vitamin C-rich foods improves the absorption of dietary iron.

SNACKING AND FAST FOOD

Teenagers often prefer snacks loaded with fat, salt and sugar: crisps, French fries, hamburgers, pizza and chocolate. These strike a poor balance between calories and nutrition; a steady diet of them is low in vitamins A and C, calcium and dietary fibre. Encourage them to choose grilled chicken (not crumbed), sandwiches or wraps with lean meats and salad or a slice of vegetarian pizza.

The occasional 'junk food' treat will do no harm, especially as children should be encouraged to enjoy food and not treat it purely as 'fuel'. But an appreciation of well-cooked, healthy food will lead to a healthy, adult attitude towards eating.

Childhood obesity and TV

Several studies have documented associations between number of hours of TV watched and the rate of obesity. Moreover, heavy TV watching has been associated with higher intakes of calories, fat, sweet and salty snacks and carbonated drinks in children, exacerbated by increased exposure to advertising for these foods.

A consumer's guide to chillies

Chilli hotness is rated in Scoville units. The hottest chilli on record is the habanero, which is rated at 100,000 to 350,000 Scoville units. By contrast, the serrano comes in at about 5,000 to 15,000 Scoville units. Scoville units are the measurement of capsaicin level (the oil that makes chillies hot). Pure capsaicin rates 16 million units. Although chillies can vary from pod to pod and plant to plant, listed below is an approximate ranking for several varieties of chillies, with '10' being the hottest:

Rank	Scoville units	Type
10	100,000-350,000	Habanero; Scotch Bonnet
9	50,000-100,000	Santaka; Chiltepin; Thai
8	30,000-50,000	Aji; Cayenne; Tabasco; Piquin
7	15,000-30,000	Chile de Arbol
6	5,000-15,000	Yellow Wax; Serrano
5	2,500-5,000	Jalapeño; Mirasol
4	1500-2,500	Sandia; Cascabel
3	1,000-1,500	Ancho; Pasilla; Espanola
2	500-1,000	New Mexico; Anaheim; Big Jim
1	100-500	Mexi-bells; Cherry
0	0-100	Mild Bells; Sweet Banana; Pimento

The following is a description of a selection of popular chillies available in most parts of the world, from the mildest to the hottest.

MILD TO MODERATELY HOT:

- **Anaheim.** These long, slender red or green chillies are among the most popular.
- **Ancho.** These dark red, heart-shaped chillies are usually dried.
- **Pasilla.** A dark greenish-red chilli, usually dried.
- **Poblano.** Green chillies with a small, tapered shape; they are usually roasted, and may be stuffed or added to a variety of dishes.

HOT:

- **Cayenne.** Long, red chillies, dried and often ground into a hot pepper spice.
- **Jalapeño.** These tapered green or red chillies are sold fresh, canned or pickled.
- **Serrano.** Small, bullet-shaped green or red chillies, often used in hot salsas.
- **Thai.** Long, thin green or red chillies with many seeds, used in Thai salads and noodle dishes.

VERY HOT:

- **Bird's eye.** Small, thin-fleshed, and usually red. Deep fiery hot, but with a sweet flavour that is excellent in curries.
- **Habanero or Scotch Bonnet.** Shaped like red, yellow or orange lanterns, these are considered the hottest of cultivated chillies.

Chillies

BENEFITS

- Rich in beta carotene and vitamin C
- May help to relieve nasal congestion
- May help to prevent blood clots that can lead to a heart attack or stroke

DRAWBACKS

- Require careful handling during preparation to prevent irritation of the skin and eyes
- May irritate haemorrhoids in susceptible people

C

A popular ingredient in Asian recipes, chillies, or hot peppers, add spice and interest to many foods; some of the milder varieties are consumed as low-calorie snacks.

The heat in chillies comes from capsaicinoids, substances that have no odour or flavour themselves but impart their bite by acting directly on the mouth's pain receptors. This results in the teary eyes, runny nose ('salsa sniffles') and sweating experienced by most people who indulge in the hotter varieties.

For people with a cold or who suffer allergies, eating chillies can provide temporary relief from nasal and sinus congestion. Capsaicin and other capsaicinoids are concentrated mainly in the white ribs and seeds, which can be removed to produce a milder flavour.

When using chillies, handle them with care. Wear thin gloves and wash all utensils well with soap and water after use. Even a tiny amount of capsaicinoids causes severe irritation if it is transferred to the eyes. Be sure to avoid handling your contact lenses after chopping chillies.

Did you know?

Milk can be a chill pill

To quell the fire from eating a hot chilli, the best antidote is a glass of milk. The capsaicinoids are fat soluble and milk (other than skimmed) contains fat. Yoghurt also douses the flames for the same reason and that is why yoghurt-based dishes often accompany some spicier menu items. A glass of water may seem logical, but in fact rates low in effectiveness since the capsaicinoids are only slightly soluble in water.

Packed with goodness

Chillies are more concentrated sources of some nutrients than peppers, and the red varieties generally have a higher nutritional content than the green ones.

They are very good sources of antioxidant, including beta carotene and vitamin C. Just one raw, red hot chilli (45g) contains about 90mg of vitamin C, more than 100 per cent of the Reference Nutrient Intake (RNI). Chillies also contain bioflavonoids, plant pigments that some researchers believe may help to prevent cancer and protect against lung disorders. In addition, recent research indicates that capsaicin may act as an anti-coagulant, and may prevent blood clots that can lead to a heart attack or stroke. It slows the growth of prostate cancer.

Incorporated into creams, capsaicin is sometimes used as a treatment to alleviate the burning pain of shingles. It is also used by many doctors as an effective treatment for the pain of arthritis. Capsaicinoids may also reduce the mouth pain associated with chemotherapy. Commercially available poultices for relief of lower back pain also contain capsaicin.

Chillies may cause ulcers or digestive problems, as well as extensive rectal and anal irritation.

Chocolate

BENEFITS

- Can elevate mood in some people
- Like other plant foods, it contains various antioxidants
- Plain chocolate is a useful source of iron, magnesium and potassium, and may lower blood pressure

DRAWBACKS

- High in calories and fat
- May trigger migraine headaches

The returning crew of Columbus's fourth voyage in 1502 brought the first cocoa beans from the New World to Europe. The Spanish combined them with vanilla and other flavourings, sugar and milk to arrive at a concoction that, as one writer noted at the time, people 'would die for'; the Aztec emperor Montezuma described it as a 'divine drink, which builds up resistance and fights fatigue'.

For the first couple of centuries, chocolate was served only as a beverage. A solid form – probably more like marzipan than today's chocolate – was touted as an instant breakfast in 18th-century France. The stimulant effects of chocolate are due to its caffeine content and made it a particularly useful food for soldiers on night watch.

The chocolate bar, first marketed in about 1910, captured the public's imagination when it was issued to the US armed forces as a 'fighting food' during the Second World War.

The source of chocolate

Chocolate is made from the beans found in the pods that grow on the cocoa tree, an evergreen that originated in the river valleys of South America. Native Central and South Americans valued cocoa so highly that they used cocoa beans as

currency. Today about three-quarters of the world's chocolate is grown in West Africa and most of the rest is grown in Brazil.

After cocoa beans are harvested, an initial phase of fermentation and drying is followed by roasting at a low temperature to bring out the flavour. Various manufacturing processes follow, depending on whether the product is to be sold as chocolate or cocoa powder.

In 1828 the Van Houten family of Amsterdam, seeking to make a better drinking chocolate, invented a screw press to remove most of the cocoa butter from the beans. Not only did it make a better drink, but they also found that by mixing the extracted cocoa butter back into ground cocoa beans, they could make a smoother, fatter solid paste that would absorb sugar; this led to 'eating chocolate'.

Components

Chocolate is not a great source of nutrients, but the dark variety does contain useful minerals.

A 30g piece of solid chocolate contains about 150kcal and about 2g of protein. The original bean has significant amounts of vitamins B and E. These nutrients, however, are so diluted as to be neg-ligible in modern processed chocolate. Sweet or semisweet chocolate contains about 30 per cent fat, or cocoa butter. Both dark chocolate and

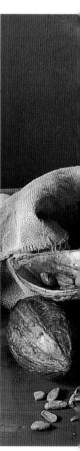

▶ **Justifying pleasure**
Plain chocolate is rich in phytochemicals which may help to protect the body against heart disease.

cocoa powder supply chromium, iron, magnesium and potassium, but fat and calories make chocolate an inappropriate source of these minerals except when used in emergency rations.

Chocolate is a solid at room temperature, but since its melting point is just below the human body temperature, it begins to melt and release its flavour components as soon as it is placed in the mouth.

White chocolate, a mixture of cocoa butter, milk solids and sugar, contains no cocoa solids. Unlike milk chocolate, white chocolate does not keep well, because it lacks the compounds that prevent milk solids from becoming rancid over time.

A chemical composition that prevents cocoa solids from quickly turning rancid made cocoa butter valuable as a long-lasting food and cosmetic oil.

The feel-good factor

Chocolate contains two related alkaloid stimulants, theobromine and caffeine, in a 10:1 ratio. Theobromine, unlike caffeine, does not stimulate the central nervous system; its effects are mainly diuretic. Commercial chocolate products contain no more than about 0.1 per cent caffeine, so a 100g slab has about as much caffeine as a cup of coffee. Unsweetened chocolate for home use is a more concentrated source of caffeine. Chocolate is also rich in phenylethylamine (PEA), a naturally occurring compound that has effects similar to amphetamine, and can also trigger migraine headaches in susceptible people.

Some people have a tendency to binge on chocolate after emotional upsets, possibly because compounds in chocolate stimulate the release of

Do one simple thing

Make dark chocolate your choice

Choose dark chocolate over milk chocolate. Dark chocolate contains more antioxidants although no less fat. Milk chocolate contains milk, which provides more calcium.

mood-elevating endorphins. However, psychiatrists think that 'chocoholics' may have a faulty mechanism for regulating their body levels of phenylethylamine; others attribute chocolate cravings to hormonal changes, such as those that take place during puberty or during the premenstrual phase.

After centuries of investigation, chocolate's famed aphrodisiac qualities can be discounted. But in its myriad modern forms, chocolate is an endless temptation and a culinary source of pleasure.

New studies

A report in the February 2003 issue of the *Journal of the American Dietetic Association* sheds some positive light on chocolate. Researchers reviewed a number of studies on possible health benefits, particularly for dark chocolate, and cocoa. They found that flavonoids in dark chocolate have some disease-fighting anti-oxidant properties – also found in red wine, and some fruit and vegetables – associated with a decreased risk of heart disease.

Chocolate is best tasted on an empty stomach. Never put chocolate in the refrigerator – the cocoa butter will separate and form a white bloom. When tasting chocolate, let it sit in your mouth for a few seconds to release its primary aromas and flavours. Chew it a few times to release the secondary aromas. Then let it rest against the roof of your mouth so you get the full flavour.

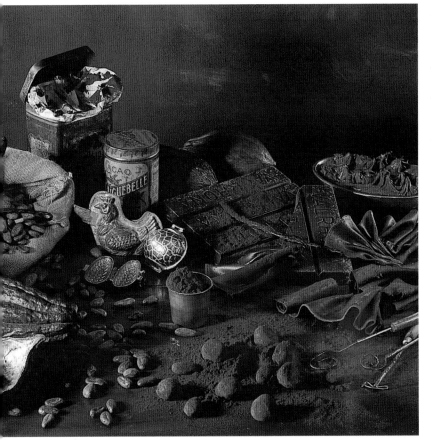

Cholesterol
The facts and the myths

By now, most people know that high levels of blood cholesterol can lead to blocked arteries. If an artery that supplies blood to your heart becomes blocked, a heart attack may occur. A blockage in an artery supplying blood to your brain means you may suffer a stroke. Still, confusion abounds over the role of diet in affecting cholesterol.

Although often portrayed as a dietary evil, cholesterol is essential to life. The body needs it to make sex hormones, bile, vitamin D, cell membranes and nerve sheaths. These and other functions fall to serum cholesterol, a waxy, fatlike compound, termed a 'lipid', that circulates in the bloodstream. The liver manufactures about a gram each day, which is all the body requires.

Dietary cholesterol is found only in animal products. The body doesn't need this cholesterol as it can make its own supplies, but anyone other than a vegetarian who excludes all animal products will consume varying amounts of it. Many factors – exercise, genetics, gender and other components of the diet – influence how the body processes dietary cholesterol. Some people can consume large amounts but have normal blood levels, while others eat very little but have high blood levels. Ready-made cholesterol in foods accounts for about 20 per cent of the cholesterol in the body, with the remaining 80 per cent produced by the liver.

GOOD VERSUS BAD CHOLESTEROL

To travel through the bloodstream, cholesterol molecules attach themselves to lipid-carrying proteins, or lipoproteins. Two types of lipoproteins are the major transporters of cholesterol: low-density lipoproteins (LDLs) carry two-thirds of it; most of the remainder is attached to high-density lipoproteins (HDLs). LDLs tend to deposit cholesterol in the artery walls, leading to atherosclerosis and an increased risk of heart disease. In contrast, HDLs collect cholesterol from the artery walls and other tissues and take it to the liver to be metabolised and eliminated from the body. This is why LDLs are often called the 'bad' cholesterol and HDLs the 'good'. A third type, very-low-density lipoproteins (VLDLs), carries a small amount of cholesterol and triglycerides.

A blood cholesterol test measures the amount of cholesterol in the blood. In the UK, this is expressed in millimoles (mmol) of cholesterol per litre, often abbreviated to mmol/l. Until recently, most blood tests for cholesterol measured only the total amount. A value below 5mmol/l is considered desirable. If the total is more than 5.1 mmol/l, LDL and HDL levels are now measured individually. LDL levels

The Mediterranean diet

Doctors have known since the 1950s that the so-called Mediterranean diet reduces the risk of premature death. The first study showed that heart disease rates can be predicted from cholesterol levels, that an intake of saturated fats increases the risk and that monounsaturated fats, mainly olive oil, reduce the risk of heart disease as well as cancer.

The same study found the lowest premature mortality rate on the Greek Island of Crete. The Cretans ate very little meat, lots of legumes and fruit, moderate amounts of fish and red wine and copious amounts of olive oil. Bread, mostly wholegrain, was an integral part of their diet. The first clinical evidence suggesting that a Mediterranean diet was advantageous in the West came in 1994 when Dr Serge Renaud in France investigated what would happen to patients who had a heart attack and then were asked to follow a Mediterranean diet.

The patients on the Mediterranean diet were encouraged to eat more fruit, vegetables and fish; less red meat; and were also asked to replace butter with margarine that was enriched in alpha-linolenic acid. The reason for this was that the traditional Cretan diet features lots of walnuts, olive oil and a vegetable called purslane, all of which are rich in alpha-linolenic acid, a compound that is thought to be protective against heart disease. It didn't take long for results to show up. After just two years, the death rate in the intervention group was reduced by 70 per cent.

Do one simple thing

Spread your bread with margarine containing plant sterols and plant stanols

Results from studies and trials indicate that people can reduce blood cholesterol by 10 per cent by using these margarines. Plant sterols can also be found in supplements.

should be below 3mmol/l; 3.1–3.9 is classified as borderline high, over 4.0 is considered high risk for coronary artery disease and a heart attack. HDL levels should be at least 1.2mmol/l, and the higher the better. In assessing cardiovascular risk, doctors calculate the LDL/HDL ratio by dividing the total cholesterol by the HDL figure. A desirable ratio is less than 4.5 and no more than 5.

HOW DIET CAN HELP

In the UK the average total cholesterol level is about 5.8mmol/l, which is too high. A diet that limits calories and restricts trans and saturated fats to 8 per cent or less is recommended to lower total blood cholesterol. Reducing the intake of saturated fats has the greatest effect on lowering LDL blood cholesterol levels.

Most people can significantly lower intake of saturated fats by cutting down on, or eliminating, fatty meats, whole milk and other full-fat dairy products, as well as tropical oils (coconut, palm and palm kernel). It's also important to lower the intake of saturated and trans fatty acids found in partially hydrogenated oils and foods containing them such as biscuits, other commercial baked goods, many snack foods and some margarines and spreads.

Tobacco should be avoided completely. Both smoking and passive smoking cause a drop in the health-promoting antioxidants such as vitamin C. Tobacco also encourages the immune system to increase LDLs.

Exercise is also important – you should try to get at least 30 minutes of moderate physical activity at least five days a week.

Eating to keep cholesterol in check

There's no doubt that what you eat influences the levels of cholesterol and other fats in your blood. Numerous studies confirm that a diet high in saturated fats tends to elevate cholesterol levels, in contrast to the low levels found in people whose diet consists largely of whole grains, fruit and vegetables. People with a family history of heart disease should be diligent in following a diet that limits the cholesterol-raising foods and emphasises the cholesterol-lowering foods indicated below.

FOODS THAT MAY LOWER CHOLESTEROL

- Wholemeal, pumpernickel, rye and multigrain breads and rolls.
- Oats and breakfast cereals that contain oat or rice bran, as well as tofu and other soya products.
- Poly or monounsaturated margarine, spreads containg plant sterols and plant stanols, olive oil and rape seed, sunflower and soya bean oils.
- Vegetables, such as sweetcorn, onions, garlic, lima beans, kidney beans and other legumes.
- Fresh fruit, such as oranges, apples, pears, bananas and dried fruit such as apricots, figs and prunes.
- Nuts such as almonds, walnuts, pecans; seeds such as sesame and sunflower seeds.

FOODS THAT MAY RAISE CHOLESTEROL

- Hard margarine and vegetable shortening, which are high in saturated fats and trans fatty acids.
- Biscuits, cakes, pastries and chocolates, especially those made with butter, saturated fat or partially hydrogenated oils.
- Full-fat dairy products, such as cheese, cream and butter; all are high in saturated fats.
- Fatty meats such as marbled beef, pork and lamb chops, hamburgers, bacon, salamis and other cold meats.
- Partially hydrogenated oils used in crisps, chips and fast foods.

STRICT DIETS FOR BEST RESULTS

Try a vegetarian diet. A low-fat diet (less than 10 per cent of calories) can lower the levels of LDL cholesterol substantially. It should be combined with a moderate amount of exercise.

Be sure to include foods that actually lower cholesterol. It isn't just what you don't eat that matters; consuming foods that have a cholesterol-lowering effect also helps. Flavonoid-rich foods, including citrus fruit and onions, are known to promote healthy cholesterol levels. Soluble fibre is also a weapon against cholesterol. It is commonly found in oats, beans and linseeds. The pectin in apples and other fruit lowers it, as does the soya protein found in tofu, tempeh and soya milk. It has been shown that regular daily consumption of carrots can lead to a reduction of LDL cholesterol levels.

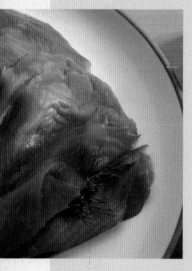

Eat fish for omega-3s. Two or three servings a week of salmon, sardines and other seafood is linked with a reduced risk of heart attacks and strokes. It was thought that the omega-3 fatty acids in fish reduced cardio-vascular risk by lowering blood cholesterol levels; however, recent studies suggest that their benefit comes from interfering with blood clotting and from possible changes in the way the liver metabolises other lipids.

Eat foods with soya protein. A large body of evidence has shown that adding soya protein to a low-fat diet helps to lower 'bad' cholesterol levels. and lowers the risk of cardiovascular disease. Soya protein is found in soya beans, tofu and soya drinks.

Did you know?

A vegetarian 'monkey diet' can lower cholesterol as well as a statin drug

According to a study at the University of Toronto published in the *Journal of the American Medical Association*, a diet modelled on the food groups that apes eat has been shown to lower high cholesterol as effectively as lovastatin, an anticholesterol drug in the statin group. The diet consists of four food groups: nuts (especially almonds), soya proteins, high-fibre foods (like oats and fruit) and a margarine with plant sterols in it.

Margarine with plant sterols. Plant sterols have been shown to help lower cholesterol levels when used as part of a heart-healthy diet. They are found in plant-sterol enriched margarines, with small quantities present naturally in vegetable oils, nuts, sesame and sunflower seeds, soya and other legumes. At one time, increasing the intake of polyunsaturated fats – corn, safflower, soya and sunflower oils – was advocated to lower cholesterol, but studies have found that large quantities of these oils may reduce levels of the protective HDLs while lowering the harmful LDLs. However, monounsaturated fats found in canola and olive oils, some nuts and avocados can cut LDLs without altering levels of beneficial HDLs.

The role of dietary cholesterol is now quite clear; it does far less harm in terms of raising the levels of blood cholesterol than eating a diet full of saturated fats does. But some experts still recommend limiting dietary cholesterol intake to 300mg a day The British Heart Foundation has suggested that people who already have high cholesterol levels should limit themselves to three eggs a week.

OTHER APPROACHES

Increasing exercise, weight loss and reducing stress can all lower cholesterol or improve the LDL/HDL ratio. Oestrogen protects women from developing coronary artery disease in their reproductive years but, according to the most recent research, oestrogen supplements taken after menopause do not offer similar protection.

Moderate alcohol intake lowers the risk of heart attack. This may be due to alcohol's ability to raise HDL, its tendency to reduce the stickiness of platelets or the presence of antioxidants in red wine. If dietary and other lifestyle changes fail to reduce blood cholesterol, drugs may be prescribed.

Chronic fatigue syndrome

EAT PLENTY OF

- Pasta, rice and wholegrain cereals and breads for complex carbohydrates
- Fruit and vegetables for vitamin C
- Foods rich in essential fatty acids such as fish, linseeds, nuts and seeds, rape seed oil and wheatgerm

LIMIT

- Caffeine, especially near bedtime

AVOID

- Alcohol

This mysterious ailment, also known as myalgic encephalomyelitis or ME, often has flu-like symptoms, no apparent cause and no proven cure. It is marked by debilitating fatigue, as well as other baffling symptoms that include headaches, muscle aches and weakness, tender lymph nodes, sore throat, joint pain, sleep that doesn't refresh, difficulty in concentrating, post-exercise exhaustion that lasts for 24 hours and short-term memory problems. There may also be a chronic or recurring low-grade fever.

There is no laboratory test for Chronic Fatigue Syndrome (CFS), so a doctor must systematically rule out all other medical causes that produce similar symptoms.

Although some claim that CFS is a relatively new disorder (it is thought to have been the 'yuppie flu' of the 1980s), doctors since the 1800s have reported similar disorders but given them different names, including hypoglycaemia (low blood sugar), chronic Epstein-Barr virus, postviral fatigue syndrome and the myalgic encephalomyelitis (ME), already mentioned. Many theories regarding possible causes have been advanced, but none has been proven. In many cases, CFS develops in the aftermath of a viral illness, such as glandular fever or the flu, but no single viral cause has been identified. Other possible contributing factors include prolonged stress, hormonal imbalance, allergies, immune system disorders and psychological problems. Some experts suggest that CFS is a group of ailments that share similar symptoms. An accurate incidence is not known, but at least two-thirds of the sufferers are women. Most CFS patients eventually recover, but it may take a year or much more to do so.

Medical treatment

Various medications are prescribed to treat CFS symptoms, but none appear to cure the disorder. Aspirin and other painkillers may alleviate headaches, joint pain and muscle soreness, and antidepressant drugs help some patients. To date, the only treatments of proven benefit are cognitive behaviour therapy and graded aerobic exercise.

Nutritional approaches

Although there is no known cure for CFS, certain nutrients in foods may help. Doctors stress the importance of a well-balanced diet.

Start with ample healthy sources of carbohydrate. Eat plenty of pasta and breads, as well as fruit and vegetables to provide energy. They also supply the vitamins needed to resist infection.

Avoid alcohol. It lowers your immunity and may worsen fatigue. Use caffeinated drinks moderately: caffeine can exacerbate symptoms because it stimulates the nervous system and can disturb sleeping patterns even more.

Eat to strengthen your immune system. Foods rich in zinc, such as seafood (especially oysters), meat, poultry, eggs, milk, beans, nuts and whole grains, as well as foods rich in vitamin C, such as citrus fruit, berries, melons, kiwi fruit, broccoli and cauliflower, may help keep the immune system working properly. A robust immune system can help to ward off certain viruses, such as flu and cold, that may possibly precede the onset of CFS.

Consume more essential fatty acids. Some of the symptoms of CFS include swollen glands and inflammation of the joints, which may be relieved temporarily by foods rich in essential fatty acids. These include fish, nuts, linseeds, rape seed oil, wheatgerm and leafy green vegetables.

One study indicates that low blood pressure may contribute to the fatigue experienced by CFS patients. Usually, blood pressure rises slightly during periods of stress or physical activity. But in some people, blood pressure remains constant or goes down, resulting in fatigue. These people may be salt-resistant and need a higher salt intake to raise blood pressure.

Five-step action plan

COPING WITH CFS

1 Obtain an accurate diagnosis, preferably from a doctor who has experience in treating CFS.

2 Keep a detailed diary of your progress, noting symptoms and how foods and activities affect your physical wellbeing.

3 Establish a sensible and balanced programme of treatment that covers diet and graded exercise.

4 Don't nap during the daytime; instead get between 7 and 9 hours of sleep each night.

5 Join a support group.

Mighty magnesium

Magnesium is associated with the contraction and relaxation of muscles. Getting more of the mineral may help to alleviate muscle tenderness in people with CFS. Good food sources include sunflower seeds, nuts, muesli and cereals containing bran.

Researchers have noted that many CFS patients have low-salt diets, which may lead to hypotension and fatigue. Symptoms improved with increased intake of salty foods.

Some alternative practitioners advocate injections of vitamin B_{12}, along with supplements of vitamins A and C, iron and zinc, to treat CFS. But a balanced diet is preferable to taking supplements. Another approach that appears hopeful is for patients to take a combination of evening primrose oil and fish oil; in one study, 85 per cent reported some improvement after 15 weeks.

Circulatory disorders

EAT PLENTY OF

■ Fish, such as salmon and sardines and other seafood, for omega-3 fatty acids

■ Citrus and other fresh fruit and vegetables for vitamin C, as well as garlic and onions

■ Wholegrain cereals, breads and pasta, plus seeds, nuts and wheatgerm

LIMIT

■ Fatty meat and poultry skin, processed meats and high-fat dairy products

AVOID

■ Smoking, alcohol and caffeine

The most common circulatory, or vascular, disorders are high blood pressure and atherosclerosis; plus a number of clotting abnormalities and diseases marked by reduced blood flow. Other circulatory disorders include aneurysms, phlebitis, intermittent claudication and Raynaud's disease.

Aneurysms

These balloon-like bulges form in weakened segments of the arteries, especially the aorta, the body's largest artery, which stems directly from the heart. Many aneurysms are due to a congenital weakness, while others are caused by atherosclerosis and high blood pressure.

A low-fat, low-salt diet is recommended. There is no specific dietary treatment for an aneurysm, but following a low-fat, low-salt diet can help to prevent those caused by atherosclerosis and high blood pressure. Consuming ample fresh fruit and vegetables will provide the vitamin C needed to strengthen and maintain blood vessels.

Intermittent claudication (leg pain)

Severe leg pain and cramps induced by walking are symptoms of intermittent claudication. A lack of oxygen due to inadequate blood flow causes the pain.
Atherosclerosis is responsible for most intermittent claudication; it is also common in those with diabetes. Adopting a very low-fat diet and an exercise programme has helped many patients. Including onions and garlic in the diet is said to improve blood flow. Patients with severe blockages, however, may require surgery to remove them.

Phlebitis

Any inflammation of a vein is referred to as phlebitis. The large, superficial veins in the lower legs are the most commonly afflicted. Although it is painful, this type of superficial phlebitis is not as dangerous as when veins located deeper in the legs become inflamed, setting the stage for the more serious thrombophlebitis. This is when clots form at the site of the inflammation; pieces may break away and travel to the heart and lungs.

Phlebitis can be treated with aspirin and other anti-inflammatory drugs and by applying warm compresses. Clot-dissolving drugs may be administered for thrombo-phlebitis; other measures may be required to prevent clots from reaching vital organs.

Eat more fish. A diet that includes several servings a week of oily fish or other sources of omega-3 fatty acids, as well as foods high in vitamin E, helps to reduce inflammation and clot formation. Gamma linolenic acid, a substance found in evening primrose and borage oils, has a similar effect; but check with your doctor first, as they may interact with prescribed drugs.

Raynaud's disease

This condition is characterised by periods of numbness, tingling and pain in the fingers and toes due to the constriction or spasms in the small arteries that carry blood to the extremities.

Typically, Raynaud's disease is set off by exposure to the cold; in some people, however, periods of stress may trigger an attack. For unknown reasons, two-thirds of all Raynaud's sufferers are women. Some victims

Do one simple thing

Eat more onions and garlic

These vegetables are especially helpful in improving blood flow. After chopping garlic, let it rest for 10 minutes prior to cooking it. This will allow the allicin and its potent derivatives to be activated and will unleash the full nutritional power of the garlic.

may also have lupus, rheumatoid arthritis, schleroderma and other inflammatory auto-immune disorders. Smoking is not a cause, but it certainly makes these conditions worse.

Get your fill of omega-3s. Eating foods that are high in omega-3 fatty acids and vitamin E may help. Avoiding exposure of the hands and feet to cold temperatures can usually prevent or minimise attacks. Of course, not smoking and avoiding passive smoking is critical.

Cirrhosis

EAT PLENTY OF

- A combination of grains and legumes instead of meat for protein
- Carbohydrates for energy
- Cereals, breads, potatoes and legumes for B-complex vitamins
- Fruit and vegetables for vitamin C

LIMIT

- Animal protein, salt and fatty foods

AVOID

- Alcohol and salty processed foods

In cirrhosis, a chronic progressive disease, normal liver cells are replaced by scar tissue. Prolonged, heavy alcohol use is the most common cause, but cirrhosis may also result from inflammation or blockage of the bile ducts, hepatitis, inherited conditions or a reaction to a drug or environmental toxin.

In its early stages, cirrhosis does not usually produce symptoms, but as the liver is increasingly infiltrated with fibrous tissue, a person may experience fatigue and nausea, and have a poor appetite. In the later stages, jaundice may develop and fine, spidery blood vessels appear on the skin. The liver damage is

Danger signs

If you, or someone you know, has the symptoms listed here, cirrhosis may be the cause and should be investigated as soon as possible: weight-loss, nausea, vomiting, jaundice, impotence and swelling of the legs.

irreversible, but the progress of cirrhosis can be arrested and the complications treated with diet and other measures.

Diet and liver repair

Stop drinking alcohol. Whether or not alcohol intake is the cause of cirrhosis, it is essential to stop drinking entirely to prevent further liver damage. Although the scar tissue cannot be replaced, the liver does have a remarkable ability to repair itself. To achieve this and regain lost weight, a daily intake of 1,900kcal-2,850kcal is necessary. Most people with cirrhosis, however, have little appetite; so frequent small meals may be more tempting than three large ones.

Eat plenty of protein. It is important to include enough protein in the diet. The recommended daily intake of protein for those with cirrhosis is 1.2g per kilogram of body weight. This is more than the amount that is recommended for healthy people.

Some evidence supports the use of vegetable protein foods such as those in soya, peas and legumes, especially for people who develop mental confusion, a condition called hepatic encephalopathy. A good supply of carbohydrates is needed.

Moderate amounts of unsaturated fats (fish, corn oil and safflower oil) also provide needed calories without overburdening the liver. The regular intake of vitamin C in the form of plenty of fresh fruit and vegetables every day will also help to strengthen the immune system.

Replace depleted vitamins and minerals. Nutritional deficiencies are common among those people with cirrhosis. Cereals, breads, pasta, and fruit and vegetables will help. Often, a doctor will also prescribe supplements.

Fluids and salt

The orderly flow of body fluids is an early casualty of cirrhotic damage. In a healthy person, the blood supply circulates through vessels in the liver; but in cirrhosis, rigid scar tissue forms on the liver, hindering the blood from passing freely.

As the blood backs up, the pressure in the supplying vessels increases, which forces plasma out of the blood vessels and into the tissues that surround the entire abdominal cavity.

People with cirrhosis often have distinctive abdominal swelling, known as ascites. The volume of blood in the vessels throughout the body is decreased, and when the kidneys register the fall in blood flow, they send out a signal for help in the form of the hormone aldosterone. Far from helping, this causes the body to retain sodium (instead of excreting it in the urine in the normal way), which in turn produces a further damming of fluid and worsens the ascites. The whole body becomes puffy and swollen, and the vicious cycle continues with other complications that arise as the blood seeks a way to bypass the obstruction in the liver. This entails increasing blood flow in vessels in neighbouring organs, such as the veins of the oesophagus.

Some cirrhotic patients suffer from varices (varicose veins) in the oesophagus, which can rupture and cause severe bleeding.

People with cirrhosis should eat little salt, especially if ascites is present, and drink about four to six glasses of fluids a day. If varices are present in the oesophagus, the food should be soft and thoroughly chewed.

Coconuts

BENEFITS

■ A useful source of iron and fibre

■ High in easy-to-digest fatty acids

DRAWBACKS

■ High in calories and saturated fats

The coconut, the seed of a palm tree that grows mostly in tropical coastal areas, yields many food and non-food products. The oil is used in vegetable shortening, some spreads and many commercial baked goods; it is also an ingredient in shampoos, moisturising skin lotions, soaps and various cosmetics. The creamy coconut flesh that lines the interior of the nut's hard outer shell is eaten raw or used to flavour ice cream, confectionery products and baked goods. Fresh coconut milk, the sweet white fluid from the heart of the nut, is served as a beverage or used as a marinade.

Dried coconut flesh, or copra, is rich in oil. In fact, more than 90 per cent of the fatty acids in coconuts are classified as saturated; remarkably, coconut oil is more highly saturated than the fat in butter or red meat. This high level of saturation results in an oil that resists turning rancid, making coconut oil ideal for commercial baking. However, saturated fats tend to raise blood cholesterol levels. So people who have high cholesterol levels or any other cardiovascular risk factors are advised to avoid products made with coconut oil. Desiccated coconut has a slightly less saturated fat than fresh coconut. On the plus side, the fatty acids in coconut are easy to digest.

Canned coconut milk and coconut cream are widely used in Thai and Indian food. In theory, the coconut cream is thicker and higher in fat than coconut milk, but in practice, the naming of the products overlaps. Read the labels of coconut milk containers carefully.

Full-fat coconut milk contains 179kcal and 17g of fat in 100ml. The same amount of reduced-fat coconut milk contains about 110kcal and 10g of fat.

Coeliac disease

EAT PLENTY OF

■ Low-fat milk, eggs, fish, meat and poultry for protein

■ Vegetables and fruit for vitamins and minerals

■ Legumes, potatoes, sweetcorn and rice for starches, minerals and protein

AVOID

■ Bread, wheat, pasta, cereals, cakes and other wheat, rye or barley products

■ Foods using wheat products as a thickening agent or coating, such as breaded or battered foods, meat loaf, sausages and other processed meats, sauces and soups

■ Beverages containing gluten, such as beer and malted drinks

■ Pizza, stuffing in a roast chicken

Coeliac disease, also known as coeliac sprue or nontropical sprue, is a disorder that is estimated to affect 1,500 people in the UK.

Typically, the disorder becomes apparent when a young child starts to eat foods containing wheat, rye, barley and other cereal grains. The problem is caused by gliadin, one of the proteins collectively known as gluten, found in these grains. Gliadin combines with antibodies in the digestive tract to damage the walls of the small intestine and interfere with the absorption of many nutrients, especially fats, iron and certain starches and sugars.

Children with the disease have such symptoms as stomach upsets, diarrhoea, abdominal cramps, bloating, mouth ulcers and an increased susceptibility to infection. Their stool is pale and foul-smelling, and it floats in the toilet bowl, indicating a high fat content. The child's growth may be stunted; some children develop anaemia and skin problems, especially a particular type of dermatitis.

Diagnosis is confirmed by an inspection of the small intestine with a special viewing instrument and an intestinal biopsy indicating abnormalities characteristic of coeliac disease. People who develop coeliac disease later in life may have had a mild or symptomless form of the disease in childhood. In unusual cases, adults with no prior history of gluten sensitivity develop

Do one simple thing

Stay the course on a gluten-free diet

When a person with coeliac disease first starts a gluten-free diet, the body's healing response time may take several weeks or months. This is because of the time it takes for the lining of the digestive system to regrow. However, the immune system will remember gluten, and any further ingestion of gluten can cause prolonged damage.

the condition after surgery on the digestive tract. Women with coeliac disease often fail to menstruate and can have problems getting pregnant.

Once the disease has been identified, patients are advised to permanently eliminate any foods that contain gluten from their diet. A dietitian can assist in planning nutritionally balanced meals that are gluten-free. Most doctors also prescribe supplements to counter any nutritional deficiencies. If anaemia is a problem, iron and/or folate supplements will also be recommended.

Avoiding gluten

Hundreds of everyday foods contain gluten: breads, biscuits, cakes, crackers, rolls, muffins, baking mixes, pasta, sausages bound with breadcrumbs, foods coated with batter, sauces and gravies, soups thickened with wheat flour and most breakfast cereals, as well as some confectionery, ice creams and desserts. Many baby foods are thickened with gluten, although most commercial first-stage foods are gluten-free.

Always read labels on packaged foods. Avoid ingredients such as flour-based binders and fillers and modified starch. Be suspicious of any label that specifies 'cornflour' because some cornflour is made from wheat starch. Beer is made from barley and should be avoided, along with malted drinks.

Outside the home, order only plain foods, such as grilled fish or meat, steamed vegetables and a baked potato – all without any sauces or dressings. Communion wafers contain some gluten, but gluten-free wafers are now available; check with your vicar or minister. Contrary to popular belief, people with coeliac disease can eat pasta, bread and other baked products, but they must look for gluten-free items,

such as rice or corn or buckwheat pasta and baked goods made with corn, rice, potato or soya flours. Gluten-free flour is now available. In general, it is better to prepare most foods at home to avoid risking exposure to gluten.

It was once believed that oats also contained the offending gliadin protein, but some analyses have shown that they do not. Doctors are now allowing patients to experiment with oat products; if they provoke symptoms, however, they should still be avoided. It is important to distinguish between pure oats and oat products that have been contaminated with wheat. To be on the safe side, it is better to have no more than 50g of oats a day.

Coffee

BENEFITS

■ Stimulates the central nervous system

■ Can help you to stay awake and alert

DRAWBACKS

■ May contribute to difficulty falling asleep and disturbed or reduced sleep

■ Drinking large amounts can cause irritability and jittery nerves

■ Large quantities increase excretion of calcium

Coffee is our major source of caffeine. In addition to caffeine, coffee contains nearly 400 other chemicals, including trace amounts of several antioxidants and one vitamin, niacin. It also contains minerals, tannins and caramelised sugar. Coffee itself has virtually no calories, although combining it with milk and sugar will add some. A dedicated coffee drinker might consider reducing caffeine from other sources – for example, giving up caffeinated soft drinks.

Did you know?

Coffee improves memory and mental function

A study on ageing revealed that coffee helped older people to think more quickly, improve their memory and reason better. Another study reported that women over 80 with a history of coffee consumption had better performance results on tests of mental function. Lifetime coffee consumption has even been linked to a lower risk of Alzheimer's disease. So regular, moderate consumption is good for you.

Possible hazards

Coffee is best consumed in moderation. The following are possible hazards linked to coffee:

- Infertility. A number of studies have found that the consumption of more than 300mg of caffeine a day is associated with a delay in conception.
- Heart problems. Caffeine prompts a temporary rise in blood pressure; it can also provoke cardiac arrhythmias in susceptible persons.
- Bone loss. In large quantities, coffee increases calcium excretion in the urine. To compensate for this loss, heavy coffee drinkers should consume extra calcium-rich foods.
- Caffeine withdrawal. Heavy coffee drinkers who stop imbibing coffee abruptly may suffer headaches, irritability and other withdrawal symptoms for a few days. Cut back gradually.
- Cholesterol problems. Cafestol and kahweol, compounds in coffee, can boost cholesterol synthesis by the liver. These are found in highest concentrations in Scandinavian and Turkish coffees, which are boiled.
- Caffeine increases the output of urine. This is a concern for men with prostate problems.

C

Decaffeinated coffee

Many people drink decaffeinated coffee to escape the insomnia and jittery nerves caused by caffeine. Decaffeinated coffee has virtually no caffeine.

Cold meats

See Smoked, cured and pickled meats

Colds and flu

CONSUME PLENTY OF

- Fruit and vegetables for vitamin C
- Garlic and chillies, which may act as natural decongestants
- Fluids to loosen phlegm

The runny nose, cough and sore throat of a cold are hard to escape; most people suffer two or three colds a year. That's why it's called 'the common cold'.

In the winter months, flu (short for influenza) inflicts a similar misery on people; what makes flu worse is the presence of fever, as well as muscle and joint aches. The complications of flu – especially pneumonia – can be serious and there are deaths from flu or its complications each year.

Colds and flu are highly contagious respiratory infections that are caused by viruses. More than 200 cold viruses (rhinoviruses) have been identified; developing immunity to one does not protect you from the others. There are fewer flu viruses, but they undergo frequent mutations – that is, they change their protein structure just a little – each year as they sweep around the globe. This is why new flu vaccines are produced yearly that protect against the prevailing strains of the virus. Doctors recommend annual flu shots for everyone over the age of 65, and those over six months of age who have disorders of the lungs or heart or other chronic diseases.

Catching the 'bug'

Colds and flu are spread when virus-laden fluid droplets are released into the air by coughing and sneezing or transferred to surfaces by touch. It is well known that cold viruses can survive on hard surfaces, such as handles, lift buttons and work surfaces; what is not so well known is that flu viruses can live on hard surfaces for up to 48 hours.

Researchers have shown that the cold virus is activated when body temperatures fall below 37°C. So it seems that the old wives' tales about catching cold have a grain of truth: if you sit in a draught, your body temperature may drop just enough to activate the cold viruses that have been biding their time in your nasal passages.

When you breathe overly dry air (especially in planes and artificially ventilated office buildings), your nasal passages may form tiny cracks that provide entry for viruses. The best defence is plenty of fluids to rehydrate the tender membranes; try using a humidifier or bending over a bowl of hot water, with a towel over your head. Make sure the water is not too hot.

You're more vulnerable to colds and flu when your immune system is depressed. Preventive steps include avoiding alcohol, getting plenty of rest and reducing stress levels.

Grandma's secret weapon

It seems that the centuries-old home remedy of the consumption of chicken soup for fighting the common cold is not just an old wives' tale. Scientists believe that a bowl of the soup may reduce inflammation of the lungs. It is thought that chicken soup slows down the activity of white blood cells that can cause the inflammation.

The role of diet

While there's no cure for colds or flu, eating properly may help to prevent them, shorten their duration or make symptoms less severe.

More than two decades of extensive research has failed to substantiate claims that megadoses of vitamin C can prevent or cure colds. While there is no evidence to suggest it will prevent you from getting sick, one study showed it can shorten the length of the cold or lessen the symptoms. Vitamin C has a slight antihistaminic effect, so drinking more citrus juice or taking a supplement may help to reduce nasal symptoms.

One of the worst effects of high fever is dehydration. During a cold or flu, drink a minimum of eight to ten glasses of fluids a day to replenish lost fluids, keep mucous membranes moist and loosen phlegm. Drink water, tea and broth. Abstain from alcohol, which dilates

▶ **Throat soother**
Add lemon and honey to hot water or weak tea to loosen mucus and ease pain.

small blood vessels and makes the sinuses feel stuffed up. Alcohol may produce adverse effects when taken with many drugs and reduces the body's ability to fight infection.

Doctors recommend eating whenever you feel hungry when you have a cold or flu. These foods may be helpful and comforting:

Chicken soup. Not only is it soothing and easy to digest, but chicken soup also contains cystine, a compound that helps thin the mucus, relieving the congestion.

Spicy foods. Hot chillies contain capsaicin that can help to break up nasal and sinus congestion. Garlic, turmeric and other hot spices have a similar effect.

Zinc's effect. Some research shows that sucking on zinc lozenges at the first sign of a cold may help to cut the cold's duration by about two days if taken early enough. Taking zinc supplements over a pro-longed period is not a good idea as getting more than 40mg a day over a long period of time can actually weaken your immune system, making it less able to fight against disease. It is important to ensure that your diet contains zinc-rich foods since zinc is important to a healthy immune system. Food sources of zinc include seafood (especially oysters), red meat and poultry, yoghurt and other dairy products, wheatgerm, wheat bran and whole grains.

When to see a doctor

Most colds and bouts of flu go away by themselves, but a doctor should be seen if you have any of the following symptoms:
- A cough that produces green, yellow or bloody phlegm.
- A severe headache or pain in the face, jaw or ear.
- Trouble swallowing or breathing.
- A fever over 37.8°C that lasts more than 48 hours.

Confectionery

BENEFITS

- Popular source of quick energy

DRAWBACKS

- High in calories and sometimes fat

- Sugary confectionery can cause tooth decay

- Liquorice may raise blood pressure in susceptible people

Confectionery offers little nutritional value, but occasional consumption of most types of confectionery should not prove harmful to any healthy person who consumes an otherwise balanced diet. A little comfort food is good now and then.

Our preference for sweet tastes is evident at a very early age and is considered to be part of human evolution. For instance, edible berries and fruit tend to be sweet as opposed to the bitter taste of many poisonous plants.

Commercial production of confectionery is generally believed to have begun when marzipan (made of almonds and sugar) was brought to Italy and Spain through trade with the Arabs and Moors during the Middle Ages. The word 'candy' is derived from the Arabic pronunciation of *khandakah*, the Sanskrit word for sugar.

The earliest European sweets were made by apothecaries who preserved herbs in sugar. These were rare treats, however, until the widespread cultivation of sugar cane and the development of large-scale refining processes in the 17th and 18th centuries.

Modern confectionery is mostly a variation on three basic forms: taffy, from the Creole French word for a mixture of sugar and molasses; nougat, from the Latin word for nutcake; and fondant, from the French word for melting (which

● **Myth.......**
Sweets make children hyperactive.
.......Reality ●
Many studies have shown that sugar does not cause hyperactivity, although some food dyes in sweets and drinks may exacerbate existing hyperactivity.

can be recognised in the texture of fudges and soft-centred chocolates and chocolate bars).

Energy highs and lows

All confectionery is packed with simple sugars – sucrose, syrups and fructose – which supply about 380kcal in a 100g serving and provide quick energy because they rapidly convert to glucose, or blood sugar. Unfortunately a rapid rise in blood sugar causes insulin levels to spike, which encourages the liver to convert sugar into fat. And when your blood sugar crashes after its high, you're likely to feel hungry again – and tired.

Additives and sensitivities

Practically all hard sweets are made with artificial flavourings and colourings. There is no scientific evidence that the rigorously tested food dyes allowed in confectionery cause allergies or adverse reactions. These additives are included in minute amounts. Some children are hypersensitive to the ingredients in sweets, but as long as sweets are not an essential part of their diet, it should be easy enough for parents to banish the offending ones.

Natural liquorice is known to raise blood pressure in certain people. The effect takes place mainly through salt retention. If you know you're hypertensive, you may be better off avoiding liquorice. Much of the 'liquorice' is now artificially flavoured and does not originate from the liquorice root.

C

Sweets and tooth decay

Sweets and sugary foods form an acid bath that is corrosive to tooth enamel and creates an environment where destructive, caries-causing bacteria flourish. The effect is less harmful if you brush your teeth regularly to remove dental plaque. Sweets that linger in the mouth are more damaging than those that are quickly swallowed.

When you can't brush after a meal, chewing sugarless gum may help to stimulate the saliva flow and flush food particles out of the mouth. 'Sugarless' chewing gums fall into two categories. Some contain artificial sweeteners and therefore are very low in calories; others contain 'sugar alcohols', such as xylitol. Although it does provide some calories, xylitol cannot be converted by bacteria in the mouth and on the teeth to acidic substances that erode tooth enamel. In rare cases sugar alcohols can cause diarrhoea and gastric problems in those susceptible.

Constipation

CONSUME PLENTY OF

- Unpeeled fresh fruit and green leafy vegetables, whole-grain cereals and wholemeal bread for insoluble fibre.
- Fluids (at least eight glasses a day)

LIMIT

- Sugar and refined starchy foods

AVOID

- Excessive use of laxatives

Many people wrongly assume that they must be constipated because they don't have a daily bowel movement. In fact, it's perfectly normal for bowels to move as often as three times a day for some people or as infrequently as once

The problem of haemorrhoids

Chronic constipation, obesity, pregnancy and an inherited predisposition are common causes of haemorrhoids – varicose veins in the anal area. Most are symptom-free, but some cause itching, pain and bleeding, especially during bouts of constipation. Straining to pass a hard stool can rupture one of the distended veins and result in considerable bleeding; more often, the stool contains small amounts of bright red blood. The blood loss itself is usually inconsequential, but any rectal bleeding should prompt medical investigation to rule out colon cancer or polyps.

Avoiding constipation and maintaining a normal weight will often eliminate haemorrhoid symptoms. Some sufferers find that curries, chillies and other hot, spicy foods increase discomfort during bowel movements; citrus fruit and other acidic foods may also be irritating.

In severe cases, chronic blood loss from haemorrhoids can cause anaemia; a doctor may prescribe iron supplements and removal of the haemorrhoids. Eating iron-rich foods can help to restore the body's iron reserves.

in three days for others. Regularity is different for everyone; an unexplained change in pattern needs investigating.

There are two common types of constipation: atonic occurs when the colon muscles are weak and lack tone; spastic (sometimes called irritable bowel syndrome) is characterised by irregular bowel movements. Atonic, the more common of the two, develops when the diet lacks adequate fluids and fibre; a sedentary lifestyle is another common cause. Spastic constipation can be caused by stress, nervous disorders, excessive smoking, irritating foods and obstructions of the colon.

▲ **Eating smart**
A diet rich in whole grains and fibre helps to relieve constipation.

Drink hot liquids

Hot liquids stimulate the bowels. Drink a cup of herbal tea, a glass of hot water with lemon or a cup of tea or coffee first thing in the morning to help to ease the effects of constipation.

Drink water. Adults should drink plenty of fluids every day, usually about eight glasses. When a low-fibre diet coincides with a low-fluid intake, the stool becomes dry and hard, and increasingly difficult to move through the intestinal tract.

Exercise. Regular exercise helps to stimulate bowel movements, and prolonged inactivity can cause constipation. Several medications, especially codeine and other painkillers, reduce the rhythmic muscle movements that push digested food through the bowel.

Use laxatives sparingly. Excessive laxative use reduces normal colon function. If a laxative is needed, one made of psyllium or another high-fibre stool softener is the best choice.

Recipe for relief

Increase intake of dietary fibre. The insoluble type of fibre that absorbs water but otherwise passes through the bowel intact is vital in preventing constipation. Fibre occurs throughout fruit and vegetables, so including the peel, stems and outer leaves, which are the parts that many cooks discard, can increase the fibre ingested. But any increase in high-fibre food consumption should be gradual to avoid excessive flatulence.

Soluble fibre found in oats, legumes, fruit and vegetables is also valuable in preventing constipation. Bacteria break down soluble fibre and use the fibre as food for their own growth and reproduction. A significant part of stool weight consists of these beneficial bacteria.

Convenience and processed foods

BENEFITS

■ Provide meals for people who don't have the time or ability to cook

DRAWBACKS

■ Many are high in fat, salt, sugar and calories

Technological advances have dramatically enhanced the quality and increased the range of processed foods. Vacuum-packed or frozen pre-cooked meals ready for the microwave; instant mashed potatoes and hot cereals; jars of prepared baby foods and packets of soup, dessert and sauce mixes are just a few of the timesaving foods that many people rely on. In addition, delicatessens and takeaway restaurants are everywhere.

Some critics blame this growing reliance on convenience foods, which are typically high in fat and calories, for the fact that more than half of all adults in the UK are either overweight or obese. As these convenience foods are a fact of life, it is important to follow the basic rules of variety, moderation and balance to work some convenience foods into a healthy, nutritious diet.

Convenience foods

Almost everyone consumes some convenience foods – usually items: from ready-to-eat breakfast cereals, canned or frozen goods, to sprepackaged heat-and-serve meals.

Nutritionally, these products do not measure up to home-cooked meals, but this varies greatly among foods. Instant soups contain a few dehydrated vegetables and many artificial flavourings, emulsifiers, fillers and preservatives.

Canned soups may be slightly more nutritious, but chilled fresh soups may be better value. As a rule, most convenience foods also contain more sugar, salt and fat than comparable dishes prepared at home.

Processing may strip vitamins and minerals from some foods, but there are exceptions in which convenience foods are actually more nutritious than their fresh counterparts.

Vegetables and many fruits harvested and quick-frozen at their peak often have more vitamins than those picked before maturity, shipped long distances and then allowed to sit on store shelves. Some enriched cereals and breads provide more nutrients than those made with the original grains.

Many food processors have been prompted by consumer demands to enhance the nutritional quality of their products by adding healthy ingredients (for example, folate to bread) or by reducing fat, sugar and salt. Although some claims of low-fat, no cholesterol and 'lite' may be misleading, an informed shopper who knows how to decipher food labelling can make healthy choices.

The price of convenience

Most convenience foods carry a higher price tag than the total cost of their ingredients. Some people, however, consider that the extra cost is worth the savings in time and effort. Still, they may worry about the nutritional value of frozen dinners, breakfast bars and other

Do one simple thing

Always add a fresh side salad

When preparing a meal consisting of processed food, like a frozen lasagna, always add a side salad. A fresh green salad provides a wide assortment of valuable nutrients.

Do-it-yourself convenience foods

A growing number of cooks are discovering that they can make their own convenience foods – all it takes is a freezer and planning. Instead of discarding leftovers, for example, make up a frozen prepackaged meal that can be popped in the microwave at a later date. This approach also allows you to control the amount of fat, salt and other ingredients.

If you are making a soup or a casserole, double the recipe and then freeze the extra portion. Similarly, buy extra fresh vegetables that are in season and freeze them for later use. Be sure to date the packages, and be careful to use the oldest first.

convenience foods. It's important to check labels and ingredient lists. A few special health or dietary items are available, but tend to be more expensive than the regular lines, even though their components may be similar.

Combining convenience foods with fresh ingredients can save both time and money while increasing interest and nutritional value. For example, you can build a tasty and nutritious meal around a frozen meal by adding a green salad and seasonal vegetables that take only minutes to prepare.

Foods for children

Most parents rely upon at least some convenience items when introducing foods into a baby's diet. Instant cereals and jars of puréed fruit, vegetables and meats may be easier than homemade baby foods.

Even more questionable are the convenience foods that many older children seem to prefer. Favourites like sausage rolls are usually loaded with fat, salt and preservatives; and children's individually packaged desserts may provide milk, but they may also be high in sugar, fats and artificial flavourings and colourings.

When feeding children, emphasise foods made with minimal amount of processing; for example, chicken is a better choice than sausage rolls, yoghurt is healthier than many desserts, porridge or wheat cereals are a wiser choice than sweetened cereals aimed at children.

Courgettes

BENEFITS

■ Low in calories

■ A good source of vitamin C and folate; also supply beta carotene

Courgettes may be dark green, pale green or also golden. Courgettes and cucumbers are members of the gourd family, but courgettes are closer cousins to pumpkins than to cucumbers. Picked and eaten while still immature, courgettes have a soft skin and tender light-coloured flesh that has a delicate, crisp, fresh flavour.

Courgettes, like squash, are about 94 per cent water, making them one of the lowest calorie vegetables. One medium courgette has about 17kcal and provides about 25 per cent of the adult Reference Nutrient Intake (RNI) for folic acid, as well as 50 per cent of the RNI for vitamin C and 22 per cent of the RNI for vitamin B_6. Although courgettes are not as high in beta carotene as pumpkin, they still contain this important antioxidant. The deeper their colour, the higher their content of beta carotene.

Courgette facts

● Courgettes, like other varieties of squash, are New World plants that were cultivated by North America's Native people long before the arrival of European explorers and settlers.

● Young, small courgettes have more flavour than larger ones.

Versatile vegetable

The subtle flavour of courgettes complements other ingredients in a variety of dishes. They are an especially suitable companion to tomatoes and a splendid addition to vegetable lasagna, marinara sauce and ratatouille. They are also delicious when grated and made into cakes and other baked goods.

Probably the best way to eat courgettes is to slice them lengthways and barbecue them until barely tender. If desired, spray them while cooking, with a little balsamic

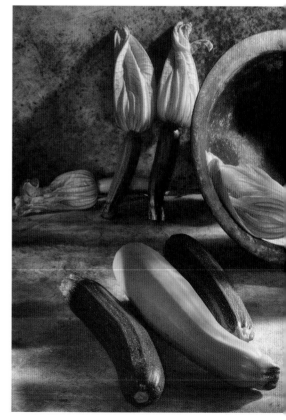

vinegar. Courgettes are tender enough to eat uncooked. Raw, they are a pleasant addition to a vegetable platter or salad, and dieters sometimes keep bags of sliced courgettes in the refrigerator for easy snacking.

Orange-coloured courgette flowers are edible and contain some of the same nutrients that are present in the vegetable. Stuffed courgette flowers are considered a delicacy – the blossoms are often stuffed with a cheese sauce or finely chopped vegetables and then dipped in a light batter and deep fried. To avoid the fat in such dishes, try sautéeing or steaming them instead.

Courgettes can grow very large, and summer gardeners will often find them in gigantic proportions. However, courgettes taste best when eaten small – ideally, 10-15cm long. As they grow larger, they are less flavoursome, and become primarily ornamental. When buying courgettes, look for specimens that feel firm and heavy when you pick them up. Although they can be refrigerated for a few days, courgettes tend to spoil quickly.

Do one simple thing

Bake a cake with courgettes

Your slice of cake can double as a small serving of vegetables, when you bake this delicious chocolate-courgette cake. Cream 115g butter and 200g caster sugar until fluffy and light. Slowly beat in 2 eggs. Sift 185g self-raising flour, 25g cocoa and ½ teaspoon cinnamon together. Add the flour mixture to the butter mixture with 60ml milk, 150g grated courgettes and 50g chopped walnuts. Spread into greased and paper-lined loaf tin, and bake at 180°C, 350°F or gas mark 4 for 40 minutes.

◀ **Popular berries**
Cranberries are at their peak when they bounce.

Cranberries

BENEFITS

- A fair source of vitamin C and fibre
- Juice helps to prevent or alleviate cystitis and urinary tract infections
- Contain bioflavonoids, that may protect eyesight and help to prevent cancer, heart disease and stomach ulcers

DRAWBACKS

- Need a large amount of sugar to make them palatable
- Not advised for people taking warfarin

Once served mostly with the Christmas turkey, cranberries are now consumed as juice, a dried snack fruit and an ingredient in some baked goods. Cranberries belong to the same family as blueberries, but unlike that fruit, they are too tart to eat raw. Even when sweetened, cranberries retain a fresh tartness that complements poultry and pork.

Cranberries are a native North American plant. When fresh cranberries are available, look for firm, bright red fruit. Cranberries are sometimes called 'bounce berries', because, at their peak, they will bounce when dropped; those that don't bounce are likely to be soft and past their prime.

Role in cystitis

Cranberry juice has long been used as a remedy for cystitis and also to prevent kidney and bladder stones. Originally, this benefit was attributed to quinic acid, a substance that increases urine acidity and prevents the formation of calcium stones. It was also thought that this acidity helped to prevent cystitis. Studies show, however, that cranberries also have a natural antibiotic that makes the bladder walls inhospitable to the organisms responsible for urinary tract infections. This prevents the bacteria from forming colonies; instead, they are washed out of the body in the urine. The same effect may help to protect against heart disease and stomach ulcers. (Blueberry juice has a similar effect on the stomach lining.)

Patients who suffer recurrent or chronic bladder infections are being advised by their urologists and gynaecologists to drink two 200ml glasses of cranberry juice daily as a preventive measure. See a doctor, however, if symptoms develop or persist; prescription antibiotics are usually necessary to cure an established urinary infection.

Commercially produced cranberry juice is high in added sugar, so it may not be suitable for certain people such as diabetics. Also, there is now good evidence that cranberries can raise blood levels of warfarin to dangerously high, potentially fatal, levels; those taking warfarin are advised against eating or drinking cranberries in any form.

Other benefits

Cranberries provide fibre, along with some vitamin C; they also contain bioflavonoids, plant pigments that help to counter the damage of unstable molecules that are formed when oxygen is used by the body. European researchers have found that anthocyanin, one of these bioflavonoids, promotes the formation of visual purple, a pigment in the eyes instrumental in seeing colour and in night vision. Other studies suggest anthocyanin has an anti-cancer effect.

Cravings

EAT PLENTY OF

■ Low-fat starchy foods to satisfy a carbohydrate craving

■ High-fibre foods to avoid feeling hungry

LIMIT

■ Foods you might crave, especially sweets, chocolates and salty items

AVOID

■ Becoming over hungry, which can lead to overindulgence

All of us occasionally have an irresistible urge for a certain food or beverage. But merely having a sudden need for a particular food does not constitute a true craving, nor does indulging in an occasional treat. A craving goes much deeper – it's an insistent desire that you can't ignore, even though satisfying it may entail some inconvenience or even danger.

Women report food cravings more often than men. Recent research suggests that hormonal changes are responsible for many food cravings, especially those that develop during periods of stress, pregnancy or different phases of a

Did you know?

Pica is the term that describes bizarre food cravings

For unexplained reasons, some people, especially children, develop intense cravings for non-food items, such as paint chips, soil, clay or laundry starch. This phenomenon is known as pica, a word which comes from the Latin term for magpie – a bird that will collect and eat almost anything.

Pica can have serious medical consequences, such as lead poisoning, intestinal obstruction, worm infestations and even death if poisonous substances are consumed.

woman's menstrual cycle when their metabolic rate rises and they tend to eat more, anyway.

Following this theory, fluctuating hormonal levels may influence the brain's production of serotonin and other chemicals – changes that can trigger an intense desire for specific foods. Under these circumstances, a person usually craves chocolate or other sweets; researchers think this is because chocolate's sweet, creamy feel in the mouth is comforting.

Carbohydrate cravings are strongly associated with obesity, but eating a diet high in wholegrain, starchy foods along with moderate amounts of protein may prevent the craving for sweets because these complex carbohydrates and protein are metabolised more slowly than sugars, thus providing a steady supply of glucose.

Carbohydrate cravings are often associated with SAD (Seasonal Affective Disorder). One study has shown that chromium supplements (600mg daily) can alleviate the carbohydrate craving in patients who are depressed.

More obsessive cravings, however, can stem from a specific illness, an addiction or a deep-seated psychological problem.

Pregnancy cravings

Pregnant women often develop strange food cravings, especially for pickles and other salty foods. In this instance, the craving reflects a physical need. During pregnancy, a woman's volume of blood doubles, and as a result she needs extra sodium to maintain a proper fluid balance. Normally, adding salt to food supplies the necessary sodium. As for other cravings, there's usually no harm in satisfying them in moderation, provided overall nutritional needs are met. But if the cravings are for bizarre indigestible items like laundry starch, soil, clay and ice, it constitutes 'pica' and may reflect a serious medical or psychological problem, and requires the attention of professionals.

A craving for ice is said to be a sign of iron deficiency; conversely, the deficiency can be caused by eating starch, clay and other substances that bind to iron and prevent its absorption. Ask your doctor if you need extra iron.

To give in or to deny?

Some experts believe that food cravings reflect the 'wisdom of the body'; we feel an urge to eat particular foods to fulfil a nutritional need. In general, however, we tend to crave foods that are not particularly nutritious, and in these cases, psychological factors are probably more influential than physical needs. For some people, food may fill an emotional void, so they turn to certain foods during periods of stress or sadness. The power of suggestion is another possible trigger, which is why just a brief whiff of a favourite food can result in an intense desire for it.

People often make the mistake of trying to deny a craving. Some may succeed, but more often than not, denial fosters an even stronger desire for the food. Unless the object of the craving poses a serious health risk (for instance, a person with high blood pressure craving salty foods), experts say it is better to satisfy the longing, but to do so in moderation. A healthier approach is to anticipate the craving and to satisfy it in advance. For example, if a woman invariably develops a strong craving for sweets during her premenstrual phase, she can lessen it somewhat by increasing her intake of starchy foods, which raise blood glucose levels. Eating more fruit, which is high in natural sugars, may also satisfy the desire for sweets.

Some medications, particularly steroids and hormonal preparations, can promote food cravings. These drug-related cravings, however, are usually non-specific; the person may simply feel ravenously hungry and crave eating in general.

Avoiding becoming over hungry can also forestall cravings for sweets or fatty foods. Hunger is the body's way of letting you know it's running short of fuel; it's a powerful instinct that is almost impossible to deny for any length of time. This is one reason why dieters often find it so hard to adhere to an over restrictive regimen; their resolve may be strong, but it's almost impossible to deny the body's instinct for self-preservation. Eating small, frequent meals is how to avert hunger and the subsequent strong cravings that can lead to overeating.

Crohn's disease

CONSUME

■ Lean meat, fish and poultry for the protein necessary for healing

■ Under a doctor's supervision, vitamin, mineral and other nutritional supplements

LIMIT

■ High-fibre foods, especially if the bowel is partially obstructed

AVOID

■ Any food that worsens symptoms

Crohn's disease is also known as ileitis. It is a type of inflammatory bowel disease that can affect any part of the intestinal tract, from the mouth to the anus. However, it most commonly attacks the colon and the lower part of the small intestine, or the ileum.

It is a chronic condition that may recur after lengthy periods of remission. Common symptoms are abdominal pain, often in the lower right area, and diarrhoea.

Typically, diseased portions of the intestine are interspersed with normal segments; fistulas (abnormal passageways between portions of the intestine) are common. The diseased portions may become obstructed, giving rise to an emergency situation.

There may also be weight loss, fever and intestinal bleeding persistent enough to cause anaemia. Children with Crohn's disease may suffer stunted growth and delayed sexual development.

There are many unproved theories about the causes of Crohn's disease. Some scientists believe that the immune system is affected by a virus or a bacterium that triggers an inflammatory reaction in the intestinal wall. Crohn's disease appears to run in families; about 20 per cent of those who have the disease have a blood relative with some form of inflammatory bowel disease.

Symptoms can flare up in periods stress, but stress doesn't appear to be the main cause.Crohn's disease is increasing in most developed countries, but is uncommon in Asia, Africa and South America.

Medical treatment

Crohn's disease has no cure, but a combination of drugs usually alleviates symptoms. As in the case of ulcerative colitis, sulfasalazine is the most popular choice. When Crohn's flares up, prednisolone is commonly used. Drugs that suppress the immune system, such as mercaptopurine or the related azathioprine can also be effective. While these drugs suppress the immune reaction that contributes to inflammation, they also increase the susceptibility to infection. Even minor infections should be reported to a doctor. If all these therapies fail to provide relief, infliximab (Remicade) has been approved as an intravenous treatment (given via a drip). This substance partially neutralises the activity of a protein called tumour necrosis factor (TNF), which is thought to be responsible for the inflammation associated with Crohn's disease. If bacterial over-growth occurs in the intestine, antibiotics will be prescribed.

Surgery is often needed to correct complications, such as an intestinal blockage, perforation and abscesses. Sometimes it is necessary to remove the diseased section of bowel; but this does not prevent recurrences in other portions of the intestinal tract.

Nutritional approaches

Nutritional deficiencies are common in people with Crohn's disease for several reasons. During a flare-up, symptoms kill the appetite, and a person is unlikely to consume enough food to maintain weight and good nutrition. Nutrition can be a problem even during periods of remission; if the small intestine is damaged by inflammation, vitamins and nutrients are not absorbed properly. Surgical removal of portions of the intestine will even further impair the body's ability to absorb nutrients from food.

Eliminate any foods that provoke symptoms. Although some doctors advise patients to avoid all fried foods, dairy products, spices and high-fibre foods, there is no specific diet for Crohn's disease. The overall objective is to consume adequate calories, protein, vitamins and minerals without exacerbating symptoms.

Try eliminating any food that seems to create problems, for several weeks, and keep a diary of your symptoms to determine whether giving it up is helpful. Eliminate only one type of food at a time, such as milk and other dairy products. Then reinstate them and watch for reactions to them.

Avoid foods high in fibre. High-fibre foods are generally discouraged during a flare-up because they may be irritating to the affected portion of the intestine, and they can also exacerbate diarrhoea.

Eat smaller, more frequent meals, and chew thoroughly. Consuming six or more small meals a day is less likely to provoke symptoms than having three large ones. Eat slowly and chew each mouthful thoroughly. This is good advice for anyone hoping to improve digestion, but it is of particular importance to those suffering from Crohn's disease.

Talk to your doctor about taking nutritional supplements. Even patients who can consume a normal diet may develop nutritional deficiencies because of the poor absorption of nutrients; thus, many patients need to take a daily multivitamin and mineral supplement. High-dose vitamins should only be taken under a doctor's supervision. Those who develop vitamin B_{12} deficiency, for example, often need to take it by injection if they lack the intestinal substances to metabolise it.

Special supplements

Those with severe symptoms or who have had extensive surgery may need a special high-calorie liquid formula, either as a nutritional supplement or as a replacement for normal meals. Again, such supplements should be prescribed by a doctor. In some cases, an elemental diet – an easy-to-digest formula – may be prescribed and can be given through a feeding tube (known as enteral nutrition) if it is thought necessary.

The most severe cases of Crohn's disease may require total parenteral nutrition (TPN), in which all nutrients are given intravenously. TPN may be used to allow the intestinal tract to rest and heal. This approach is also beneficial in treating a child whose growth is being stunted by inadequate nutrition. Because it can be administered at home, TPN allows for a more normal lifestyle.

Cucumbers

BENEFITS

■ Low in calories

Cucumbers belong to the same plant family as melons and pumpkins. Varieties of cucumber include apple (white skin and pale flesh), common or English (green skin, white flesh), Lebanese (small with green skin and greenish flesh) and telegraph (long with green skin and white flesh).

Lebanese cucumbers have twice as much vitamin C as other varieties and telegraph cucumbers have the highest content of potassium. If served unpeeled, a 100g cucumber provides about 1g of fibre and all varieties have less than 12kcal per 100g. One reason for their low calorie-count is that cucumbers are about 95 per cent water.

Folk healers often recommend cucumbers as a natural diuretic, but any increased urination is probably due more to their water content rather than to any inherent substance.

Cucumbers are used mostly as a salad ingredient. They can also be used to make pickles and relishes; cucumber juice contains some alpha hydroxy acids, which improve the effectiveness of facial masks, and other cosmetic products.

In many countries cucumbers are an important staple; worldwide, they rank ninth among vegetable crops and have multiple uses. In India and Central Europe, for example, cucumbers are diced and mixed with herbs and yoghurt to serve as a salad. Thai salads also use cucumber freely. When eaten with hot, spicy foods, cucumber has a cooling, refreshing effect.

◀ **Multipurpose vegetable**
Cucumbers are eaten whole, pickled, are put into salads and are used to make relishes, as well as a variety of cosmetic products.

Currants

BENEFITS

- Fresh currants are an excellent low-calorie source of vitamin C and potassium
- High in bioflavonoids

DRAWBACKS

- Fresh currants are highly perishable and are available for only a few weeks in summer

The several varieties of fresh currants – black, red and white – are actually berries that are related to gooseberries. The fruit sold as dried currants is a variety of grape.

Redcurrants are the most often available, usually for only a short time during summer. Blackcurrants lead both the red and the white types of currant in nutritional value. A 100g portion of fresh, black currants provides a whopping 200mg of vitamin C, as well as 270mg of potassium. This compares with 40mg of vitamin C and 280mg of potassium in 100g of red currants (also good amounts of these essential nutrients). All types of fresh currant are low in calories – about 200kcal and 3g of fibre in 100g. Currants are also a good source of fibre, providing about 2g per 100g.

Because they are quite tart, fresh currants are not usually eaten raw; instead, they are used in baking or to make jams and sauces. Diluted and sweetened blackcurrant juice is a refreshing beverage that is very high in vitamin C. The juice can be fermented and made into cordials.

Medicinal uses

All varieties of currant are rich in bioflavonoids, pigments that are thought to boost the antioxidant effects of vitamin C; they also help to inhibit cancer growth and may possibly prevent other diseases.

Blackcurrants have long been valued for their antibacterial and anti-inflammatory properties, which are thought to come from anthocyanin, a bioflavonoid in the berry skins. In Scandinavia, a powder made from dried blackcurrant skins is used to treat diarrhoea, especially that caused by *E. coli*, a common cause of bacterial diarrhoea. Blackcurrant syrup often used to ease the inflammation of a sore throat.

Cystic fibrosis

CONSUME PLENTY OF

- Fish, poultry, eggs, meat and other high-protein foods for growth
- Starchy foods and a moderate amount of sweets for energy
- Fat (as much as can be tolerated) for extra calories
- Salt to replace that lost in sweat
- Fluids to prevent constipation

AVOID

- Low-calorie products

Cystic fibrosis is a genetic disease afflicting more than 7,500 babies, children and adults in the UK.

Cystic fibrosis affects the glands that produce mucus, sweat, enzymes and other secretions. The most serious consequences of the disease occur in the lungs, pancreas and intestine, all of which can become clogged with thick mucus. As the lungs become congested, they are especially vulnerable to pneumonia and other infections. When the ducts that normally carry pancreatic enzymes to the small intestine become clogged, difficulty in breaking down fats and protein is the result, along with a number of other digestive problems. Abnormal amounts of salt are lost in sweat and saliva, which can lead to serious imbalances in body chemistry. At the moment there is no cure for cystic fibrosis, although scientists are testing gene therapy as a means of correcting the underlying genetic defect. Meanwhile, a combination of an enriched diet, vitamin supplements, replacement enzymes, antibiotics and other medications, and regular postural drainage to clear mucus from the lungs serves as the best treatment, and has greatly improved the outlook for people with cystic fibrosis. Life-expectancy is now better, and with good treatment there is an 80 per cent chance of surviving to the late 40s.

Nutritional needs

Since diet is critical in managing cystic fibrosis, the treatment team usually includes a clinical dietitian. To grow properly, children who have cystic fibrosis typically need to consume many more calories than are normally recommended.

In the past it was difficult to meet these markedly increased energy demands because of the body's inability to digest and absorb fats and protein. The development of improved enzyme preparations to supplement or replace those normally produced by the pancreas has helped to solve this problem. These supplemental enzymes, which may be in the form of tablets, capsules or powder, must be taken with every meal and snack to aid digestion.

Eat larger portions and lots of snacks. There is no special diet for sufferers of cystic fibrosis; rather, the child is encouraged to take larger portions during meals and have more frequent snacks. Babies with the disease may be given a formula that contains predigested fats.

Eat more protein. For older children, high-protein foods, such as meat, poultry, fish, eggs and milk, are emphasised – and as much fat as the child can tolerate to ensure the intake of the extra calories. Vitamin and mineral supplements are often necessary as well, but should be taken only under the supervision of a doctor.

Consume more sodium. Salt is also an essential part of the diet because cystic fibrosis affects the sweat and salivary glands, causing them to excrete abnormal amounts of sodium and chloride in perspiration and saliva. This situation can be especially critical during hot weather or exercise, when it may be necessary to consume extra salt. Otherwise, adding moderate amounts of salt to flavour foods should be sufficient to maintain adequate sodium levels.

Prescribed supplements. If digestive problems develop, despite taking enzymes, supplements of predigested fats may be prescribed and, in some cases, high-calorie supplements may be necessary. Usually these can be taken by mouth, but in severe cases they may be administered at night

◀ **Extra nutrition**
An omelette made with herbs and cheese; and stir-fried prawns, meat or chicken, with vegetables and a generous portion of noodles, provide good amounts of nutrients, protein and calories.

through a feeding tube. Intravenous feeding is rarely necessary, but if required, it can be given at home.

Some people with cystic fibrosis may also develop diabetes if the pancreas becomes so clogged that it can no longer make adequate insulin, the hormone needed to metabolise carbohydrates. In such cases, insulin injections are added. Constipation and even intestinal obstruction are common in cystic fibrosis. It's important to consume adequate water and other fluids. A doctor may prescribe a laxative to prevent constipation.

Dietary differences
Parents often find it difficult to deal with the dietary recommendations for a child with cystic fibrosis.

Above all, it's important to understand that the nutritional needs of a person with cystic fibrosis are very different from those of a healthy person. A high-calorie diet with as much protein and fat as can be tolerated is necessary. Prescription enzymes that improve absorption of fats and protein have made a big difference in living with cystic fibrosis.

Fats provide more calories per unit than other nutrients, so they are a critical source of energy. The body also needs fat in order to absorb vitamins A, D, E and K.

In the absence of diabetes, it's not necessary to restrict sugary foods. These simple carbohydrates are more easily absorbed than starches. However, sweet snacks should be accompanied by plenty of protein to provide balance and the amino acids needed for growth, immune function and for the repair and maintenance of body tissue.

People with cystic fibrosis can become vegetarian or even vegan, but it can be difficult to achieve the right balance of protein and calories, so they should seek dietary advice.

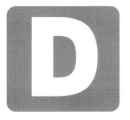

D

Dates

BENEFITS

- A good source of potassium
- A source of iron, niacin and vitamin B₆
- High in fibre

DRAWBACKS

- High sugar content and stickiness promote tooth decay

Date palms are among the world's oldest trees – they have been grown in North Africa for at least 8,000 years. Prized for their sweet fruit, these desert trees are extraordinarily fruitful, producing up to 200 dates in a cluster.

Fresh dates are classified by their moisture content into three categories: soft, semi-soft and dry. Most commercial varieties are semi-soft, which are marketed fresh, as well as dried, after part of their moisture has been evaporated.

With about 60 per cent of their weight coming from sugar, dried dates are one of the sweetest of all fruits: 100g of dried dates contain about 227kcal. The same amount of fresh dates has 107kcal. Dried dates provide potassium; 100g provide

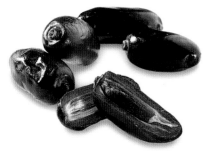

700mg, more than a comparable amount of other high-potassium foods, such as bananas and oranges. They also provide 15 per cent of the Reference Nutrient Intake (RNI) of magnesium, 14 per cent of niacin and 28 per cent of vitamin B₆, as well as 4g of fibre. Fresh dates give 33 per cent of the RNI for vitamin C.

Dates contain tyramine, an organic compound found in aged cheese, certain processed meats, red wine and other products. Anyone taking monoamine oxidase (MAO) inhibitors to treat depression should avoid dates, because tyramine can interact with these drugs to produce a life-threatening rise in blood pressure. In some people, tyramine can also trigger migraine headaches.

It's important to brush your teeth after eating dates. Both the dried and the fresh fruit are very sticky, and because of their high sugar content, they can lead to dental decay if they cling to teeth.

Dental health

CONSUME PLENTY OF

- Calcium-rich foods, such as milk, yoghurt and cheese
- Fresh fruit and vegetables for vitamins A and C, and for chewing in order to promote healthy gums
- Tea, which is a good source of fluoride

LIMIT

- Dried fruit and any sticky foods that lodge between the teeth

AVOID

- Sweet drinks, confectionery, crisps and snacks containing refined carbohydrate
- Sipping acidic drinks very slowly

In addition to brushing, flossing and using a mouthwash, a healthy diet (with natural or added fluoride)

protects teeth from decay and keeps the gums healthy. Tooth decay (cavities and dental caries) and gum disease are caused by colonies of bacteria that constantly coat the teeth with a sticky film called plaque. If plaque is not flossed or brushed away, these bacteria break down the sugars and starches in foods to produce acids that wear away the tooth enamel. Plaque also hardens into tartar, which can lead to gum inflammation, or gingivitis.

A well-balanced diet provides the minerals, vitamins and other nutrients essential for healthy teeth and gums. Fluoride, occurring naturally in foods and water, or added to the water supply in some areas, can be a powerful tool in fighting decay. It can reduce the rate of cavities by up to 40 per cent.

Dental health guidelines

Start well by eating healthily during pregnancy. Make sure that your children's teeth get off to a good start by eating sensibly during your pregnancy. Calcium is very important because it helps to form strong teeth and bones, and so is vitamin D, which the body needs in order to absorb calcium.

You need lots of calcium for healthy teeth and gums. Dairy products (full-fat or low-fat), fortified soya and rice beverages, canned salmon or sardines (with bones), almonds and dark green leafy vegetables are all excellent sources of calcium.

You need vitamin D to help to absorb the calcium. Vitamin D is obtained from moderate exposure to the sun. It is also present in butter, margarine and fish such as salmon.

Fluoride is key. To a large extent, cavities can be prevented by giving children fluoride in the first few years of life. Fluoride may be supplied through fluoridated water (very few UK water companies add fluoride to their water supply, however), beverages made with fluoridated water, tea and some fish, as well as many brands of toothpaste and some mouthwashes. Fluoride supplements are available for children who don't have access to fluoridated drinking water. It is wise to check to see if the water supply in your area is fluoridated. Excess consumption of fluoride can cause mottling of the teeth.

Also needed are phosphorus, magnesium, vitamin A and beta carotene. In addition to calcium and fluoride, minerals needed for the formation of tooth enamel include phosphorus (richly supplied in meat, fish and eggs) and magnesium (found in whole grains, spinach and bananas). Vitamin A

Do one simple thing

Chew gum sweetened with xylitol

Chew it for at least 5 minutes within 5 minutes of finishing a meal. Gum sweetened with xylitol helps to counter harmful bacteria in the mouth, which promote cavities. A study showed that people who chewed this gum after meals had far fewer cavity-causing bacteria in their mouth 5 minutes afterwards than people who chewed other gums or no gum at all.

also helps to build really strong bones and teeth. Good sources of beta carotene, which the body turns into vitamin A, include orange-coloured fruit and vegetables and the dark green leafy vegetables.

Children's teeth are vulnerable to decay, so parents should:
- Provide a good diet throughout childhood;
- Brush children's teeth until they're mature enough to do a thorough job by themselves (usually by six or seven years old);
- Supervise twice-daily brushing and flossing thereafter;
- Never put babies or toddlers to bed with a bottle of milk (which contains lactose, a natural sugar), juice or other sweet drink;
- Never dip dummies in honey or syrup.

The sugar factor

Sucrose, most familiar to us as sugar, is the leading cause of tooth decay, but it is not the only culprit. Although sugary foods are major offenders, starchy foods (such as crisps and crackers) also play an important part in tooth decay. When starches mix with amylase, an enzyme in saliva, the result is an acid bath that erodes the enamel and makes teeth more susceptible to decay. If starchy foods linger in the mouth the potential for damage is all the greater.

Be careful when eating dried fruit. Dried fruit can have an adverse effect on teeth, because it is high in sugar and clings to the teeth. Even unsweetened fruit juices can contribute to tooth decay – they are acidic and contain relatively high levels of simple sugars.

Fresh fruit, especially apples, are better choices. Fresh fruit, although both sweet and acidic, is less likely to cause a problem, because chewing stimulates the saliva flow. Saliva decreases mouth

acidity and washes away food particles. Apples have been called nature's toothbrush because they stimulate the gums, increase saliva flow and reduce the build-up of cavity-causing bacteria. A chronically dry mouth also contributes to decay. Saliva flow slows during sleep; going to bed without brushing the teeth is especially harmful. Certain drugs, such as those used for high blood pressure, reduce saliva flow.

Helpful foods

You can protect your teeth by concluding meals with foods that do not promote cavities and may even prevent them. For instance, cheese helps to prevent cavities if eaten at the end of a meal. Chewing sugarless gum stimulates the flow of saliva, which decreases acid and flushes out food particles. Rinsing your mouth and brushing your teeth after eating are important strategies to prevent cavities. Take care with drinks. Diet soft drinks have no sugar but their high acid levels can cause erosion of tooth enamel. Sports drinks are also acidic and are potentially damaging, especially if sipped slowly. Using a straw and consuming an acidic drink over a short time period is the safest strategy to avoid dental erosion.

Gum disease

More teeth are lost through gum disease than through tooth decay. Gum disease is likely to strike anyone who neglects oral hygiene or eats a poor diet. Particularly at risk are people with alcoholism, malnutrition or AIDS/HIV infection or who are being treated with steroid drugs or certain cancer chemotherapies. Regular brushing and flossing help to prevent puffy, sore and inflamed gums. Gingivitis, a very common condition that causes the gums to redden, swell and bleed, is typically caused by the gradual build-up of plaque. Treatment requires good dental hygiene and removal of plaque by a dentist. Left untreated, gingivitis can lead to periodontitis – an advanced infection of the gums that causes teeth to loosen and fall out. There may be more serious consequences of gum disease. Studies show a link between poor oral health and heart disease. Bleeding gums apparently provide an entry port for bacteria or viruses that can cause heart problems. Women with tooth or gum problems are also more likely to give birth to premature babies.

Bleeding gums may also be a sign that your intake of vitamin C is deficient. Be sure that your diet includes plenty of fresh fruit and vegetables every day; munching on hard, fibrous foods, such as a celery stick or carrot, stimulates the gums.

Depression

CONSUME

- A balanced diet including complex carbohydrates, oily fish and food sources of vitamins B_6 and B_{12} and folate

LIMIT

- Alcohol, which can be a depressant

- Caffeine, which can interfere with sleep and mood

AVOID

- Foods and drinks that contain tyramine (if you are taking MAO inhibitors)

Throughout his life, Sir Winston Churchill lived in dread of visits by the 'black dog', as he called his bouts of paralysing depression. Other writers, seeking to describe the anguish of clinical depression, have told of trying to find their way through a thick, yellow fog or being kept from the sunlight by a trailing black cloud. Clinical depression

Fish oils: a cure for depression?

Could eating more oily fish be a simple way to help to alleviate depression? Research points to 'yes'. Researchers have known for some time that rates of depression are lower in countries where lots of fish is consumed and higher in countries where little fish is eaten. Recently experts have noted that some people who suffer from depression have markedly low levels of omega-3 fatty acids, which are normally found in high concentrations in the brain.

These fatty acids are abundant in fish, especially salmon, trout, swordfish, fresh tuna and mackerel. Low fish consumption and low levels of a potent form of an omega-3 fatty acid called DHA have both been shown to be linked with higher rates of post-partum depression.

Recently, a flurry of research studies has supported the notion that consuming more omega-3 fatty acids can help to stabilise the mood. When researchers fed omega-3 fatty acids to piglets, the fatty acids had the same effect as the anti-depressant Prozac – they significantly increased levels of the neurotransmitter serotonin. New studies in people have shown that omega-3 fatty acids can help symptoms of depression as well as bipolar disorder.

More research is needed, but meanwhile, there's no harm in adding two or three fish meals to your weekly diet. People who don't like fish, should try fish oil supplements. Talk to your doctor before taking them, though, since they can thin the blood. Linseeds, rape seed oil and walnuts are other sources of omega-3 fatty acids.

is quite different from the normal 'down' reaction to disappointment. Depression is a serious disorder. It can strike out of the blue and – for a few of the more fortunate sufferers – can disappear just as mysteriously. Many sufferers can benefit from medications to lift their mood.

One of the signs of depression is a dramatic change in eating patterns. Some people lose all desire to eat; others develop voracious appetites, especially for carbohydrates. People with depression typically have little energy. Other common signs of depression include an unshakeable feeling of sadness, inability to experience pleasure,

early awakening or awakenings throughout the night, insomnia, excessive sleepiness, other sleep disorders, inability to concentrate and indecisiveness. Feelings of worthlessness or guilt may be accompanied by recurrent thoughts of death.

Anyone who has some or all of these symptoms nearly every day for more than two weeks may be suffering from major depression.

People over the age of 65 are four times more likely to suffer from depression than younger people; however, elderly sufferers do not always exhibit the classic signs. Instead, they may show signs of dementia, complain of aches and pains and appear agitated, anxious or irritable.

Researchers estimate that almost a third of widows and widowers meet the criteria for depression in the first four weeks after the death of a spouse. Half of these people are still clinically depressed after a year. If you notice symptoms of depression in someone, try to persuade the person to see a doctor.

People with Parkinson's disease, stroke, arthritis, thyroid disorders and cancer often suffer from depression. They may feel depressed because of the diagnosis of a serious illness or the underlying disease has itself triggered a chemical change in the brain. Depression can also be a side effect of many medicines taken for other disorders; these include beta-blockers for hypertension, digoxin and other drugs for heart disease, indomethacin and other painkillers, corticosteroids (including prednisone), anti-parkinsonism drugs, antihistamines and oral contraceptives and other hormonal agents.

Dietary factors

People with depression often fail to take care of themselves, neglecting their appearance and eating irregularly. Nutritious food is needed to cope with any disease, but unfortunately, depressed people are especially likely to be careless about their nutrition. The resulting poor nourishment may impede

Did you know?

Chocolate is a mood enhancer

The naturally occurring substance in chocolate called phenylethylamine (PEA) has been found to elevate endorphin levels and to act as a natural antidepressant.

their recovery. On the other hand, eating the right foods can actually help to stabilise mood.

Eat a diet that emphasises carbohydrates. Meals that contain carbohydrates have been associated with a calming, relaxed effect. These foods allow the amino acid tryptophan to enter the brain where it is then used to make serotonin. Feel-good food choices include pasta, breads, grains, cereals, fruit and juices.

Limit sugar consumption. When some sugar-sensitive people eat a lot of sweets, they may experience an energetic 'high' followed by a 'low' with weakness and 'jitters' when the sugar is metabolised.

Get a lot more of B vitamins. Vitamins B_6, B_{12} and folate may all help certain forms of depression. Vitamin B_6 has been shown to give some relief to women suffering from PMS-related depression. Part of this may be due to the role of B_6 in helping to convert tryptophan to serotonin in the brain. B_6 sources are meat, fish, poultry, whole grains, bananas and potatoes.

Other research has found that many depressed people are deficient in folate and B_{12}. Folate is found in green leafy vegetables, orange juice, avocado, salmon, lentils, corn, asparagus, peas, nuts and seeds. B_{12} is found in all animal foods and fortified soya and rice beverages.

Turn to tryptophan. Found in poultry and milk and other animal products, this amino acid is needed to make the mood-critical neuro-transmitter serotonin. Research indicates that tryptophan can help to induce sleep and may play a role in treating some types of depression. Tryptophan is licensed in the UK for use in cases of depression resistant to standard antidepressants. Its trade name is Optimax. It should only be used under specialist supervision. However, you can obtain tryptophan

from food. Besides poultry, good amounts of the amino acid are found in nuts (including peanuts) eggs and pumpkin seeds.

Drug-food interactions

Antidepressant drugs in the class called monoamine oxidase (MAO) inhibitors are only rarely used in th UK now; they can have serious side effects when taken with certain foods, especially those containing tyramine and other amines. Alcohol should be avoided altogether. These drugs include isocarboxazid and tranylcypromine (Parnate). If you are taking one of these drugs, your blood pressure could rise dangerously when you eat foods rich in tyramines.

As a general rule, all protein-rich foods that have been aged, dried, fermented, pickled or bacterially treated should be cut from the diet. Foods that are rich in tyramine include all aged cheeses, dry fermented sausages such as pepperoni, salami, pastrami, smoked or pickled fish, non-fresh meat or poultry, tofu and soya products including soy sauce, beer and ale, any overripe or fermented fruit or vegetable, broad beans, sauerkraut, bananas, soups containing meat extracts or cheese, gravies and sauces containing meat extracts, yeast extracts and meat extracts, protein dietary supplements and certain wines (including Chianti and champagne). Coffee, tea, colas, chocolate, yeast, yeast extracts, broad bean pods, fava beans and ginseng contain small amounts of tyramine but are generally safe enough if taken only occasionally.

Antidepressants and weight

Another class of antidepressant drugs, called selective serotonin reuptake inhibitors, can reduce the appetite, leading to a slight but progressive weight loss. These drugs include fluoxetine (Prozac), sertraline (Lustral), and paroxetine (Seroxat). If you are taking one of these drugs, you may need to make a special effort to maintain your optimum weight during treatment.

Tricyclic antidepressants, which can cause weight gain, include imipramine, and nortriptyline (Allegron). If you are overweight to begin with, or gain weight while taking any of these drugs, ask your doctor to suggest an alternative.

The herbal preparation St John's wort is used increasingly; recent evidence suggests it is as effective as a mild antidepressant, and has fewer side effects; but it may interact with prescription drugs.

Diabetes

EAT PLENTY OF

- Regular meals and snacks to avoid blood sugar level fluctuations

- A balance of carbohydrate, protein and unsaturated fat at each meal

- Low-fat, high-fibre foods to achieve and maintain a normal weight

LIMIT

- 'Empty calorie' foods such as sweets and snack foods, which can contribute to obesity.

- Saturated fats and foods made with hydrogenated fats.

About 1.4 million people in the UK have diabetes, which is a serious metabolic disease that affects the body's ability to derive energy from blood sugar, or glucose. Diabetes results when the body cannot produce or properly use insulin, a hormone

The weight connection

The prevalence of Type 2 diabetes is increasing as the population (particularly of developed countries) becomes increasingly overweight. Not every overweight person will get diabetes, but 85 per cent of those with Type 2 diabetes weigh more than they should. Extra fat, especially abdominal fat in the 'apple-shape' body, is associated with insulin resistance. Newly diagnosed, overweight people with Type 2 diabetes may banish the disease by adopting a healthier lifestyle to reach and maintain their ideal weight. Even if they don't reach their ideal weight, any loss makes the disease easier to control with diet and exercise alone.

needed for glucose metabolism. Because all human body tissues need a steady supply of glucose, diabetes can affect every organ. Blood vessels and nerves can become damaged, leading to heart disease, kidney failure, blindness and other complications.

▶ **Keeping control**
Diabetes does not demand special meals, just a healthy diet. Clockwise, from top, are pasta with vegetables, a baked potato topped with a vegetable medley, and poached salmon on wholegrain bread.

Two types of diabetes

About 25 per cent of diagnosed diabetes cases are Type 1, also called insulin-dependent diabetes, which often develops in children. In this auto-immune disease, the body's mechanisms for protecting itself

D

D

from foreign organisms are turned against its own tissue. Type 1 diabetes often develops after an infection, such as chickenpox, so researchers think that after destroying the invaders, the immune system keeps attacking; but having no worthy targets, turns on body tissue. As a result the cells that produce insulin in the pancreas are destroyed. People with Type 1 diabetes must take insulin daily and also control their diet and physical activity strictly to maintain near-normal blood glucose levels.

The most common type of diabetes, responsible for 75 per cent of cases, is Type 2, or non-insulin-dependent diabetes. Once termed adult-onset diabetes, this type used to occur in older adults who were overweight, who despite having adequate or even high levels of in-sulin, cannot use the hormone properly. However, with the increasing level of obesity being seen in British children, Type 2 diabetes is beginning to occur in greater numbers in youngsters. The early symptoms of Type 2 diabetes may go undiagnosed until there is a heart attack or stroke. So thousands of people may have Type 2 diabetes but not know it. They may not experience any symptoms, but the disease may be

● **Myth.......**
People with diabetes have to give up sweet desserts.
.......Reality ●
An occasional sweet treat is fine, with the best choice being a dessert that contains fibre and has a low glycaemic index.

damaging the heart, blood vessels, nerves, kidneys, eyes and other organs. While much of this damage is permanent, it can be prevented with early treatment. If you could be at risk – if you are overweight, have a family history of diabetes, or had raised blood sugar in pregnancy – your GP may wish to check your blood glucose levels at intervals.

For most people with Type 2 diabetes, diet and exercise alone can be effective; some may also need oral medications to improve the effect of their own insulin, and a few may need insulin injections.

Diet strategy

Diet is key to managing diabetes. An appropriate diet can help to maintain optimal blood glucose levels and prevent or delay the long-term complications of diabetes. It may be advisable to avoid coffee with meals as at least one study suggests that, in people with Type 2 diabetes, caffeine

appears to interfere with the body's ability to manage blood sugar. As well as managing blood glucose, they should consider cholesterol levels and high blood pressure.

Reduce saturated fat intake to protect against heart disease. An overweight person needs to focus on weight loss by decreasing calorie intake and, at the same time, increasing levels of daily activity.

Fats

A diet low in fat, and especially low in saturated fat, is the most important aspect of a diabetic diet. All fats contribute to obesity, and saturated fats increase the risk for cardiovascular diseases, which occur in 15 per cent of those with diabetes, compared with 2.5 per cent of those without diabetes. Saturated fats occur in animal fats and hydrogenated vegetable fats used in many fried foods, snacks, baked goods and prepared meals. Unsaturated fats found in liquid vegetable oils, nuts and avocado are good for the heart and are the fats of choice for those with diabetes. The omega-3 fats in seafood are also beneficial for the heart. The general recommendation is that fats should contribute no more than 30 per cent of the daily calories, with saturated fats not more than a third of total fat, and preferably even less.

Carbohydrates

Once thought of as simple sugars and complex carbohydrates (starches), carbohydrates are now rated according to their glycaemic effect. The glycaemic index (GI) measures how quickly carbohydrate in a food is converted to blood glucose compared with the same amount of carbohydrate taken as glucose. Foods with less than 10g of carbohydrate per serving do not have a GI as they do not influence blood glucose levels. Research shows

Pregnancy-related diabetes

Gestational diabetes can complicate pregnancy for both mother and baby. The effects of hormonal changes and weight gain during pregnancy increase demands on the pancreas and can lead to insulin resistance. Gestational diabetes can strike any expectant mother but is most likely in those who are over 30 years of age and overweight, as well as those who have had a previous baby weighing more than 4kg or a family history of gestational or Type 2 diabetes.

All women should have a blood test for diabetes between the 24th and 28th weeks of pregnancy. If gestational diabetes is diagnosed, the mother should modify her diet and monitor weight gain carefully; she may require daily insulin injections for the rest of the pregnancy. This type of diabetes usually disappears almost immediately after childbirth, but women who've had it are at high risk for Type 2 diabetes in later years.

that low GI foods create less stress on blood glucose and are the preferred options for those with diabetes.

The GI (on its own) should not be the sole basis for choosing one carbohydrate food over another; the overall nutritional contribution the food makes is also important. Within a food group, low GI foods that are high in nutrients are the best choice. For example, low GI, nutritious choices of breakfast cereal include wholegrain cereals (such as rolled oats or muesli), or bran-based cereals with mixed grains.

The GI of a meal depends on the GI of each of the components, so adding milk (low GI) to a cereal such as wholewheat breakfast biscuits (medium GI) will reduce the total GI of the meal. Highly processed cereals such as cornflakes and popped rice have a high GI.

Among breads, the low GI choices include wholegrain breads (with 'bits' of grain), sourdough loaves (even if the flour is white) and fruit breads. Their GI is only marginally lower than white bread but the higher content of fibre and nutrients in the wholegrain loaf makes it a better choice than white bread. Other examples of low GI food choices include peas, beans, lentils and other legumes (including canned varieties), most fruit (apples, pears, oranges, kiwi fruit, stone fruit), sweet potatoes, peas and sweet corn, milk, yoghurt and all types of pasta.

Evidence that weight loss is a powerful preventive medicine

A major clinical trial studied a large group of overweight people at high risk for Type 2 diabetes. Researchers found that those who lost modest amounts of weight cut their diabetes risk by 58 per cent. People over the age of 60 cut their risk even more. It was found that losing just 5 per cent of body weight is enough to make a difference.

What's new?

A deficiency of chromium, a trace mineral, has been associated with reduced glucose tolerance. Chromium is found in foods such as wheat bran, whole grains, chicken breast and mushrooms. Processed and refined foods such as white bread, white rice, pasta, sugar and sweets all contain little chromium.

Some research of chromium supplements shows that they may have a beneficial effect on blood-glucose control for those with diabetes, but other research shows no benefit. If you choose to take a chromium supplement, take no more than 200mcg per day – this dosage is considered safe.

High GI foods include refined cereals, rice cakes, savoury crackers, soft drinks, snack foods, sweets, watermelon and floury potatoes (waxy ones have a medium GI). Green salad leaves and many salad vegetables have too little carbohydrate to have a GI.

The idea that people with diabetes must avoid all sugar is no longer considered valid. However, the usual diet consumed in the UK has more sugar than advisable for most people with diabetes.

Foods containing sugar should be chosen on the basis of their GI and overall nutritional contribution to the diet. For example, an apple crumble with a topping made from a small amount of unsaturated spread combined with a little sugar, rolled oats and wholemeal flour would be a more suitable diabetic dessert than a high-fat apple pie.

A sweetened yoghurt (with its low GI plus calcium and protein) would be more suitable than jelly (that has a high GI and no essential nutrients).

Soluble fibre – the kind in apples and other fruit, oats and legumes – may help to lower blood-sugar levels (it also helps to lower cholesterol). And insoluble fibre, found in whole grains and many vegetables, helps you feel full on fewer calories.

Protein

Choose nutritious protein sources. There is no research to support an increased or decreased protein intake for uncomplicated diabetes, so the recommended amounts are also appropriate for adults with diabetes. High-quality protein foods (lean meats, meat substitutes and lower-fat dairy foods) should supply up to 20 per cent of daily calories.

Diarrhoea

CONSUME PLENTY OF

- Water, mineral water, herbal teas, weak tea, ginger ale, broth or sports beverages to replace lost fluids, salts and minerals

- Skinless baked potatoes, boiled or poached eggs and other bland foods as the bowels return to normal

- Bananas for potassium, and apples to cleanse the digestive system

AVOID

- Fruit juices

- Most other foods, especially salads, fruit and whole grains, until bowel function normalises

- Alcohol, which dehydrates, and caffeine, which stimulates the bowel, for at least 48 hours after the symptoms disappear

Acute infectious diarrhoea is one of the world's most common ailments. An estimated 5 billion cases occur every year, and diarrhoea and the common cold are frequent causes for absences from work. Although diarrhoea causes fatalities – due to dehydration – it is seldom a threat in affluent, well-nourished societies, except to such vulnerable groups as babies, the elderly and invalids.

In developing countries this is not the case; however, many deaths have been prevented with the use of a homemade rehydration fluid that has been promoted through the World Health Organization (WHO).

The definition

Diarrhoea – the frequent passage of loose, watery stools – is not a disease but a symptom of an under-lying problem. It is most commonly brought on by food poisoning, especially among travellers.

Transient looseness can be caused by overconsumption of laxative foods (such as prunes), heavy use of sugarless chewing gum sweetened with sugar alcohol (such as sorbitol) and non-prescription indigestion remedies containing magnesium. Emotional stress that causes irritable bowel syndrome may disrupt the normal bowel pattern with alternating constipation and

diarrhoea; similar symptoms occur in ulcerative colitis and Crohn's disease, both inflammatory bowel disorders. In many instances, however, diarrhoea develops without any identifiable cause. Unless the problem persists or recurs often, this is not a cause for concern.

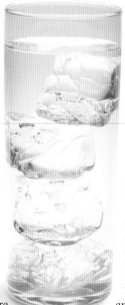

Dietary management

Most cases of diarrhoea are minor and short-lived and usually they can be managed at home with simple dietary measures.

Stop solid food and rehydrate. Start by eliminating all solid foods and sipping warm or tepid drinks to prevent any further dehydration. Drinking half a cup of fluid every 15 minutes or so is usually enough. Suitable drinks include water, mineral water, herbal teas, weak tea and ginger ale. Clear broths also help to replace the salts and other minerals lost. You can make your own rehydration fluid by mixing a teaspoon of salt and 8 teaspoons of sugar into a litre of water. Drink about a litre of this mixture every two hours.

Slowly introduce low-fibre foods. When you feel like eating, start with the BRAT diet – bananas, boiled rice, apples and toast. After about 48 hours, start to introduce bland foods such as cooked carrots,

boiled potatoes and poached or boiled eggs. Apples and other fruit high in pectin (a soluble fibre) help to counteract diarrhoea. Cooked carrots are also high in pectin. Try them puréed. Although fruit and vegetables can usually be tolerated fairly well, do not eat fatty foods until the bowel movements have returned to normal. Other suitable foods include savoury biscuits and chicken-rice soup, which will help to replenish depleted sodium and potassium.

Avoid milk products until the symptoms disappear. Some of the organisms that cause some types of diarrhoea can temporarily impair the ability to digest milk.

Recurrent diarrhoea

Some people have recurrent or chronic diarrhoea because they are unable to absorb a particular nutrient. For example, in people who have a lactose intolerance, the sugar in milk passes intact into the colon, where it is fermented by bacteria, producing hydrogen gas, along with water retention, bloating and diarrhoea. As a general rule, in all cases of recurrent or chronic diarrhoea, you should see your doctor as soon as possible.

Over-the-counter remedies

Non-prescription anti-diarrhoeal drugs may give some relief when diarrhoea has no obvious cause or is due to a minor illness, such as a flu, but many doctors believe that you will heal faster by letting nature take its course. Never use a non-prescription anti-diarrhoea product for more than two days without consulting your doctor.

When to call the doctor

Mild diarrhoea can usually be self-managed. But call your doctor promptly for any of the following:

▪ Diarrhoea that lasts more than two days (one day for a child under two, a frail elderly person, or someone with diabetes) or if it worsens during that time.

▪ The appearance of blood, mucus or worms in the faeces.

▪ Severe abdominal pain.

▪ Diarrhoea that is accompanied by vomiting or fever.

C A U T I O N

Apple juice is often thought of as bland and hence appropriate for people with diarrhoea, but it contains natural sorbitol, which has a laxative effect. Drinking too much fruit juice of any kind is often the cause of diarrhoea in toddlers.

Dieting
Keeping the weight off

There's no easy way to lose weight. Whether you decide on a high-protein diet, a low-fat diet or some other approach, experts agree that the only way to shed excess weight is to cut the total numbers of calories you consume and/or burn more calories through exercise. Simple enough to understand – but often much more difficult to do.

Despite becoming more and more obsessed with diets and dieting, we've become fatter and fatter. Obesity in the industrialised world is reaching epidemic proportions. Well over half of the adults in the UK are overweight or obese (overweight is defined as having a Body Mass Index [BMI] of 25 or more; obesity is defined as having a BMI of more than 30). It seems that even as diet books and low-fat foods fly off the shelf, the essential messages about how to lose weight safely and permanently aren't sinking in.

REAL WEIGHT LOSS

The 'secret' to losing weight is this: burn more calories than you eat. When the body uses more energy than it takes in (remember, food equals energy), it depletes its fat stores. In other words, eat less and your body will burn fat for energy. Of course, what you eat is important, too. A diet based solely on cabbage soup won't provide the nutrition your body needs – and you'll get tired of it soon enough and return to your old eating habits with a vengeance.

Any weight-loss plan needs to centre on foods you can keep eating for a lifetime – and of course it helps if those foods will also help to protect you from cancer and other diseases. After all, it's not all about losing weight. A diet that is high in meat and low in fruit (Atkins, for example) may lead to short-term weight loss, but is not in keeping with current nutritional wisdom. Excessive meat consumption has been linked with a variety of diseases and a high-fruit diet protects against cancer. Fruit, vegetables, wholegrain foods, low-fat dairy products and lean protein are the cornerstone of healthy eating, whether or not you're trying to trim your waistline. The foods that your body can easily do without – the ones packed with calories – are the ones to cut back on. That means cakes, biscuits, fatty meats, whole milk, cream sauces, snacks and the like.

When people want to lose weight, they usually want instant results. Most people who go on crash diets to shed weight fast usually end up putting it back on just as quickly – and they often put back more than they lost. Experts suggest a goal of losing up to 0.5kg a week. To lose this amount, you would need to consume 500 fewer calories a week or use up 500 more a week in exercise.

People who exercise in addition to eating less keep off the most weight for the longest time. Work up to accumulating at least 30–60 minutes of moderate exercise (such as fast-paced walking) a day. By exercising you'll raise your metabolism so that you burn more calories, even as you sleep. Exercise also helps you feel better mentally and physically, and may help you to stick to your plans.

TIPS FOR TAKING IT OFF

Countless people try the latest fad diets, only to go off the diet when it stops working and eventually try another one, and so on. They would be wiser to follow these basic tips for losing weight safely, naturally and permanently.

EAT BREAKFAST, AND DON'T SKIP MEALS. Eat more often to avoid a completely empty stomach, which can make you overeat at your next meal. Researchers have discovered a hormone called ghrelin that is secreted by the stomach. When your stomach is empty, your ghrelin levels surge, which makes you run for the nearest food. Instead of skipping meals, plan to divide your three meals into four to six small meals or snacks, spaced 3 to 5 hours apart.

CHOOSE CARBOHYDRATES CAREFULLY. Despite what the popular media might have you believe, you don't need to avoid carbohydrates in order to lose weight. But you should shy away from carbohydrate foods that have little nutritional value, such as sugar, soft drinks, confectionery, biscuits and cakes.

These foods are quickly turned into glucose by the body, and the influx of glucose causes a rapid rise in the hormone insulin, whose job it is to escort glucose out of the bloodstream and into cells. A surge of insulin is followed by a glucose 'crash', which leaves you hungry in no time.

Instead of poor-quality carbohydrates, focus your attention on carbohydrates found in wholegrain foods as well as in vegetables and fruit. To avoid insulin spikes, forgo meals that are made up mostly of sugars or starches without fibre (think snack foods and soft drinks). Instead of white toast with jam for breakfast, have wholewheat toast with a tomato or banana.

EAT FOODS WITH A LOWER GLYCAEMIC INDEX. The GI or glycaemic index indicates the rate at which carbohydrate-rich foods are digested. Foods with a high GI are digested faster and are converted into glucose, leaving you hungry again. They include sweets, biscuits and soft drinks – avoid them if you're trying to lose weight. Foods with a low to medium GI include pasta, lentils, wholegrain bread and apples.

CHOOSE BULKY FOODS. Foods that don't leave you hungry are higher in bulk and lower in calories. Any food that contains plenty of fibre, water or air is a 'bulky' or 'high-volume' food. These include high-fibre fruit and vegetables as well as beans. Instead of eating crisps, choose water-dense grapes. Instead of a glass of orange juice, have an orange, which is far less energy-dense and contains fibre that juice lacks. If you're making chilli con carne, add more beans to bulk it up without adding a lot of calories. Instead of crisps, try air-popped corn. Other low-energy, high-volume foods to favour are soups. Studies show that people who start a meal with soup eat less at that meal and later in the day. Just be sure to avoid cream soups, which are high in calories.

WATCH OUT FOR LOW-FAT FOODS. Some low-fat foods, such as low-fat dairy products, are a real boon to dieters. But food manufacturers often remove fat from biscuits and other treats only to replace that fat with sugar. So check the label before you indulge with abandon; a serving may contain just as many calories as the higher-fat original version.

CAUTION

Beware of any diet regimen driven by an obvious profit motive. Fad diets don't work in the long term. Be wary of so-called 'fat blockers' and 'starch blockers'; their claims to absorb fat and block digestion of starch have not been proven. Nor should you be tempted by herbal weight-loss products sold over the internet; many are packed with stimulants such as ephedrine that can provoke cardiac arrhythmias and other serious side effects.

Cutting saturated fat from your diet and replacing it with unsaturated fat makes sense, as your body needs some fat to function well. Replace some of the meat you eat with fish or poultry. Remove the skin from poultry before you cook it, and banish the frying pan in favour of steaming, grilling, baking or barbecuing. Choose lean cuts of meat and also trim off visible fat. And stay away from sausages, bacon and salami.

Don't attempt to cut all the fat out of your diet. The type of fat you eat is more important than the quantity you eat. Research has shown that people are able to stay on a diet longer and are better able to maintain their weight loss when their diets allow at least some foods that contain unsaturated fat – for example, nuts and olive oil.

DOWNSIZE YOUR PORTIONS. We have become used to bigger and bigger portions both at home and when we eat out. If your fast-food restaurant offers super-size or 'value meals', think twice about where those extra calories will end up!

At restaurants, order a starter rather than a main course. When eating at home, check the portion size of foods you enjoy. If your pasta portion has grown to two cups, cut it back to one and a half, and your waistline will start to show the difference. To fool your eye into thinking you're getting more food, use a smaller plate for your meal or a smaller bowl instead for your pasta.

DRINK PLENTY OF FLUIDS – ESPECIALLY WATER. An adequate liquid intake is essential. Bottled or tap water are both good choices. Fluids quench your thirst and reduce your appetite as well. Fruit juice is healthy, but adds calories without fibre. Coffee or tea is fine. If you take it with sugar or milk, use skimmed milk and an artificial

Do one simple thing

Eat more calcium-rich foods

Evidence suggests that calcium may stimulate fat loss by suppressing hormones that cause fat to be stored rather than burned. Adding calcium-rich foods such as milk, yoghurt or other dairy products to a low-calorie diet therefore may make it easier for your body to mobilise fat stores and burn fat.

Did you know?

Eating some fat helps you to stay on a diet

Researchers at Harvard Medical School and Brigham and Women's Hospital in Boston studied people on two weight-loss diets. Both diets contained the same number of calories but one was low in fat and the other higher in monounsaturated fats, such as olive oil, rape seed oil, peanuts and other nuts. The researchers found that those on the higher-fat regimen (45 to 60g added fat per day) were able to stay on their diet longer and were better able to maintain their weight loss.

sweetener. Allow yourself to have an occasional glass of wine or beer if you wish, but be aware that they add about 120kcal per glass.

DON'T DEPRIVE YOURSELF. Let yourself have small portions of your favourite high-calorie foods once in a while so that you don't get frustrated and end up bingeing.

KEEP YOUR EYE ON THE MIRROR. Most people on a diet want to see a lower weight reflected on the bathroom scales. But remember, while you're losing fat, if you're exercising, you may be adding muscle, so your weight might remain the same for a while. Instead of relying totally on the scales, check your reflection in the mirror, your clothing size, your energy level and the notches on your belt.

NEVER FAST. Fasting, even when plenty of water is consumed, can be very dangerous; it may lead to lowered blood pressure and heart failure. Also, weight loss achieved by fasting is rarely sustained once normal eating is resumed. If you must fast, make sure it is under medical supervision and do it for no longer than necessary.

Digestive disorders

CONSUME PLENTY OF

- Fresh fruit, vegetables, wholegrain products and other high-fibre foods to help digestion

- Fluids (usually six to eight glasses of water, juices or other non-alcoholic fluids daily)

LIMIT

- Coffee, tea and other sources of caffeine

- Refined carbohydrates

- Fried foods and other high-fat foods

AVOID

- Any foods or beverages that provoke a flare-up of symptoms

Digestion refers to the overall process by which food is broken down mechanically and chemically and is converted to forms that can be absorbed into the bloodstream and delivered to cells. Only water, salt, simple sugars such as glucose and some other small molecules can be absorbed unchanged. Starches, fats and proteins must be broken down into smaller molecules before they can be used. Specific proteins called enzymes play a significant role in the breakdown of food.

The digestive process actually begins in the mouth. As food is chewed, it is mixed with saliva, which moistens it and supplies enzymes that start breaking down carbohydrates. Once the food has been sufficiently chewed, it is carried through the oesophagus, which has a ring of muscles at its base that relaxes to open the passage to the stomach. The ring should normally close to prevent food and stomach acid from returning to the oesophagus. In some cases the ring fails to close properly and food is regurgitated, a process that is referred to as reflux; this can occur in people with a hiatus hernia. Reflux can cause indigestion and heartburn, the most common digestive disorders.

When food reaches the stomach, it is churned by the stomach's muscular walls and broken down into smaller pieces. In addition, the stomach walls secrete gastric acid and an enzyme called pepsin that begins the breakdown of protein. Special mucus-producing cells within the stomach ordinarily prevent it from digesting its own tissues with these strong digestive juices. If these mechanisms fail for any reason, an ulcer can arise.

By the time the food leaves the stomach, it has already been converted into a semi-fluid called chyme. Digestion continues in the duodenum, the start of the small intestine, where bile from the liver and enzymes from the pancreas break down fats, carbohydrates and proteins. The intestine is a muscular tube that moves food with rhythmic contractions known as peristalsis. The 6m long small intestine is lined with millions of hairlike projections called villi. These have surface membranes that allow the digested nutrients to pass through them and into the tiny blood vessels they harbour. Amino acids from proteins and glucose from sugars are absorbed directly into the bloodstream for delivery to cells throughout the body. While smaller fat molecules also go into the blood, larger ones enter the lymph system.

Fibre and other undigested waste products move into the large intestine, or colon, where much of the water they contain is reabsorbed. That's one reason it is important to drink enough water, juices and other non-alcoholic fluids a day; otherwise, the faecal mass moving through the colon may become dehydrated, resulting in constipation. Fibre absorbs large amounts of water, and it, along with some of the starches from vegetables and fruit, provides the bulk that helps to stimulate the muscles of the colon.

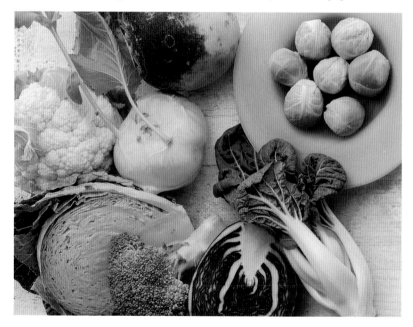

◀ **Eat plenty of fresh vegetables**
Vegetables are low in fat, low in calories and are excellent sources of fibre, which is essential for a healthy digestive system.

Depending on the contents of a meal and a person's individual metabolic rate, it may take from 2 to 6 hours for a meal to be fully digested and its nutrients absorbed. Simple sugars are broken down rapidly and may enter the bloodstream just minutes after eating. Starches require about an hour or longer to be digested; proteins need 2 to 3 hours. Fat takes from 4 to 6 hours to be digested and absorbed. For this reason, protein and fat will satisfy hunger for longer periods of time than sugars and carbohydrates will. It takes another 8 to 36 hours for the undigested waste to move through the colon.

The intestine has a remarkable ability to heal itself. It replaces its lining every 72 hours and reacts swiftly to expel harmful substances. However, a diet high in refined and nutritionally deficient foods, usually found in Western countries, can lead to digestive problems ranging from unpleasant but minor episodes of indigestion to more serious disorders such as diverticulitis.

Digestive disorders

The digestive system has a relatively small repertoire of symptoms, principally nausea, vomiting, pain (such as heartburn), bloating, cramping, diarrhoea, constipation and excessive flatulence. The onset of such symptoms may simply reflect a normal response to an unusual meal or be associated with some lifestyle factor, such as eating an improper diet or dealing with the stresses of daily life. Excitement, disappointment, fear, anxiety and other strong emotions can cause some upset in the digestive system. This should not cause alarm if it is transient.

The digestive system's limited set of distress symptoms means that the same symptoms may also reflect any one of a number of very serious

Do one simple thing

Cook with healing herbs

Some herbs are known to help troubled digestion. Ginger, for example, has been shown to ease nausea. Many of the herbs and spices traditionally used in cooking aid digestion, so use plenty of mint, dill, caraway, horseradish, bay, chervil, fennel, tarragon, marjoram, cumin, cinnamon, ginger and cardamom. Chamomile tea or Angostura bitters, a tincture of the bitter gentian root, may also help. A small amount of bitters can promote digestion and alleviate flatulence.

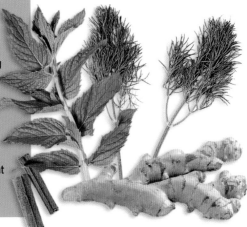

▼ **Herbs and spices**
Cinnamon, mint, dill and ginger are some of the herbs and spices that can help digestion.

disorders, including gastritis, or inflammation of the stomach lining; problems in the intestine, such as ulcerative colitis or Crohn's disease (both are inflammatory disorders); diverticulitis, an inflammation and infection of small sacs protruding from the intestinal wall; irritable bowel syndrome, a functional disorder that affects movement within the intestine; or cancer anywhere in the digestive tract. Similarly, nausea and vomiting may be triggered by an adverse reaction to a medication, emotional upset, mild viral infection, ear disorder, migraine headache and motion sickness, as well as other serious disorders, including a heart attack and intestinal obstruction.

Malabsorption disorders

A similar group of symptoms, especially diarrhoea and bloating, also indicate a malabsorption problem, which occurs when the digestive tract is unable to properly utilise one or more components of the diet. Depending on the severity of the problem, the person may experience weight loss, muscle wasting and show evidence of vitamin and mineral deficiencies. While some malabsorption

problems are congenital, others may occur because of illness or its treatment. Problems may arise from the digestive tract itself, or from disorders of the heart and blood vessels, the endocrine glands or the lymph system.

Some malabsorption conditions involve a single nutrient, as in coeliac disease, when the body is unable to absorb gluten, or lactose intolerance, when the body is unable to digest lactose, the sugar in milk. Others involve an array of nutrients. For example, in cystic fibrosis, enzymes needed to digest protein, carbohydrate and fat are either missing completely or are present only in reduced amounts.

People with malabsorption problems may be in danger of malnutrition. They may avoid certain foods to prevent symptoms, and not get adequate nutrients. Or the side effects of the disorder may lead to malnutrition. For example, when fat is not properly absorbed, it is discharged from the body as waste and takes with it the fat-soluble vitamins A, D, E and K.

A dietitian can plan meals to help with malabsorption problems, and a doctor or dietitian may recommend vitamin and mineral supplements.

Diverticulitis

CONSUME PLENTY OF

- Fresh fruit and vegetables
- Wholegrain cereals and bread
- Fluids (water, juice, milk, soup and tea)

LIMIT

- Refined carbohydrates, such as biscuits, cakes and sweets

Diverticula are small pouches that form in the wall of the large intestine, creating a condition called diverticulosis. The specific cause remains unknown, but the disease occurs most often in people aged over 60 and who are overweight. Weakening of the intestinal wall as a person ages is believed to contribute to the formation of the pouches. As pressure builds up in the large intestine – for example, during a bout of constipation – the weakened areas balloon outward into pouches.

The pouches or sacs are not a problem in themselves, producing no symptoms until they become infected or inflamed – which can occur when waste flowing through the intestine is diverted into one of the sacs and becomes impacted. The resulting condition is called diverticulitis, or inflammation of the diverticula. It can be painful and serious, and may lead to complications, such as abscesses, intestinal obstruction or perforation of the intestinal wall. In addition to abdominal cramps and pain, other symptoms of diverticulitis include gas, flatulence, fever and rectal bleeding. Constipation may alternate with diarrhoea, in some cases.

Diverticulitis occurs primarily in the industrialised Western world, where diets that are high in fat and low in fibre are common. Inadequate consumption of dietary fibre can cause stools to become hard and compact, resulting in constipation. This may provoke unnatural contractions of the large intestine, which in turn leads to the formation of diverticula.

The role of dietary fibre

A diet rich in vegetables and wholegrain cereals may help to prevent diverticulitis. The ailment is known to be less common among vegetarians than those who include meat in their diet.

◀ **Foods to avoid during an acute attack** Any foods that have hulls, seeds, strings or other fibrous parts can become trapped in the diverticula, leading to inflammation and other intestinal symptoms.

Vegetarian diets are typically higher in fibre-rich foods, such as vegetables, fruit, cereals and grains. However, excessive fibre, taken as unprocessed bran, can create other digestive problems; for example, studies have suggested that it can irritate the colon. It is important to increase fibre intake gradually, giving the body a chance to get used to it. If you have diverticular disease, do not start taking fibre supplements without first discussing this with your doctor.

To date, there is no scientific evidence to support the association between nuts and seeds and inflammation of the diverticula. People with diverticular disease consuming a diet low in fibre demonstrate more disease symptoms than those consuming a liberal diet (including nuts and seeds).

However, foods with indigestible particles such as corn, nuts and seeds may need to be avoided during an acute attack of diverticulitis. In addition, people may find that certain foods cause inflammation and pain and so should avoid them.

Drink plenty of water. Along with a high-fibre diet, increased fluid intake (six to eight glasses a day) may help to produce bulky, soft stools that move easily through the intestinal tract.

If you have diverticular disease, it is important to avoid constipation, which can increase your risk of a diverticulitis flare-up.

Eating to boost energy
A new mindset

In our fast-paced, high-stress society, fatigue and even exhaustion have become the norm. More sleep, of course, is the best answer. But the right diet can also help to fuel your body for the long haul and keep your energy levels from flagging throughout the day.

WHERE DOES ENERGY COME FROM?

The major components of all foods – proteins, fats and carbohydrates, – are the nutrients that provide calories and so give you energy. The human body converts carbohydrates to glucose, its most important source of energy. Glucose is the 'blood sugar' that rises after eating carbohydrates. A rise in blood sugar triggers your pancreas to release insulin, a hormone that helps glucose enter the body's cells. Once inside the cell, glucose supplies the energy to fuel your body. A certain amount of glucose is converted to glycogen and stored in the muscles and liver. Your body draws on liver glycogen stores whenever your blood sugar drops. Once glycogen stores are full, excess glucose is converted to fat.

Protein can also be converted to energy but is a less efficient source than carbohydrates. While fats are the most concentrated source of calories, they are actually a less efficient source of energy than carbohydrates because they take longer to digest and metabolise.

Despite some extravagant claims, vitamins don't provide energy. They are needed, however, to power many of the metabolic processes that lead to energy production. A diet that includes an ample supply of vegetables, legumes, fruit and wholegrain products will provide adequate vitamins and minerals. Fruit also provides sugars that are converted to energy.

SEVEN STRATEGIES FOR HIGH-ENERGY EATING

Eating for optimal energy breaks many of the 'rules' people commonly believe – for instance, that carbohydrates are bad, that snacking is a no-no, and that sugar is a good pick-me-up. These seven simple steps will put you on the right path.

1. EAT BREAKFAST. This is the meal that sets you up for the day, replenishing your body's energy supply after a night's fast. You will feel lethargic if you force your body to keep going all morning without any fuel. Eat a sustaining breakfast such as wholemeal toast, wholegrain cereal, porridge, or fresh fruit and yoghurt. Studies have shown that children who eat breakfast concentrate better, are more creative and behave better; this may apply to adults as well.

2. GET ENOUGH IRON-RICH FOODS. Iron-deficiency anaemia is one of the most common nutritional deficiencies in the world. Iron is essential for producing haemoglobin, the main component of red blood cells. Haemoglobin carries oxygen to your body's cells where it is used to

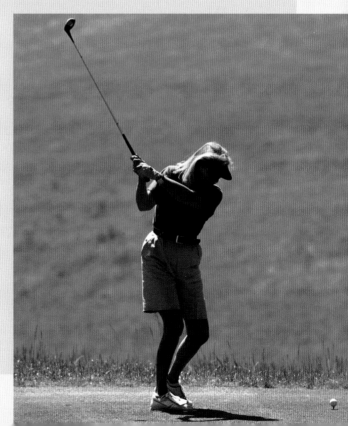

produce energy and perform essential metabolic functions. If your iron stores are low, your red blood cells can't supply as much oxygen to the cells. The results of iron deficiency are fatigue, low energy and difficulty in concentrating. The best food sources are oysters, mussels, red meats, offal, iron-fortified cereal products and wholegrain breads, dried fruit, green leafy vegetables, beans, tofu, nuts and seeds.

There are two kinds of iron in our food: haem and non-haem. Haem iron, found in red meat, chicken and fish, is better absorbed than the non-haem iron found in enriched cereals, some dark green vegetables, beans, eggs, nuts and seeds.

You can help your body to absorb non-haem iron by eating the food with one that contains vitamin C. For example, if you want to increase the absorption of iron from a bowl of iron-enriched cereal (such as wheat biscuits), have a banana, some strawberries or a glass of orange juice.

3. FOCUS ON COMPLEX CARBOHYDRATES. Carbohydrates found in breads, grains, cereals, fruit, starchy vegetables and sweets are digested and end up as the simple sugar, glucose.

CAUTION

Increasing your iron intake comes with an important caution. Do not take iron supplements unless you know you are iron deficient and cannot correct the deficiency with an appropriate diet. Too much iron can cause constipation, and excessive doses can be toxic, especially for the 1 in 300 people who have haemochromatosis and store excess iron. If you think that you are tired because of an iron deficiency, check with your doctor.

This glucose provides fuel for your brain, muscles and other body tissues. Choose complex carbohydrates in wholegrain breads and cereals, lentils, legumes and starchy vegetables since they are digested slowly and serve as a steady fuel supply for body and brain. In addition, they provide many important vitamins, minerals and plant chemicals to keep your body well nourished.

4. GO EASY ON THE SIMPLE SUGARS. Sweets and soft drinks, for example, may give you a quick rise in energy but this is usually followed by a 'crash' that leaves you tireder than ever.

5. EAT SMALL AMOUNTS OF FOOD THROUGHOUT THE DAY. Small meals and/or snacks throughout the day stave off hunger and keep blood sugar steady; low blood sugar is a common cause of afternoon fatigue. Lunch is also an important way to refuel for the afternoon. A sandwich, soup, cheese and crackers, yoghurt with fruit or a bean dip and vegetables all make the nutritional grade. Just be sure to eat less at mealtimes if you're snacking between meals.

6. STAY HYDRATED. Most people need at least six to eight glasses of fluid a day to stay properly hydrated. If you exercise, drink more. Water regulates your body temperature, transports nutrients to your body and carries waste away. Fatigue is one symptom of mild dehydration. If you sweat heavily during exercise or in extreme heat, you may not be able to depend on thirst as an indicator of your fluid needs and you could be mildly dehydrated without knowing. You should get in the habit of consuming fluids regularly, even if you are not active. Fluids can come from water, tea, coffee, juice, sports drinks, milk, soup or watery foods such as lettuce, cucumbers and fruit.

7. GO EASY ON CAFFEINE. The proper amount of sleep is vital for staying energetic. Caffeine is a stimulant that fights with adenosine, a chemical that helps to induce sleep. The more caffeine you drink, the less adenosine is available for making you drowsy – and your sleep may suffer as a result.

The Glycaemic Index

Some carbohydrate-rich foods are digested and absorbed into your bloodstream quickly while others are broken down more slowly. The Glycaemic Index (GI) is a tool developed to measure how different carbohydrates affect your blood sugar after they are eaten and digested.

Foods with a low to medium GI such as rye bread, brown rice, bulghur wheat, oats, lentils, apples, pears and yoghurt cause a slower, more gradual rise in blood sugar, take longer to digest and so release energy more slowly, leading to more consistent energy levels. Foods with lower GIs are better for blood-sugar control in diabetes and may help with weight loss.

High-GI foods such as sweets, many snacks, sports drinks, cornflakes and watermelon are more quickly absorbed and so provide a quicker source of energy.

For athletes or other active people, high-GI foods can be a source of quick energy to aid short-duration sports performance and recovery, while lower-GI foods are better for endurance events. (For more on this, see *Glycaemic Index*.)

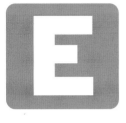

Ear disorders

CONSUME PLENTY OF

- Garlic, onions and chillies when mucus is a problem, plus vitamin-rich foods

LIMIT

- Foods high in saturated fats

Ear problems should never be ignored. Whether you experience dizziness, earache or pain, consult your doctor.

Glue ear is a common condition in children. It is the result of a build-up of sticky mucus behind the eardrum. A possible link has been found between it and bottle-feeding. When a child is breastfed, the action of sucking on the breast exercises a muscle that helps to open the Eustachian tube, which connects the middle ear to the back of the throat and drains away any fluid. In bottle-feeding the muscle is not as well exercised.

There are two main kinds of hearing loss: one is usually caused by something in the ear such as fluid, wax, a burst eardrum or a disease such as otosclerosis; the other is nerve deafness and is usually age-related (about 30 per cent of people aged over 60 have some hearing loss) or it may be the result of acoustic trauma, infections, tumours, drugs or diseases such as multiple sclerosis or Ménière's disease. There are also congenital causes. Vitamin A and thiamin are thought to help to repair damaged cell tissue in the ear and strengthen the auditory nerve. Vitamin A is found in liver and as beta carotene in apricots, carrots, mangoes and spinach; wholemeal bread contains thiamin. It may be advisable to avoid dairy products and eat garlic, chillies, onion and horseradish which help to reduce mucus production, although there is no scientific proof that these measures will be effective.

Ménière's disease may respond to a low-salt diet.

Eczema

CONSUME PLENTY OF

- Oily fish and evening primrose oil

AVOID

- Foods that trigger or worsen eczema
- External causes, such as wearing woollen clothing next to the skin

Eczema is an itchy, scaly rash often caused by sensitivity to foods, certain chemicals or environmental conditions such as dryness. It affects one in five children and 1 in 12 adults in Britain, and has increased threefold over the past 30 years.

Two common types of eczema are contact eczema, which develops in people who are sensitive to certain irritants, and atopic eczema which often runs in families, along with a tendency to develop asthma, hay fever, urticaria or hives.

Do one simple thing

Drink three cups of oolong tea to avoid eczema

One study suggests that consuming 3 cups of oolong tea a day relieves the symptoms of eczema. It is believed that the polyphenols found in the tea act as antioxidants and suppress allergic responses.

The role of diet

Certain foods can trigger eczema. Common culprits include eggs, dairy products, nuts, seafood, soya products, wheat, yeast and certain food additives.

Some babies develop eczema when their mothers stop breast-feeding and introduce formula milk, which may indicate an intolerance to cow's milk. If the baby develops eczema while the mother is still breastfeeding, the mother should consider consulting a dietitian about her own diet, since babies rarely react badly to mother's milk. Cow's milk can cause eczema in babies and small children; a few may be able to tolerate goat's milk or soya-based products. Most children out-grow sensitivities by the age of four.

Consume more antioxidants. Dryness may cause eczema by triggering the formation of free radicals and so may be countered by antioxidants such as beta carotene. Preliminary studies indicate that foods rich in beta carotene can improve eczema. Brightly coloured fruit and vegetables including apricots, mangoes, carrots, pumpkin and sweet potatoes are good choices.

Eat foods rich in essential fatty acids. Foods like vegetable oils, fish, and linseeds may decrease swelling by helping to generate hormone-like substances called prostaglandins, which reduce inflammation.

Another excellent source of essential fatty acids is evening primrose oil.

Get enough vitamin B$_6$. Some researchers believe a diet rich in vitamin B$_6$ protects against sensitivity rashes. Good sources include fish, legumes, brown rice, wheatgerm and meat (especially pork), peanuts, avocados and potatoes.

Dip into the yoghurt. If you have an infant with eczema, try adding probiotics to his or her diet, through either yoghurt or supplements.

E

A recent Finnish study found that eating the probiotic *Lactobacillus acidophilus* halved the incidence of eczema, compared with infants who were receiving a placebo. It is safe to use *L. acidophilus at an early age.*

Try adding a container of live-culture yoghurt to your own daily diet, if you are not allergic to dairy products. Although no studies have been done yet to prove its efficacy, yoghurt may work just as well for adults as it does for babies.

Environmental triggers

Chemicals in the environment probably trigger eczema more often than foods do. Common offenders include nickel, which is often used for making costume jewellery and latex, which is used in household and industrial rubber gloves.

People sensitive to wool should also try to avoid skin-care products based on lanolin, the natural oil that is found in wool.

It makes sense to avoid known triggers. If your rash is worse in either hot or very cold weather, avoid extremes of temperature. Buy only soaps, detergents and toilet papers that are free of dyes and perfumes.

Eggs

BENEFITS

■ An excellent source of protein, vitamins A, D and the B group, zinc and iron

■ A source of the antioxidants lutein and zeaxanthin

DRAWBACKS

■ Yolks are high in cholesterol

■ A common cause of food allergy

The egg is one of nature's best designs, providing all that a developing chick requires. Its protective shell is strong enough to support the mother hen's weight as heat is transferred from her body to the chick, and also supplies all the chick's dietary requirements of protein, vitamins and minerals.

Despite concerns about their high cholesterol content, eggs remain a popular and inexpensive source of nourishment. Eggs are a nutrient powerhouse. Like other animal proteins, those supplied by eggs contain all the essential amino acids. In one egg you get protein, vitamins A, D and the B group, zinc and iron. Eggs are also an excellent source of vitamin B_{12}, which is essential for proper nerve function. Because vitamin B_{12} is found only in animal products, vegetarians can rely on eggs as an important source of this vitamin.

Eggs are a good source of the antioxidants lutein and zeaxanthin, linked to a reduced risk of age-related macular degeneration, which is a leading cause of loss of vision in older adults. Lecithin – a natural emulsifier found in eggs – is rich in choline, which helps to move cholesterol through the bloodstream, as well as aiding fat metabolism.

Choline is also an essential component of cell membranes and nerve tissue. Although the body can make enough choline for its normal needs, it has been suggested that dietary sources may be helpful in reducing the accumulation of fat in the liver, as well as repairing some types of neurological damage. Choline is thought to be important for early brain development and may improve memory later in life.

The cholesterol issue

A large egg (70g) contains 106kcal, 7.8g of fat, 2.2g of saturated fat and 266mg cholesterol. Studies show that for most healthy people, it is saturated fat (found in fatty meat, chicken skin, full-fat dairy products and coconut and hydrogenated vegetable oils) and trans fats (found in processed and snack foods) that have the greatest effect on blood cholesterol levels. In general, the cholesterol we get from our food (and that includes eggs) is not an important factor in raising blood cholesterol. It is far mor important to cut down on saturated fats in your diet.

There is no recommended limit on how many eggs people eat. So, as long as you are eating a normal, balanced diet, you need to cut down on eggs only if you have been told to do so by your doctor or a dietitian for a specific reason. But the British Heart Foundation has suggested that those with high cholesterol should eat no more than three eggs a week.

In this case, as only the yolks of eggs contain cholesterol, egg whites need not be restricted. In fact, the whites can be used to replace whole eggs or just the yolks in many recipes without detriment to their taste or texture. For example, you can replace one whole egg with two whites, or you can substitute beaten whites instead of a whole egg to coat foods for frying.

Eggs rich in Omega-3

Omega-3 enhanced eggs are laid by hens fed a diet high in omega-3 fats, so their yolks contain omega-3s, the polyunsaturated fats that are associated with lower risk of heart disease and stroke. These eggs are low in saturated fat and are a better source of vitamin E than regular eggs.

▶ **Eggs of the world**
Chicken eggs are most often used in our homes, but in other parts of the world, quail, duck and goose eggs are eaten as well.

Confusing egg labels

Labels such as 'farm' or 'country-fresh' can conjure up misleading images; the hens that laid the eggs may well have been raised in cages. Eggs labelled as 'free range' can be applied to any battery hens with daylight access to open-air runs and palatable vegetation and shade. The terms 'barn' or 'perchery' are equally misleading. These are often laid by hens in cramped barns. There are no significant differences in protein, mineral or vitamin content between free-range eggs and eggs from caged hens but free-range hens that eat green material may have higher levels of carotenoids.

Always open the carton to inspect eggs before you buy them. Reject cracked eggs and run your fingers across the top of the eggs to ensure none are stuck to the bottom of the box. It is a myth that brown eggs are more nutritious than white ones. Both are equally nutritious; they simply come from different breeds of chicken.

Egg facts

- Eggs age more in one day at room temperature than in one week in the refrigerator.
- Egg yolks are one of the few foods that contain vitamin D, which is normally obtained from sunshine. So, in winter, it is helpful to keep up your egg intake.

Storing eggs

Keep eggs in the main part of the refrigerator, which is cooler than the shelves on the inside of the door. Store the pointed end of the egg down, so that the yolk remains centred in the shell away from the air pocket at the larger end. Refrigerated eggs can be kept safely for up to three weeks.

Did you know?

Eggs are a 'complete protein' food

Protein is composed of 20 different amino acids. Nine of these amino acids cannot be made by the body. These nine are considered essential amino acids and must come from food. Those foods that contain all nine essential amino acids are called 'complete protein' foods.

Test for freshness

To check if an egg is fresh, place it in a bowl of cold water. Fresh eggs sink; stale eggs will float because air will have entered and increased the size of the air cell.

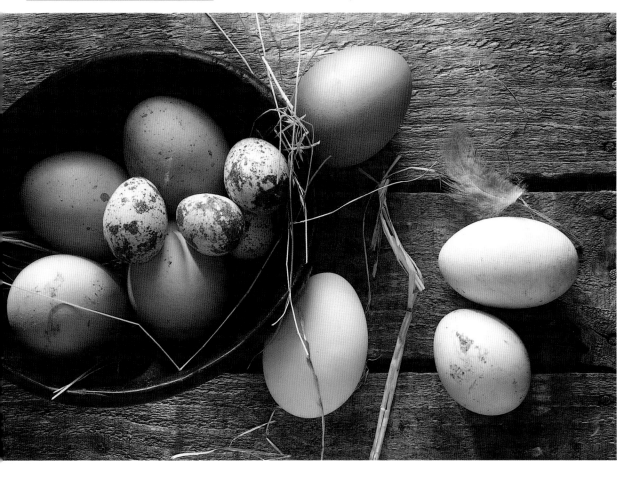

The salmonella scare

One egg in 7,000 may be found to harbour salmonella bacteria, which can be passed on by the hen or can enter through cracked shells. Although the risk of food poisoning is relatively low these days, it is best to avoid eating raw or partly cooked eggs. People at special risk include the frail elderly, young children, pregnant women and anyone with lowered immunity due to illness.

Foods to avoid are Caesar salads, fresh mayonnaise, egg-based sauces and dressings, mousses and ice cream as they can all contain raw or partly cooked eggs.

To be certain that eggs have been cooked for long enough, boil them for at least 4 minutes, poach them for 5 minutes or fry them for 3 minutes. Both the yolk and the white should be firm. Omelettes and scrambled eggs should be cooked until firm and not runny.

Another way to tell a fresh egg from an old one is by breaking the shell and tipping the contents onto a plate: a fresh egg has a high, rounded yolk and the white is thick and gel-like. In an older egg, the yolk will be flatter and the white will be thin and spread widely.

Allergies and eggs

Eggs are among the foods most likely to trigger allergic reactions. People who are allergic to eggs should be on the lookout for obvious sources, such as sauces and mayonnaise, pancakes and bakery items, as well as ice cream. They should always check food labels, which must declare the presence of all ingredients derived from eggs. Those allergic to eggs should also avoid flu shots and other vaccines incubated in eggs.

Energy bars

BENEFITS

- Convenient and portable
- Some are sources of protein, fibre, carbohydrates, vitamins and minerals

DRAWBACKS

- Many are high in calories, sugar and/or fats

Energy bars – the words conjure up visions of high-performance athletes going the distance on the strength of a single bar. These bars have come into the mainstream and are sold in supermarkets, gyms and health-food shops. People eat them as a performance enhancer, a snack, a high-energy, nutritional pick-me-up, a meal replacement and even a weight-loss tool.

The word energy means the capacity for work or vigorous activity. In the nutrition world, the word energy is synonymous with calories. The truth is that all foods give you energy. Just because a food is called an energy bar, it does not mean that eating it will make you more energetic.

Energy bars are not magic foods, but if you're a serious athlete, working out for a long time, or engaging in an endurance sport such as a triathlon or marathon, they can help.

If you're trying to increase your calorie intake to support an endurance event and have eaten your full food allowance, energy bars can provide the extra calories along with other important nutrients. They're portable, non-perishable and may be handier, at times, than yoghurt, fruit or other high-energy snacks.

Many athletes find nibbling them helpful during a long run, and they have proven to be popular with rowers, cyclists and sailors. Energy bars also come in handy for all-day sports events when other foods are not available.

While endurance competitors may reap benefits, energy bars aren't much help for recreational athletes. They won't provide extra performance, build muscle or increase stamina. That has to come from training. If the extra calories provided by these energy bars are not 'burned', they can quickly lead to weight gain.

For busy people on the go, these products can be a handy midday snack or a pre or post-workout snack if you don't have access to fruit, bread or yoghurt.

What's in a bar?

All bars are not created equal, and it is important to examine what you are eating and determine if it is right for you. There are high-carbohydrate bars, high-protein bars, breakfast bars, brain-boosting bars, meal-replacement bars, diet bars and more. Some are nutritious and some are not.

Look for bars that are low in saturated or trans fats. A giveaway for the presence of trans fats is the term 'hydrogenated fat' on the label. Some bars are a good source of fibre – aim for 3g to 5g – and offer some vitamins and minerals.

High-protein bars can be helpful for vegetarian athletes, long-distance runners, and people who require high-protein diets. Go for bars with protein sources such as whey, soya, casein or nuts and seeds.

The meal-replacement bars are sometimes used by people trying to lose weight, but should not be used on a regular basis. If you are using the bar as an occasional meal replacement, look for the bars with at least 10g to 15g of protein.

If you are an athlete, try different bars during your workouts before you use them in a competition.

Everyone's system is different, so it's important to find what works best for you before you are in a race.

While energy bars may appear to have the same vitamins and minerals found in fruit, vegetables and grains, they don't contain the phytochemicals, bioflavonoids and natural fibre found in foods. They also contain more calories from added sugars and fats.

Epilepsy

AVOID

- Alcohol

- Any food that appears to trigger attacks or may interact with anticonvulsants

One in every 200 Britons has some form of epilepsy, recurrent seizures triggered by abnormal electrical impulses in the brain. Some seizures are so mild and fleeting that they are barely noticeable; others last for several minutes, during which the person falls down and is convulsed. The frequency of seizures also varies; some people with epilepsy suffer many seizures each day, while others may go for months between episodes. Medication keeps 80 per cent of sufferers free from seizures.

Neurologists generally discount any link between diet and epilepsy, with some exceptions. People with epilepsy who have migraine headaches that are triggered by certain foods often cease to have seizures when the offending foods are eliminated.

Some people with diabetes suffer seizures when their blood sugar levels drop suddenly. Large amounts of alcohol consumed in a short time can cause seizures. Although the evidence is sketchy, there have been rare reports of aspartame triggering seizures in those with epilepsy.

The high-fat diet

A rigid diet that appears to halt seizures in children whose attacks cannot be controlled by drugs has been hailed as a recent break-through. In reality, however, the diet dates to the early 1900s, when doctors devised a dietary treatment for epilepsy based on the ancient observation that seizures ceased during periods of prolonged fasting. Fasting is hardly a practical long-term treatment for chronic seizures, but researchers found that a high-fat diet mimicked fasting metabolism without starvation.

The ketogenic diet. With the development of effective anti-convulsant drugs, the dietary treatment was dropped. But now a dietary treatment for some cases of severe epilepsy is occasionally used. After about 24 hours of fasting, or 48 hours on a low-carbohydrate diet, the body depletes its reserves of glucose and starts to burn stored fat for energy. However, burning fat in the absence of glucose gives off waste products called ketone bodies, which build up in the blood and are excreted in the urine. Very high blood levels of ketones can upset body chemistry, and even lead to a coma and death. But at lower levels they may eliminate some seizures. Carefully structuring the diet by allowing only a sprinkling of carbohydrates can result in a therapeutic level of ketones in the bloodstream.

This regimen, called the ketogenic diet, appears to work best in young children, especially that 20 per cent whose seizures are not adequately controlled by drugs. The diet provides about 75 per cent of the calories generally recommended for healthy children, and most of these come from fats. Protein is added to allow for growth, but carbohydrates are kept to a minimum. Fluid intake is restricted.

The diet must be carefully tailored to the patient and followed exactly: even a small deviation can bring on seizures. It can be difficult to follow, but after two to three years, most patients can go back to eating normally and still be seizure-free.

Unfortunately, studies show that the long-term use of this diet leads to raised blood cholesterol.

Eye disorders

CONSUME PLENTY OF

- Carrots, sweet potatoes and dark green vegetables for beta carotene

- Citrus and kiwi fruit for vitamin C

- Salmon, sardines, herring and dairy products for vitamin A

- Nuts, seeds, seed oils and avocados for vitamin E

- Seafood, meat, poultry, wheatgerm and beans for zinc

- Leafy greens, peas, sweetcorn and peppers for lutein and zeaxanthin

LIMIT

- Saturated and trans fats

The role of antioxidant nutrients and bioflavonoids in vision loss and other degenerative problems associated with ageing is becoming increasingly clear. With advancing age, there is an increase in the body's production of free radicals, those unstable molecules that form when the body uses oxygen. Free radicals can cause eye damage similar to that resulting from exposure to radiation, and can also contribute to such disorders as cataracts and macular degeneration.

Age-related disorders

Cataracts develop when the lens, the transparent membrane that allows light to enter the eye, yellows,

E

hindering the passage of light rays through it. Vision becomes hazy, cloudy or blurry; if untreated, the lens may become completely opaque, resulting in loss of vision.

Although ageing is the most common cause of cataracts, they can occur at any time of life, even in infancy. Smoking and diabetes can hasten their development. But a diet that provides ample antioxidants – in particular, vitamins C and E and the carotenoid lutein – appears to slow their progression.

At least one study has shown that the prevalence of cataracts was significantly lower in people who took vitamin C supplements for at least ten years but other studies have not confirmed these results. Some antioxidants may ward off the damage done by free-radicals.

Macular degeneration, another eye disease that is usually associated with ageing, is one of the most common causes of loss of vision among older people. It entails a gradual, painless deterioration of the macula, the tissue in the central portion of the retina. The first symptom is usually blurring of central vision but eventually peripheral vision also becomes limited. The cause of macular degeneration is unknown, but recent research suggests that a diet high in antioxidant nutrients may help to prevent or slow the disorder.

Lutein and zeaxanthin are two antioxidants that may help. These carotenoids are the dominant pigments in the macula of the eye and are thought to help to filter out some of the harmful light that can damage the retina.

Lutein is found in green leafy vegetables such as broccoli, kale and watercress, as well as in sweetcorn, peas and egg yolks. Greens, red peppers and sweetcorn are excellent sources of zeaxanthin.

One clinical trial involved more than 3,500 people aged 55 to 80 who already had at least one symptom of age-related macular degeneration. Some were treated with zinc alone, some took the antioxidant vitamins C, E and beta carotene, some took that mixture plus zinc. Those who took the antioxidants plus zinc had the lowest risk of developing advanced stages of macular degeneration.

Research also shows that a diet high in saturated or trans fats increases the risk of age-related macular degeneration. Scientists theorise that saturated fats may clog the arteries in the retina in the same way that they contribute to atherosclerosis in larger blood vessels, such as the coronary arteries. Eating fish more than once a week significantly reduces the risk.

Diabetic retinopathy

There are certain similarities between macular degeneration and diabetic retinopathy – the infiltration of the retina with tiny ruptured blood vessels – which suggest that antioxidant nutrients may also be beneficial in this common complication of diabetes. Diet is critical in maintaining tight control of blood glucose levels, which also reduces the risk of diabetic retinopathy.

Night blindness

The eyes need vitamin A or its precursor, beta carotene, as well as bioflavonoids, to make the pigments that absorb light within the eye. A deficiency in vitamin A, or a failure to utilise it properly, impairs the eye's ability to adapt to darkness and leads to a condition known as 'night blindness'.

This does not entail a total loss of night vision, but rather difficulty in being able to see well in dim

▼ Vitamin A improves night vision
Apricots and other fruit of a deep orange colour, such as mangoes and melon, are rich in carotenoids, some of which is converted to vitamin A – essential for good night vision.

lighting, such as at twilight or dawn when natural light is at its strongest.

Vitamin A deficiency is rare in the Western world, but it remains a major problem in many developing countries. Offal, margarine, butter and other full-cream dairy products are good sources of vitamin A. Dark yellow or orange foods, such as carrots, sweet potatoes, apricots and dark green leafy vegetables, are the richest sources of beta carotene, that the body converts to vitamin A.

Failing night vision should not be self-treated with vitamin A or beta carotene supplements; the problem may stem from a digestive or malabsorption disorder that prevents the body from using the vitamin. Treatment of the underlying cause usually cures the night blindness. An exception is night blindness caused by retinitis pigmentosa, a genetic disease. However, recent research suggests that vitamin A may, in fact, slow the progressive vision loss of this incurable disease.

Conjunctivitis

Also called pink eye, conjunctivitis is an irritation or infection of the delicate membrane that lines the front of the eyeball and eyelid.

Viruses are responsible for most conjunctivitis, but in recurring cases an allergic reaction may be the cause. Soreness and reddening may signal a lack of riboflavin, found in milk, whole grains and offal.

Fast food

Eating on the run

Fast-food restaurants are widespread throughout the United Kingdom, some even being established in hospitals. According to market research statistics, up to 50 per cent of Britons are eating fast food at least once a week.

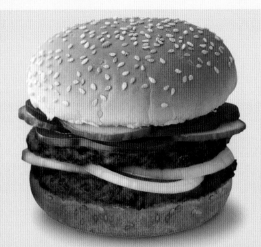

Britain is ranked in the top 10 countries in the world for fast-food consumption. Some critics blame this passion for fast food (which is typically high in fat, sugar, salt and calories) and the super-sizing of portions for the increasing incidence of excess weight and obesity, especially in children and teenagers.

In 1995, an original burger, fries and cola at McDonald's in the USA contained 520kcal. Now a super-size value meal contains an incredible 2,225kcal in the USA and about 1,260kcal here. UK fast food portions have increased in size by 30 per cent over the past decade. Many fast-food chains often advertise 'combo' meals that offer reduced prices if you buy multiple items. Some fast-food establishments are now offering some lower-calorie, healthier options, but the overwhelming majority of the foods we eat at fast-food chains – the burgers, fries, hot dogs, fried chicken and pizza – are loaded with fat, salt and calories, and have very little fibre.

Most fast food is high in saturated fat. Fried foods – especially French fries – also tend to contain significant levels of trans fats, which are now believed to be as bad as – or even worse than – saturated fats for your health.

Fast-food chains like McDonald's have made commitments to reduce saturated fats in their products and to introduce more nutritious menus or food items. Many fast-food establishments have added a variety of healthier choices to their menus, including salads, sandwiches, soups, low-fat frozen yoghurts and juices. Some chains also provide a nutritional analysis on their web sites or make copies available in their restaurants to help nutrition-conscious diners eat healthily.

THE SAFETY FACTOR

Occasionally, an outbreak of food poisoning is traced to a prepared-food outlet. Any meal that is mass-produced and then allowed to stand for any length of time is vulnerable to contamination. Especially deadly, particularly to young children, is a type of *E. coli* infection contracted by eating undercooked contaminated beef.

It is not wise to buy fast food and then wait several hours before eating it. Any food that is not consumed straightaway should be refrigerated, and then thoroughly reheated before it is eaten. If you're eating in a restaurant, refuse any precooked item that looks as if it has been sitting around for a while.

WHEN YOUR HECTIC LIFESTYLE NEEDS A LITTLE HELP FROM FAST FOOD

Many of us lead such busy lives that we often eat on the run, sometimes in the car. It is possible, however, to make your fast-food choices a little lighter just by being careful which toppings you choose on your menu item. When making your selection, keep the following in mind:

HAMBURGERS: Basic hamburgers contain about 225kcal, with about 16g of fat, while whopper burgers weigh in at about 450kcal, with 50g of fat. Choose a basic hamburger with no extras and have it with fresh onion, tomato and lettuce.

F

FRENCH FRIES: Of course we all want fries with that, but we must be prepared to pay the nutritional price. Just small-sized serving of French fries delivers about 200kcal and 10g of fat. A large order of fries from major chains provides almost 490kcal with an enormous 23g of fat, and much of it saturated or trans fat. If possible, skip the fries, or eat them rarely. Fries cooked in vegetable oil may still be high in saturated fat. If there is a choice, order wide, large-cut chips. They are usually slightly lower in fat than the skinny ones because there is less total surface area for the oil to cling to. Do not add extra salt; add a little vinegar instead. Vinegar has no fat and virtually no calories.

HOT DOGS: The traditional hot dog contains 400kcal and 18g of fat. Typically, 45–50 per cent of the calories come from fat. Eat hot dogs only occasionally, and stick with mustard, relish and onions for toppings.

FISH AND CHIPS: In their raw state, fish and potatoes are two healthy foods. But when they're deep-fried they soak up fat like a sponge. A typical portion of fish and chips contains about 700kcal and 49g of fat. You could always eat the fish and leave the batter – that would save about 283kcal and 21g of fat.

Cod with no batter has only 165kcal and 2g of fat; add the batter and it's 448kcal and 23g of fat.

Did you know?

North Americans love fast food

They consume more than 7 billion hot dogs each year, and the average North American has more than 100 orders of fries and approximately 150 slices of pizza annually.

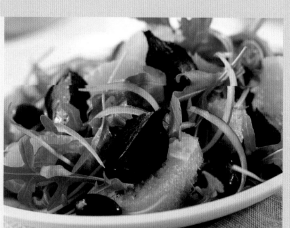

Salad – is it always the healthier choice?

You probably think a salad would be the healthier choice at a fast-food restaurant. It can be – but not always. You might be surprised to hear that a salad, complete with dressing and toppings, often contains more calories and fat than many of the more traditional fast-food choices. For example, a typical Caesar salad can easily clock up a whopping 500kcal and 30g of fat – about the same as a small burger and fries.

Some salads can be healthy and some of the new salad offerings from fast food outlets are making an effort to reduce calories and fats. A flame-grilled chicken salad, without dressing, will usually have about 200kcal and 7g of fat. But if you have the proffered sachet of dressing, you are adding about 70kcal and 6g of fat.

Many salads now available from fast-food outlets certainly offer a better choice, but take care that you don't go in intending to have the salad and then succumb to the burgers and fries.

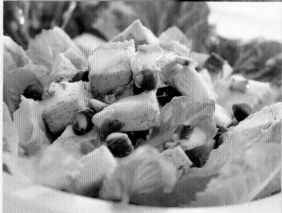

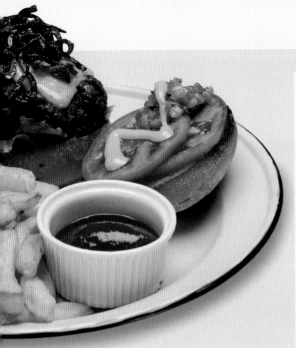

A large portion of chips has 502kcal and 13g of fat. Then there's the mushy peas – they add a modest 65kcal and only 0.5g of fat. Fish cakes contain about 220kcal and 13g of fat each.

PIZZA: There's no question that pizza is one of our all-time favourite fast foods. Unfortunately, it is also a major source of fat. A 35cm commercial pizza has anywhere from 40 to 95g of fat. Calories depend on the toppings. When eating pizza, try the following:

Stick to one slice. One or two slices of pizza served with a side salad will boost the nutrition of your fast-food meal while decreasing your intake of fat and calories.

Load up on vegetable toppings. They have the least calories and fat, and the most nutrients. Lean meats like chicken and ham are better choices than fatty sausages and pepperoni.

Cut down on cheese. Ask for less cheese. If your toppings are grilled vegetables, chicken or seafood and herbs, try having no cheese at all.

Fast-food hunting?

The suggestions in the following chart can help you to avoid bad choices and enjoy the most nutritious and delicious types of fast food.

BEST PICKS	GO EASY ON
JAPANESE Teriyaki beef, chicken or prawn; yakitori chicken; miso soup; stir-fries; sushi; sashimi; noodle soup dishes	Tempura dishes
ITALIAN Pasta with tomato or marinara sauce; green salads; pizza with lots of vegetables and light on cheese; minestrone soup	Pasta with cream sauces; double cheese pizza with fatty-meat toppings, cream sauces
MEXICAN Chicken fajitas, enchiladas, soft-shell beef taco, bean burrito (cut down the sour cream and cheese); salsa	Nachos and cheese, guacamole, refried beans, fried taco shells
GREEK Lean souvlaki or chicken kebab with salad, dressing on the side; tzatziki (cucumber in yoghurt)	Stuffed pastry
BURGERS Plain or veggie burger with lettuce, tomato, beetroot and onions; grilled chicken on a bun	Fries, onion rings, mayonnaise, bacon and cheese toppings
ASIAN Soups; mixed vegetables; steamed rice, steamed dim sum; stir-fries; noodles with seafood, chicken or beef	Chicken wings, any deep-fried dishes
SANDWICHES Turkey, chicken breast, lean corned beef; grilled vegetables; egg sandwiches; salad vegetables	Sausage or salami salad with mayonnaise
CHICKEN Roast chicken sandwich or wrap, grilled chicken, barbecued chicken (remove skin)	deep-fried, or nuggets, or fingers, stuffing; chicken skin

F

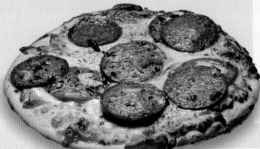

Fats

Facts and fallacies

The role of fats in the diet has excited much controversy and debate in recent years. Eating too much of certain types is harmful but others - in small amounts - are vital for the body and can help to prevent disease.

Dietary fats are the most concentrated source of calories. Weight for weight, they contain more than twice as many calories as carbohydrate or protein; 25g of fat has 225kcal.

Fats make food tasty; they give it a smooth creamy texture and impart flavour and smell. Certain fats are essential for childhood growth, healthy development and regulating the body's metabolism. The Department of Health in Britain has suggested that fats should provide around 35 per cent of total calories; in the United States, however, the recommended level is 30 per cent.

Surveys have shown that the typical Western diet derives 40 per cent or more of its energy from fat. This is divided almost equally into visible oils, spreads and meat fat and the invisible fats which are present in foods such as cheese, milk, meat products, biscuits and nuts. A high-fat diet is likely to lead to obesity because fatty foods are so rich in calories. Obesity and high intakes of certain types of fat can contribute to ailments such as atherosclerosis, heart disease and forms of cancer.

Some fats, like those found in fish and olive oil, actually lower our risk of heart disease. The trouble is, these aren't the fats we tend to crave.

DIFFERENT TYPES OF FAT AND WHY WE NEED THEM

Eating too many fats and oils of any kind may prove harmful, but excluding them from the diet deprives the body of important nutrients. Dietary fats from oily fish, fish oils, vegetable oils and full-fat dairy products, supply the fat-soluble vitamins A, D, E and K and are also required to absorb them. The body needs at least 25g of fat a day to absorb these fat-soluble vitamins and also beta carotene which the body can convert into vitamin A.

When fats are removed from dairy products, the foods lose much of their vitamin A content. Low-fat yoghurts, skimmed milk and cottage cheese are poor sources of vitamin A; the vitamin is added to margarines to make them more nutritious.

While fat intake can often be sensibly reduced in adults, the diets of children under five should not be similarly restricted. They need a wide choice of foods to make sure they obtain enough calories and vitamins, as well as all the essential fatty acids; these are vital for healthy growth and development.

THE ESSENTIAL FATTY ACIDS

Fats are made up of fatty acids. There are two main types - saturated and unsaturated. Fats rich in saturated fatty acids, such as butter and lard, tend to

Did you know?

Essential fatty acids, like alpha-linolenic acid, help to keep heart disease at bay

Alpha-linolenic acid, an essential fatty acid found in linseeds, rape seed and soya oil, has been shown to provide numerous health benefits, including helping your heart to keep a strong and regular beat. One study showed that in men, the heart-protective effect achieved by consuming this fat was even more significant than reducing saturated fats. Another study showed that women who consumed the most alpha-linolenic acid had a significantly lower risk of dying from heart disease.

be solid at room temperature; fats rich in unsaturated fatty acids, such as vegetable oils, tend to be liquid. The unsaturated fatty acids can be subdivided into monounsaturated and polyunsaturated.

The body can make its own saturated and mono-unsaturated fats from carbohydrates, alcohol or proteins. However, it cannot make certain poly-unsaturated fatty acids (essential fatty acids) which must be supplied by foods that contain them.

Polyunsaturates come in two forms: the omega-6s derived from linoleic acid and found in vegetable oils such as sunflower oil and corn oil, and the omega-3s derived from linolenic acid and found in vegetable oils such as soya bean, rapeseed and linseed oil, in walnuts, leafy vegetables and in oily fish such as sardines, herring, mackerel, tuna and salmon.

Omega-6 fatty acids are needed as part of the make-up of all cells in the body and to produce hormone-like substances called eicosanoids which help to control a wide range of functions including inflammation and blood flow. Deficiency in omega-6 fatty acids (sometimes found in babies fed on skimmed milk and patients unable to absorb fats) can lead to poor growth, skin problems, blood clots, and an impaired immune system.

An adult requires about 4g omega-6 fatty acids a day (equivalent to two teaspoons of sunflower oil or a handful of almonds or walnuts); more may offer some protection from heart disease. A daily limit of 25g is suggested as very high intakes may be harmful because they increase the production of free radicals.

Omega-3 fatty acids are needed in smaller amounts (about 1-2g) per day, found in 100g of herring, 1 to 2 teaspoons of linseed or rape-seed oil or a handful of walnuts. They are needed as structural components of the brain and the retina of the eye. They reduce inflammation and the tendency of blood to clot, and have also been shown to be helpful in the treatment of a wide range of chronic diseases.

WHY SOME FATS SHOULD BE RESTRICTED.

Medical research and population studies have borne out the theory that high intakes of saturated fats which occur naturally in meat and dairy foods increase blood cholesterol levels and the risk of coronary heart disease. But manufacturers also take 'healthy' unsaturated oils and convert them into trans fats by hydrogenation, which converts them into semi-solid fats. Hydrogenating vegetable oils helps to extend their shelf life but by changing the nature of the fat they also change the way it behaves in the body. Although, chemically, trans fats are still unsaturated fat, in the body they behave as if they were saturated fats. In fact, research suggests that they are even worse than saturated fat. Not only do they increase levels of LDL 'bad' cholesterol in the blood in the same way that saturated fats do, but they also reduce levels of HDL 'good' cholesterol.

One study which tracked the diet of over 80,000 female nurses

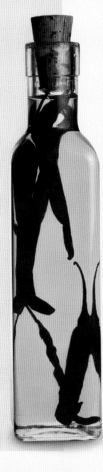

found that those women who ate the most foods high in trans fats were over 50 per cent more likely to suffer from heart disease compared with women who rarely ate these fats.

Although trans fats are found naturally in small amounts in meat and dairy products, over 70 per cent of the trans fats in our diet are the artificially created trans fats created by hydrogenation. The main source of these fats are processed foods like biscuits, cakes, pastries, meat pies, sausages, crackers, ice cream and some confectionery such as chocolate bars. Because trans fats are less likely to turn rancid, hydrogenated oils are also often used for deep-frying in fast-food restaurants. All packaged foods sold in America must list levels of trans fats on the nutrition panel on the label, although in the UK at the moment there is no legal requirement to give information about trans fats.

What you can do is to look at the ingredients list. If a product lists 'hydrogenated fat' or 'partially hydrogenated vegetable oils' in the ingredients list you can assume it contains trans fats and the higher up the list of ingredients it appears the more it will contain. However, there is absolutely no way of knowing what type of fat is used in take-away foods and in the foods you eat in restaurants and cafés.

The good news is that many retailers and manufactures are removing hydrogenated oil from their products. While it's true that our average intake of trans fats in the UK is well below the maximum safe target of no more than 2 per cent of our total energy (this works out at more than 4.4g for women and no more than 5.6g day for men) many experts feel that they only really safe intake of trans fats is zero. Replacing both trans and saturated fats with naturally occurring monounsaturate-rich fats (such as olive oil) or polyunsaturate-rich fats (sunflower oil) lowers blood cholesterol levels. These unsaturated fats are also the major dietary source of vitamin E which

Action plan to reduce your fat intake

■ Limit meat to 90–120g per serving. Buy lean cuts and trim all visible fat before cooking. Buy extra-lean minced beef, or better still, select a lean cut and ask the butcher to mince it for you.

■ Remove the skin from poultry before eating it. In some instances, this can be done before cooking.

■ Don't buy prebasted chicken or turkey; it's often injected with coconut oil, butter or other fats.

■ Barbecue, bake, grill or roast meat, fish and poultry. Use a roasting rack to drain off the fat as the meat cooks.

■ Cook casseroles and soups in advance; chill and skim off the congealed fat, then reheat thoroughly.

■ Avoid fried foods. Use a nonstick pan and vegetable oil spray for sautéeing. Sauté in broth, wine, tomato or fruit juice, or use a small amount of olive oil.

■ Buy semi-skimmed or skimmed milk, fat-reduced cheese, cottage cheese and yoghurt.

■ Toss salad with fat-free dressings or make your own with lemon juice or vinegar, mustard, herbs and spices. If oil is called for, use olive oil.

■ Cook rice in stock; flavour it with chopped fresh herbs and spring onions instead of butter.

■ Mash potatoes with low-fat yoghurt or skimmed milk; add chives and parsley for extra zip.

■ Choose broth-based soups instead of cream soups.

■ Spread sandwiches with mustard, horseradish or chutney instead of butter or margarine.

■ Choose English muffins, bagels or pitta instead of croissants, muffins, doughnuts or Danish pastries.

■ Serve sorbet or frozen yoghurt instead of premium ice cream, or consider other low-fat dessert alternatives, such as fresh fruit.

■ Measure oil, don't estimate it. The tablespoon of olive oil you drizzle over salad or put in your frying pan contains 11g of fat and about 99kcal. If you measure it, you will use less.

■ Gram for gram, fat contains twice as many calories as proteins or carbohydrates do, which explains why foods that contain a lot of fat always contain a lot of calories. Let this guide you when choosing food in restaurants and cooking at home. Always go for the lowest-fat option.

■ Reduce the fat in baking quick breads and muffins by substituting puréed apple, banana or other puréed fruit for part of the fat.

■ Order your cappuccino or latte 'skinny', which means it is made with semi-skimmed or skimmed milk.

Choose your oil carefully

All fats are a mixture of saturated, monounsaturated and polyunsaturated fatty acids (though we usually call them by the name of the fatty acid they have the most of). Look for the least saturated (red), and a good mixture of everything else. Polys (yellow and green) lower cholesterol, while monos (blue) only lower cholesterol if you eat them in place of saturated fats. Alpha-linolenic acid (green) is an omega-3 polyunsaturated fat that may protect the heart. Rape seed and soya oil are good sources. Many researchers recommend a mix of alpha-linolenic acid and linoleic acid (yellow). (Linoleic is a polyunsaturated omega-6 fat.) If you don't want the details, just stick with rape seed for cooking. It is among the lowest in saturated fat and it has a good mix of alpha-linolenic and linoleic acids.

Type of fat (1 tablespoon) — **Fat (grams)**

Type of fat	Saturated	Monounsaturated	Linoleic acid	Alpha-linolenic acid	Other
Rape seed oil	1.0	8.2	2.8	1.3	0.7
Safflower oil	1.4	2.0	10.6		
Sunflower oil	1.4	2.7	8.9	0.1	0.6
Corn oil	1.7	3.3	7.9	0.1	0.6
Olive oil	1.8	10.0	1.1		0.5
Sesame oil	1.9	5.4	5.6		0.7
Soya bean oil	2.0	3.2	6.9	0.9	0.6
Groundnut oil	2.3	6.2	4.3		0.7
Cottonseed oil	3.5	2.4	7.0	0.1	0.7
Chicken fat	3.8	5.7	2.5	0.1	0.7
Lard (pork fat)	5.0	5.8	1.3	0.1	0.6
Beef dripping	6.4	5.4	0.4		0.5
Palm oil	6.7	5.0	1.2		0.7
Butter	7.2	3.3	0.3	0.2	0.5
Cocoa butter	8.1	4.5	0.4		0.6
Palm kernel oil	11.1	1.6	0.2		0.7
Coconut oil	11.8	0.8	0.2		0.8

Fat (grams)

Legend: ■ Saturated ■ Monounsaturated ■ Linoleic acid ■ Alpha-linolenic acid — Polyunsaturated — ■ Other

may protect against heart disease and atherosclerosis. A low intake of animal fats and a high intake of olive oil is thought to contribute to the low rate of heart disease in Mediterranean countries. The Inuit people of Greenland also have a low incidence of heart disease; medical experts believe that this is because the fish and marine animals which they eat in large quantities are high in the omega-3 fatty acids, DHA and EPA.

High intakes of fish oil may also protect against cancer of the breast, bowel and pancreas which are linked with obesity and excessive total fat intake. The omega-3 polyunsaturated fatty acids that fish oils contain have been shown to inhibit tumour growth in animals. In several human studies, fish oils appear to protect against cancer of the colon.

CHANGING YOUR FAT INTAKE

It is wise to spread butter more thinly or to replace it partly with a low-fat spread or soft margarine that is high in polyunsaturates and low in trans fats. Semi-skimmed or skimmed milk should be used in place of full-cream milk (but not in infants' diets).

Some days, eat nuts and oily fish for protein rather than foods which contain animal fats. When eating meat, choose lean cuts and trim off the excess fat. Stewing or grilling is healthier than frying.

Use olive oil for cooking, rather than other vegetable oils and hard fats, to reduce your intake of omega-6 and saturated fatty acids.

Carefully inspect food labels. Some manufacturers already specify polyunsaturated, monounsaturated and saturated fat contents of prepared foods. The hydrogenated fat content will soon also have to be declared.

STRIKING A BALANCE

Studies show that the type of fat you eat may be as important as how much fat you eat. Lowering saturated fats seems a clear principle to work on. It's when you come to balance the intake of the omega-3s and omega-6s in your diet that it gets a little complicated. Although both are essential fatty acids, which your body cannot make on its own, the ratio of omega-6s to omega-3s is too high in many of our diets. Although omega-6s do not increase the level of LDL 'bad' cholesterol, when eaten in excess, they may decrease the levels of HDL 'good' cholesterol. They appear to contribute to the production of some cell-damaging free radicals. You can shift you ratio by getting more omega-3 fatty acids from fish and other sources.

Omega-3s provide linolenic acid and omega-6 fats provide linoleic acid. These acids are both essential to health and have to be provided by the foods we eat.

NEW POSSIBILITIES

The properties of 'conjugated linoleic acid', or CLA are being researched. This is a polyunsaturated fat that may be very beneficial to health. It is found in small amounts in dairy foods and meat. CLA may help to reduce body fat, increase muscle mass and even inhibit the growth of certain cancers. More research is needed before an increased intake of CLA can be recommended.

Seven sources of beneficial fats

- Olive oil, especially extra virgin
- Rapeseed oil
- Fish and seafood
- Nuts
- Seeds
- Linseeds
- Avocados

Fennel

BENEFITS

- Leaves are a source of folate and vitamin B
- A source of potassium and fibre
- Low in calories and good for digestion

DRAWBACKS

- The oil in fennel seeds can irritate skin
- High in nitrates

Filling, yet low in calories – only 12kcal per 100g – fennel is ideal for people trying to lose weight.

Although it has a distinctly different flavour, its stalks can be mistaken for celery. Both vegetables are members of the parsley family. Fennel is much more nutritious than celery, however; 100g contains 10kcal. An 80g serving of fennel is a useful source of potassium and fibre and also contains vitamin B and folate; the leaves contain vitamin C. Like celery, fennel can be high in nitrates.

The sweet, liquorice-like flavour of fennel is similar to the flavour of anise. It goes especially well with fish; for a delicious change, try baking fish on a bed of fennel stalks. All parts of the plant are edible, and it can be prepared in many ways: raw in salads or braised or sautéed as a side dish. Stuffed fennel bulbs are a delicious vegetarian dish; the chopped leaves make a colourful and nutritious garnish for a number of other vegetable dishes.

Doctors through the ages have prescribed fennel for a variety of reasons: to stimulate milk production in nursing mothers; to aid digestion and prevent bad breath; to treat kidney stones, gout, liver and lung disorders. Ancient healers often prescribed the seeds to prevent obesity; modern herbalists advocate fennel tea as a diet aid.

Fennel seeds are one of our oldest spices; they are also used to make a refreshing tea that is said to alleviate bloating, flatulence and other intestinal problems. They should be avoided during pregnancy.

▶ **A cousin of celery**
Fennel may look like celery with a fat bulb, but it has its own distinctive flavour that is an asset to a variety of dishes.

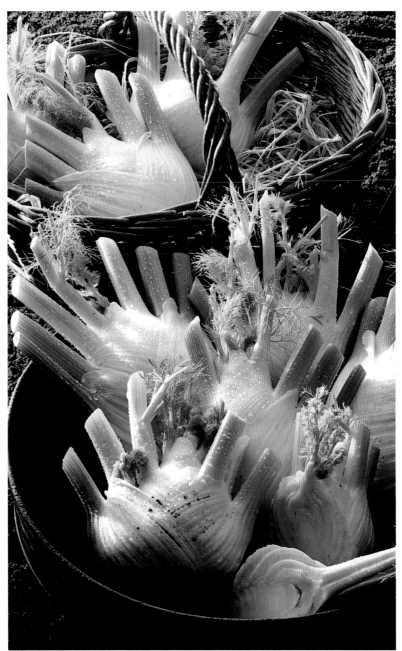

Fever

TAKE PLENTY OF

- Fluids
- Frequent small, light, bland meals

Although normal body temperature is generally spoken of as 37°C, human temperature tends to vary over the course of the day, from

F

about 36.4°C in the morning to about 37.5°C in the late afternoon – and what's normal for one person can vary above or below the average temperature by as much as one degree. Minimal increases may simply be caused by hot weather or being bundled up in too much clothing, but most people can feel a difference in their body temperature that they will call a fever once it reaches 38°C or 38.5°C. With a fever, you may feel cold at first, then hot, then cold again, as your body strives to fight off infection or heal an injury.

Fever is not a disease in itself, but rather a symptom of some underlying problem, most commonly an infection. Depending on the cause, a fever is often accompanied by other symptoms, such as sweating, shivering, thirst, flushed skin, nausea, vomiting and diarrhoea.

A fever alone may not require treatment – it is one of the body's natural ways of fighting disease and, generally, should not be suppressed unless it is very high, is causing distress (especially in a child) or there is a risk of febrile convulsions. If the fever is mild, and there are no other problems, keep up fluid intake and get plenty of rest.

Consult a doctor if:

- An infant under three months old has a fever that is higher than 38°C and lasts for more than 24 hours.
- A child or adult has a fever above 39°C lasting for more than three days.
- Fever is accompanied by a rash which does not disappear when firm pressure is applied with a glass.
- Fever is accompanied by persistent vomiting, diarrhoea, severe pain, drowsiness, confusion or fits .
- A child or adult has a fever of 38.5°C that is accompanied by severe headache, nausea and vomiting, a stiff neck, change in alertness or hypersensitivity to light.

When fever-lowering medication is indicated, either ibuprofen or aspirin may be effective. There is a junior formulation of ibuprofen. Aspirin should never be given to anyone under the age of 16 without a doctor's approval; aspirin given during a viral infection increases the risk of developing Reye's syndrome, a potentially life-threatening disease affecting the brain and liver.

Keep in mind that children's fevers can rise rapidly, and that even a high temperature over 39°C does not necessarily reflect the severity of an illness.

Nutritional needs

Drink lots of fluids. Sweating, the body's response to high temperature, results in the loss of fluid, which is worsened if there is diarrhoea or vomiting. So it is important to drink at least eight glasses of fluid daily to prevent dehydration. If a feverish person does not feel thirsty, it may be easier for them to sip a bit of fruit juice diluted with an equal volume of water every few minutes rather than to drink a whole glass at once. Or the person, especially if a child, can be given an ice lolly to suck on.

Warning: Feverish infants can become dehydrated very quickly, because they have a large body surface in proportion to their fluid volume. When babies have high temperatures, breastfeed them often or give them frequent bottles of plain water or a commercial infant rehydration solution (ORS). All chemist shops stock ORS preparations, but if an ORS is unavailable, give diluted juice or diluted flat lemonade. Do not add salt, as too much can be hazardous.

Don't starve a fever. The saying 'feed a cold and starve a fever' is a misinterpretation of the more sensible 'feed a cold to <u>stave</u> a fever'. If anything, you need more calories

than normal if you have a raised temperature because your metabolic rate rises as the fever rises. So even if you don't feel like eating, eat.

Fibre

BENEFITS

- Helps prevent constipation
- Relieves the symptoms of diverticulosis and haemorrhoids
- May help to reduce risk of colon cancer
- Soluble fibre plays a role in lowering elevated blood cholesterol levels
- Useful as a means of controlling weight

DRAWBACKS

- Too much fibre from unprocessed bran can cause bloating, flatulence and other digestive problems
- Excessive fibre may interfere with the absorption of calcium, iron, zinc and other minerals

All plant foods and their products contain some fibre – such as pectins, cellulose and gums that make up their cell walls – which is not digested. This indigestible part is called dietary fibre (or roughage). The effects of fibre appear to have been known since Biblical times, but it has only been in recent years that scientists have begun to understand its importance in the daily diet as a means of preventing disease and maintaining good health.

Research suggests that the typically low-fibre diets that are consumed in Western industrialised countries may contribute to such widespread illnesses as coronary artery disease, diabetes and various diseases of the large intestine, including cancer.

The Department of Health in the UK suggests the amount of fibre consumed in the average British diet should increase by at least 5g a day to about18g. That is an increase of about 40 per cent. They advise more complex carbohydrate foods, as well as fruit and vegetables.

Dietary sources

Most dietary fibre comes from wholegrain cereals, grains, fruit, vegetables, dried beans, peas and other legumes, nuts and seeds. The outer layer of a grain, which contains the most fibre, is removed in the refining process. This explains why whole-grain products, such as brown rice and wholemeal bread, are good sources of fibre.

Fibre falls into two categories: soluble and insoluble. Most plants contain both kinds of fibre although certain foods are richer in one than the other. The soluble fibres dissolve in water and become sticky. These are found in lentils, legumes, oat bran, oatmeal, psyllium, barley and pectin-rich fruit such as apples, pears, strawberries and citrus fruit. Insoluble fibre does not dissolve, passing through the digestive tract largely unchanged. It is found in wheatbran, whole-wheat products, brown rice, vegetables such as legumes and sweetcorn, pulses and nuts of all kinds.

Increasing fibre intake

- Use wholegrain cereals and breads, wholemeal pasta and brown rice.
- Eat at least two servings of fruit and three servings of vegetables daily, leaving skins if possible.

F

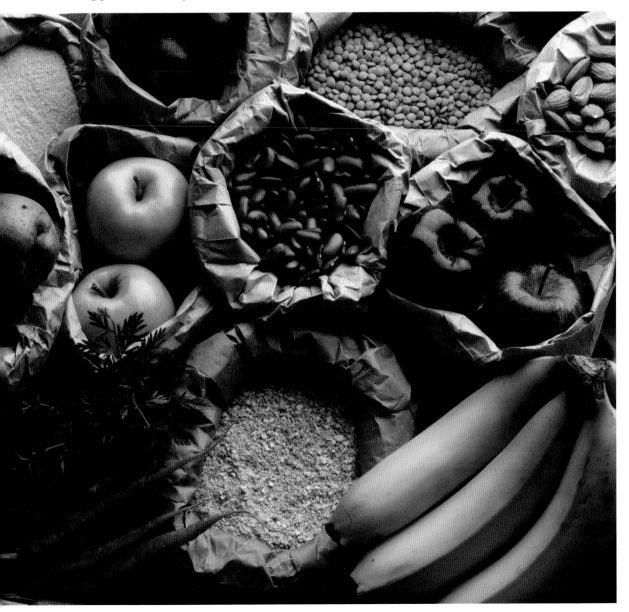

Foods that contain more than 3g of fibre

- small can baked beans
- 3 heaped tablespoons lentils
- 3 tablespoons red kidney beans
- 3 tablespoons peas
- medium bowl bran cereal
- bowl of muesli
- 2 slices wholemeal bread
- 50g prunes
- 3 dried figs
- 1 pear

- Eat breakfast: it is one of the best fibre opportunities of the day. You can get up to 50 per cent of your daily fibre requirement by eating wholegrain cereal, wholemeal toast and fruit.
- Snack on high-fibre fruit such as pears, berries or apples, and dried prunes or apricots.
- Serve vegetables raw or steamed. Eat high-fibre vegetables such as sweetcorn, peas, potatoes (with skin on), sweet potatoes, broccoli, Brussels sprouts and turnip.
- Try bulghur wheat or barley and other high-fibre grains.
- Add extra wheatgerm or bran to muffins, pancake batter or as a crispy coating for chicken or fish.
- Include beans and pulses in your diet, regularly. Try lentil soups, stews or casseroles.
- Have beans for lunch. One cup of baked beans contains 9g of fibre. Eat it with a slice of wholemeal bread for another 3g of fibre and you are two-thirds of the way to your suggested daily amount.
- Eat more salads. Add nuts, seeds or kidney beans to salads.
- Choose baked goods that are made with wholemeal flour, bran, oats, raisins or sesame seeds.

Role in good health

As it passes through the digestive tract, insoluble fibre acts as a sponge, absorbing many times its own weight in liquid. The result is that stools are softer and bulkier and are able to pass through the intestine more rapidly and be expelled more easily, thus decreasing the likelihood of constipation. This quick passage through the intestine also helps to prevent bowel disorders, such as diverticulosis and haemorrhoids, which can occur from the increased pressure that is created by hard stools. It is also thought that the faster passage of food through the intestine may protect against cancer of the colon by reducing contact with cancer-causing agents. In addition, some researchers speculate that the increased water content of high-fibre stools is also protective because it dilutes these carcinogens. This theory is unproved, however, and it is believed that there may be other substances in high-fibre foods that protect against cancer. Two important studies published in 2003 show that a high intake of dietary fibre is associated with a lower risk of colorectal cancer.

Some of the soluble fibres are able to lower blood cholesterol levels; in turn, this decreases the risk of

Did you know?

High-fibre diets can lower cholesterol

A recent study underscores more reasons for you to fill up on fibre. The study concluded that adding 10g of soluble fibre to one's diet was as effective in reducing blood cholesterol levels as lowering fat intake (less than 30 per cent of kilojoules from fat). In addition, the drop-out rate of study participants was only 13 per cent over six months, suggesting that people found it easier to stay on a high-fibre diet than on a fat-reduced diet.

A little fibre makes a big difference

One analysis of 67 different studies concluded that for every gram of soluble fibre you add to your diet, you can expect a decrease in LDL ('bad') cholesterol of 0.05mmol/l.

coronary artery disease and heart attacks due to atherosclerosis, which is the build-up of fatty plaque in the arteries.

Although insoluble fibres have little or no effect, some soluble fibres also help to control blood-sugar levels in people with diabetes. Increasing fibre will not cure diabetes, but a diet that is high in complex carbohydrates and fibre can allow some people with diabetes to better manage their blood sugar.

Because it is filling, eating fibre is helpful when you're trying to lose weight or control it. It provides a comforting feeling of fullness, although this tends to wear off as it passes through the digestive system. The best way to use fibre for weight loss is to consume a balanced diet that also includes modest amounts of protein and fat in each meal. Because the body metabolises these more slowly than fibre, you will not become hungry again as quickly.

How much is too much?

Increasing the amount of fibre in the diet should be done gradually. A sudden increase from 10g to 18g a day, for example, can provoke such unpleasant symptoms as bloating and flatulence. Consuming a large amount of fibre at once can lead to abdominal cramps or even a bowel obstruction, particularly among older or sedentary persons who may already have rather sluggish bowel function.

Fibre pills are not a good alternative to getting fibre through what you eat. Pills and other types of supplements lack the other nutrients and substances found in high-fibre foods, and it is possible that these, too, are instrumental in disease prevention, not just the fibre itself.

Too much unprocessed wheatbran and other insoluble fibres can stop the digestive system from absorbing some minerals properly, particularly calcium, iron and zinc. However, this is rare and is unlikely to occur unless more than 40g to 50g of fibre per day are consumed.

It may be that fibre is directly anti-carcinogenic. Wheatbran, for example, binds nitrite, making it unavailable to form cancer-causing nitrosamines. Fibre may prevent carcinogens from entering cells.

Figs

BENEFITS

- A source of vitamin B$_6$, potassium, calcium and iron
- High in fibre

DRAWBACKS

- Fresh figs spoil quickly
- The high sugar content in dried figs and their stickiness can contribute to tooth decay
- Can cause diarrhoea
- May be contaminated by moulds and their toxins

Figs have provided sugar, fibre and nutrients in the Mediterranean diet for at least 6,000 years.

Figs are not actually fruit, but flower receptacles. They bud like other fruit blossoms on the bare branches. The true fruits are the seedlike

▶ **Fresh figs are divine**
But dried figs are also quite delicious and available year-round.

achenes that develop, along with the inconspicuous flowers, inside the fleshy bulb.

Neither bees nor wind contribute to the pollination of figs. Most figs are self-pollinating but the old-fashioned Smyrna figs are pollinated by a unique species of wasp, only about 3mm long, which pollinates the flowers as it enters and exits through the small pore on the rounded end of the fig. Commercial fig growers foster this symbiotic relationship by tying wild figs containing wasp eggs to the branches of their cultivated trees. This method of ensuring fertilisation has been used at least since it was recorded in ancient times by a pupil of Aristotle.

Traditionally, figs were ripened by rubbing their skins with oil, which stimulated production of the maturing agent, ethylene. Commercial fig growers no longer follow this practice, as it detracts from the taste of the fruit.

Most of the figs we see for sale are dried. Although relatively high in calories – about 45kcal a fig – dried figs are a highly nutritious snack food, and a fig contributes about 15 per cent of the Reference Nutrient Intake (RNI) for calcium and iron, as well as 7g of fibre, 500mg of potassium and some magnesium and vitamin B$_6$. Eating dried figs with a

citrus fruit or another source of vitamin C increases the absorption of their iron.

Fresh figs bruise easily and do not travel well. They are available for a short time only after they are harvested in late summer or early autumn. Examine the figs carefully before buying them; the fruit should be soft but with no bruises or signs of mould.

Both fresh and dried figs are high in pectin, a soluble fibre that helps to lower blood cholesterol. Figs may also have a laxative effect, so they are good for people who suffer from chronic constipation; in others, however, eating too many can provoke diarrhoea.

Because dried figs tend to stick to teeth, it's important to remember to brush your teeth after eating them.

Fish

BENEFITS

- An excellent source of complete protein, iron and other minerals
- Some are high in vitamin A
- Contains omega-3 fatty acids

DRAWBACKS

- Some may contain mercury

Although a portion of fish is a gold mine of concentrated nutrients, supplying between a third and a half of the protein we need daily, in Britain today, we eat far less fish than we used to; a decline in fish consumption was one of the major dietary deteriorations seen in the 20th century; there are important health benefits to be gained from eating more fish and less meat.

The average Western diet's protein choices of red meat and dairy products come packed with large quantities of saturated fats. In contrast, fish and shellfish are rich in protein with fewer calories, and much less fat per serving than most meats. The fats in fish are high in polyunsaturates, which remain liquid even when chilled. (If fish had a lot of saturated fat, it would congeal into a solid mass and prevent them from moving in their cold-water habitat.) And despite the fact that some shellfish do contain cholesterol, they are low in saturated fats and are unlikely to increase blood cholesterol levels.

Health benefits

Eating fish two to three times a week has been strongly linked to a decrease in the rate of heart disease. Scientists first noted that coronary artery disease was virtually non-existent among the people of Greenland, the Inuit and Japanese fishermen. What these three groups had in common was a diet that relied heavily on fish for protein. When researchers looked at the effects of diet in other populations, they found that men who ate fish regularly two or three times a week were much less likely to suffer heart attacks than men who didn't.

In the recent Physicians Health Study, male participants who ate fish at least once a week were 52 per cent less likely to die of a heart at-tack than men who ate fish once a month or less. It's not yet known whether the effect is due to one fac-tor or many, but evidence so far points to the beneficial action of fish oils, which are rich in a type of un-saturated fatty acids known as omega-3s. These fatty acids decrease the stickiness of blood platelets, making it less likely that they will clump together to form clots. They also increase the flexibility of red blood cells, enabling them to pass more readily through tiny vessels, reduce inflammation of the artery walls and lower the levels of triglycerides in your blood.

Where are the omega-3s?

All seafood contributes omega-3 fats, with the richest sources being swordfish, salmon (fresh and canned), mackerel, mullet, trout, fresh tuna, sardines and herrings.

A study of more than 43,000 men, published in 2003, showed that men who ate about 85-140g of fish one to three times a month were 43 per cent less likely to have an ischaemic stroke, the most common type of stroke, caused by blood clots.

The human body uses omega-3 fatty acids to manufacture chemicals called prostaglandins that play a role in many processes, including inflammation and other functions of the immune system. Several studies have found that a diet that includes fish oil equal to the amount in a 230g daily serving of fish, could relieve the painful symptoms of rheumatoid arthritis.

Researchers believe that the beneficial effect was due to omega-3 fats, especially eicosapentaenoic acid (EPA). This fatty acid seems to promote the production of forms of prostaglandins and other substances that are less active in inflammation than those derived from saturated and polyunsaturated fats. The anti-inflammatory effects of omega-3 fats are being studied as a possible treatment for Crohn's disease and ulcerative colitis.

Some studies also suggest that people who eat fish regularly are less likely to suffer from a decline in age-related thinking skills such as memory. Other studies link low levels of omega-3s to higher rates of depression.

A study from Australia involving more than 3,500 older adults found that eating fish just one to three times per month appeared to protect participants against age-related macular degeneration, the leading cause of vision loss in older adults.

Nutritional value

All fish are rich in nutrients, especially protein, niacin, vitamin B_{12}, zinc, magnesium and more. Cod, haddock, salmon, sardines and swordfish are particularly rich in vitamins A and D. In addition, the bones in canned salmon and sardines are an excellent source of calcium.

Fish are high in protein because they carry a massive bulk of muscle on a much more spindly skeleton than land animals do. Contrary to popular belief, it's not necessarily true that the darker the flesh, the oilier it is; the dark colour is, in fact, due to the presence of myoglobin, a pigment that stores oxygen in the muscles. The flesh of salmon and trout gets its appealing pink colour from astaxanthin, a carotenoid pigment derived from the insects and crustaceans the fish feed on.

There is very little difference in omega-3 content between farmed fish and those caught in the wild, but farmed fish contain more total fat and calories as well as having higher toxin levels. Farmed fish should be eaten no more than once a month to avoid risk from toxins.

How much is enough?

There is mounting evidence of fish-linked cardiovascular benefits and long-standing advice is to include at least two servings of fish a week. Some experts suggest up to three servings of fish a week are needed to provide the benefits attributed to omega-3 fatty acids. On average, people in the UK eat a third of a portion of oily fish a week, and seven out of ten eat none.

Fish oil supplements may be advisable for some people, but check with your doctor first since they can 'thin' the blood. Look for a

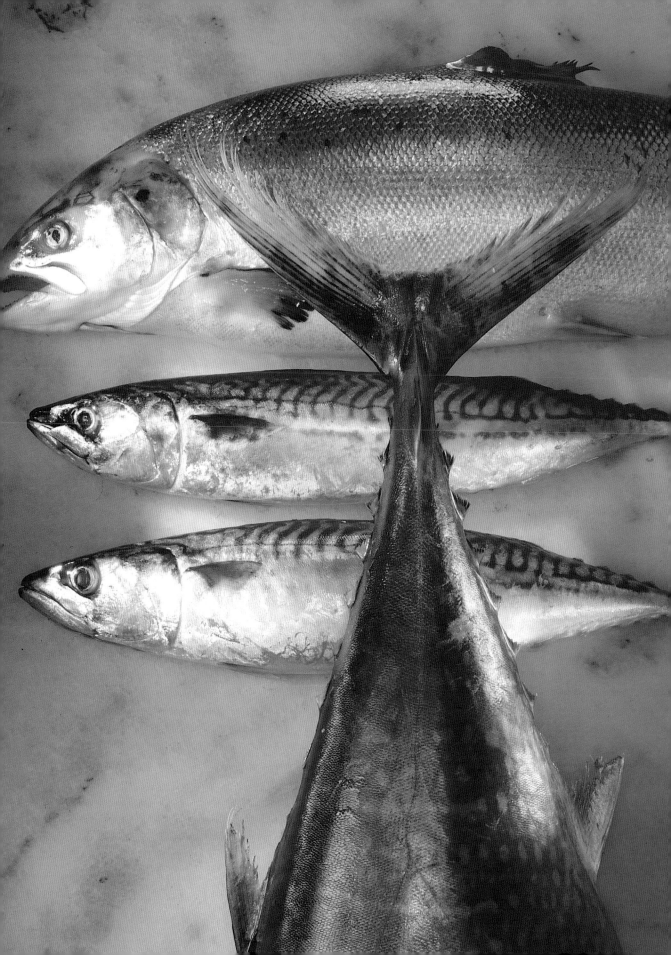

Fish facts and food values

NUTRIENTS PER 100G	DID YOU KNOW?
WHITE FISH, SUCH AS COD, HADDOCK, PLAICE. SKATE, SOLE AND WHITING	
Kcal: 95-123 Protein: 19-23g Fat: 0.8-1.3g Iron: 0.1-0.8mg	These fish are rich in vitamin B_{12}.
OILY FISH, SUCH AS HERRING, MACKEREL, SALMON, TUNA AND TROUT	
Kcal: 107-214 Protein: 18-24g Fat: 2.5-7.5g Iron: 0.8-1.5mg	Oily fish are an excellent source of omega-3 fatty acids and vitamin B_{12}.
CANNED FISH, SUCH AS ANCHOVIES, SARDINES AND TUNA	
Kcal: 107-286, depending on whether the fish is canned in oil or water. Protein: 18-25g Fat: 2.1g (tuna in water) to 15g (sardines in oil) Iron: 0.5mg (tuna in water) to 2.7mg (sardines)	Canned tuna contains only small amounts of omega-3 fatty acids. Canned salmon and sardines, eaten with the bones, are good sources of calcium. Anchovies are high in sodium and purines; they should be avoided by those with gout or high blood pressure. Similarly, sardines contain purines and should not be consumed by people with gout.
SMOKED FISH, SUCH AS SALMON, MACKEREL AND KIPPERS	
Kcal: 83-226 Protein: 18-23g Fat: 1g (cod) to 30g (mackerel) Iron: 0.5-1.2mg	Smoked fish, while tasty, tend to be packed with sodium; thus, they should either be consumed occasionally in very small amounts or avoided entirely by people with high blood pressure.
FROZEN FISH FINGERS	
Kcal: 202 Protein: 10g Fat: 11.5g Iron: 1.1mg	Fish fingers are an extremely popular frozen food product, especially with children, who might not otherwise be willing to try fish. However, as they are crumbed, they tend to be high in fat. To lower the fat content, try baking them in an oven rather than frying them in oil, and serve them with tomato ketchup which is low in fat and offers benefits from lycopene.
CAVIAR, BLACK AND RED; LUMPFISH OR SALMON ROE	
Kcal: 95-155 Protein: 10-20g Fat: 5.5-7.6g	Beluga caviar is the highest quality caviar, and also the most expensive; the sturgeon that produce these eggs can weigh as much as 1,600 kg and live for up to 100 years old. Caviar is highly perishable and should be bought fresh, stored in a refrigerator, and served in a tub of ice. It is high in sodium. This delicacy should be avoided by those with high blood pressure.

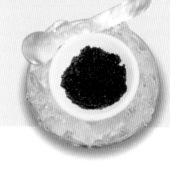

product with a combination of DHA and EPA (two omega-3 fatty acids). Fish liver oil capsules, which are a concentrated source of vitamins A and D can be toxic when taken in large amounts for long periods. Fish body oils, on the other hand contain less of vitamins A and D, but more omega-3 fatty acids and may relieve symptoms of psoriasis.

Health risks

Oily fish, such as fresh herring and mackerel, must be cooked or processed soon after they are netted. If kept too long before cooking they are susceptible to bacterial growth, which can cause scombroid poisoning, characterised by a rash and stomach upset. This is reflected in the expression 'Holy mackerel': it harks back to the days when the fishmarkets in Cornwall were given a special licence to open on Sundays to sell the night's catch while it was still fresh.

Shellfish from waters polluted by human waste bring a threat of viral hepatitis and bacterial infections that can cause severe gastrointestinal upset. Oyster farms are required to meet strict health standards to ensure that their products are safe, but bacterial contamination may still occur. The old rule of eating raw oysters only when there is an 'R' in the month may have some validity since bacteria are more likely to survive in warmer waters.

Coastal waters in some parts of the world are, at times, tinged red by a species of algae (*Karenia brevis*) in a phenomenon known as 'red tide'. Shellfish from red tide areas should not be eaten because they concentrate a toxin produced by the algae. Eating contaminated shellfish brings on symptoms of poisoning within 30 minutes: facial numbness, breathing difficulty, muscle weakness and sometimes partial paralysis.

Fugu: dining with death

The Japanese specialty fugu – puffer fish, or blowfish – can turn a dinner into a fatal game of Russian roulette. The ovaries, roe and liver of the puffer fish contain a deadly toxin. A slip of the knife during preparation can allow this poison to contaminate the flesh. This toxin, tetrodotoxin, is so powerful that consuming just a drop quickly brings on paralysis, followed by death. Fugu is never served in Japanese homes, and restaurant chefs must undergo long apprenticeships before they are entrusted with preparation of the dish. Despite these precautions, fugu is the major cause of fatal food poisoning in Japan, causing dozens of deaths every year.

Large, long-lived fish, such as tuna, shark, king mackerel and swordfish, may accumulate heavy-metal contaminants – especially mercury – which are toxic to the human nervous system and can be harmful for children and unborn babies. The amount of mercury in tinned tuna is now monitored routinely. Children under 16, pregnant and breastfeeding women and those planning a pregnancy, should avoid shark, swordfish and marlin and should have no more than two tuna steaks or four medium-sized cans of tuna a week.

Other chemical pollutants such as PCBs were reported in fish liver oils from the Baltic Sea, but levels are low in fish from the Atlantic and Pacific Oceans. Most commercially available fish oils are monitored for these pollutants and their levels are no cause for concern.

Most food experts emphasise the nutritional benefits of fish for pregnant women and young children, noting that their omega-3 fatty acids are important for the development of the central nervous system in babies, before and after they are born.

Freshwater fish may also be vulnerable to contamination. In the mid 1990s about 10 per cent of farmed salmon in the UK was found to contain residues of a potentially toxic pesticide. Elsewhere freshwater fish have suffered from accidental spillage of industrial and agricultural chemicals into rivers and streams. Many of the Great Lakes of North America have been contaminated with cadmium and mercury from industrial waste. This makes fish from these waters unsafe to eat.

Buying fish

Regulations to ensure that the processing of fish is safe and sanitary and that companies can easily detect potential problems and move quickly to react, prior to the food coming to market, are rigorously upheld. But when it comes to choosing your fish, here are some guidelines:

• When buying fresh fish, look for bright, glossy skin; clear, bulging eyes; tight scales; and firm flesh. There should be only a clean, briny aroma – no whiff of iodine, ammonia or strong 'fishiness' should be present. You should buy fish only at markets that store them with ice.

• Buy canned tuna packed in water; as oil-packed tuna is higher in calories and the oil is usually vegetable or olive oil, that doesn't contain the beneficial omega-3s.

Cost and preparation

Although some fresh fish can be expensive, it is economical to use. If you buy a whole fish, you can use the head and bones to make stock for low-fat soup. Combine fish with carbohydrates to stretch a small amount: a single poached salmon steak can be flaked into spinach noodles, or fillets of cod can be mixed with herbed mashed potatoes for a family meal of fish cakes. Fish needs little preparation, and cooks quickly. Steaming, poaching, baking, barbecuing and grilling all preserve flavour without adding calories. Avoid dishes that demand lavish amounts of buttery sauces that spoil the low-fat value of the fish.

Laboratory studies suggest that smoking and pickling fish can produce compounds that may be carcinogenic if eaten too often or to excess.

Flatulence

CONSUME PLENTY OF

■ Yoghurt made with live cultures

■ Peppermint and fennel teas

LIMIT

■ Fatty foods

■ Beans and other legumes, onions, broccoli and other members of the cabbage family, and any other foods that exacerbate the problem

■ Fruit and fruit-based sweeteners, such as sorbitol and fructose

AVOID

■ Milk if you are lactose intolerant

■ Carbonated drinks, chewing gum, and drinking straws, which all encourage swallowing air

■ Unprocessed bran and high-fibre laxatives

Excessive wind, or flatulence, causes uncomfortable abdominal bloating, which can be relieved only by bringing up the wind from the stomach (burping) or expelling it through the anus. Although it is embarrassing, this experience is the natural result of intestinal bacteria acting on undigested carbohydrates and proteins. The average person has more than 13 episodes a day, more if the diet is high in fibre. Sometimes flatulence is due to a medical disorder: excessive wind may be a symptom of chronic constipation or a stomach ulcer. If the problem is severe and persists, it could be a symptom of food allergies, irritable bowel syndrome (IBS), Crohn's disease or intolerance to milk. Ask your doctor's advice if you suspect your flatulence falls into any of these categories.

Flatulence seems to worsen with age, and some individuals are simply more susceptible to it than others. Eating smaller portions, chewing food thoroughly, and not gulping liquids should minimise episodes. Some experts also believe that reducing the amount of air in the digestive tract may help to prevent flatulence, so they advise against drinking carbonated beverages, chewing gum or drinking through a straw, which promotes swallowing air.

Some foods are notorious wind producers; topping the list are those that produce wind when fermented by intestinal bacteria. Soya beans, kidney beans, lentils and dried peas can all result in increased wind.

Soak dried beans first. Except for lentils and split peas, which do not need to be presoaked, soaking dried beans for 4-8 hours before cooking them in plenty of water helps to reduce the indigestible sugars, raffinose and stachyose, that cause wind. Canned beans should be rinsed thoroughly to remove the sugars that cause wind.

Cooking vegetables from the cabbage family. Many people also experience excessive flatulence after eating onions and Brussels sprouts, broccoli, cauliflower and other members of the cabbage plant family; you may be able to reduce

flatulence by adding such spices as anise, ginger, rosemary, bay leaf and fennel seeds during cooking. Some cooks add kombu seaweed to cooking water for the same purpose. This product is available in Asian markets and health-food shops.

Increase fibre intake very gradually. Passing wind can be an uncomfortable side effect of a well-intentioned move towards eating a healthier, high-fibre diet. Try to increase fibre intake gradually, and avoid unprocessed bran and laxatives. In addition, sorbitol, fructose and some other types of sweetener can cause quite a degree of flatulence in some people.

Other approaches. A cup of peppermint or fennel tea after a meal sometimes helps to improve digestion and reduce flatulence. Some people find that eating yoghurt made with live cultures cuts down on flatulence. Yoga, particularly the knee-to-chest pose, is also said to alleviate the condition.

Flax

See Linseeds

Flour

BENEFITS

■ A concentrated source of carbohydrate

■ Can provide B vitamins and fibre when whole-grain flour is used

DRAWBACKS

■ Substantial vitamins, minerals and fibre can be lost during milling

People have been grinding various seeds, as well as dried fish and other foods, to make flour for thousands of years. Initially, the seeds were roasted and ground between two

stones to make them easier to eat; water was added to the flour, and the paste baked into a type of crude bread. As agricultural societies developed, they devised increasingly sophisticated methods of grinding and sifting grains and seeds. Today, huge, fully automated mills are responsible for producing tonnes of flour, which are then transformed into breads, pasta, pastries and other baked goods and thickening agents and other food additives.

Nutritional value

Generally, flour is a more concentrated source of calories than its source material because moisture has been removed. For example, 500g of potato flour has 1,785kcal, compared with 320kcal in 500g of raw potatoes; a cup of cornmeal has about 560kcal, while a cup of cooked sweetcorn has only 159kcal. This increased density of calories is the reason food relief organisations often prefer to provide flour made from grains, legumes, tubers or dried fish rather than the raw products.

On the other hand, nutrients are lost in flour milling and processing. Wheat flour, which is our most common variety, is milled by using steel rollers to crack the grain. The bran and germ are then sifted out and the remaining part of the seed (the endosperm) is passed through a series of rollers and sifters to make a fine, powdery product. Removing the bran and germ from wheat reduces the fibre and the amounts of many vitamins and minerals found in the whole grain. Because of this depletion, white flour in the UK is enriched with calcium, thiamin, iron and niacin. Some bakers add vitamin B as well.

Wholemeal flour, which is made by restoring the germ and bran at the end of the process, provides more fibre, protein, vitamin E and trace minerals than white varieties

▶ **Full of flavour**
By combining wholegrain and refined flours, bakers can produce a tastier, more nutritious product that still has a fine texture.

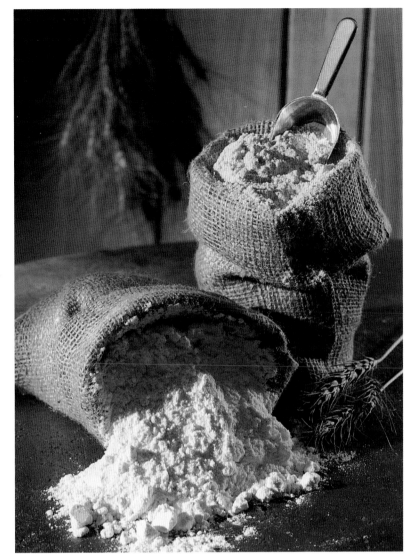

do. Depending upon the type of flour, other ingredients are added; these include salt and baking powder to make self-raising flour or extra gluten for special products.

Stoneground wholemeal flour is made by grinding whole wheat grains rather than recombining the flour with wheatgerm and bran. Stoneground flour has higher levels of most nutrients and antioxidants but because it tends to have a higher content of unsaturated fats, it goes rancid more quickly than ordinary wholemeal flour.

Types of flours

Almost any type of grain or seed can be ground into flour, although those with a high fat or moisture content may first be defatted and roasted or dehydrated.

Because most grains lack gluten, the protein that makes flour ideal for baking, they are usually mixed with varying amounts of wheat flour, which is high in gluten. Some of the more common flours include the following:

Amaranth is higher in protein, including the amino acid lysine, than most other flours.

Arrowroot, made from maranta root, is an easily digestible flour.

Barley, a soft, bland flour, is used for baked goods.

Buckwheat, made from the same seeds as kasha, is high in lysine.

Chestnut, made from ground chestnuts, has a distinctive flavour but can be used in baking.

Chickpea, widely used in Indian breads and batters, is a good source of protein and vitamins. It becomes bitter if kept for too long.

Cornmeal is not as nutritious as many other types of flour, but it

provides a complete protein when it is combined with beans and other legumes.

Fish flour, produced from whole dried defatted fish, contains very high levels of calcium and protein and is used in aid programmes in some developing countries.

Oat, high in soluble fibre, is used mostly in cereals and breads.

Potato, or farina, made from steamed and dried potatoes, is used extensively in baking and is a common thickening agent.

Rice is manufactured mostly from broken polished grains; typically, this flour is used to make noodles,

biscuits, gluten-free products and unleavened baked goods. It is made in brown and white versions.

Rye is high in fibre as long as the bran and germ have been retained. It is usually combined with wheat flour to form a mixture used in bread-baking.

Soya, made from soya beans, is often used with wheat flour to increase the protein content of baked goods.

Triticale is a hybrid of wheat and rye and is also high in protein; triticale may be mixed with wheat flour to increase its nutritional content.

Food and fitness

To boost endurance

Regular physical activity does wonders for your health, your shape and your mood. No matter what your age, health and level of fitness, there's a form of exercise to suit you.

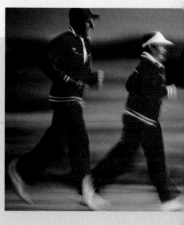

Exercise burns fat; it also keeps bones healthy, improves cardiovascular performance, enhances digestion, tones the muscles and the skin and increases your chance of getting a restful night's sleep. In addition to its physical benefits, endurance exercise activates the brain to release endorphins, morphine-like natural painkillers that soothe pain and create a sense of emotional wellbeing. Endorphins are responsible for the 'runner's high' that many athletes experience. They help to explain why exercise has a positive impact on your state of mind and your ability to manage stress.

EXERCISE IS ENERGISING

The paradox of exercise is that by using energy you can increase energy. By improving the heart's performance and ability to pump blood, aerobic exercise makes your body more energy-efficient, and you consume less oxygen when going about normal daily activities. In effect, it is like tuning up a car's engine and getting better petrol consumption. If you are unused to regular exercise, however, you may feel a bit stiff or sore and tired at first. Start slowly, perhaps adding only 10 minutes of activity three times a week, and gradually build up the intensity and length of your workout. After a few weeks of following a regular exercise routine, most people report a surge of energy.

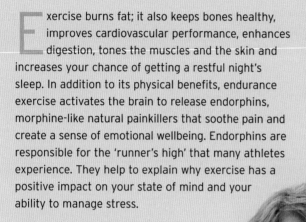

EXERCISE BURNS FAT

In this sedentary society you need to take regular exercise to keep your body trim and improve your health. If you eat more food than your body uses up in energy, the surplus calories are stored as fat. The only way to lose weight and keep it off is to combine a healthy calorie-controlled diet with regular aerobic exercise, such as brisk walking, jogging, cycling, swimming or aerobic dancing. By speeding up your breathing and raising your heart rate, aerobic exercise helps to burn body fat. Undertaking an exercise programme, however, doesn't give you a licence to eat all the French fries, chocolate and pastries you can lay your hands on. On the contrary, a balanced diet is essential to provide the energy you need to sustain a regular exercise programme.

MOVE IT TO LOSE IT

It's been proven that when you exercise aerobically, your body first burns the glucose that is circulating. It then turns its attention to the glycogen that is stored in the muscles and the liver, as well as to some fatty acids. Thus, an exercise or training session that lasts longer than about 20 minutes burns more fat and helps to shed weight and keep it off. Endurance training increases the amount of fatty acids being burned. Therefore, the best way to promote the burning of fat is steady and sustained effort, in which you exercise for long periods – at least 25 to 30 minutes at a time – at 30 to 40 per cent of your maximum capability.

FUEL FOR SPORT

The food you eat fuels your performance, at the gym, on the playing fields or even at home and work. The right combination of food and exercise will give you the added edge. Here are some fitness tips:

1. Carbohydrates are the body's preferred source of fuel for physical activity and are an integral part of an athlete's training program. Breads, grains, cereals, pasta, fruit and starchy vegetables provide powerful fuel for muscles and speed up the restocking of muscle fuel after exercise. If you aren't eating enough carbohydrates, you will tire more quickly. The amount of carbohydrate required depends on an individual's personal requirements. Athletes training heavily can need from 7g to 10g of carbohydrate for every kilogram of body weight. Check the chart on the right to work out just how much carbohydrate you should be getting every day, if you intend getting fit.

2. Fluids are critical to high performance. During high activity, fluid loss increases the risk of cramps, heat exhaustion or heat stroke. Drink before, during and after an event as part of your exercise routine. Drink lots of fluids even on days when you aren't working out. Water, sports drinks, fruit and vegetable juices or mineral water are good choices. Cold water or sports drinks are recommended for workouts or training sessions of more than an hour, and competitions. Alcohol and caffeine should only be counted as a small part of your hydrating fluid intake. Drink 400–600ml liquid 2 hours before a workout and 150–350ml every 15 to 20 minutes during exercise.

3. Time your meals. If you're running a race or competing in an event, have a high-carbohydrate, low-fat meal 2 to 3 hours beforehand. Eat foods you're familiar with and that you digest easily. Fruit, yoghurt,

Sports drinks

There is a lot of hype about sports drinks, and some athletes and other exercisers spend a great deal of money buying them every year. They get into the habit of drinking them even when they're not exercising – which is expensive and the extra calories are fattening. When you exercise, your body runs low on fluids, salt and calories. As long as you can replace these, there is no need for an expensive sports drink. You could do just as well with a bottle of your favourite, drink, whether it is cola, iced tea, lemonade or just plain water. Exercise for about 25 minutes, and your endurance can be increased with fluids. Go on for about 45 minutes, and you need a little sugar in the drink – such as fruit juice. If you keep going for several hours, you need to replace lost salt, too, and that can be done with a few salted peanuts. And to replace calories, it doesn't matter what you eat as long as it isn't too indigestible.

What does a high-carbohydrate diet look like?

A 60kg (9st) athlete training 2 to 4 hours daily would need about 420g to 600g of carbohydrate per day. Use these numbers to total your carbohydrates for the day:

FOOD	GRAMS OF CARBOHYDRATE
3 pancakes (150g)	50
1 large potato (200g)	26
1 cup cooked rice	45
1 medium bagel	42
200g flavoured yoghurt (low fat)	26
1 cup cooked pasta	40
1 pitta bread	33
2 slices of bread	30
1 cup apple juice	27
1 banana	22
30g sultanas	25
1 apple	20
1 cup cereal	20
2 rice cakes	16
1 tablespoon jam	14
1 cup milk	12

Meeting your protein needs

An endurance athlete needs 1.2g to 1.4g of protein per kilo of body weight per day. So, a 70kg (11st) athlete would need 84g to 98g of protein per day. The table of approximate protein values, below, shows how easy it is to meet your requirements and enjoy a varied diet.

FOOD	Grams of protein
85g canned tuna	22
150g cooked meat or fish	42
¼ roasted chicken	44
1 cup cooked lentils	14
100g firm tofu	10
60g almonds	12
1 cup milk	9
200g yoghurt, low-fat, natural	14
30g Cheddar cheese	8
1 egg	6
1 cup rolled oats	4
1 slice bread	3
1 cup cooked pasta	6

a smoothie, bread or a bowl of cereal are good choices. If you have food in your stomach when you exercise, blood is diverted away from your digestive tract to your working muscle, leading to cramps and a heavy feeling. If you exercise first thing in the morning, you have enough reserved energy from the day before to sustain 60 to 90 minutes of exercise. If you find it difficult to eat breakfast before an early morning workout, have a carbohydrate-rich snack the night before. If you exercise later in the day and it has been longer than 4 hours since your last meal, have a snack 45 to 60 minutes before you begin. Your food choices may vary depending on the time of day, the sport you are doing, and the level of intensity of your workout. You'll learn which food combinations work best.

4. Try carbo loading before endurance events. Carbohydrate loading is appropriate for athletes entering marathons, triathlons or long-distance bike races. For events that last less than 90 minutes non-stop, a regular high-carbohydrate diet is sufficient. Loading involves reducing training somewhat three to four days before a race and increasing carbohydrates to 70 to 80 per cent of total calories during this time.

5. Replenish carbohydrate after exercise. After an energetic workout, it is important to replenish the glycogen in muscles. Eat a high-GI, carbohydrate-rich meal/snack within 30 minutes after exercising. This is when your muscles are most receptive to new carbohydrates. Eating high-GI, carbohydrate-rich foods within the first 1 to 4 hours after a hard workout is especially important if you are doing two or more events in a day. Foods like watermelon, bread or rice crackers are also easy to eat. Sports drinks or diluted juices are good sources of carbohydrate immediately after exercise if you don't have an appetite for solid foods. They will also help you to rehydrate.

6. Replace the sodium and potassium lost during exercise with food. Eat potassium-rich fruit and vegetables including bananas, oranges, melon and tomatoes. Replace the sodium lost through sweat by lightly salting your food after exercise.

7. Physical activity may increase your need for some vitamins and minerals. However, if you are eating enough calories to meet the demands of your activity and the calories are coming from nutritional foods, you probably don't need any supplements. Supplements won't give you added energy unless you are deficient to begin with.

8. No need for more protein. Protein is important to help to build and repair body tissues and muscle. Many athletes believe that because muscles are made of protein, eating

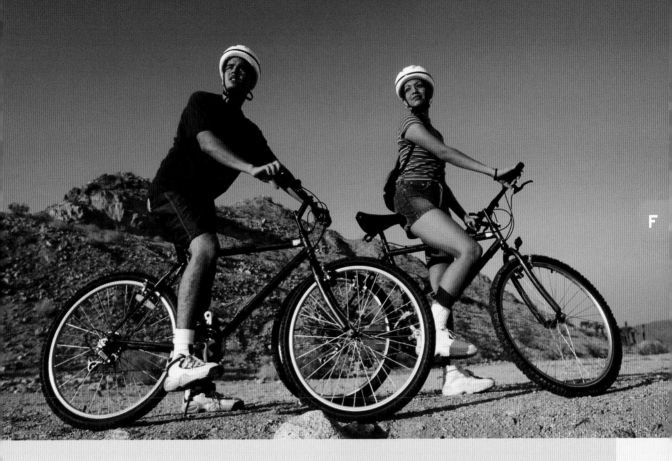

F

large servings of protein foods will help to build larger muscles. This is not true. Training, and not protein supplements, is the best stimulus for muscle growth. Athletes do have an increased protein requirement, but this can be met easily by a well-planned and well-balanced diet. The best way to build muscle is to eat enough food to replace the energy used during the day. The daily protein recommendation for endurance athletes is 1.2 to 1.4g per kilogram of body weight, whereas for resistance and strength-trained athletes it can be as high as 1.6 to 1.7g per kilogram of body weight per day.

CREATING A PERSONAL PROGRAMME

■ Don't try to cram exercise into an already crowded schedule. Instead, substitute it for a less important activity, such as watching television. Increase your daily exercise by walking at least part of the way to and from work, or try taking a walk or working out at lunchtime.

■ Choose an exercise you enjoy. Try cross-training to ward off boredom. Take a brisk walk one day, go to the gym and lift

When eating to train, consume plenty of:

■ Starchy foods, such as pasta, legumes, brown rice, potatoes and wholegrain breads, for complex carbohydrates to provide a steady source of energy

■ Fluids, before, during and after exercise

■ Fruit and vegetables for vitamins and minerals, especially potassium

■ Vegetables and legumes for vitamins and minerals

■ Lean meat, fish, poultry, eggs, low-fat dairy products and milk, and other high-protein foods to maintain muscles

weights the next. Enrol in a yoga class for stretching and flexibility, or go swimming.

■ Whatever your exercise plan, begin slowly and build gradually. Anyone who is over 40, over-weight or who suffers from high blood pressure, heart, bone or joint disease, diabetes, or who is a smoker, should see a doctor before embarking on any sort of exercise routine.

■ If you prefer to exercise alone, go to a gym and try all the equipment. Then consider buying a suitable exercise machine to use at home.

Food poisoning

F

CONSUME PLENTY OF

- Diluted sweetened drinks to replace lost body fluids and provide energy

AVOID

- Overhandling any food
- Having raw and cooked foods touch, such as on food preparation surfaces
- Raw eggs, such as in mayonnaise, sauces, mousses, cold desserts or unbaked cake batters
- Old leftovers or foods that are past their expiry date

The incidence of food poisoning in the UK is alarming: more than 79,283 notified cases in 2005, but probably nearly 5 million when unreported cases are included.

In all, more than 250 diseases can be spread through contaminated food. The term 'food poisoning' is now generally applied to illness (most often gastroenteritis, but some nervous system complications) resulting from bacterial or viral contamination of food. Bacteria, including those that can cause food-borne illness, are found naturally all around you. They are invisible, so you cannot rely on sight or taste to detect them. Bacteria can cause disease either through their rapid multiplication inside the body (bacterial infection) or through toxins that they may produce (bacterial intoxication).

Heat destroys bacteria in food, but toxins, such as those produced by staphylococcal organisms, are heat stable and not affected by cooking. Infestation with parasites from raw or contaminated meat and fish can also cause food poisoning. The strict regulations that now control food processing and the use of additives, offer considerably more protection than in the past. However, there remain many opportunities for contamination to occur along the trail of harvesting, processing, packing, transporting and displaying food for sale. Most cases of food poisoning are caused by bacterial contamination, usually traceable to faulty handling and preparation in the home, in restaurants, or food-service outlets. The micro-organisms that are most often responsible are *Clostridium botulinum, Clostridium perfringens, Escherichia coli, Listeria monocytogenes, Salmonella* strains and *Staphylococcus aureus.*

Typical symptoms

Food poisoning usually causes nausea and vomiting, diarrhoea and cramps, headache and sometimes fever and prostration. The infection can be serious in vulnerable people, especially in infants and young children, people with chronic illness (including HIV, AIDS and other immune system disorders) and the elderly. Call a doctor if someone you know in these groups has symptoms of food poisoning. Otherwise, most cases clear up without medical help.

Botulism is a rare but grave form of food poisoning caused by a nerve toxin from *C. botulinum*. Symptoms of nerve and muscle impairment are double vision and difficulty in speaking, chewing, swallowing and breathing; any of these call for immediate medical attention.

The body rids itself of the organisms that cause food poisoning through vomiting and diarrhoea. Unpleasant though they may be, it's best to let nature run its course. Don't tax your digestive system with food until it's able to handle it. Prevent fluid depletion by sipping water or a mixture of apple juice and water, or weak tea. When your system has settled down, gradually reintroduce foods. Start with bland foods, such as dry white toast, jelly, chicken and potatoes.

Simple precautions

Foods of animal origin are the most susceptible to contamination. The muscles of healthy animals are free of bacteria, but they provide a rich culture medium for the growth of bacteria picked up in handling and processing. The skin prevents bacteria from entering the flesh of a living animal, but micro-organisms can be transferred from the skin to the muscle when the carcass is cut up. Animal foods with skin, such as fish and poultry, are the most prone to spoilage, because bacteria may remain on the skin despite thorough washing after slaughter. Vegetables can also carry bacteria and should be washed thoroughly.

Be careful when handling meat, fish, shellfish and poultry. Wash hands thoroughly with hot water and soap before starting any food preparation, and repeat as necessary throughout the process. Also, remove rings, and make sure fingernails are clean both before and after food preparation. Clean the whole area afterwards, in cases of splashes of contaminated juices.

Use hot, soapy water to thoroughly wash food preparation surfaces, such as chopping boards and counter tops. Never allow cooked food to touch an unwashed surface where traces of raw food remain. Wash plates and utensils used for raw meat or poultry before using them for cooked meat or other food. Wash and sterilise your meat thermometer after each use.

Did you know?

Antibiotics can prolong symptoms

For most common causes of food poisoning, your doctor will not prescribe antibiotics. Antibiotics can prolong diarrhoea and actually keep the organism in your body longer.

Always keep raw foods away from other foods, and separate starchy foods and dairy products to prevent cross-contamination. Ensure that raw foods don't contaminate cooked foods, either directly by contact or indirectly (if meat juices touch other foods). Put raw foods in sealed containers.

Wet and microwave your dishcloth for 2 minutes daily. This will stop cross-contamination and the spread of bacteria. Change tea towels daily – they harbour germs.

Keep food refrigerated. If you don't intend to eat food immediately after preparing it, refrigerate or freeze it. Never leave food sitting at temperatures between 7°C and 60°C, which are ideal for bacterial growth.

Discard food that smells bad or is discoloured. Don't use food from damaged cans or containers. Never taste foods that look 'off'. Never buy or use a can if the ends are bulging. This is most likely caused by the pressure of gases produced by bacterial metabolism.

You cannot see or smell most bacteria that might make you sick. Tasting is risky and won't tell you if a food is unsafe. For some bacteria, such as certain varieties of *E. coli*, even a tiny taste may make you sick. That is why the best advice is: When in doubt, throw it out!

Good versus bad germs

It may seem puzzling that the yeasts and bacteria used in fermentation produce healthy foods, while some of their relatives cause various forms of sickness. The reason is that the beneficial bacteria (for example, *Lactobacillus acidophilus* and *L. bifidus* in some yoghurts) inhibit the growth of unwanted organisms, crowding out potentially harmful members of the *Clostridium*, *Bacillus* and *Streptococcus* families. Clearly, not all bacteria are alike; some are dangerous, while some are helpful.

What's your poison?

If you have symptoms of food poisoning, try to work out when and where you ate a suspect meal: prompt reporting could prevent a mass outbreak. If a fever develops or the symptoms persist for more than a couple of days, consult your doctor.

MICRO-ORGANISMS	SYMPTOMS
CAMPYLOBACTER JEJUNI Infection usually stems from contact with infected animals or contaminated food (in many cases, from raw or undercooked poultry).	Fever, nausea, abdominal pain and diarrhoea, which may be bloody. Symptoms typically come and go; they appear within 2 to 6 days and can last from 1 to 10 days.
CLOSTRIDIUM BOTULINUM (BOTULISM) Home-canned foods; improperly packed and sterilised canned products; and contaminated vegetables, fruit, fish and condiments. More rarely it is found in beef, pork, poultry, milk products, honey and garlic bottled in oil.	Within 18 to 36 hours, double vision and difficulty with muscular coordination, such as chewing, swallowing, breathing and speech. Progressive muscle weakness and paralysis can lead to respiratory failure and death.
CLOSTRIDIUM PERFRINGENS Often associated with meat such as mince or a casserole kept over a low heat.	Severe diarrhoea, abdominal pain, bloating and flatulence appear in 8 to 24 hours.
ESCHERICHIA COLI (E. COLI) Undercooked beef or unpasteurised milk. Many cases are traced to contaminated mince, but a few have been linked to rare roast beef. Often found in fast-food outlets.	Bloody diarrhoea and vomiting. In severe cases, seizure, paralysis and even death. Symptoms appear within 12 to 72 hours. Patients may require hospitalisation.
LYSTERIA MONOCYTOGENES Organism found in the soil and intestinal tracts of humans, animals, birds and insects. Infection usually follows eating contaminated cold deli meats, pre-cooked chicken, pâté, prepared salads, oysters, prawns, sushi, soft cheeses, soft-serve ice cream, raw goat's or cow's milk. Alarmingly, it can reproduce at refrigerator temperatures.	Fever, headache, aching joints and fatigue, usually within anything from 4 hours to several days after ingestion. Lysteria can be especially dangerous during pregnancy as even if symptoms are mild in the mother, miscarriage, or, rarely, stillbirth may result. Although the incidence of lysteria poisoning is uncommon, it is potentially serious. The elderly and the unwell are also at risk.
SALMONELLA Infected meat-producing animals; under-cooked poultry; and raw milk, eggs and egg products; unrefrigerated cooked foods.	Within 8 to 36 hours, nausea, abdominal pain, diarrhoea, vomiting and fever; symptoms typically last 1 to 4 days.
STAPHYLOCOCCUS AUREUS Commonly spread by food handlers with skin infections who transmit the organism to such foods as custards, cream-filled pastries, milk, processed meat and fish; poison is caused by a toxin rather than the bacterium.	Severe nausea and vomiting. There may be also diarrhoea, abdominal cramps, headache dizziness and fever. Shock, prostration and electrolyte imbalance may occur in extreme cases. Symptoms can occur within minutes or up to 6 hours later.

Food safety

Storage and preparation

The techniques used to clean, store and prepare food in your home, not only affect its taste, texture and nutritional value, but are also instrumental in preventing spoilage and food-borne illness.

By using the proper methods to prepare and store foods, you can keep them wholesome and nutritious; preserve their appearance, taste and texture; and use them economically. Exposure to heat, light, moisture and air can cause some foods to spoil; many lose flavour, texture and nutritional value if kept too long. Improper handling and storage also raise the possibility of food poisoning.

Use the 2-hour rule in your home and while shopping. Refrigerate or freeze all perishables within 2 hours of purchase or preparation. If the weather is hot, reduce that time to an hour. The highest risk foods are meat, fish, shellfish, poultry, eggs, dairy products, mayonnaise mixtures and moist foods such as poultry stuffing. It is especially important that these foods be handled carefully and most importantly, kept at the right temperatures – keep hot foods hot, and cold foods cold.

FOOD STORAGE

Heat and humidity greatly increase the risk of food spoilage, so you should never store foods in warm places, such as near the stove or refrigerator. To minimise the risk of contamination and accidental poisoning, always keep food and cleaning products in separate areas in your kitchen.

Even canned foods deteriorate with time, so you should stack cans in the order of their date of purchase so that the oldest can is used first. Practise 'first in, first out' for all food products. Store them well away from moisture in a 10°C to 21°C temperature range. Dry goods should be kept in a cool, dry place and used before their expiry date.

Always read labels carefully. They often contain important storage information and recommended 'use by' dates. When in doubt about shelf life, call the company (many have free numbers). Remember, when in doubt about any food, toss it out! It's not worth risking your health.

GRAINS AND NUTS

Grains, flours and other foods packed in materials easily penetrated by insects – for example, cardboard boxes, paper bags and cellophane packages – should be transferred to plastic, metal or glass containers with tight-fitting lids. (Even then, insect eggs in the flour or grains may hatch. To kill the eggs before storage, put the product in a microwave oven set on 'High' for 2 to 3 minutes.) Under normal storage conditions, the shelf life of white flour is about one year from the time it is milled. Flour can be frozen for long-term storage if carefully wrapped in moisture and vapour-proof material.

Wholegrain flours spoil within a few weeks because their fats turn rancid. Storing them in a freezer extends their life.

Cake mixes last about a year at room temperature, after which time the quality starts to decline.

Bread, cereals and crackers are normally best kept in closed containers at room temperature. Cereals, like other foods made from grains, should be stored in a dark place because they will lose riboflavin if left exposed to light.

Yeast breads will keep for a few days if wrapped in plastic or foil and stored in a cool, dark place, such as a bread box. In hot weather, refrigeration may be required

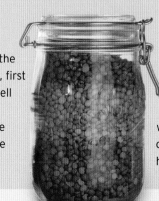

carrots, beetroot, parsnips and turnips, will help to conserve vitamins by preventing the tops from drawing them up from the roots.

When stored below 4°C, potatoes develop a sweetish taste from the conversion of starch to sugar; the sweetness disappears when the tubers are returned to room temperature. Store potatoes in the dark, preferably in a brown paper bag, because exposure to light causes poisonous alkaloids, such as solanine and chaconine, to form.

Freezing raw fruit and vegetables causes the water they contain to form ice crystals that break down cell membranes and walls, resulting in a mushy texture and a loss of nutrients. Deterioration of fruit and vegetables can also be caused by enzymatic activity; blanching prevents this. Immerse vegetables for a few seconds in rapidly boiling water to deactivate their enzymes, then plunge them into cold water to stop the cooking process.

to prevent mould. Unshelled nuts can be kept at room temperature for three to six months; shelled nuts may become rancid unless refrigerated or frozen. Discard any that smell musty or are mouldy.

Baking powder generally lasts 12 to 18 months. To test for freshness, mix 1 teaspoon baking powder with ⅓ cup hot water. If it foams vigorously, it still has rising power. Store tightly covered in a dry place. Make sure measuring utensils are dry before dipping into the container.

Bicarbonate of soda should be stored tightly covered in a dry place. If using as an odour catcher, change it four times a year.

FRUIT AND VEGETABLES

Raw fruit and vegetables slowly lose their vitamins when kept at room temperature, but tropical fruit deteriorates rapidly if stored in the cold. Most produce is best stored at about 10°C; if refrigerated, put it in the crisper section; the restricted space slows down moisture loss. Avoid storing fruit and vegetables for long periods in sealed plastic bags; they cut off the air supply, causing the produce to rot. Paper and cellophane are better storage materials, because they are permeable. Keep juice in a small container so that vitamins are not lost through exposure to oxygen.

Where winter temperatures average –1°C or less, fruit and vegetables bought in bulk can be stored in a cool basement or cellar. Carrots, cabbage and lettuce keep well at about 0°C. Wash produce before using.

Leave the stems on berries until you're ready to use them, and refrigerate peas and beans in their pods. Cut the green tops off root vegetables, such as

Food storage and preparation tips

- To store fresh herbs, wash them and stand them upright in a glass containing 2.5–5cm of cold water. Cover with a plastic bag and refrigerate.
- To freeze berries, place them in a single layer on a flat tray, freeze, then pack into airtight containers.
- Fruit, vegetables and grains left to soak in water can lose vitamins and minerals. Wash vegetables and fruit under running water to remove soil, insects and water-soluble pesticides just before using them.
- The skins of fruit and vegetables do contain important nutrients, but they also are more likely to be tainted with bacteria or pesticide residues. Many nutrients are lost when potatoes are peeled, but carrots store toxins near the skin, so peeling them is important. Always discard the coarse, outer leaves of many green vegetables for the same reason.
- Store cottage cheese upside down in its original container. It will keep for longer.
- Eggs are porous and will absorb refrigerator odours. Store them in their carton, not in the refrigerator door compartment.
- Before returning an opened ice-cream carton to the freezer, press its own plastic film onto the surface of the ice cream to prevent ice crystals from forming.
- Acid foods, such as rhubarb, cabbage and soft fruits can become tainted if stored in aluminium foil.
- Wrap cheese and meats in only the sort of cling film that says it is suitable for this use; many types are not.
- When reheating or cooking food in the microwave, don't let cling film come into contact with the food.

F

Handling meat and fish safely

- Wash poultry under cold running water and then pat it dry with paper towels before preparation. Some experts recommend washing it with diluted vinegar in order to reduce the risk of bacterial contamination.
- Rinse fish and pat dry.
- Use a meat thermometer to ensure that the food reaches a safe temperature in the middle. This is the only way to tell if your food has reached a high enough internal temperature to destroy harmful bacteria.
- A thermometer in a rare roast or grilled steak should register 60°C. Bacteria exist only on the surface of raw meat. Therefore, roasts and steaks can be eaten rare, providing the surface of the meat is well cooked.
- Minced meats or poultry should always be well cooked and reach a temperature of 70°C. Poultry is cooked when the leg joints move easily and the juices run clear. Fish should flake easily with a fork when it is cooked. Pork should have no pink colour.
- Never refreeze minced meat or poultry.
- When basting or applying a sauce during grilling or barbecuing, brush the sauce on the cooked surface only. Be careful not to recontaminate fully cooked meat or poultry by adding sauce with a brush previously used on raw or undercooked foods.

All produce should be wrapped air-tight to prevent freezer burn, which causes dry patches that have a rough texture and 'off' taste. Frozen vegetables should be cooked straight from the freezer; thawing encourages the destructive activity of residual enzymes and micro-organisms. Do not refreeze foods that have been thawed.

Canning preserves foods by the rapid heating of hermetically sealed containers. The heat destroys micro-organisms and stops enzyme action, and the vacuum seal prevents contamination. An improperly canned food may cause serious food poisoning. Cans and jars that have dents, bubbles, damaged seals or gas escaping on opening must be discarded.

Surprisingly, some commercially processed foods may be more nutritious than fresh (although they may have added sugar or salt). Produce for freezing or canning is often harvested in peak condition and processed quickly to preserve its appearance and nutritional value. Many fresh fruits and vegetables, on the other hand, are picked before ripening and matured in cool rooms; they never reach peak flavour. Look for vine and tree-ripened varieties, and buy them in season.

MEAT, POULTRY AND FISH

- Store meats and fish in the coldest part of the refrigerator. Store meat in special freezer bags or wrap designed to eliminate 'freezer burn'.
- Shellfish cannot be kept more than a few hours at refrigerator temperature, but they last two or threedays on ice or at a temperature below 0°C.
- Cold meats stay fresh until their expiry dates if they are refrigerated unopened in their original vacuum-sealed bags. Once opened, they should be rewrapped in an airtight bag and used within days.
- Cured and smoked meats are best stored in their original wrappings; make sure that cold meats bought from the deli counter are wrapped well and used within a day or two. Meat that shows any discolouration, an off smell or any sign of mould must be discarded.
- Never defrost meat, poultry or fish at room temperature. Defrost all foods on the bottom shelf of the refrigerator. If using the microwave to defrost, cook food immediately after it is thawed.

DAIRY PRODUCTS

- Fresh milk and cream should be tightly sealed in order to prevent tainting by odours from other strong-smelling foods. Milk retains its nutritional value better in cartons, because exposure to light destroys some of the vitamin A and riboflavin.

Thermometer know-how

1 Take the temperature of thin foods like burgers within one minute of removal from heat, larger cuts like roasts, after 5 to 10 minutes.

2 Insert thermometer stem/indicator into the thickest part of the food, away from bone, fat or gristle.

3 Leave thermometer in food for at least 30 seconds before reading temperature.

4 When food has an irregular shape, like some beef roasts, check the temperature in several places.

5 Always wash the thermometer stem thoroughly in hot, soapy water after each use.

- Store nonfat powdered milk in a tightly closed container at room temperature in a place where it's not exposed to light.
- Keep soft cheese and butter tightly covered and refrigerated. Because of concerns about chemical contamination, some people keep plastic materials away from fatty foods, including cheese and butter. Foil is a good wrapper. Butter freezes well in its original wrapping.
- Hard cheeses. Refrigerate Cheddar cheese and other hard cheeses. Very hard Parmesan will keep well if covered and placed in a cool, dark cupboard in the winter. Refrigerate during summer.

OILS

Storage times vary according to the oil and method of processing; some companies claim they can be stored up to one year opened and two years unopened, depending on the oil, and recommend refrigerating after opening. Oils that have a shorter storage life include walnut, sesame, hazelnut, rape seed and almond oils. These are better stored in the refrigerator. Check the label for storage information. Fats turn rancid on exposure to air and pick up odours from other foods. Store tightly sealed oils in a dark cupboard or the refrigerator. Exposure to light and warm temperatures robs oils of vitamins. The cloudiness that forms in some refrigerated oils clears at room temperature. Margarine, like butter, should be well covered and refrigerated; stores for future use may be frozen.

Spices and herbs

The average shelf life of spices and herbs, properly stored, can be one to two years for leafy herbs, two to three years for ground spices and four years for whole spices. Air, light, moisture and heat speed up both flavour and colour loss. Store in a tightly covered container in a dark place away from sunlight, such as inside a cupboard or drawer. For open spice rack storage, choose a site away from light, heat and moisture. Avoid storing above or near the refrigerator, dishwasher, microwave, cooker, sink or a heating vent. Check freshness of spices and herbs by look, smell and taste. A visual check for colour fading is a good indicator of flavour loss.

Cold storage times

PRODUCT	Refrigerator (4°C)	Freezer (-18°C)
Bacon	7 days	1 month
Butter	1–3 months	6–9 months
Chicken or turkey, whole	1–2 days	1 year
Commercial mayonnaise	2 months	Don't freeze
Eggs, fresh, in shell	3–5 weeks	Don't freeze
Minced beef, turkey, veal, pork, lamb	1–2 days	3–4 months
Sausages, unopened package	2 weeks	1–2 months
Sliced meats, unopened package	2 weeks	1–2 months
Margarine	4–5 months	1 year
Milk	7 days	3 months

You can refrigerate commercial mayonnaise after opening it. Use homemade mayonnaise as soon as it's made; however, discard leftovers to reduce the risk of food poisoning by *Salmonella* bacteria.

SUGARS

Honey, golden syrup and molasses keep well at room temperature, as they are too sugary for bacteria to thrive in them. However, natural maple syrup and artificially flavoured syrups are susceptible to moulds – refrigerate after opening. Also refrigerate opened jams and spreads.

White sugar, left unopened in its original package, can be kept for many years in a cool, dry place. Store sugar in an airtight container or freezer bag.

Brown sugar should be stored in an airtight container to retain its moisture and prevent it from hardening. Tightly close the bag or transfer it to an airtight container. If your sugar hardens, place a slice of apple or orange in the container to help bring back its original consistency. Or heat the hardened sugar for 20 to 30 seconds in the microwave just before using it.

182 ■ Fruit

Fruit

BENEFITS

- Excellent sources of vitamin C, beta carotene and potassium; lesser amounts of other vitamins and minerals

- Contain various phytochemicals, which may protect against cancer and other diseases

- High in fibre and low in calories

- A source of natural sugars that provide quick energy

DRAWBACKS

- Some provoke allergic reactions and asthma attacks in susceptible people

For much of human history, fruit has been a favourite food, and with good reason: fruit is tasty, easy to digest, a good source of quick energy and packed with vitamins and minerals.

Anthropologists theorise that apes and early humans alike favoured sweet-tasting fruit, because both species discovered that they were less likely to be poisonous than those that were bitter. Early hunter-gatherers foraged for wild fruit and berries, but as agrarian societies developed, humans learned to cultivate fruit-bearing bushes and trees. Humans also developed methods of drying many fruits so that they could still be enjoyed during their off-season.

Nutritional value

Today, fruit is appreciated for its nutritional value as well as for its pleasing flavour.

Fruit is rich in phytochemicals. Numerous studies demonstrate that people who eat ample amounts of fruit (health experts recommend at least two to three servings a day) enjoy a reduced incidence of many diseases including cancer, heart

Did you know?

Eating pears and apples may help you to shed weight

One study suggests that adding pears and apples to your daily diet may help you to lose weight faster. Researchers studied the impact of fruit intake on overweight women who ate just 300g per day of apples or pears, while following a low-calorie diet. They found that the women who ate fruit lost more weight than the women who didn't.

attacks and strokes. A large study found that men and women who ate five to six servings of fruit and vegetables every day had a lower risk of ischaemic stroke, the most common type of stroke. Another large Harvard study found that those who ate eight or more servings a day of fruit and vegetables had a lower risk of heart disease compared to those who ate fewer than three servings.

Researchers believe that the high amounts of antioxidants, possibly including vitamins A and C (in the form of its precursor, beta carotene), in most fruit protect against these and other diseases.

Antioxidants work by preventing the cell damage caused by free radicals, unstable molecules that are released when the body uses oxygen. Fruits are also high in phyto-chemicals that may help to prevent or retard tumour growth.

Citrus fruit is among the richest sources of vitamin C. Nutritionists recommend at least one daily serving of a vitamin C-rich food such as an orange, grapefruit, tangerine or other citrus fruit. A serving is one medium-size fruit or a 150ml glass of pure juice. Other fruits that are high in vitamin C include all types of melon, kiwi fruit, strawberries,

raspberries, mangoes and papaya. Cranberry juice is another excellent source of vitamin C.

Brightly coloured fruit is high in beta carotene. Fruit with orange or deep yellow flesh – including apricots and mangoes – gets its colour from the yellow-orange pigment beta carotene, which the body converts to vitamin A. Other carotene pigments, such as lycopene in guavas and pink grapefruit, or bioflavonoids such as quercetin in grapes and apples, are thought to protect against heart disease. In fact, recent studies indicate that quercetin or resveratrol may be the ingredients in wine responsible for the noted reduction in heart disease and stroke among moderate wine drinkers. Many fruits are high in potassium,

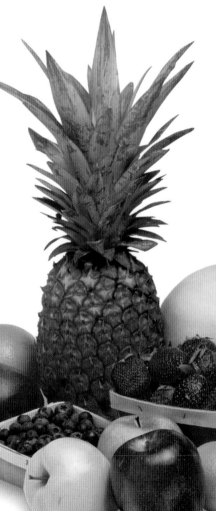

an electrolyte that is essential to maintaining a proper balance of body fluids. Adequate potassium also appears to reduce the risk of developing high blood pressure. People taking diuretic drugs, which increase the excretion of potassium in the urine, are advised to eat extra servings of bananas, melons, apricots and dried fruit to maintain adequate levels of this mineral.

Most fruit is low in calories and high in fibre, a fact that enhances its appeal to people who are weight conscious. Apples, pears and many other fruits contain pectin, a soluble fibre that helps to regulate blood cholesterol levels. Berries, citrus and dried fruit are especially high in both soluble and insoluble fibres.

The pesticide issue

Because fruit trees are particularly vulnerable to a variety of worms, flies and other destructive insects, many growers use pesticide sprays to keep them in check. Many people worry that residues of these pesticides pose a substantial health risk. The use of these chemicals is controlled by law and must meet specific safety standards. Experts agree that the health benefits of eating fruit outweigh any risk. Even so, fruit should be washed well before eating, and some

fruit should be peeled. Ones that should be peeled include apples that have been sprayed with a wax to extend their shelf life and to make them more attractive. The wax itself is harmless, but it seals the skin and prevents pesticide residue from being washed away.

Citrus fruit is often coated with fungicides and other pesticides that are used to prevent mould growth and fruit fly infestation. Ordinarily, this would not pose a problem because the peels are discarded. But if you are using the zest of fresh citrus peels, wash the fruit well. This is also a good precaution when squeezing the juice from citrus fruit. Do not use any form of soap when washing produce. You may consume the soap residues.

Imported fruit may be more hazardous than that grown locally, since pesticides that may be banned in the UK may be used abroad. There are safety standards for imported foods, which are also subject to inspection, but not every batch of imported food can be tested for pesticide residues. It's a good idea to be extra diligent about washing imported fruit and other produce before eating it.

People who are uncomfortable eating foods that have been treated with pesticides can now choose from a wide range of organic produce that has been

grown without the use of pesticides. The disadvantages of organic produce, is that it is more expensive and doesn't look as perfect as foods that have been grown using pesticides.

12 ways to eat more fruit

1 At breakfast, top your cereal with sliced bananas, kiwi fruit, fresh berries or dried fruit such as sultanas or apricots and drink a small glass of juice.

2 Keep the fruit bowl full and easily accessible.

3 Carry single-serving packs of dried fruit for snacks at work.

4 Pack your briefcase, backpack or glove compartment with easy-to-carry fruit such as apples, pears, bananas, mandarins or dried fruit.

5 Make a smoothie with yoghurt, milk, or soya milk mixed with a fresh or frozen berries.

6 Mix a bowl of low-fat yoghurt with fruit.

7 Add 1 cup fresh or frozen berries to pancake batter. Top pancakes with stewed apples or rhubarb compote instead of syrup.

8 In restaurants, order fruit as a dessert.

9 Don't throw out overripe bananas. Freeze them and use them for banana smoothies.

10 Add fruit such as apples, pears, melon and orange sections to green salads.

11 Try something new like dried cranberries or sliced mango.

12 Add chopped dried apricots to couscous, salads and tabboulehs.

Functional foods

Enhanced for health

The link between diet and health continues to grow, and researchers have begun looking at benefits that certain foods may provide beyond their basic nutritional value. Recent years have seen a growing interest in functional foods – that is, foods that have specific components, naturally occurring or added, that may reduce the risk of certain diseases. Whole as well as fortified, enriched or enhanced foods can fall into this category.

Unmodified whole foods such as vegetables and fruit are the simplest example of a naturally occurring functional food. For example, broccoli, carrots or tomatoes may be considered functional foods because they are very rich in compounds that have been linked with reduced risk of various diseases. Modified foods, including those fortified with nutrients or enhanced with specific phytochemicals or botanical extracts, are also functional foods. There is now hope that these can play a role in preventing and treating conditions such as cancer, diabetes, high blood pressure, heart disease, arthritis and other disorders.

First developed by the Japanese, the functional-food market is now one of the fastest-growing segments of the food industry in the UK, the United States and Japan. In many other countries, such as Canada, Australia and New Zealand, its growth has been made slower because of current regulatory constraints.

Some types of fortified functional foods have been around for decades. For example, we fortify margarine with vitamin D to prevent vitamin D deficiency diseases such as rickets. We add iodine to salt to prevent goitre. But the recent explosion of research into the role of food, nutrients and disease has resulted in huge interest by food companies to develop and market foods as medicine. Supermarkets are becoming filled with foods that are enriched with disease-protecting compounds.

In the pipeline are discussions about adding a number of functional elements to foods and drinks in the the UK. Flax is already added to bread and cereals.

Many areas of controversy surround functional foods. Those not in favour of them believe that they will distract people from eating healthy diets. Others believe that there is plenty of evidence to show that

The link between diet and disease

Proportion of disease onset linked to diet	
Atherosclerosis	50%
Hypertension	50%
Stroke	50%
Type 2 diabetes	50%–70%
Coronary heart disease	40%
Cancer	35%–50%

Definitions

FUNCTIONAL FOODS: Foods or food components that have shown benefits in reducing the risk of disease beyond basic nutritional functions. Other terms that have been used interchangeably with functional foods are designer foods, medicinal foods and pharma foods.

FORTIFIED FOODS: A type of functional food that has been enhanced, or fortified, with nutrients or other food components, to help to prevent or treat disease. Calcium-fortified orange juice is an example of a fortified food. Fortified foods can also be called enriched or enhanced foods.

NUTRACEUTICALS: Products isolated from food and sold in medicinal forms to help to prevent or treat disease, such as omega-3 fatty acids, or phyto-oestrogens.

certain functional foods could be the counterbalance to the prevalence of chronic disease and the cost of treatment. Here are some of the food components that are the focus of current research.

■ **OMEGA-3 FATTY ACIDS.** These have been linked to the treatment and prevention of a large variety of diseases, including heart disease and stroke, lupus, diabetes, inflammatory bowel disease, arthritis, and breast, colon and prostate cancer. Foods containing omega-3 fatty acids include oily fish and all seafood, fish oils and linseeds. Some eggs and some types of milk now contain small amounts of omega-3 fatty acids.

■ **SOYA PROTEIN.** Research supports the role of soya protein in the reduction of blood cholesterol levels. It remains unknown whether the effect comes from the isoflavones (hormone-like plant compounds) in soya or some other components – perhaps sterols. Isoflavones are now being studied for their potential anti-cancer properties. They may also protect against osteoporosis. Soya protein can be found in soya beans, tofu, tempeh, soya cereals and soya beverages.

■ **PROBIOTICS AND PREBIOTICS.** Probiotics are active bacterial cultures that may help to restore gut function and improve immune response. They are found in yoghurt and other fermented foods. Prebiotics are substances that stimulate the growth of specific beneficial bacteria in the colon. Fructo-oligosaccharide and inulin, both of which are found in chicory (endive) root, are good examples. They can be extracted from the root and added to foods.

■ **LUTEIN.** This carotenoid (a type of antioxidant) is believed to help to counter age-related macular degeneration, the main cause of vision loss in older people. It is in foods such as eggs, corn, spinach, kiwi fruit, oranges, broccoli and Brussels sprouts.

■ **PSYLLIUM.** Psyllium is added to some heart-healthy cereals and other foods for its cholesterol-lowering soluble fibre. It also helps to soften stools and cleanse the intestinal tract.

■ **OATS.** They are rich in a cholesterol-reducing soluble fibre, which is known as beta-glucan.

When in doubt, stick with nature's functional foods

As researchers and food companies continue to look at new ways to link food products with disease prevention and treatment, remember that nature has provided us with an abundance of functional foods. Fruit and vegetables, as well as whole grains, legumes, nuts and seeds are examples of foods naturally packed with phytonutrients that we know can lower the risk of cancer, heart disease, hypertension and many other chronic diseases. No matter what the future of functional foods brings, you can't go wrong sticking with the basics.

■ **PLANT STEROLS AND STANOLS.** These cholesterol-lowering compounds, which are extracted from soya beans and are also found in nuts, seeds and wheatgerm, are added to some margarines such as Benecol and Flora Pro activ.

■ **BROCCOLI.** This vegetable contains sulphoraphane, which has been shown to have anti-cancer properties. Some people are unable to benefit from this as they lack a gene to help them to retain it in the body. British researchers are breeding a type of 'super broccoli' with higher than normal levels of sulphoraphane to help these people to retain enough.

■ **BLACKCURRANTS.** Increasing the starch levels in a blackcurrant bush's leaves, increases the amount of vitamin C in the fruit, the following year.

■ **GINGER AND CHILLIES.** They are being investigated for potential to reduce certain cancers.

■ **CURCUMIN.** This is the natural yellow pigment in turmeric and is being looked into for potential benefits in reducing cholesterol, improving cardio-vascular health, relieving inflammatory bowel diseases and fighting cancer. Research is still at an early stage.

F

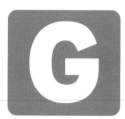

Gallstones

EAT PLENTY OF

- Small meals at regular intervals
- Breakfast daily

AVOID

- Weight gain
- Excessive alcohol

The gall bladder seems to serve no purpose other than to store and concentrate bile, a substance that is produced by the liver to digest fats in the small intestine. Removing it has little effect on digestion in most people. Bile fluid contains high levels of cholesterol and bilirubin, both of which precipitate as crystals to form stones; these may be as fine as beach sand or as coarse as river gravel. Most gallstones are hardened cholesterol; the rest are made up of bilirubin plus calcium.

Gallstones are most common in overweight middle-aged women. They also tend to run in families. Women, especially those who have borne children, are thought to be particularly vulnerable to developing gallstones because of the high levels of blood cholesterol and bile that develop late in pregnancy and in the weeks following childbirth. It is believed, too, that progesterone and oestrogen, occurring naturally or taken in oral contraceptives, may play a role in gallstone formation. Crash weight-loss diets are believed to be another precipitating factor;

many people appear to develop gallstones after a period of weight loss and gain, or after a single dramatic weight loss.

Many people have no symptoms. For some, however, the presence of gallstones can cause pain in the upper right abdomen when the gall bladder contracts to release bile after a meal, and inflammation of the gall bladder (cholecystitis) that brings on sudden, severe pain extending to the back and under the right shoulder blade, with fever, chills and vomiting. If the stones obstruct the flow of bile, the skin and the whites of the eyes become jaundiced. Untreated, stones lodge in the bile duct and cause the liver or pancreas to become inflamed.

For frequent painful attacks, the usual treatment is the surgical removal of the gall bladder, called cholecystectomy. Medications have been used with mixed success to dissolve gallstones, but the stones often recur if the person stops taking the drug. Another option is a procedure called lithotripsy, which uses shock waves to break up the gallstones.

Gallstones and nutrition

Eat small, frequent meals – especially breakfast. For years, people with gallstones have been warned to eliminate fats and cholesterol from their diets, based on the observation that most stones are formed of cholesterol. In fact, there's little evidence that a low-cholesterol diet will lower the risk of gallstones. Some clinicians even claim that the occasional fatty meal causes the gall bladder to empty itself, which may be beneficial.

Although a diet high in fibre and low in fats is recommended for general health, there are no scientific grounds for believing that high fibre intake can favourably influence

cholesterol metabolism, at least as far as gallstones are concerned. It is known, however, that the bile is more likely to form stones after the long period of fasting that occurs overnight, while we sleep. Because of this, some doctors recommend that people with gall bladder problems should eat a substantial breakfast, which will cause the bladder to empty itself and flush out any small stones and stagnant bile. Other doctors go even further, and advise patients to eat frequent small meals to maintain this filling and emptying cycle.

Consume plenty of starchy foods with lots of fruit and vegetables. People with gallstones should avoid foods that cause them discomfort. Their diet should emphasise starchy foods, with lots of fruits and vegetables, moderate servings of protein and small amounts of fat. Alcohol should be used in moderation, if at all, especially if the gall bladder disease also affects the liver and pancreas.

Game and game birds

BENEFITS

- Low in fat and calories, compared with untrimmed meat from farm animals
- Excellent sources of protein
- Rich in B vitamins
- Rich in iron
- Good source of phosphorous and they contain potassium

DRAWBACK

- Danger of biting or swallowing lead shot in wild game

Because of their harsh environment, wild game can rarely afford to build up the fat reserves that are typical of many domesticated animals. Hence there is little or no fatty tissue to be trimmed from game. But once the meat has been trimmed, lean cuts of both game and domesticated animals have a similar fat and calorie content. Like all meat, game and game birds provide abundant amounts of protein and are rich sources of B vitamins and iron. They are also good sources of potassium, which is needed for the maintenance of all cells, and phosphorus, which is essential for healthy bones and teeth.

Rabbit, hare, venison and a wide range of game birds are available in good butchers and larger super-markets throughout the year, now. Prices are often very reasonable during the shooting season (which varies for different game species), while at other times – when only frozen game is available – it can be very expensive.

Much of the game sold in Europe is wild, but in the United States hunters are usually not allowed to sell their quarry, so most retail game has been farmed. With wild game any risk of contamination by anti-biotics, artificial growth hormones or pesticides is minimal. Reared game, however, is not always clear of these chemicals.

Tough old birds

As game and game birds tend to be more active than domesticated animals, their meat tends to be tougher. This is mainly due to the collagen of their muscles being more resistant to breakdown during cooking than the collagen found in meats from domesticated animals. It is important, therefore, that game meats are prepared and cooked in the correct way. Hanging game helps to tenderise it and improve its flavour. If you are unsure how long you should hang game, ask your local butcher for guidelines. The age of the animal and the temperature of the room can make a difference. In cold conditions pheasants may need to be hung for as long as two to three weeks, but if it is warm, a day or two may be enough. Game birds that have been frozen should not be hung after they have been thawed. Roasting is the best way of cooking all young game birds. A hot oven gives a brown, crispy skin – but game should never be overcooked. Rabbit is best cooked in a traditional stew and venison usually needs long, slow cooking for tender and flavoursome meat.

Although lead is an accumulative poison and you should try to avoid ingesting any pellets, swallowing one by mistake will not normally cause any ill effects. Remove the lead shot from wild game as you prepare it for cooking, and warn any diners that there may still be some in the meat because lead shot can damage teeth.

Garlic

BENEFITS

- May help to lower high blood pressure and elevated blood cholesterol
- May prevent or fight certain cancers
- Antiviral and antibacterial properties help to prevent or fight infection
- May alleviate nasal congestion

DRAWBACKS

- Causes bad breath
- Can cause indigestion, especially if eaten raw
- Direct contact irritates the skin and mucous membranes

Herbalists and folk healers have used garlic to treat myriad diseases for thousands of years. Ancient Egyptian healers prescribed it to build physical strength, the Greeks used it as a laxative and the Chinese traditionally used it to lower blood

What is in your game pie?

Wild game is generally considered healthier than farmed meat. If you bag your own, there is the benefit of physical exertion while out hunting. The chart below gives details of game's nutritional benefits. The recommended daily allowance for phosphorus is 550mg; for potassium 3,500mg; and for iron 8.7mg.

FOOD PER 100g	FAT (g)	SATURATED FAT (g)	PROTEIN (g)	PHOSPHORUS (mg)	POTASSIUM (mg)	IRON (mg)
Roast venison	6.4	2.0	35	290	360	7.8
Stewed rabbit	7.7	1.7	27.3	200	210	1.9
Stewed hare	8.0	2.0	29.9	250	210	10.8
Roast pheasant	9.3	4.0	32.2	310	410	8.4
Roast grouse	5.3	0.5	31.3	340	470	7.6
Roast partridge	7.2	2.0	36.7	310	410	7.7
Roast pigeon	13.2	2.0	27.8	400	410	19.4

G

CAUTION

GARLIC AND OIL PRODUCTS

Some people like to store chopped garlic in oil, but these preparations are potentially dangerous if the garlic has not been thoroughly cleaned. Minute amounts of adhering soil can harbour spores of the *Clostridium botulinum* bacterium that can germinate and cause botulism, a deadly form of food poisoning. This can occur without any evidence of spoilage such as 'off' odour, taste or appearance. Buy only commercial preparations of chopped garlic that contain preservatives such as salt or acids.

pressure. In the Middle Ages, eating quantities of garlic was credited with providing immunity to the plague. But just because garlic has been used for a long time does not mean that it has been used effectively for a long time. Current research on garlic has curbed the optimism fostered by earlier studies.

Louis Pasteur, the 19th-century French chemist, was the first to demonstrate garlic's antiseptic properties, information that was put to use during both World Wars by the British, German and Russian armies. Since then, numerous studies have confirmed that garlic can be effective against bacteria, fungi, viruses and parasites. Today, many herbal treatments prescribe garlic to help to prevent colds, flu and other infectious diseases.

The study of garlic

Garlic has been intensively studied in recent years, with more than 500 papers having been published in medical journals since the mid 1980s. The subject of most of these studies has been the sulphur compounds that form when allicin undergoes a variety of chemical reactions. Allicin is not found in fresh garlic but forms when cells

are disturbed by cooking, cutting or chewing. Ajoene, allyl sulfides, S-allyl cystein (SAC) and other products of this allicin cascade have been associated with anti-cancer, anti-clotting, antifungal, anti-hypertensive, antioxidant and cholesterol-lowering effects.

Some garlic supplements tout their allicin 'content'. This is not valid because allicin is an unstable substance. Claims about 'allicin yield' or 'allicin potential' are more appropriate, but not much. Manufacturers usually determine 'yield' by mixing crushed tablets with water and measuring the amount of allicin released. This is not an appropriate model for what happens in the body.

Garlic supplements must be kept from contact with stomach acid since it would immediately destroy alliinase and hinder the release of allicin. This is usually done by encapsulating in gelatin or coating the pill with cellulose or polyacrylic acid derivatives that dissolve only in the less acidic conditions of the intestine. A test for allicin release, which simulates the conditions encountered by a pill as it travels through the digestive tract was applied to garlic supplements, with astounding results. More than 80 per cent of products tested released less than 15 per cent of their claimed allicin potential. Clearly they do not deliver a therapeutic allicin dosage. Whether garlic is therapeutic at all can be determined only by human trials. It may be impressive to learn that some garlic extract retards

cholesterol oxidation in cells; but that does not mean this happens in the body. Numerous studies of garlic's effects on health have been carried out. Early studies suggested a cholesterol-lowering effect and received much publicity.

Unfortunately more sophisticated studies curtailed the initial optimism. When researchers analysed the results of the garlic studies, they found, much to their disappointment, that garlic's ability to reduce cholesterol was minimal, and the effect on blood pressure was insignificant. Still, some companies keep promoting supplements based on the early studies.

Effect on heart disease

While garlic may not reduce cholesterol, it may still have an effect on heart disease. Ajoene, one of the breakdown products of allicin, may reduce the risk of heart attacks by preventing the formation of blood clots.

Promising studies on garlic and cancer

The situation is more encouraging with respect to cancer, perhaps because most studies investigated the effect of raw or cooked garlic instead of supplements. A meta analysis showed that consuming an average of six or more cloves a week lowered the risk of colorectal cancer by 30 per cent and stomach cancer by 50 per cent when compared with the consumption of less than one clove a week. Even the risk of prostate cancer may be reduced. A National Cancer Institute study of men in Shanghai showed that eating a clove of garlic a day reduced the risk of prostate cancer by more than 50 per cent.

There is a caveat to this type of study, though. Consumption of specific foods is determined by means of questionnaires and people's memories may not be all that reliable. Furthermore, heavy garlic consumption may simply be the hallmark of a mostly vegetarian diet.

There is no consensus, however, on how much garlic should be consumed to make use of its anti-cancer effect, and neither is there agreement on whether cooked or dried garlic confers the same benefits imparted by eating garlic raw. It does seem clear though, that to activate garlic's full nutritional power, it should be chopped or crushed and then left to stand for about 10 minutes before cooking. This allows allicin and its potent derivatives to be activated. While there is no guarantee that garlic will have an effect on health, it will have an effect on the breath.

Treating garlic breath

Eating parsley after eating garlic might help to reduce the unpleasant odour, possibly because of its chlorophyll content. Garlic may cause indigestion, especially if eaten raw. Handling raw garlic can irritate the skin and mucous membranes. Garlic (both fresh and supplements) may enhance the effects of blood-thinning medications, so talk to your doctor before using it, if you are taking such medication.

Gastritis

CONSUME

- Regular meals with a balance of starchy foods, fruit, vegetables and low-fat protein

AVOID

- Fatty foods, chocolate, alcohol, caffeine and peppermint, which can cause acid reflux

- Spicy foods if they irritate you

- Frequent use of aspirin, nonsteroidal anti-inflammatory drugs (NSAIDs) or other arthritis pain relievers

An inflammation of the stomach lining, gastritis is usually signalled by indigestion, either with or without bleeding in the digestive tract. Acute gastritis often develops when people are subjected to sudden stress, such as from extensive burns or other severe injury or illness; it may also develop after surgery, leading to stress ulcers and severe intestinal bleeding.

Chronic inflammation can occur with long-term use of certain medications (such as aspirin, anti-inflammatory and arthritis drugs), gastrointestinal disorders (for example, Crohn's disease), alcoholism or viral infections. It has recently been discovered that many cases of gastritis are caused by a bacterium, *Helicobacter pylori*. This organism has also been linked to peptic ulcers and is the only germ that is currently known to be able to survive in the acidic environment of the human stomach.

Gastritis is more common with age and most sufferers complain of indigestion, heartburn, nausea and belching. Other people have no noticeable symptoms, which can be dangerous if gastritis is caused by erosion of the stomach lining with bleeding – normally a result of aspirin or other anti-inflammatory medication.

Usually, people with acute gastritis caused by illness or injury have already been hospitalised for treatment of their underlying condition; therefore, symptoms of gastritis are managed in the course of their intensive care.

Avoid spicy foods. Although foods are not usually the cause of gastritis, people with symptoms should avoid spicy foods, which can irritate the stomach lining. They should also avoid fatty foods, chocolate, drinks with caffeine, decaffeinated coffee, peppermint and alcohol. These foods relax the valve between the stomach and oesophagus and make it easier for the stomach contents to back up into the oesophagus, causing further irritation.

If you need a pain reliever, ask your doctor to prescribe a non-irritating alternative to aspirin or other nonsteroidal anti-inflammatory drug (NSAID). For gastritis caused by *H. pylori*, the doctor may prescribe antibiotics. Antacids can sometimes soothe the irritation until the inflammation subsides.

Gastroenteritis

See page 192

Genetically modified foods

GMs – benefit or hazard?

The availability of genetically altered foods continues to be a hotly debated issue with powerful lobbies on both sides. Maize that resists attacks by insects, rapeseed crops that tolerate herbicides and cheese that can be made without using animal rennet have been some of the processes introduced by genetic modification, but some people worry that possible long-term effects may not have been adequately assessed.

For centuries, food growers have attempted to improve plants and animals by bringing out desirable traits while suppressing less desirable ones, in order to produce increasingly abundant foods. This was a slow process and took years; however it is much faster now with the relatively recent discovery of the ability to genetically modify plants, animals and micro-organisms. Genes can now be moved from one organism to another in order to increase resistance to pests and disease, increase the ability to adapt to environmental conditions, improve flavour or nutritional value, delay ripening or increase shelflife. This is called 'genetic engineering' – and is highly controversial worldwide. Crops that have been genetically modified are known as GM foods or GMOs (genetically modified organisms).

The production of GM foods is high in the United States and Canada. To date, each of these countries has approved at least 40 plant varieties derived by genetic modification. Soya beans, corn and canola (rapeseed) are the most widely produced GM crops, supplying a number of ingredients used in highly processed foods (about 70 per cent of them contain some GM ingredients).

IMPROVING ON NATURE

There are, undoubtedly, benefits to genetically modifying crops, and research botanists are able to add desirable hereditary traits to almost any plant, including producing more nutritious foods while at the same time increasing the plant's resistance to pests. For example, maize that has increased high-quality protein but resists the corn-borer weevil; or a type of rapeseed that synthesises more of the unsaturated fatty acids of the oil it provides. Soya beans can be modified to become resistant to herbicides, so crops can be sprayed to remove weeds. And rice can be enriched with beta carotene by adding one gene from a daffodil and another from a bacterium. Agricultural scientists are also trying to alter plants to make them more productive or more able to withstand adverse growing conditions, such as drought. This type of genetic engineering has tremendous potential in overcoming world food shortages; conceivably, arid desert areas could one day produce drought-resistant grains and GM plants may even help the world to survive global warming.

Cheese producers have also benefited from genetic modification. The traditional way to make cheese involves using rennet, extracted from calf stomachs to curdle milk. But chymosin, the major enzyme in rennet can also be produced through genetic engineering. Cheese made with it is therefore acceptable to vegetarians and tastes the same as normal cheese.

THE DOWNSIDE

Not all experiments have been as successful: in the early 1990s, genetically modified tomatoes were introduced. They were bred to stay firm after harvest, which meant they could ripen fully on the vine. However, the skins were so delicate that they were easily damaged, and were removed from the market in 1997. Another controversial development, the use of growth hormones in cows in the USA to make them produce more milk, was declared unsafe by the United Nations Food Safety Agency in 1999 as it posed cancer risks. The hormone is still used in the USA.

Some people are concerned that there may be other unforeseen consequences.

Allergic reaction. If a gene that produces a protein that causes an allergic reaction is introduced to a food plant, a person who is allergic to that protein will react adversely. Although companies have to state whether altered food contains any suspect allergens, unknown allergens may slip through.

Increased toxicity. Genetic modification may enhance natural plant toxins in unexpected ways.

Herbicide resistant weeds. Once modified crops are planted, their genes may be carried by wind, water or animals to related species (including weeds), causing them to be herbicide resistant as well.

Unintended harm to the organism. Animals subjected to genetic engineering do not fare as well as plants. Sheep injected with genetically engineered hormones to increase wool growth, for example, become more vulnerable to the heat. Chickens and pigs treated with special growth hormones develop painful bone and joint problems. There are also ethical issues involved in tampering with animal genes.

Resistance to antibiotics. As part of the genetic modification of organisms, marker genes are used to check if the desired gene has been successfully embedded. These marker genes are usually resistant to antibiotics and, over time, could contribute to the already growing problem of antibiotic resistance.

ECOLOGICAL CONCERNS

Insecticide-producing maize is said to kill butterflies as well as insect pests, and concerns have been raised about the effects on soil quality and wildlife. GM plants may cross-pollinate with others growing nearby so that pesticide resistance is transferred to other species with unknown consequences.

Although use of genetically modified species in the UK is tightly regulated, in 2000 it was discovered that a small proportion of oilseed rape grown in the UK and Europe contained low levels of a GM variety. It was believed to have occurred because the original seed stock from Canada was grown too close to a genetically modified crop.

IT'S A QUESTION OF BENEFITS VERSUS RISKS

The potential benefits of genetic modification are numerous. Sweet potato is an important crop in Africa but is very susceptible to feathery mottle virus. Inserting genes from chrysanthemums that have naturally insecticidal compounds called pyrethrins has the potential of increasing yields dramatically. The use of pesticides on cotton has already been reduced by incorporating a gene that protects it from insects. While there are environmental concerns about pollen drift and crossbreeding with non-GM plants, no adverse health effects have been reported.

LABELLING

European Commission legislation that came into force in 2004, requires all GM products to be traceable throughout the chain, from farm to table, and ensures that all food and feed containing or produced from GM organisms is suitably labelled.

Foodstuffs imported from the USA may well contain genetically modified organisms, but as the USA and Canada do not label these foods, it is impossible for the customer to know. Foods from Australia and New Zealand are labelled 'genetically modified' if they contain organisms that have been altered in any way.

Gastroenteritis

CONSUME

■ Fluids, such as chicken broth or clear soup, for rehydration

■ Solid foods gradually, as symptoms subside

AVOID

■ Alcohol and caffeine, which stimulate the lower bowel

■ High-fibre foods, which may irritate an inflamed bowel

■ Frequent use of aspirin or other anti-inflammatory painkillers

■ If travelling abroad: unpeeled fruit and vegetables, uncooked foods, unboiled tap water and ice cubes in drinks

■ Milk and dairy products

Gastroenteritis is extremely common; it affects about 20 per cent of people every year. Symptoms include diarrhoea, vomiting, fever and abdominal pain brought on by inflammation of the stomach and lower gastrointestinal tract.

It has many causes: infection with a virus, bacterium or parasite; ingestion of toxic substances; an allergy to or intolerance of food; and some medications, often antibiotics, that alter the normal bacterial population of the lower tract.

People with eating disorders, such as anorexia and bulimia, may develop gastroenteritis as a result of laxative abuse.

Viral infection is most often responsible and can be transmitted via contaminated food, especially through infected and unhygienic food handlers. It can be passed on from person to person, making it contagious. Bacterial infection is due to food poisoning through contaminated food. Dairy products and seafood, especially those past

their 'use by' dates, can be culprits. Thanks to clean water supplies, gastroenteritis due to cholera and typhoid fever is now rare in the developed nations. By contrast, gastroenteritis caused by parasites, can strike in any country. Parasites can be transmitted in a variety of ways, such as through unsanitary food handling, contamination of drinking water and close physical contact with an infected person.

When vomiting and diarrhoea persist longer than 48 hours, your doctor may prescribe a medication to quell nausea, as well as an antibiotic if it seems advisable. If diarrhoea is bloody, your doctor may investigate the possibility of a parasitic infection or bacillary dysentery.

Gastroenteritis is often referred to as 'stomach flu'. Provided that the infecting organism is a bacterium or virus and not a parasite, symptoms usually clear up within a few days. But in babies, the elderly and people with a suppressed immune system, gastroenteritis usually needs medical attention. Dehydration is a danger; it is vital to keep the patient's fluid intake up, especially in children.

Rehydration solutions are better than water alone. You can buy them in pharmacies or make your own by dissolving 8 teaspoons of sugar and one of salt in a litre of water. While the symptoms last, take two glasses of rehydration solution every hour. Other soothing fluids are teas made from raspberry leaf, ginger or cinnamon. Sipping ginger ale can help to calm any surges of nausea. Don't drink alcohol or beverages with caffeine; they stimulate the digestive tract and can actually worsen diarrhoea.

Try the BRAT diet. This diet – based on bananas, boiled rice, apples and dry white toast – often helps to relieve symptoms. Eat small amounts of these for 48 hours.

Reintroduce solid foods slowly. As your bowel settles down, try small portions of other bland foods. Basically, you can eat any food that you feel like, but you should keep portions small, avoid fried foods and don't overtax the digestive system with fibre that could be irritating to an inflamed bowel.

A virus by any other name

In recent years outbreaks of an illness called the Norwalk Virus have made the news. In fact, Norwalk is viral gastro-enteritis and has the same symptoms. It is most often caused by contaminated food or water. Cruise ships, swimming pools, recreational lakes, wells and even municipal water supplies may become contaminated and cause out-breaks. Shellfish and salad ingredients are the foods most likely to be culprits. Fortunately, the virus doesn't multiply in food and is destroyed through cooking. Stick to well-cooked food and bottled drinks without ice, especially when travelling, to avoid this illness.

After about 48 hours you should be able to tolerate foods such as steamed or boiled potatoes, cooked vegetables (carrots are kind to stomachs) and a boiled or poached egg. Leave dairy foods until last; the fat in cheese may be difficult to digest and stays in the stomach longer than other foods. Some infections can temporarily interfere with your ability to digest lactose, the sugar found in milk. Strangely, many people find they can tolerate yoghurt even when other dairy foods provoke digestive problems. Keep up your fluid intake with water and juices, and resume a normal diet when you feel ready.

Because some drugs can cause severe gastroenteritis, contact your doctor if any digestive upset occurs while you are taking an antibiotic or other medication. The doctor may decide to switch you to another medication or therapy.

Ginger

BENEFITS

- May prevent motion sickness
- Can help to quell nausea, including nausea in early pregnancy
- Ginger wine may help to relieve menstrual cramps

DRAWBACKS

- Raw or sweet ginger may irritate oral tissue and other mucous membranes

The Chinese were using ginger to flavour food in the 6th century BC, and Arab traders introduced the spice to the Mediterranean before the 1st century AD. Transported from the Middle East to Europe by the Crusaders, ginger was an ingredient in almost every recipe found in a 1390 cookbook that was compiled at the English royal court. Spanish settlers brought ginger to the New World in the 1500s.

The Zingiberaceae family includes ginger and two other popular spices – cardamom and turmeric – as well as the banana, an unlikely distant cousin. Cardamom is widely used in tropical cuisines; in addition, it lends fragrance to Scandinavian breads and pastries.

Turmeric, a major ingredient in commercial curry powders, is also used in Asia to dye fabrics yellow and in Western countries to improve the colour of some foods.

Do one simple thing

Relieve a cold with ginger tea

A comforting way to relieve the chills and congestion of a cold: make ginger tea with a teaspoon of freshly grated ginger, the juice of half a lemon and a teaspoon of honey, topped up with boiling water. Let it stand for 10 minutes before drinking.

▶ **Root remedy**
Adding a slice or two of peeled raw ginger to bean dishes is said to reduce the flatulence these foods often cause.

Popular folk remedy

Ginger has a long and honoured tradition in folk medicine, and was traditionally used to protect against respiratory and digestive infections, and to ease the flatulence and griping pains of indigestion.

Modern research is exploring the scientific basis for ginger's effects.

Cancer. Studies have shown that beta ionone, a terpenoid found in ginger, has anti-cancer properties.

Nausea and motion sickness. Various forms of ginger have been used to counter the nausea and vomiting of motion sickness. This practice is particularly well established in Germany, where it is an approved treatment for motion sickness and heartburn. A recent study found that ginger was as effective as prescription medication in preventing motion sickness, without causing the drowsiness that the drug sometimes does.

Sipping flat ginger ale or sucking pieces of crystalised ginger, which has a more concentrated flavour, may help to quell spells of nausea due to morning sickness, food poisoning, gastroenteritis or chemotherapy. Ginger is also available in capsule form for those who find that it irritates the mouth.

Pain. Because ginger blocks the pro-inflammatory prostaglandins (hormone-like chemicals), it may also be useful in helping people who suffer from the pain of:

- Migraines. They are thought to be caused by inflammation in blood vessels in the brain. At least one study suggests that taking ginger at the first sign of a migraine can help to reduce the symptoms.
- Arthritis. Prostaglandins contribute to joint swelling in people with arthritis. Studies have shown that people with either osteoarthritis or rheumatoid arthritis experienced less pain and swelling when they took powdered ginger daily.

Glandular fever

CONSUME PLENTY OF

- Fruit and vegetable juices for vitamins and minerals
- Milkshakes or smoothies for calories, minerals and vitamins
- Soups for easy nourishment
- Soft foods to soothe a sore throat

AVOID

- Alcohol

A common disease, glandular fever, or mononucleosis, is caused by the Epstein-Barr virus which is passed on in the saliva by coughing, sneezing or kissing. Otherwise, most people who have only casual contact with an infected person do not become infected.

Glandular fever is most common in adolescents and young adults in their early 20s and can be quite debilitating. They generally have fatigue, fever, severe sore throat and swollen lymph nodes. Loss of appetite, headaches and general achiness are common. The fever and sore throat may be misdiagnosed as tonsillitis as the symptoms are similar. If the sore throat is treated with ampicillin, an antibiotic similar to penicillin, the person with glandular fever develops a rash. The spleen – and, less often, the liver – may become enlarged. In very severe cases the patient may develop jaundice.

The symptoms typically last for a week or two, and most people are able to return to work at that time. In a few cases, however, recovery may take several months, as a low-grade fever, poor appetite and fatigue persist for weeks after the other symptoms have disappeared. Sometimes fatigue persists for months or even years.

One of the best ways to avoid glandular fever, especially for young people, is to avoid kissing or sharing cups or mugs with people who have had the infection recently.

The role of diet

If you are diagnosed with glandular fever, aim to give your immune system the best possible chance of fighting the illness.

Consume lots of immune-boosting nutrients. A well-balanced diet can aid recovery and boost the strength of the immune system. Stimulate a poor appetite with several light, appetising meals rather than a few larger ones.

Drink at least eight glasses of water or juice daily. During the acute phase, when fever may be high, it's important to drink plenty of liquids in order to prevent dehydration. During recuperation, juices have the added benefit of providing vitamins and other beneficial, immune-boosting nutrients. Milkshakes, smoothies and fruit juices diluted with water will help to soothe a sore throat and will also provide calories for energy, along with useful minerals and vitamins.

Try soft foods and foods with fibre. Stewed fruits supply soluble fibre, which helps to prevent constipation. Soups are nutritious and easy to drink. Soft foods, such as tofu, scrambled eggs, cottage cheese and yoghurt, are easily swallowed, even by someone with a sore throat. Fruit and vegetables can be puréed to make them easier to swallow, if necessary; serve puréed vegetables as a sauce over rice or soft noodles. Herbal teas made from peppermint or elderflower are soothing, and gargling with tepid salt water can relieve a sore throat. Avoid alcohol, which weakens the immune system and can further damage the liver.

Supplements of vitamin C and vitamin B complex may be a good idea until you have recovered.

Treatment

See a doctor if you think you have glandular fever, since blood tests are necessary for a definitive diagnosis. Rest is an important part of recovery. Take aspirin or some other nonsteroidal anti-inflammatory drug (NSAID) to ease symptoms. As the disease is a viral and not a bacterial infection, it should not be treated with antibiotics; people suffering from glandular fever must let it run its course. Recovery time varies greatly: it is usually about three weeks, but it can take months.

Long-term complications are rare, but activity and exercise should be limited until you feel your strength returning and the doctor says the spleen has returned to its normal size. Contracting glandular fever increases the risk of Hodgkinson's disease in later life.

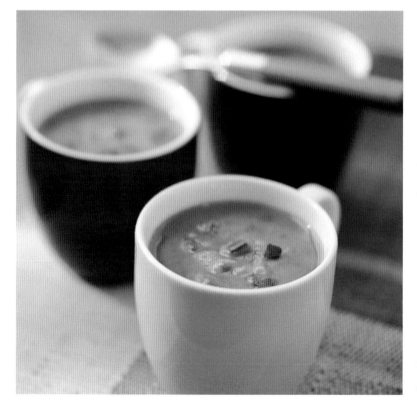

◀ **Softly does it**
Soft foods such as soups, particularly home-made ones, are nutritious and easy on a sore throat. They also provide much-needed fibre.

Glycaemic Index
An evolving story

Despite its growing popularity as a tool to help people to improve their health, there are still many controversies and misconceptions surrounding this food classification system.

The Glycaemic Index (GI) is a classification of carbohydrate foods according to the effect they have on the level of blood sugars compared with an equal quantity of pure glucose. Regulating blood sugars is a key strategy in preventing and controlling certain diseases, particularly diabetes.

Over 20 years ago, researchers at the University of Toronto studied more than 50 carbohydrate-rich foods and their effect on blood glucose. The Glycaemic Index was developed by measuring how much a person's blood glucose increased 2 to 3 hours after eating a carbohydrate-rich food compared with a reference food, which was either pure glucose or white bread. Subsequent studies have shown large variations if white bread is used as a reference food, consequently only glucose is recommended for the comparison.

A food that is digested and absorbed quickly has a high GI value, causing a rapid increase in blood sugar. A food that is digested and absorbed slowly has a low GI value. Foods are rated into three categories. They can have a low GI (55 or less), an intermediate GI (56–69) or a high GI (70 or more). There are currently 750 foods with published GI values.

GLYCAEMIC INDEX AND HEALTH

We used to believe that foods high in sugar, such as cakes and biscuits, sweets and ice cream, were harmful for people with diabetes because they were quickly digested, leading to a rapid rise in blood sugar. Complex carbohydrates like potatoes, rice and pasta were thought to break down more slowly, resulting in a more gradual rise in blood sugar. But some sweet foods actually have a lower Glycaemic Index than many starchier foods. Considering the GI of a food, as well as its overall nutritional contribution, provides a more useful guide for planning a diabetic diet than merely considering whether the carbohydrate present is complex (from starches) or simple (from sugars).

Factors that affect the Glycaemic Index

Some processing methods and nutrients can affect the GI value of a food.

FACTOR	MECHANISM	EXAMPLES
COOKING OR PROCESSING STARCH	Changes the structure of starch and the granules become swollen (gelatinised). Less-gelatinised starch has a lower GI.	Al dente pasta has a lower GI than overcooked pasta or canned spaghetti.
SUGAR	Prevents gelatinisation of starch.	Frosted flakes have a lower GI than corn flakes.
FIBRE	Slows down interaction between starch and enzymes.	Rolled oats, beans, lentils, apples have lower GIs.
PROTEIN AND FAT	Slows down rate of carbohydrate digestion.	Foods containing fat and protein, like milk and legumes have low GIs.
ACID IN FOODS	Slows rate of digestion and absorption.	Vinegar, lemon juice and acidic fruits lower the GI.

Researchers are also testing whether a low-GI diet may help to lower the risk of developing diabetes and heart disease in healthy people.

In sports nutrition, high-GI foods are often used as a source of quick energy to help short-duration sports performance and recovery, while low-GI foods have been used in endurance sports. An interesting theory in another area of research is that low-GI foods may aid in weight loss because they take longer to digest and they help to control insulin levels. The hormone insulin promotes the storage of fat and also inhibits the breakdown of stored fat for energy.

CAUTION

Don't rely on half the story. If you look only at their GI figure, carrots seem to be a food to avoid as they have almost the same GI as sugar – very high. But, in fact, a carrot has just 4g of carbohydrates and when the formula for determining the GL (Glycaemic Load, see below) is used, carrots come up as winners!

CURRENT CONTROVERSIES

Although many large health organisations, including the World Health Organization and diabetes organisations, support the use of the GI for people with diabetes, some question its value. The trouble stems from the difficulty in applying the GI system in a practical and understandable way to help people improve their health.

One of the biggest issues is that many foods that are considered healthy choices have a higher GI than foods that are considered to be nutritionally less desirable. For example, mashed potatoes have a higher GI than table sugar, and it is confusing to find that packaged wholemeal bread has almost the same GI as white.

This is where the concept of Glycaemic Load (GL) comes in. It assesses the effect of carbohydrate foods on blood sugar by taking into account the GI and the quantity of carbohydrate (GL = GI x grams of carbohydrate per serving). The GI tells you how rapidly a particular carbohydrate turns into sugar. It doesn't tell you how much of that carbohydrate is in that food. Both have an important effect on blood sugar. For example, the carbohydrate in watermelon has a high GI. But there isn't a lot of it, so the GL is relatively low. However, most foods that have a low GL have a low GI. One unit of GL is approximately the glycaemic effect of 1g of glucose. A Glycaemic Load less than 80 for a whole day is considered low; a GL over 120 for a day is considered high.

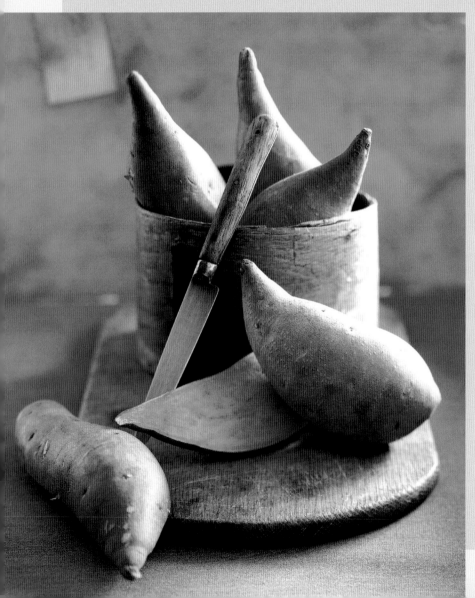

◀ **Sweet version of a classic**
Boiled sweet potatoes have a GI of 44 (compared with mashed white potatoes which have a typical GI of 80) and are also loaded with beta carotene.

◀ **Low GI lentils**
Lentils not only have a low GI, but they are rich in protein and high in fibre. They make excellent meat substitutes and are great hunger-busters, which makes them ideal for people with diabetes.

OTHER ISSUES

GI values vary from one study to another, for many reasons. Values are determined by measuring blood sugar responses after particular foods are eaten. But one person's glycaemic response can differ considerably from another's. It may vary even in the same person from day to day. Even the state of food can change its GI. For example, small differences in a banana's ripeness can alter its GI. And the GI of boiled potatoes can be increased by 25 per cent just by mashing them.

In addition, when you combine foods (adding butter or sour cream to a potato, for instance, or having the potato with a serving of meat) the GI of the combined foods becomes much different from the GI of the potato by itself. The reason is that fat and protein slow gastric emptying, making the GI of the whole dish different from the GI of just a single food.

Only foods that have at least 10g of carbohydrate per serving have a GI. Most vegetables and herbs do not have enough carbohydrate to have any effect on blood glucose. It is therefore incorrect to describe foods such as broccoli, spinach, lettuce, tomatoes or avocados as 'low GI'. Their GI is zero.

THE BOTTOM LINE

Remember that the GI is only one measurement of a food and its contribution to health. Some high-GI foods, such as potatoes, contain many essential nutrients and are good sources of energy.

▶ **Red grapes**
Grapes have a low GI, but the red variety has the extra advantage of being rich in antioxidants.

Glycaemic Index (GI) and Glycaemic Load (GL) of some common foods

FOOD	GI	SERVING SIZE	GL
BREAD AND GRAINS			
Bread, light rye	68	40g	12
Bread, multigrain sliced	43	35g	6
Bread, sourdough	54	35g	8
Bread, soya & linseed	36	40g	6
Bread, white sliced	71	30g	9
Bread, wholemeal sliced	70	30g	8
Cereal, corn flakes	77	30g	19
Cereal, natural muesli	40	60g	9
Cereal, wheat biscuits	68	30g	3
Rice, basmati, boiled	58	150g	24
Rice, brown, boiled	66	150g	32
Rice, short grain, white, boiled	83	150g	35
Spaghetti, white, boiled	38	180g	17
DAIRY			
Milk	31	250ml	4
Yoghurt, low-fat fruit	33	200ml	11
LEGUMES			
Baked beans in tomato sauce	48	150g	7
Chick peas, boiled	28	150g	8
Lentils, red, boiled	26	150g	5
FRUIT			
Apple, 1 medium	38	150g	7
Banana, 1 medium	52	120g	12
Orange, 1 medium	42	150g	6
Orange juice	53	250ml	9
STARCHY VEGETABLES			
Potato, new, boiled	56	150g	13.7
Parsnips, boiled	95	80g	7.8
Sweet potato, boiled	44	150g	11
Peas, boiled	48	80g	3
MISCELLANEOUS			
Sports drink	78	250ml	14
Cola soft drink	53	250ml	12
Muesli bar	61	63g	17

G

Gooseberries

BENEFITS

- A good source of vitamin C and bioflavonoids

- Some potassium, iron and vitamin E

- High in fibre, low in calories

DRAWBACKS

- Their tartness is usually offset with large amounts of added sugar

Gooseberries are prized for their acidic tartness and are made into pies, jams, spreads and sauces for poultry and fish. Some are made into vinegar. New, sweeter-tasting varieties have been developed, which are more palatable for eating raw and are slightly larger than the cooking varieties.

Both fresh and cooked goose-berries have many nutritional benefits. They are high in fibre, and 100g of cooked gooseberries contain 11mg of vitamin C and 140mg of potassium. They are also rich in bioflavonoids.

Gooseberries retain their nutrients well when stewed, although 100g of berries stewed with sugar will have 54kcal compared with 19kcal in 100g of raw berries. Their tart flavour, however, means that extra sugar is often added; and consequently, when they are served with cream, or whipped into a gooseberry 'fool', they become a high-calorie dessert.

Folk healers in the past used gooseberry juice to treat liver and intestinal disorders. They also believed that a tea brewed from the plant's leaves was a remedy for menstrual and urinary tract disorders – such as 'gravel' in the urinary tract. Old herbal medicine books refer to the fruit as fever-berries and recommend it for inflammatory disorders. However, there is no scientific evidence that gooseberries or their leaves have any special medicinal qualities.

Gooseberries carry fungi that are transmitted to pine trees and other types of fruit bushes. As a result, efforts are now under way to develop more disease-resistant strains of gooseberries.

▲ **A berry of many hues**
Although green gooseberries are the most familiar, some of the more than 700 varieties are red and different shades of blue.

Cape gooseberries are small, golden berries inside a papery skin which looks like a Chinese lantern. They can be eaten raw or made into jam

Gout

CONSUME PLENTY OF

- Fluids to dilute the urine and prevent the formation of kidney stones

- Fresh fruit and vegetables for vitamins, minerals and dietary fibre

AVOID

- Offal, game, anchovies, sardines, herring, meat extracts and other high-purine foods

- Alcohol, especially beer

- Diuretics and aspirin-based drugs

- Skipping meals, crash diets

Marked by swelling, inflammation and excruciating tenderness in the joints, gout most commonly affects the joints at the base of the big toe, other foot joints, knees, ankles, wrists and fingers. The slightest touch – even that of a bedsheet – may be unbearably painful during an attack. Gout affects 16 men in every 1,000,

Gooseberry facts

- The origin of the name 'gooseberries' has nothing to do with geese, even though their acidic flavour goes well with roast goose. Instead, the term comes from the Old English words for the berries – 'groser', 'grosier' and 'grozer'. Gooseberries have been cultivated in Europe, and especially in England, since the 15th century.

- Gooseberries have been known by many names over the years including fever-berries, carberries, feaberries, goosegogs and honeyblobs.

- There are some 50 different species and more than 700 varieties of gooseberry. Although the gooseberry originated in Europe and western Asia, the United States and Canada now have the most species.

but only three women in 1,000, and seldom before menopause.

Gout has had an undeserved reputation for being the penalty for high living and overindulgence. In fact, it is a type of arthritis that is caused by an inherited defect in the kidney's ability to excrete uric acid. This waste product of protein metabolism comes both from the digestive process and from the normal turnover of cells.

When deposits of uric acid crystals build up in the synovial fluid that surrounds the joints, the body's immune system tries to eliminate these crystals through the process of inflammation; unfortunately, this causes attacks of intense pain that can continue for days or even weeks if the condition is left untreated. Over time, uric acid crystals gather in lumpy deposits under the skin of the ears, the elbows and near the affected joints.

An attack usually occurs suddenly and unpredictably. Fortunately, there are now several drugs available that will stop the pain. The first line of treatment is nonsteroidal anti-inflammatory drugs (NSAIDs) which should be started as soon as pain strikes. Colchicine, a drug derived from the autumn crocus flower, has been used to treat gout since the 6th century, but is considered too toxic to be widely used. It causes severe nausea and diarrhoea. However, used at a low dose, colchicine is well tolerated and is sometimes used as an effective method of preventing the recurrence of pain.

Other, less toxic drugs, such as allopurinol (Zyloric), are given on a long-term basis to prevent the onset of attacks; a flare-up is likely if these drugs are stopped, however.

To reinforce the beneficial effect of drug treatment, people with gout should make dietary changes to help to reduce their production of uric acid, and possibly to lose weight.

Managing gout with diet

Lose weight gradually. Many people who have gout are obese; losing weight – especially fat around the abdomen – often prevents future attacks. Weight loss should be gradual, however, because a rapid reduction can raise blood levels of uric acid and provoke gout.

Fasting increases the blood levels of uric acid. Therefore, people with gout should avoid skipping meals. High-protein, low-carbohydrate diets should also be avoided since these diets encourage the formation of ketones, metabolic by-products that hamper the body's ability to excrete uric acid.

You may have to modify your drug therapy. Gout may be brought on by using aspirin or diuretics for high blood pressure. These medicines may interfere with normal kidney function and the elimination of uric acid. Your doctor may change treatment if you experience severe joint pain while on a drug therapy.

Avoid foods that are high in purines. Foods high in naturally occurring purines promote over-production of uric acid in people with gout. High-purine foods include anchovies, sardines, liver, kidney, brains, meat extracts, herring, mackerel, scallops, game and beer; these should be avoided completely. Some vegetables such as peas, asparagus, cauliflower, mushrooms and spinach contain purines and were once forbidden, but recent research shows they have no adverse effects for gout sufferers if eaten in moderation. This is thought to be due to the wide range of anti-inflammatory compounds found in these vegetables.

Consume plenty of liquids. Try to drink 2–3 litres a day to dilute the urine and prevent kidney stone formation. Although beer is the only alcoholic drink known to be high in purines, any alcohol can interfere with the elimination of uric acid. With alcoholic drinks, gout sufferers should drink only wine and only in small amounts. Caffeinated drinks can also increase the production of uric acid and impair its removal from the body.

Eat fish rich in omega-3s. The omega-3 fats in oil-rich fish such as salmon and tuna have been found to reduce pain and inflammation in people with rheumatoid arthritis and may have a similar benefit in gout, but this may be countered by the purine content of the fish. Gout sufferers may find that fish-oil supplements, which contain omega-3 fatty acids, can offer some relief for painful swelling of the joints.

Gout sufferers also may have hypertension, heart disease, diabetes and high blood cholesterol. Counselling by a State Registered Dietitian may help in designing appetising, healthy meals that strike a balance between these health concerns and the enjoyment of a variety of food.

The truth about cherries

Cherry juice – especially black cherry juice – is an old folk remedy for gout that's still popular today. But does it work? Nothing definitive has been proven. However, a study published in the *Journal of Nutrition* in June 2003 reported that eating cherries did indeed lower uric acid levels in the urine of the women in the study, which could explain any anti-gout effect.

Eating pineapple or taking bromelain, an anti-inflammatory enzyme found in pineapple, is also said to work against gout, but it has not been shown that bromelain can be absorbed intact into the bloodstream, and it will almost certainly be destroyed by acid in the stomach.

G

▶ **Whole grains**
Grains such as wheat, barley and oats can be added to soups and baked goods such as muffins to give foods a nutritional boost.

Grains

BENEFITS

■ An excellent source of starchy carbohydrate and dietary fibre

■ A good source of thiamin, niacin, other B vitamins and iron

■ More economical than meat, fish and other diet staples

DRAWBACKS

■ Grains lose some nutrients and fibre during processing

■ Gluten in some grain products provokes malabsorption symptoms in people who have coeliac disease

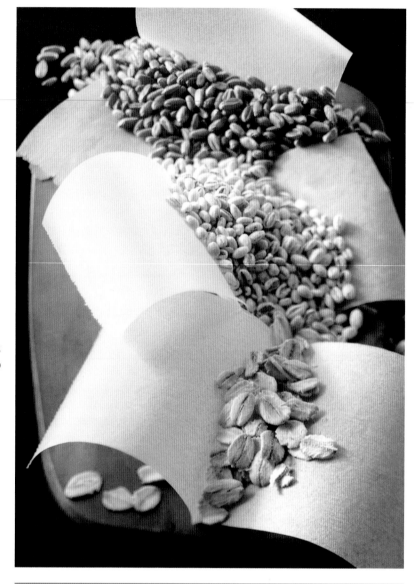

In this era of the low-carbohydrate diet, the health benefits of whole grains are sometimes overlooked. Since prehistoric times, grain products have been one of the basic foodstuffs of agrarian societies. Almost every culture has a staple grain around which its cuisine is centred. Today, thanks to modern agricultural techniques and efficient transportation, we can sample a huge variety of grain products.

Despite access to this proliferation of grains from around the world, we still tend to make the greatest use of our native wheat, which is ground into flour and made into bread and other baked goods. To a lesser extent, we also eat maize, rice, oats, barley and millet, as well as many exotic grains.

Whole grains are rich in complex carbohydrates, fibre and many vitamins and minerals. They are also low in fat, and when eaten in combination with beans and other legumes, grains are a good source

The whole truth

WHOLE VERSUS REFINED GRAINS

Many of the valuable nutrients in grains are contained in their germ and their outer covering which are removed during refining. In contrast, products made from whole grains retain most of their nutritive value; their high fibre content also adds texture and is filling. White flour is fortified with thiamin, iron and calcium and many breakfast cereals are fortified with iron, riboflavin, folate and niacin. Despite the additions, refined products still have fewer vitamins, minerals and dietary fibre than wholegrain products. Whole grains contain more B vitamins, vitamin E and an assortment of phytochemicals including lignans, saponins and plant sterols.

When shopping for wholegrain breads and cereals, read labels carefully. Look for the words 'wholemeal flour' as the first ingredient. Remember that a product that is simply labelled 'wheat flour' is usually made from white flour.

of complete protein. Nutritionists urge us to eat more grain products as a healthy substitute for high-fat foods, and recommend we include plenty of grain-based foods, such as breads, cereals, pasta and rice in our diets, along with dried beans, peas and other legumes.

Diabetes, heart disease and cancer protection

There is a growing awareness of the importance of the quality, as much as the quantity, of grains included in the diet. An increased consumption of whole grains may reduce the risk of developing Type 2 diabetes and cardiovascular disease.

Data obtained from the Physicians Health Study, in which more than 86,000 male doctors participated, showed a significant reduction in the risk of death from cardiovascular disease and death from all causes in the men eating the greatest quantity of wholegrain cereals compared with those of the men eating the fewest servings of wholegrain cereals.

The Iowa Women's Health Study followed almost 35,000 women aged 55 to 69 and found that the more whole grains eaten, the lower the risk became of dying from heart disease.

Another study found that adults with the highest intake of whole grains were 35 per cent less likely to develop Type 2 diabetes than those with the lowest intake. There is also growing evidence that eating whole grains instead of refined varieties can reduce your risk of developing cancer.

Common grain products

Barley, a staple food in the Middle East, is used in the West in the form of malt, by brewers and distillers. It is a source of soluble fibre and also contains B vitamins and minerals such as zinc and magnesium. Pearl barley is used mainly in soups,

---

How grains are processed

The methods in which grains are processed vary according to the specific grain and geographic area. The following techniques are used in industrialised countries.

CRACKING. The grains are put through machines that crack or break them into smaller pieces, which cook more quickly than whole seeds.

EXTRACTING OILS. The oil-bearing germ of the grain is pressed or heated to extract the oil.

EXTRACTING STARCHES. The grain is first soaked in a solution containing sulphur dioxide or sodium hydroxide, ground to remove the bran and then spun in a centrifuge machine to separate out the starch.

FLAKING. The grains are cooked, dried and rolled through machines to produce flakes of the desired shape and size. Sugar and flavourings may be added to make cereals.

MILLING. The grains are sent into grinders or rollers to remove the hulls, bran and seed germ; at this time, they may also be cracked or crushed into meal or flour.

PARBOILING. The grains (usually rice but sometimes wheat) are boiled in water before milling.

POLISHING AND PEARLING. After the hulls are removed, an abrasive is used to shape the kernels.

PUFFING. The grains are placed in hot rotating cylinders, or puffing guns. Alternatively, the grains are milled and made into a dough that is puffed in an oven.

ROLLING. The grains are compressed between large rollers to flatten them, as in rolled oats, or to convert them into flakes.

SHREDDING. The grains (usually wheat) are cooked, dried and then squeezed through a grooved cylinder to form long strands.

---

stews and casseroles, and offers plenty of carbohydrate, but vitamins and fibre are lost in its production. Barley contains some gluten.

Bulghur wheat is cracked and roasted whole-wheat kernels; it has a nutty flavour and can be used to make taboulleh, pilaf or stuffing.

Couscous is made from durum wheat, the hardest type, which also contains the most gluten. Couscous cooks rapidly and is light, making it an ideal starchy accompaniment for quick meals.

Maize, or corn, is gluten-free, so people with coeliac disease can eat products such as popcorn, cornflour, breakfast cereals and corn syrup.

Millet is also a gluten-free grain and can be made into tasty flat breads, used in pilaf or as a stuffing. Toasting millet in a dry skillet before cooking it adds a nutty flavour.

Oats are used in breakfast cereals and baked goods. Oat bran is high in soluble fibre, which may help to lower blood cholesterol levels. It may also help the body utilise insulin more efficiently, an important asset in controlling diabetes. Oats do not contain gluten, but oat products may be contaminated with wheat.

Quinoa, (pronounced *keen-wa*) is an ancient grain that is lower in carbohydrate and higher in protein than most other grains. This fluffy grain is sold either as whole grain or as pasta and is great in salads. It is well-tolerated by people on gluten-free diets.

Rice is the staple food for about half the world's population. Brown rice is preferable, because it is unrefined and high in B vitamins and fibre. It also has some iron and zinc. Long-grain brown rice is closer in taste to refined white rice.

Short-grain brown rice has a heartier texture and a nuttier flavour. White rice is stripped of its outer layers and is mostly starch with a little protein. It also supplies some vitamins and minerals.

Rye contains gluten, which is the reason rye bread and pumpernickel breads are not suitable for those with coeliac disease. It is used in some crispbreads.

Wheat is one of the most widely consumed grains in the world. If, during milling, the bran (outer husk) and germ (located at the base of the grain) are removed, the end product is less nutritious than if left whole. Wholegrain wheat or whole wheat is a better choice, containing the bran as well as the germ of the wheat. The germ of the wheat kernel is a concentrated source of many nutrients including vitamin E, B vitamins, iron, zinc, magnesium, potassium and fibre.

Grapefruit

BENEFITS

- High in vitamin C and potassium

- Pink and red varieties contain beta carotene and lycopene, both powerful antioxidants

- Low in calories

- Contain bioflavonoids and other plant chemicals that help to protect against cancer and heart disease

DRAWBACKS

- Can provoke an allergic reaction in people sensitive to citrus fruit

- Grapefruit juice can reduce the effectiveness of certain medications

Delicious and nutritious – it's easy to understand why grapefruit is no longer just a breakfast option. Half a grapefruit provides 30g of vitamin C – 70 per cent of the adult Reference Nutrient Intake (RNI) for vitamin C; it also has 1560mg of potassium. The pink and red varieties have more vitamin C than the yellow, and are also high in beta carotene, which the body converts to vitamin A.

A cup of unsweetened grapefruit juice has 47mg of vitamin C, which is more than 100 per cent of the RNI, and most of the other nutrients found in the fresh fruit. In the past, many people shunned the unsweetened grapefruit juice because of its tartness, but a naturally sweet juice can be made by using the red or pink grapefruit.

Over the years a number of fad diets have promoted the grapefruit as possessing a unique ability to burn away fat. There is no truth in the claim; no food can do this. People following grapefruit diets lose weight because they eat little else – a practice that can lead to nutritional deficiencies. Even so, grapefruit is worth including in a sensible weight-loss diet; a serving contains only about 24kcal, and its high-fibre content satisfies hunger.

Grapefruit are especially high in pectin, a soluble fibre that may help to lower blood cholesterol. Recent studies indicate that grapefruit contain other substances that prevent disease. Pink and red grapefruit, for example, are high in lycopene, an anti-oxidant that seems to lower the risk of prostate cancer. Researchers have not yet identified lycopene's mechanism of action, but a 6-year Harvard study of 48,000 doctors and other health professionals

CAUTION

Grapefruit should not be used if you are taking certain medications. Compounds in the grapefruit can enhance the effects of some drugs, possibly resulting in adverse effects. Drugs to watch out for include some blood-pressure lowering medication, as well as drugs prescribed for anxiety, depression and elevated lipids. Check with your doctor or pharmacist if it is safe to consume grapefruit.

has linked ten servings of lycopene-rich foods a week with a 50 per cent reduction in prostate cancer.

Other protective plant chemicals found in grapefruit include phenolic acid, which inhibits the formation of cancer-causing nitrosamines; limonoids, terpenes and monoterpenes, which induce the production of enzymes that may help to prevent cancer; and bioflavonoids, which inhibit the

▶ **Instead of white, buy pink or red grapefruit**
Pink or red pomelo grapefruit are high in lycopene, an antioxidant associated with reduced risk of prostate cancer.

action of hormones that may promote tumour growth. Some people with rheumatoid arthritis, lupus and other inflammatory disorders find that eating grapefruit daily seems to alleviate their symptoms. This may be because plant chemicals block the prostaglandins that cause inflammation.

Those people who are allergic to other citrus fruit are likely to react to grapefruit, too. The sensitivity may be to the fruit itself or to an oil in the peel.

Grapes

BENEFITS

- High in pectin and bioflavonoids
- Contain phytochemicals that may reduce risk of heart disease, cancer and strokes
- A fair source of iron and vitamin C
- Black grapes supply antioxidants

DRAWBACKS

- Dried grapes (raisins and sultanas) treated with sulphur dioxide may affect sulphite-sensitive people
- Natural salicylates may provoke an allergic response

One of the oldest and most abundant of the world's fruit crops, grapes are cultivated on six of the seven continents. Most of the 60 million tonnes grown worldwide annually are fermented to produce wine. Grapes are also made into jams and spreads, used in cooking and eaten raw as a snack food.

Dessert grapes are eaten whole and fresh, or turned into wine. Grapes used for dried fruit have skins that slip off easily and are used mostly to make jams, spreads and juice. Dessert grapes are a light, appetising food, sweet and relatively non-fattening: a handful, weighing around 80g contains about 48kcal and provides good amounts of potassium and a little vitamin C.

Another reason for eating grapes is found in research on the disease-prevention role of bioflavonoids and other plant chemicals. Anthocyanins found in purple grapes have many potential health benefits including lowering heart disease and cancer risk. Grapes contain quercetin, a plant pigment that is thought to regulate the levels of blood cholesterol and also reduce the action of platelets, blood cells that are instrumental in forming clots. Some researchers theorise that it is quercetin that lowers the risk of heart attack among moderate wine drinkers although most attribute the protection to resveratrol in grape skins, a phytochemical that is linked to a reduction of heart disease as well as a lowered risk of cancer or stroke. Grapes also contain ellagic acid thought to protect the lungs against environmental toxins.

To reap the full benefit of grapes, it is best to select purple varieties, which seem to contain the highest concentration of bioflavonoids that neutralise harmful free radicals. Commercially grown grapes may be sprayed with pesticides; they should always be washed before being eaten. People with asthma should

Grape facts

- Grapes were first cultivated about 7,000 years ago by the Egyptians. New varieties were developed by the Greeks and Romans and eventually introduced into Europe.
- *Vitis vinifera*, a species of European grape, gave rise to some 10,000 different cultivars, including almost all of those used to make wine and our most popular table grapes: muscat, purle cornichon, red globe, ribiers, Thompson seedless and Waltham cross.
- When a grape blight threatened to wipe out the European wine industry in the early 1800s, the vines were revived with grafts of disease-free American varieties.
- California is now the world's leading producer of raisins and sultanas, with South Africa a close second.

Did you know?

Sultanas or raisins?

Sultanas are dried seedless sultana grapes and raisins are dried black-skinned grapes. In North America, however, sultanas are known as raisins. Grapes are around 80 per cent water whereas sultanas and raisins have only about a fifth as much water. This makes sultanas and raisins a more concentrated source of fibre, iron, potassium and calories. It takes about 2kg of fresh grapes to produce 400g of sultanas or raisins.

either avoid raisins or sultanas or look for those that have not been treated with sulphur. Grapes naturally contain salicylates, compounds similar to the major ingredient in aspirin. Salicylates have an anticlotting effect and may partly account for the benefits of wine with respect to heart disease. However, people who are allergic to aspirin may react to grapes and grape products.

The polyphenols and tannins in red grapes may trigger migraines in susceptible people.

Guavas

BENEFITS

■ An excellent source of vitamin C

■ High in pectin and other types of soluble dietary fibre

■ Provide potassium and beta carotene

DRAWBACKS

■ Fresh fruit is expensive and not widely available

■ Sulphites in dried guavas may provoke an asthma attack or allergic reaction in susceptible persons

A small tropical fruit that originated in southern Africa, and South America, the guava is now grown in southern Mexico, Central America, the Caribbean, Florida, California, Hawaii and southern Asia. The fruit can be round, ovoid or pear-shaped and ranges in size from 2.5 to 10cm in diameter. The thin skins, which vary in colour from pale yellow to yellow-green, are usually edible. Most varieties have meaty, deep pink flesh, although some are yellow, red or white. Ripe guavas have an unmistakeable fragrant, musky aroma and a sweet flavour. By weight, guavas have four times as much vitamin C as an orange:

one medium guava (about 100g) provides 230mg, compared with 70mg in an orange. One guava also contains 230mg of potassium and 4g of fibre, much of which is in the form of pectin, a soluble fibre that may lower high blood cholesterol as well as promoting good digestive function. Folate and beta carotene are also present, with potassium which can help in regulating blood pressure.

About half of the guava fruit is filled with small, hard seeds that are fully edible, and are as high in vitamins as the fruit's flesh. They also contribute fibre. In making guava jelly, the seeds are strained out, and little fibre remains.

A versatile fruit

With only about 26kcal in a fresh guava, the fruit makes an easy, interesting, non-fattening dessert. Simply cut the fruit in half, scoop out the seeds and the flesh. A dash of lime or lemon juice contrasts nicely with the sweet flavour. Alternatively, you can peel, seed and chop or slice guavas to add to a fruit salad. Pureed guava flesh in combination with orange or other citrus juice makes a refreshing drink or cold summer soup. Unripe guavas are a little too tart and astringent to be eaten raw, but can be blended and cooked with defatted meat juice to make a low-calorie sauce for roasts and poultry dishes.

▶ **Exotic fruit**
The acid-sweet taste and pungent aroma of guavas evoke images of a tropical paradise. Although the entire fruit is edible when fully ripe, many people discard the seeds and skins.

Most guavas in the UK will have been imported. When selecting guavas, choose fruit that is firm but not hard. A guava is ripe when the skin yields slightly when pressed. As with almost any fruit, flavour is best when the guava is allowed to ripen on the tree, but green mature fruit will ripen at room temperature. Placing the fruit in a brown paper bag with a banana or apple will hasten ripening.

Gourmet sections in supermarkets carry increasing numbers of guava products – jams, jellies, dried sheets, nectar and a type of fruit paste called guava cheese.

Even after losing about 25 per cent of its vitamins in the canning process, canned guavas in syrup are still an excellent source of vitamin C, vital for the production of collagen and healthy tissues.

Dried guavas may be treated with sulphites, which may provoke asthma attacks or allergic reactions in susceptible people.

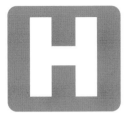

Haemorrhoids

TAKE PLENTY OF

- Apples, pears, beans, oats and cooked green leafy vegetables for their soluble fibre
- Wholemeal bread and brown rice for insoluble fibre
- Water

CUT DOWN ON

- Refined carbohydrates

AVOID

- Curries and other hot and spicy foods

Haemorrhoids – itching or painful, swollen veins in anal tissue – are usually caused by prolonged bouts of constipation or restricted blood flow to the abdomen caused by sitting for long periods. Obesity is another factor that frequently exacerbates haemorrhoids – more usually known as piles. They often occur during pregnancy, especially if there is a family predisposition to the problem.

Straining to pass a stool because of constipation is often the result of eating excessive amounts of refined foods which contain little or no fibre, and not drinking enough water or other liquids.

Help from fibre

To treat mild cases of haemorrhoids, make a few changes to your diet: eat plenty of foods that contain soluble fibre such as oats, fruit and vegetables, as well as whole grains and brown rice for insoluble fibre; and try to drink at least 2 litres of water daily.

Following a diet which includes these foods may help to prevent people getting haemorrhoids in the first place. The soluble fibre found in oats is particularly good for treating constipation because it helps to ease bowel movement by creating softer stools. Hot and spicy foods, such as curries, should be avoided as these usually exacerbate the condition and increase the discomfort of bowel movements. If dietary changes don't help, fibre supplements, stool softeners, creams or suppositories may be used.

In persistent cases, the bleeding that occurs may cause an iron deficiency which can lead to anaemia. Good food sources of iron include liver (but not for pregnant women), pulses, nuts and dark green vegetables. The vitamin C in fresh fruit improves iron absorption.

If rectal bleeding is persistent, consult a doctor, as this can indicate cancer of the rectum. More severe cases of haemorrhoids may be treated with injections or rubber band ligation; surgery is less common nowadays.

Hair and scalp problems

EAT PLENTY OF

- Fruit and vegetables, especially dark green leafy vegetables, carrots and sweet potatoes
- Shellfish, red meat and pumpkin seeds for zinc and iron
- Vegetable oils, nuts and oily fish for essential fatty acids

Baldness and dandruff are among the most pervasive hair and scalp problems. Hair loss may be either the result of illness or a normal genetic response to testosterone.

Dandruff – excessive scaling of the scalp – may be due to stress or a chronic or recurrent skin disorder, such as seborrheic dermatitis, but the most likely cause is infection by *Pytyrosporum ovale* fungus. This fungus is found naturally on the scalp but some people are more affected by it than others. It feeds on the skin's natural oils and causes irritation and shedding of dead skin.

Hair is composed of the protein keratin. Other nutrients that contribute to hair and scalp health include niacin, biotin, zinc and vitamins A, B_6 and C. A varied diet based on the basic food groups should provide ample amounts of these nutrients. Because hair is inert material, shampoos and rinses enriched with protein or other nutrients cannot affect hair growth or make hair 'healthier'.

Hair loss

A healthy human head has from 80,000 to 150,000 hairs, each of which passes through three phases of growth independently of all the others. At any time, 90 per cent of the hairs are in the growing stage (anagen), which lasts from one to five years. Growth is followed by a resting phase (telogen); this ends after a few months, after which the hair is shed (catagen) to allow new growth. A daily loss of 50 to 200 hairs is a normal part of the cycle.

Although baldness is mediated by hormonal factors, it tends to run in families; risk may be deduced from the number of bald males among the members of both parents' families. Male pattern balness cannot be changed or affected by diet.

Abnormal hair loss may be precipitated by metabolic disorders (including diabetes, thyroid disease and crash diets); damage to hair shafts caused by harsh treatments;

H

•Myth.......
Hair analysis cannot determine nutritional deficiencies – any such claim is worthless.

.......Reality ●
Scientific analysis of hair can confirm the presence of certain toxic elements – even years later. (Hair analysis was used 150 years after Napoleon's death to confirm that he suffered chronic arsenic poisoning.)

stress brought on by illness, such as alopecia areata, an auto-immune condition which causes patchy hair loss; the hormonal changes of pregnancy; and medical treatment, including cancer chemotherapy.

When diet is involved, the cause may be a deficiency of iron, biotin, zinc or protein; shellfish and red meat should help to restore levels.

Vitamin A plays a delicate role: it is important for healthy sebum production, and a deficiency may cause dry skin and dandruff; but too much can promote hair loss.

Hair loss due to stress or drug treatment is generally temporary. Hair that falls out during a crash diet soon regrows once nutrition returns to normal. Hair lost in patches usually grows back without treatment, but in some instances, corticosteroid injections may be needed. The only medicines for baldness are minoxidil (Regaine), a topical medicine which is effective in only about 15 per cent of people, and finasteride (Propecia), an oral prescription drug. Neither drug is available on the NHS.

Did you know?

Some foods promote dandruff

Some people's dandruff improves when they shun foods that cause the face and scalp to flush; typical offenders are hot liquids, heavily spiced foods and alcohol.

Dandruff

Many people have dandruff, especially in winter, when the scalp may be dry. But a small number of people have a hereditary tendency to develop skin problems that are triggered by a sensitivity to specific foods. Because the offending food varies from one person to the next, the only reasonable advice is to avoid foods that seem to make dandruff worse. Some cases may respond to linseed oil, which may help itchy skin conditions such as psoriasis and eczema. Take 1-2 teaspoons a day. It may take several weeks or months to take effect.

To control mild dandruff, doctors usually recommend shampooing, at first daily until the dandruff is under control, followed by twice weekly for maintenance. Dandruff shampoos contain zinc pyrithione, coal tar or selenium sulphide, all of which work as exfoliants to hasten the shedding of the dead cell layer from the scalp. If these do not work well, try shampoos that contain the antifungal medication ketoconazole.

Diet can help

Many of the causes of hair and scalp problems can be lessened with diet. People who suffer from stress may be short of B vitamins which can be obtained from wholegrain cereals, oily fish, yeast extracts, peas, natural yoghurts, eggs and milk.

A deficiency in vitamin A can be helped by eating two or three eggs a week and a portion of liver (not if you are pregnant). Also eating carrots, green leafy vegetables, sweet potatoes and dried apricots will provide beta carotene, which the body metabolises into vitamin A.

Hamburgers

See Fast food

Hay fever

EAT PLENTY OF

■ Seafood and other foods high in omega-3 fatty acids for their anti-inflammatory effect

AVOID

■ Honey and bee pollen capsules

■ Any food in the same plant family as sunflowers (the Compositae family)

■ Fermented foods or those with moulds if fungi spores trigger symptoms

Hay fever is a seasonal allergy triggered by the inhalation of pollen or, less commonly, moulds. Medically known as seasonal allergic rhinitis, the name 'hay fever' is a misnomer: hay itself is not the culprit, nor is there a fever.

Reactions to dust mite, cat dander and moulds are perennial allergic rhinitis, and can cause the sneezing, runny nose, tearing eyes, itchiness of hay fever symptoms.

Stay away from foods in the sunflower plant family. Although foods aren't ordinarily associated with hay fever, people with certain types of seasonal allergies may experience symptoms after eating particular foods. For example, plants in the sunflower, or **Compositae,** family which includes a broad variety of herbs and vegetables may have a reaction.

Watch out for honey. Pollens or contaminants in some foods can also trigger the onset of hay fever symptoms. This may be true of honey, which may harbour bits of pollen, and bee pollen capsules, a food supplement and natural remedy that is sold in health-food shops. However, there is reasonable evidence that eating honey that is natural, unprocessed and made near to where you live, early in the season, may actually help to reduce both the severity and frequency of the attacks. It seems that local honey has the right pollen mix for local conditions and, taken early enough, may even act as a natural 'vaccination' against the area's pollen.

Eat more omega-3s. There is no special diet that will alleviate hay fever symptoms, although some recent reports suggest that eating seafood and other foods that are high in omega-3 fatty acids may reduce the inflammation that is part of an allergic reaction. More research is necessary to confirm this, but consumption of fish is still an important part of a varied and balanced diet.

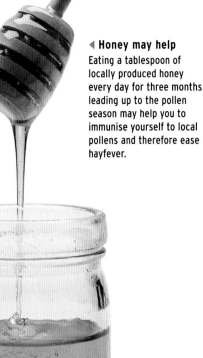

◀ **Honey may help**
Eating a tablespoon of locally produced honey every day for three months leading up to the pollen season may help you to immunise yourself to local pollens and therefore ease hayfever.

Mould

In some people seasonal allergies are triggered by mould spores instead of (or in addition to) pollen. Typically, these people suffer a flare-up of hay fever symptoms when it is cool and damp. Many mould spores grow in dark, moist indoor areas, especially in basements, shower recesses, refrigerator drip trays and rubbish bins.

Symptoms generally occur after inhaling the spores, but in some people eating foods and beverages that harbour moulds also provokes a flare-up.

Items that should be avoided:
- Alcoholic beverages, especially beer, wine and other drinks made by fermentation processes.
- Cheeses, especially blue cheese.
- Mushrooms of all kinds.

- Processed meats and fish, including frankfurters, sausages and smoked fish.
- Sauerkraut and other fermented or pickled foods, including soya sauce.
- Vinegar and products made with it: salad dressings, tomato sauce, mayonnaise and pickles.

Dust mites

Dust mites are thought to be a common cause of hay fever and asthma. The *Dermatophagoides pteronyssinus* mite lives in house dust, especially in coastal areas. It doesn't bite but certain proteins in its secretions and faeces often trigger allergic symptoms in susceptible people. Dust mites tend to congregate in beds, upholstered furniture, shaggy rugs and carpets and also in soft toys. House mite numbers can be reduced by using special dust mite-resistant covers for pillows and quilts or washing bed linen and soft toys each week in hot water. You can also try adding eucalyptus or tea-tree oil to the washing water. You should try to avoid sheepskin or woollen underlays and as far as possible, keep the house dry and well ventilated. Avoid carpets and rugs. Chemical sprays, negative ion generators and electric blankets are no help. Efficient air filters may remove some pet dander.

Pet dander

Cats and dogs constantly shed old skin cells or dander, that carries all sorts of allergenic proteins. About 15 per cent of adults and up to 50 per cent of children in the UK are allergic to pets, yet research suggests that having a cat or dog in the house may actually prevent the development of allergies, even in children genetically predisposed to them. Exposure to dogs appears to be even more effective than exposure to cats.

◀ **Go easy on the blue cheese**
Most semi-soft ripened cheeses, such as blue veined cheese, contain moulds that are recognised as common producers of allergic reactions in sensitive people.

Herbs for health

Enhance your diet

Herbs in the diet and herbal remedies are becoming increasingly popular as more and more people rediscover the value of natural ingredients and natural cures, and question the side effects of pharaceutical drugs.

Herbal medicines are viewed as the precursor of modern pharmacology, in fact, many of today's powerful drugs are derived from plants. Like drugs, however, herbs are not always safe in unskilled hands. Nevertheless there is much wisdom in the general approach of herbal medicine and there are usually fewer side effects. In addition, some ailments, such as eczema, appear to respond to herbal remedies where orthodox medicine has little to offer.

The medicinal value of herbs, known to earlier civilisations through a combination of observation, trial and error, is being rediscovered and confirmed by modern scientific tests. But while research continues to investigate the uses of new plants, many doctors and scientists still do not acknowledge the healing power of herbs, preferring instead to rely on 'tried and tested' pharmaceutical drugs. Yet our knowledge of herbs can be traced back to the Ancient Egyptians, whose priests routinely practised herbal medicine. A papyrus, dating from 1500 BC, lists hundreds of medicinal herbs – including many that are still in use today.

Most herbal medicines are still exempt from the normal product licensing requirements for medicines. Since 2005, depending on their use, herbal products have been sold in three ways: as food (with no health claim and no product licence); as herbal remedies licensed under the EU Directive on Traditional Medicinal Products (a simple registration scheme, requiring evidence of traditional use and safety); or as herbal medicines (with a medicinal-use claim, backed up by a full product licence and proven to meet stringent criteria for for quality, efficacy and safety).

THE HOME HERBALIST

Many herbs can be bought in the form of tea bags, from health food shops and supermarkets, or you can make your own herbal drinks. (If pregnant or taking medication, consult your doctor first.)

Teas and infusions are the same thing; made from flowers or leafy parts of the plants, they can be used as drinks or gargles. Use 1 teaspoon of dried herbs, or 2 teaspoons of fresh herbs, to a cup of boiling water. Pour boiling water over the herb and leave, covered, for between 5 and 10 minutes. Strain and drink, while hot, without milk or sugar. Add a little honey, if desired.

For medicinal purposes, drink 1 cup, three times a day. Decoctions, made by boiling roots or barks in water, can be used in a similar way. It is important to remember, when using fresh herbs, flowers, bark or roots, to make infusions or decoctions, you should wash them extremely thoroughly first.

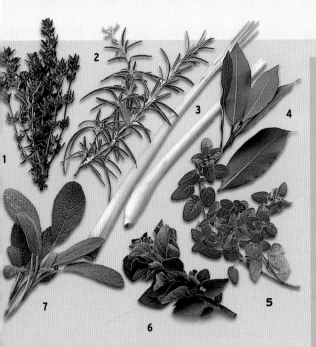

▲ Favourite herbs for the kitchen
When used generously in cooking, many herbs pack enough anti-oxidant power to help to protect your health. Instead of extra salt, look to their pungent flavour to enhance the appeal of your meals. Common culinary herbs are: 1. thyme. 2. rosemary. 3. lemongrass. 4. bay leaves. 5. marjoram. 6. oregano. 7. sage.

HERBS IN THE DIET

Most herbs have both culinary and traditional medicine uses. Generally, herbs have little nutritional value because of the small amounts used.

BASIL. The classic accompaniment to all tomato dishes, and important in Italian cooking. Basil is a natural tranquilliser and is said to calm the nervous system. It may also aid digestion and ease stomach cramps. Basil tea may relieve nausea.

BAY. An essential ingredient of the seasoning, *bouquet garni*, used in soups, casseroles and stews. Bay is used to stimulate and aid digestion.

BORAGE. As a tea or tisane, it is used against rheumatism and respiratory infections. Its leaves may be eaten in salad.

CHERVIL. This winter herb has a unique flavour a little like parsley with a hint of aniseed. It is used to stimulate digestion.

CHIVES. Mainly grown for culinary use, these tiny members of the onion family can stimulate the appetite as well as aid digestion during convalescence.

Antioxidants found in culinary herbs

Culinary herbs are healthy seasonings in the kitchen as well as natural and abundant sources of healing chemicals.

US Department of Agriculture (USDA) scientists recently carried out a scientific study on 27 culinary and 12 medicinal herbs. The study revealed that many well-known herbs are a good source of natural antioxidants – the compounds that play an important role in neutralising free radicals. In fact, the total phenolic contents of many herbs in the study were higher than those reported for berries, fruits and vegetables.

Although we might have to eat more herbs to get the equivalent total amount of antioxidants that are more easily consumed in fruits and vegetables, supplementing a balanced diet with herbs may be beneficial to our health.

In decreasing order of antioxidant activity, they include several oreganos, sweet marjoram, rose geranium, sweet bay, dill, thyme, rosemary and sage.

The culinary herbs with the highest antioxidant activities are the oreganos, which belong in the mint family. In fact, this study showed that their extremely high phenolic content and oxygen radical absorbance capacity (or ORAC) make their total antioxidant activities higher than those of tocopherol (found in vitamin E).

There are several types of oregano and they all have in common the flavour and scent that come from the essential oil carvacrol, a simple phenol they contain in varying amounts. What capsaicin is to peppers, carvacrol is to oregano; it imparts the savoury, pungent, warming sensation to the tongue. Carvacrol is not specific to oreganos and can also be found in sweet marjoram. In addition to carvacrol, high levels of rosmarinic acid contribute to the oreganos' antioxidant capacities.

CORIANDER. The pungent leaves are used in curries, salads and sauces. In herbalism, small, fresh bunches are eaten as a tonic for the stomach, and heart. Both the seeds and the leaves are used for strengthening the urinary tract and for treating urinary tract infections.

DILL. Widely used in pickles, soups and fish dishes. Dill has proved itself to be effective in the relief of gripes and flatulence.

FENNEL. The feathery leaves, which taste like aniseed, are often added to stuffings or sauces for fish. Both the seeds and the leaves can be used to aid digestion and help to prevent insomnia, excessive wind, nausea and vomiting.

MINT. The leaves of many varieties are used in cooking – for savoury dishes such as lamb, but also in desserts; subtle apple mint will bring out delicate

● **Myth.......**
Basil causes cancer.

.......Reality ●
Estragole, a naturally occuring compound in basil, causes cancer when it is fed to test animals in large doses and therefore can be accurately labelled as a carcinogen. The dose of estragole ingested from even vast quantities of basil in food is too small to cause concern.

H

flavours. Mint aids digestion, and a hot infusion can help at the start of a cold.

OREGANO. Also known as wild marjoram, this herb is widely used in stuffings and pizzas. It is thought to aid digestion and relieve the symptoms of colds, coughs and flu when used as an infusion – but it must not be used during pregnancy.

PARSLEY. This attractive and widely used herb is one of the most nutritious garnishes, containing useful amounts of vitamin C and iron. Fresh parsley makes a good breath-freshener.

ROSEMARY. Used with lamb and chicken dishes, throughout the Mediterranean, it is said to act as a stimulant to both the circulatory and nervous systems, and may help to soothe the digestive system, relieving indigestion and flatulence. Drinking a weak infusion of rosemary may help with the relief of nervous headaches, neuralgia and colds. Rosemary also makes a good antiseptic gargle.

SAGE. Purple or red sage is used in stuffings with pork and venison. Herbalists claim that sage can aid the digestion of rich, heavy foods and calm indigestion. Sage may also be used as a gargle to ease sore throats and sage tea is recommended for indigestion, anxiety and excessive sweating.

THYME. This herb is used widely in cooking for its aromatic flavour and in medicine as an antiseptic. An infusion can be used as a herbal gargle or expectorant for coughs and catarrh.

MYTH OR MEDICINE?

Traditional Chinese healers and Ayurvedic practitioners continue to use ancient herbal remedies sometimes combined with modern

◄ **The varied uses of liquorice**
Although mainly used as an adrenal tonic, liquorice can also be used to treat digestive problems, such as bloating and flatulence, as well as skin inflammation, such as erythema, and infections.

◄ **Keep colds at bay**
Echinacea is thought to help strengthen the body's immune system and increase its resistance to infection, particularly to influenza. Echinacea is also widely used to ease the common cold and other upper respiratory tract infections.

medical treatments. In the West, most medicines are synthesised, including many that were originally made from herbs. But there are exceptions: digitalis, the oldest effective heart medication, is still made from foxglove; morphine and codeine are derived from opium poppies; and vincristine, used to treat leukaemia, comes from the Madagascan periwinkle.

Ginseng is the most famous medicinal plant of China, used as a cure-all and tonic for the body. Panax ginseng is said to stimulate the nervous system and strengthen the immune system. Ginseng comes in various types – Chinese, Korean and Siberian. Ginseng is known as an adaptogen, which means it reacts to individuals according to their needs: it may help to calm a stressed person or stimulate someone who is tired.

Echinacea is also valued for its immune system benefits and its natural antibiotic properties and ginkgo biloba helps with mood and mental faculties.

The roots of valerian contain a compound that eases anxiety and promotes sleep. The herb helps to relax the gastrointestinal tract, making it useful in the treatment of conditions such as diverticulitis and irritable bowel syndrome which are worsened by stress.

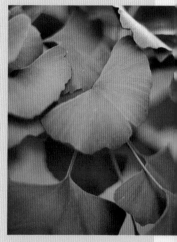

▲ **Improve memory**
Research has shown that ginkgo biloba may counteract declining mental faculties by improving concentration and memory and reducing mood swings. It is also thought to strengthen the veins and reduce bleeding in capillaries.

Herpes

EAT

■ A well-balanced, nutritious diet, with plenty of whole grains, fresh fruit and vegetables and high-quality protein for a strong immune system

LIMIT

■ Alcohol and caffeine

AVOID

■ Smoking

■ Excessive sun exposure

A common and highly contagious infectious disease, herpes is caused by strains of the *herpes simplex* virus and is experienced as painful and itchy blisters. Type 1 herpes, or oral herpes, causes cold sores or fever blisters around the mouth.

In some cases, this type of herpes infects the eyes and can result in blindness or, even more seriously, can spread to the brain and result in life-threatening *herpes encephalitis*. Type 2, or genital herpes, is sexually transmitted and causes sores in the genital and anal areas. Engaging in oral sex with an infected person can cause mouth and throat blisters that are difficult to differentiate from Type 1 herpes. Both types are often transmitted by people who are unaware that they are infected.

Regardless of the type or location, herpes blisters usually rupture into open weeping sores that crust over

The yoghurt approach

Anecdotal evidence suggests that *Lactobacillus acidophilus*, found in yoghurts containing 'active' or live cultures and also sold in capsules, may help to prevent recurrences of cold sores. You may need to take supplements to get enough.

and eventually heal within a few days or weeks. Some people also experience a mild fever, swollen lymph nodes and fatigue. Even after healing, the virus remains dormant in the body; some people never have another attack, while others have repeated but milder eruptions sporadically throughout their lives.

Recurrences may be triggered by hormonal changes, physical or emotional stress, fever, exposure to the sun or other environmental factors. Certain foods and drugs can precipitate recurrences. If you have frequent attacks, analyse your lifestyle and try to discover what may trigger attacks.

Although there is no known cure for herpes, some sufferers have reported relief when taking lysine, an amino acid supplement usually sold in health-food shops. To help to reduce the frequency of herpes attacks, some advocates of natural medicine recommend taking 500mg to 1,000mg of L-lysine daily, on an empty stomach. This amino acid is also found in meat, fish, chicken and dairy products. In more severe herpes cases, doctors prescribe acyclovir, an antiviral medication that can be taken orally or used as a cream. It can shorten the duration of an attack and help to prevent a recurrence, as can famciclovir (Famvir). Zinc supplements and aloe vera can also alleviate the symptoms of both types.

Warning: A pregnant woman who has had herpes should inform her obstetrician immediately. An active infection may be transmitted to the baby during delivery and can cause blindness, retardation or even death. A caesarean delivery can help to prevent transmission.

Self-care

Warning symptoms are usually a tingling, sensation. If you have this before an outbreak of oral herpes,

Do one simple thing

Eat foods rich in lysine

Foods high in the amino acid lysine, found in meat and fish, milk and dairy products, may help to reduce the frequency of herpes attacks.

prompt use of aspirin and ice packs sometimes forestalls the recurrence. Once the lesions appear, compresses of cold water or milk may ease the discomfort. Avoid kissing anyone or sharing cups, glasses, utensils or toothbrushes during outbreaks.

For genital outbreaks, warm baths or saltwater compresses can help to ease inflammation. Keep the infected area clean and dry. Wash your hands after contact with the sores to avoid spreading it to other parts of your body. Type 2 herpes is very contagious; those infected should never have sexual contact with non-infected persons during an attack. Latex condoms may lower, but cannot entirely eliminate, the risk of sexual transmission. Avoid sharing towels and flannels.

Eat a nutritious diet. To help to prevent recurrences, strengthen your immune system to resist disease by eating a well-balanced diet with plenty of whole grains, fresh fruit and vegetables and get enough protein. Don't smoke; avoid excessive alcohol and caffeine. Balance your lifestyle with regular exercise and adequate rest to alleviate stress. Avoid excessive sun exposure, and always wear a sunscreen to protect your skin.

There is controversy around the use of vitamin C to help this condition; it has been seen to help in some studies, but there is concern that large doses can prove acidic and actually exacerbate the situation. It may be safer to eat plenty of red grapes and use lemon balm and peppermint oil instead.

H

Hiatus hernia

CONSUME

- Small, frequent meals
- High-fibre foods, such as wholegrain cereals and breads, fresh fruit, salads and raw or lightly cooked vegetables

LIMIT

- Coffee and alcohol, including wine, especially before bedtime

AVOID

- Gaining excess weight
- Large meals and carbonated beverages
- Fatty foods, chocolate and peppermint
- Alcohol and smoking
- Any food that produces symptoms

Under normal circumstances, the hiatus is a small opening in the muscular diaphragm where the oesophagus meets the stomach. A hiatus hernia develops when the opening widens and allows the upper part of the stomach to protrude upwards through the hiatus. Some hiatus hernias are present at birth. Most of them, however, develop during life as the opening of the hiatus becomes stretched, as a result of pregnancy or excessive weight gain, both of which place upward pressure on the stomach. Severe coughing, vomiting, straining when moving the bowels or sudden physical exertion may also stretch the hiatus.

Although hiatus hernias are common, occurring in almost half of the population, most people are unaware of the condition because they don't experience symptoms. A hiatus hernia is usually diagnosed after recurring bouts of indigestion and heartburn, typically as a result of acid reflux into the oesophagus. The condition is usually not considered serious. There are

exceptions where frequent exposure to stomach acids causes severe oesophageal damage. In such cases, surgical treatment is necessary.

Dietary approaches

Avoid large meals that overly distend the stomach. Eat four or five small meals spread over the course of a day. In addition, try to avoid carbonated drinks, which may increase discomfort. After eating, don't lie down, stoop or bend over for at least an hour; this may promote reflux. Don't eat or drink anything for at least 2 hours before going to bed at night, when attacks are most likely to occur.

Avoid substances that relax the diaphragmatic muscle. Alcohol, including wine, is one such muscle relaxant; you should avoid any alcoholic beverage in the evening.

Avoid spicy and acidic foods. Eliminate foods that tend to irritate your stomach or provoke a bout of indigestion. The culprits vary from one person to another, but common offenders include spices, onions, garlic, pickles and vinegar. Regular or decaffeinated coffee increases stomach acidity, as does tobacco. Chocolate and peppermint tend to relax the hiatal sphincter; fatty foods stay in the stomach longer than other foods and can also provoke

Tips for dealing with hiatus hernias

- Don't lie down after you eat. Try to wait at least 2 hours before taking a nap or going to bed for the night.
- Don't exercise straight after eating. Walking is fine, but wait 2 to 3 hours before strenuous exercise.
- Don't wear tight-fitting clothes. They put extra pressure on your stomach.
- Relax. Stress slows down the digestion, which makes acid reflux worse. Try deep breathing, yoga or meditation to deal with daily stress.

indigestion. Small sips of water or a warm herbal tea may help when you feel a bout of regurgitation coming on, but avoid antacids that contain peppermint.

Eat lots of fibre and drink plenty of fluids. Constipation can worsen a hiatus hernia because straining distends the abdomen. Eat plenty of high-fibre foods, such as wholegrain cereals and breads, as well as fresh vegetables and fruit. Daily exercise and an adequate fluid intake are also important.

People who experience frequent night-time symptoms of a hiatus hernia can try raising the head of their bed 10–15 cm.

If lifestyle modification and conservative medical treatment do not alleviate symptoms, prescription drugs or even surgery may be recommended to reposition the stomach below the diaphragm and to narrow the hiatal opening.

Hives

AVOID

- Foods that have previously caused hives or other allergic reactions
- Foods and medications coloured with tartrazine (additive E102) if you are sensitive to this additive
- Foods that contain salicylate if you are allergic to aspirin

Medically known as urticaria, hives are the itchy red welts that develop as a result of reactions to foods and other provoking substances. For example, certain medications – aspirin, as well as penicillin and related antibiotics – can cause hives in some people. Even those without known allergies can develop hives after being stung by an insect or touching stinging plants, such as nettles. Hives may be accompanied by other symptoms of allergy, including swelling of the eyes and other parts of the body. Many food allergies provoke swelling and itching of the lips and mouth. It is important to distinguish between chronic (ongoing) urticaria and acute urticaria which could develop into anaphylaxis, a potentially fatal medical emergency.

Warning: If an attack of hives is accompanied by swelling of the mouth, tongue or throat and difficulty breathing, speaking or swallowing, get medical help immediately. These symptoms may signal anaphylaxis.

Well-known causes of hives

The blotchy rash of hives can follow ingestion of almost any food, but among the most common causes are shellfish, nuts and berries. A person who is allergic to aspirin (acetyl-salicylic acid) should also be wary of foods that contain natural salicylates including apricots, berries, grapes, raisins and other dried fruit, tea and foods processed with vinegar. Among the other well-known triggers of hives are emotional stress; exposure to the, sun, heat or cold (even ice cubes in drinks); and viral infections.

Hives generally develop within hours after exposure to a trigger, but in unusual cases, they may appear several days later. This delayed reaction can make it difficult to identify the offending substance. Delayed reactions are most common with medications; if you develop a rash while taking any drug, report it to your doctor immediately. A drug allergy may develop abruptly after months or even years of taking a medication. Always mention your sensitivity to the pharmacist and any doctor who prescribes for you.

Check food labels to avoid tartrazine. Although food additives are often blamed for causing allergic reactions, only tartrazine (additive E102), a common colouring agent, has been found to cause hives – and in fewer than 1 in 10,000 people. All product labels must list food colourings; people who are sensitive to tartrazine should read labels on food products, medications and vitamin supplements.

Dealing with hives

An outbreak of hives may fade within minutes or persist for days or weeks. If you can link a particular food to hives, avoid it and consult a doctor. When hives persist for more than a few days, a doctor may prescribe an antihistamine, as well as a lotion to reduce itching and relieve inflammation. If you get hives repeatedly, the doctor may suggest that you keep a food diary to help you to identify, eliminate and then slowly try to reintroduce culprit foods.

Eat foods that are high in niacin. Since hives are triggered by the release of histamines, it may be useful to increase consumption of foods that are high in niacin (vitamin B_3), which is believed to inhibit histamine release. Good sources of niacin include poultry, seafood, seeds and nuts, whole grains and fortified cereals. Choose these carefully, however, because, some foods that are good sources of niacin are among those that tend to provoke an allergy.

Avoiding the culprit foods that trigger an allergic reaction is the safest way to prevent an outbreak of hives or anaphylaxis.

If you have had a severe allergic reaction to any substance, ask the doctor whether you need to carry special medication to be used if the reaction occurs again. It's wise to carry a tag or card that specifies your sensitivity to alert emergency medical personnel should you become incapacitated.

Honey

BENEFITS

- A source of quick energy

- Adds flavour to foods and beverages and improves the shelf life of baked goods

DRAWBACKS

- Contamination with *Clostridium botulinum* spores may be dangerous for babies under a year old

Our inborn taste for sweet foods led Stone Age humans to forage for the sweetness of honey. Although bees were first domesticated in artificial hives in Egypt and India about 4,500 years ago, it wasn't until about AD 1000 that beekeepers began to understand the interplay between bees and flowers that is required to produce honey.

Honey was the staple sweetener in Europe until the 1500s, when granulated sugar (more easily stored and transported) became available. But sugar could not entirely replace honey's more complex flavours, and it is still a popular food. To make

H

Nature's balm

In the days before antibiotics, doctors sometimes treated wounds with honey. Why? Honey has considerable antibacterial properties. It's still considered an excellent wound dressing and it dries to form a natural bandage. Several studies of surgical wounds have shown that honey speeds healing. Some manufacturers even sell honey-infused dressings for hard-to-heal wounds. Manuka honey, from New Zealand has remarkable antiseptic qualities; it even inhibits the growth of the antibiotic-resistant bug, MRSA and *Heliobacter pylori*, which causes stomach ulcers.

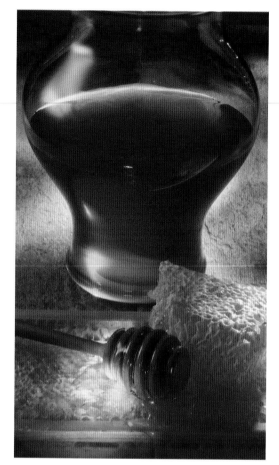

The liquid honey that is sold in supermarkets is removed from the comb by centrifugation, pasteurised, strained, filtered and bottled. Solid honeys are put through controlled crystallisation before packaging. Raw honeys that have not been heated have more flavour and higher levels of antibacterial properties.

Honey production

Australia produces the widest range of honeys in the world. New Zealand also produces a wide range of honeys, including the famous one from the nectar of the manuka tree (*Leptospermum scoparium*). The flavour of honey depends on which flowers the bees have visited. Acacia honey is mild and suitable for cooking; chestnut honey has a distinctive, almost bitter taste.

Honey can contain naturally occurring toxins from plants. Bees that collect pollen from rhododendrons, for example, can produce a toxic honey that can cause paralysis. There is also some concern over pyrrolizidine alkaloids in honey made from bees that have foraged on ragwort.

Honey as food

Despite all the claims that honey is a wonder food, its nutritional value is limited; honeys are mostly sugars – fructose and glucose, with some sucrose. Some types provide minute amounts of B complex and C vitamins. Honey does contain some antioxidants, however, but fruit and vegetables are usually better sources. Some new studies are looking into the antimicrobial and wound-healing properties of honey.

Weight for weight, honey contains fewer calories than sugar – 288 as opposed to 394 per 100g – because a quarter of it is water. A tablespoon of honey weighs more than the same volume of sugar because of its water content. Honey can be substituted for sugar at the ratio of 1 measure of honey for every $1\frac{1}{4}$ units of sugar; the liquid in the recipe may need to be decreased, however. Breads and cakes that are sweetened with honey stay moist longer than those that are baked with sugar, thanks to the

500g of honey, bees take nectar from 2.5 million blossoms. Even when flowers are plentiful, a bee colony may make 40,000 trips and fly more than 55,000 miles to produce 500g of honey.

From flowers to hives

Plants and bees have a symbiotic relationship. Bees gather nectar, carrying pollen with them from one flower to another, ensuring cross-fertilisation. The bees concentrate the flower nectar into honey, which is stored in their hives. The pollen, provides young worker bees with protein and vitamins similar to the nutrients in dried beans and peas.

While it is food for bees, pollen does nothing for humans that legumes can't do better, and it may trigger life-threatening allergic reactions in susceptible people.

Propolis power

Bees also collect a waxy substance called propolis, which they use as a sort of cement or sealant when making their hives. Propolis, like honey, has also long been used in folk medicine for its healing properties. But its composition varies greatly, making it difficult to test claims for its therapeutic powers. It consists of around 50 compounds, including fatty acids and flavonoids, known to have anti-inflammatory, anti-fungal and antibacterial effects. It is also claimed to have antioxidant and anti-tumour properties, to boost immunity, and to help in healing burns and ulcers.

Recent research suggests that extracts of propolis can dramatically enhance the activity of several antibiotics. Combined with echinacea and vitamin C, it may be useful for preventing and treating upper respiratory tract infections in children. Propolis may even be active against antibiotic-resistant organisms, including the MRSA 'superbug' responsible for many cases of hospital-acquired infection.

water-attracting (hygroscopic) properties of honey. Honey is also healthier than sugar when it comes to Glycaemic Index, too. It is a 'moderate-release' carboydrate with a GI figure of 60, making it an ideal energy source. It also makes a soothing drink for sore throats, with lemon juice and hot water.

Risk for babies

Spores of *Clostridium botulinum* have been found in some honeys. While not dangerous to adults and older children, infants should not be fed honey because it can cause serious illness in the first year of life.

Hyperactivity

CONSUME

■ A variety of foods to provide a nutritionally complete diet

LIMIT

■ Caffeinated beverages

■ Foods that contain large amounts of food additives and preservatives.

AVOID

■ Self-treatment with high-dose vitamins and minerals

■ Diets that eliminate entire food groups

Hyperactivity or attention deficit hyperactivity disorder (ADHD) is more common in boys than in girls. Parents often describe the hyperactive child as being in perpetual motion – always on the move, disruptive, impulsive and unable to concentrate. Many researchers theorise that an imbalance in brain chemistry is responsible for their abnormal behaviour, but a precise cause has not yet been identified.

In recent years, diet has been suggested as a possible cause of hyperactivity – a claim discounted by many experts. Dozens of studies have failed to prove that diet plays any role in hyperactivity. And yet, many parents and even some doctors believe that, at least for some children, there is a link.

It is now recognised that, in a few children, identifying foods that they cannot tolerate, and then removing them from the diet, can help.

The diet hypothesis was first proposed in 1973 by Benjamin Feingold, a Californian allergist, who blamed hyperactivity on sensitivity to certain food additives and salicylates, compounds found in fruit, some vegetables and in aspirin. Dr Feingold recommended eliminating from the child's diet all foods that contain certain preservatives and artificial flavours and colours, as well as any natural sources of salicylates. Half of his hyperactive patients improved on this diet, and many doctors and parent groups supported it.

Foods low in salicyclates include bananas, peeled pears and papaya. Vegetable include cabbage, peas, lettuce and potatoes. Poultry, meat, fish, eggs and cereals are low, too.

Although some reports suggest that an additive-free diet helps a few children, Dr Feingold's finding of marked improvement in a significant percentage of cases has not been duplicated in scientific studies. Some paediatricians advise parents to try eliminating foods that are especially high in preservatives, dyes and other additives – for example, processed meats and some commercial baked goods – to see if there is any improvement. But avoiding all foods that contain natural salicylates is more difficult; there is some evidence that this helps, but it could lead to an inadequate diet and deficiencies of vitamin C, beta carotene and other nutrients. You should consult a dietitian if you wish to try a low-salicylate diet on your child.

Caffeine has also been linked to hyperactivity. Experts doubt that it causes the problem, but it may add to the restlessness of a hyperactive child. In any event, eliminating caffeine from a child's diet is a good idea.

Orthomolecular therapy, which is the use of markedly high doses of vitamins and minerals to treat behavioural and other problems, is advocated by some practitioners for hyperactivity. There is no evidence that this helps, but it has been shown that self-treating with megadose vitamins and minerals can cause serious nutritional imbalances and toxicity.

Sugar cleared as the culprit

Hyperactivity has often been blamed on a high intake of sugar. Again, there is no scientific proof of this. In fact, one study conducted by the National Institute of Mental Health in the United States found that children given a sugary drink were less active than a control group that ingested only sugar-free drinks. Some researchers theorise that the calming effect noted in the group given drinks containing sugar may be related to the fact that sugar prompts the brain to increase the production of serotonin, a chemical that reduces the brain's electrical activity. Even this is not a reason to give children lots of sweets – sugar provides calories but it is devoid of other beneficial nutrients; it also promotes tooth decay.

Hypoglycaemia

CONSUME
- Small meals that provide a balance of protein, carbohydrates and fats

LIMIT
- Carbohydrate-only (especially high-GI) meals and snacks

AVOID
- Consuming alcohol without food

Glucose is the body's major source of energy; it is also the only form of energy that the brain can use effectively. During digestion and metabolism, the liver converts all of the carbohydrates and some of the protein in a meal into glucose, which is then released into the bloodstream. In response to rising blood glucose levels, the pancreas secretes extra insulin, the hormone that enables cells to use the sugar to produce energy.

Hypoglycaemia, or low blood sugar, occurs when the amount of insulin in the blood exceeds that needed to metabolise the available glucose. It is seen often when a person with diabetes takes too much insulin, but it can also occur in other circumstances, such as too much alcohol; taking large amounts of paracetamol or aspirin, beta blockers and some anti-psychotic drugs; or when tumours develop that secrete insulin.

Reactive hypoglycaemia
This condition occurs when blood sugar levels plummet 1 to 2 hours after a meal. Symptoms include

dizziness, headache, trembling, hunger, palpitations and irritability. Many people who experience vague, unexplained symptoms assume that they have reactive hypoglycaemia, but the condition is not common. This is because the human body has a very sensitive feedback system that controls insulin secretion.

Reactive hypoglycaemia can be diagnosed only by monitoring blood glucose levels after ingestion of a known dose of glucose.

Eat small, frequent meals with a mix of carbohydrates, fats and protein. A diet made up mostly of carbohydrates may produce mild symptoms of hypoglycaemia even though the blood sugar levels are usually in the low–normal range.

Here's what happens: a person may skip breakfast or have only high-GI carbohydrates – for example, a cereal bar or a sweet roll. The pancreas will secrete a fair amount of insulin to process the glucose in this meal, but because the meal contains little protein or fat, which are metabolised more slowly, the body will burn the glucose in 2 or 3 hours.

Sensing a need for more energy, the brain sends out strong hunger signals. A sweet snack will satisfy this hunger and provide a quick burst of energy, but the pancreas will pump out enough insulin to quickly metabolise the glucose again.

If this is repeated a pattern is established. The cycle can be broken by eating regular meals that include small amounts of protein and fats and low-GI carbohydrates. These take longer than sugars to be digested and converted into glucose, and they allow for a steady release of energy. Avoid having a breakfast of white toast and jam, for instance, and have a wholegrain toast with cheese instead.

Include foods in your diet that have a lower GI such as beans, oats, wholegrain bread, pasta, apples and citrus fruit since they are absorbed more slowly. Choose whole grains and wholemeal bread over refined grains (such as white bread) as often as possible.

You may also want to consume foods with a low glycaemic load (see chart, page 197).

Insulin overdose
A much more serious type of hypoglycaemia occurs when a person with diabetes takes more insulin than is needed to metabolise the available glucose.

The onset of symptoms of an insulin reaction – hunger, tingling sensations, sweating, faintness, impaired vision, mood changes, palpitations and a cold, clammy sensation – can be reversed by immediately eating a spoonful of sugar or honey, sucking on a glucose sweet or drinking a sugary drink. Do not ignore insulin reactions.

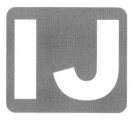

Ice cream

BENEFITS

- A source of calcium
- Provides protein and digestible, high-calorie nutrition during an illness

DRAWBACKS

- High in saturated fat and sugar

Products labelled as ice cream must be made with a minimum of 10 per cent cream, milk or butter fat. Manufacturers may add various other ingredients, as well as enough air to increase its volume. Usually, the least expensive ice creams contain the minimum 10 per cent fat and the maximum air, while the premium commercial brands have more fat and less air.

It is fat that gives ice cream its smooth texture; manufacturers of reduced-fat and low-fat ice confections and frozen yoghurts compensate for the lack of fat by increasing the sugar – by up to twice the amount – and by not beating in as much air. Therefore, although these products contain less fat, in the end they are not necessarily lower in calories.

Both soft ice cream and iced confections are 3 to 10 per cent fat and 30 to 50 per cent air. Sorbets are usually made with a small amount of milk fat and milk solids or, sometimes, egg white. Fruit ices, on the other hand, tend to be made with fruit pulp or juice, sugar and water, with the possible addition of pectin or ascorbic acid. The calories in these products vary greatly, so be sure to check the nutrition panel, and remember to check whether the stated serving is the amount you actually consume.

Ice cream has some calcium and protein, as well as small quantities of vitamin A and riboflavin. The price you pay for these nutrients, however, is a large helping of

Did you know?

An ice cream cone can have as many calories as a main meal

Watch what you put into your cone, as well as on it. Choose regular instead of premium ice creams; small instead of medium or large cones; single instead of double or triple scoops; and avoid toppings. There is such a wide variety of tempting toppings available – chocolate, caramel or hot fudge syrups; chocolate sprinkles; marshmallows; nuts and whipped cream – that you can easily add 75-100kcal with toppings alone. And beware of the cone you choose: a regular single cone has 18kcal, a sugar cone has about 40kcal while a large waffle cone has up to 83kcal. What could start out as a simple 110kcal dessert can end up having as many calories as a main meal. You can probably check the calorie and fat content of well-known brands; the content of ices bought from a stand may be harder to establish.

saturated fat, with its adverse implications for heart disease, some cancers and other conditions. Fruit sorbets – which are high in sugar but fat-free – are a much better choice when you want to finish off a meal with a frozen dessert. Low-fat frozen yoghurt is a good substitute for ice cream; a half cup of frozen yoghurt topped with fresh fruit and toasted wheatgerm can satisfy cravings for a frosty treat and supply useful amounts of calcium, vitamins and fibre at the same time.

Additives. Storing ice cream presents a problem in the form of 'heat shock'. When ice cream is removed from the freezer, its surface melts. When the ice cream is refrozen, ice crystals form, possibly resulting in a crunchy texture. This problem can be countered by including various permissable additives that sop up the water that forms as ice cream melts and prevent it from refreezing into crystals. Guar gum or locust bean gum, from plant sources, are usually used for this purpose. Other additives used in ice cream include emulsifiers such as lecithin, mono- and diglycerides or polysorbates that make for a smooth texture by dispersing the fat globules.

Immune system

Your body's secret weapon

The immune system protects the body from attack by micro-organisms, abnormal cells and chemicals. Its army includes macrophages, T cells and B cells. Most often, the external threats are infections caused by invading bacteria, viruses and fungi, while abnormal or cancerous cells pose the major internal threats. In addition, this complex system oversees the repair of tissues that are injured by wounds or disease.

Once in a while the immune system mistakes a harmless foreign substance for an enemy, resulting in an allergic reaction, such as hives, hay fever or asthma. Less commonly the immune system – mistaking an internal signal – attacks normal body tissue, leading to an auto-immune disease, such as Type 1 diabetes, rheumatoid arthritis or lupus.

The most remarkable characteristic of the immune system is its 'memory' for foreign substances and organisms. Confronted with a virus or other invading organism, it creates an antibody that will recognise it and mount an attack against it at any future encounter. This mechanism, called acquired immunity, is what makes vaccinations work.

SYSTEM FAILURE OR WHY WE GET SICK

If the immune system is such a wonder, why do we get sick? The simplest explanation is that often there is a lapse between the time an invading organism enters the body and the time the immune system conquers it. In the interim the invader can make its mark, killing cells. How sick you become depends largely on how strong a defence your immune system can launch. Infection, cancer and other illnesses develop if the immune system is weakened by any number of stressors, including viruses and other invading organisms, malnutrition and the consequences of ageing. Fortunately, antibiotics and sulphonamides drugs can wipe out most bacterial infections in otherwise healthy people; progress is also being made in the development of antiviral drugs. Doctors may lower immunity to treat an auto-immune disease or to prevent rejection of donor organs.

DIETARY INFLUENCES

The right diet is critical to a strong immune system. The following are the building blocks you need to keep your defences strong. It's best to get them from food. Supplements are usually not necessary unless you are taking therapeutic doses for a specific condition.

PROTEINS ARE CENTRAL TO THE PROPER FUNCTIONING OF THE IMMUNE SYSTEM. The amino acids they provide are used to make anti-bodies and other immune compounds that attack foreign invaders and prevent infection.

OMEGA-3 FATTY ACIDS HELP IN IMMUNE FUNCTION. Omega-3 fatty acids, abundant in fish and other seafood, are especially beneficial in controlling inflammation and the harmful effects of rheumatoid arthritis and other auto-immune disorders. Research suggests that omega-3 oils help to reduce acute inflammation, which occurs as part of the immune response to attack or injury. Omega-3s activate parts of the immune system that rein in attack cells to stop them when they have completed their task .

VITAMIN E IS A T CELL ENHANCER. Vitamin E, in oils, nuts and seeds, margarine and avocados, may increase T cell activity and help to produce antibodies.

Did you know?

Even a strong immune system isn't foolproof

Made of a strand of genetic material, viruses are so simple that they aren't even considered living things. Yet they can trigger illnesses, from the common cold to life-threatening SARS, by overtaking the genetic machinery of cells within the body. Once in command, they direct those cells to produce more viruses, which, if not stopped, can overwhelm vital organs. The best strategy is to prevent exposure to the virus in the first place.

VITAMIN C TO FORTIFY. Vitamin C, found in many fruits and vegetables, helps to build and maintain mucous membranes and collagen, as well as strengthen the blood vessel walls, and is thought to enhance the function of the immune cells. Vitamin C supplements may help to reduce the duration of a cold. Red peppers and kiwi fruit are excellent sources of vitamin C. Up to 200mg daily is needed to increase disease-fighting antibodies.

VITAMIN A IS KEY. Found in liver, fish, milk, cheese and eggs, vitamin A reduces the incidence and severity of infectious illnesses by helping to keep mucous membranes healthy and intact and may also increase antibody response and white blood cell proliferation. Beta carotene, once consumed, can be converted to vitamin A in the body.

ZINC IS A TRACE MINERAL, WHOSE MANY IMPORTANT FUNCTIONS, INCLUDE SUPPORTING IMMUNITY. A deficiency of zinc has been associated with slow wound healing. The best food sources include seafood (especially oysters), meat, poultry and liver, as well as eggs, milk, beans, nuts and whole grains. But too much supplementary zinc can actually depress the immune system.

SELENIUM IS A TRACE MINERAL ESSENTIAL FOR A STRONG IMMUNE SYSTEM. The best sources of selenium are seafood, Brazil nuts, some meats and fish, as well as wheatbran, wheatgerm, oats and brown rice.

IRON IS AN ABSOLUTE MUST. Iron is required for the manufacture of B cells and T cells and ensures that cells get the oxygen they need to function properly and resist disease. Best sources are red meat, legumes, green vegetables, tofu, eggs, dried fruit and enriched cereals.

ANTIOXIDANTS TO PROTECT AGAINST FREE RADICALS. Research suggests that the antioxidant properties of carotenoids, such as lycopene (found in tomatoes and tomato products) and beta carotene (found in orange, red and yellow plant foods and dark green vegetables) may protect immune cells from destructive free radicals – the molecules that can harm cells and damage the DNA.

ENEMIES OF THE IMMUNE SYSTEM

There are many factors that can have an adverse effect on the immune system: excessive intakes of alcohol and caffeine; ingestion or inhalation of heavy metals such as cadmium, lead and mercury; and tobacco smoke or other forms of pollution in the air. When pollutants or toxic substances are absorbed by the body, they threaten the effectiveness of minerals and vitamins in the food and are sometimes described as anti-nutrients.

More immune boosters

- Garlic and onions may stimulate the fighting power of macrophages and T cells because of their powerful sulphur compounds, which may also block enzymes that allow organisms to invade healthy tissue.

- Some studies suggest that moderate exercise may help to improve immune function, especially in people who were previously sedentary.

- Probiotics, the friendly bacteria found in some fermented milk products such as yoghurt and probiotic drinks, may help to improve immune responses against viruses.

- Blueberries, blackberries and grapes contain anthocyanins, powerful antioxidants that have potent immune-stimulating properties.

- Some evidence shows that shiitake mushrooms may boost immunity, but the practical significance of this is unknown.

- Certain whey proteins, sold as nutritional supplements, specially processed to provide a high dose of the amino acid cysteine, may enhance immune function. Cysteine is used by the body in the synthesis of glutathione, one of the most important compounds of the immune system.

- EGCG, a powerful antioxidant compound found in green tea, may have the ability to inhibit the growth of cancer cells as well as neutralising harmful free radicals.

Impotence

CONSUME PLENTY OF

- Foods rich in zinc, such as seafood (especially oysters), meat, poultry, eggs, milk, beans, nuts and whole grains

LIMIT

- Alcohol and saturated fats

AVOID

- Nicotine and all drugs except those prescribed for you

Although psychological factors certainly affect male sexual function, recent studies show that two-thirds of cases of impotence have physical factors. Diabetes, atherosclerosis, paralysis or, less commonly, hormonal imbalances are among the organic causes of impotence. The use of alcohol, nicotine, illegal substances, as well as prescription medications can lead to impotence. Nicotine impedes the blood flow by constricting small arteries, including those that bring blood to the penis.

Medications that commonly cause impotence include acid-suppressants for ulcers, antihypertensives, antidepressants and sleeping pills. In most cases, an alternative drug can be prescribed.

While diet may not have much of an effect on impotence, medications can help. The most popular drug is sildenafil citrate (Viagra), which boosts the activity of an enzyme, cyclic guanosine monophosphate (cGMP), which is the key to achieving an erection.

Is there a link between alcohol and impotence?

Alcohol should be taken in moderation. A high blood level of alcohol interrupts the relay of messages along the nervous system; heavy alcohol consumption over an extended period modifies the normal pattern of hormone production, which may affect sexual function.

Dietary factors

Zinc is absolutely key. Zinc is among the minerals thought to be essential to good reproductive health. While zinc intake may not have a direct effect on potency, it may be important for male sexual health, since very high levels are found in the seminal fluid. Good sources of zinc include seafood (especially oysters), meat, poultry, eggs, milk, beans, nuts and whole grains. Zinc supplements are not recommended; in high doses they can interfere with the absorption of calcium and copper.

Watch your weight. Men should be careful to maintain a normal weight; obesity predisposes a person to diabetes, which is one of the leading causes of impotence. Studies have shown that obesity puts men at greater risk for erectile dysfunction. Also, a diet low in saturated fats helps to prevent atherosclerosis, the build-up of fatty plaque that clogs not only the large vessels around the heart but also the penile artery.

Indigestion and heartburn

TAKE

- Small meals at regular intervals

LIMIT

- Alcohol, caffeine and coffee in all forms

AVOID

- Fatty foods
- Eating within 2 hours of bedtime
- Tobacco use of any kind

Almost everyone suffers from indigestion occasionally, but for some, it is a daily trial. The most common symptom of indigestion is heartburn, a burning chest pain

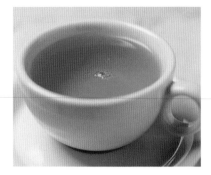

▲ **Drink chamomile tea**
Chamomile has been used for centuries for digestive disorders. Chamomile tea soothes inflamed or irritated gastrointestinal tissue and reduces the spasms of griping pain.

that occurs when stomach acid and other contents flow backwards, or reflux, into the oesophagus. Unlike the stomach, the lining of the oesophagus has no protective lining of mucus-producing tissue, so the acid produces irritation and even ulcerations. Obesity and pregnancy may also lead to heartburn because of increased intra-abdominal pressure, which tends to force the stomach fluids back up into the oesophagus. A hiatus hernia is another possible cause.

Heartburn caused by reflux can usually be controlled with a few lifestyle changes. Certain foods and beverages can trigger an attack, either by promoting stomach acid secretion or by relaxing the sphincter muscle. You should start with adopting a low-fat diet that includes a balance of protein, starches and fibre-rich vegetables and fruit. (Fatty foods take longer to digest and thus slow down the rate of the food emptying from the stomach.) Coffee, regular and decaffeinated, promotes high acid production; so does strong tea, carbonated drinks and other sources of caffeine. Some fruits can also cause problems in a few people. There is no evidence that spicy foods – except possibly, red and black pepper – cause indigestion, but people who find that a spicy meal is followed by discomfort would be better off avoiding such seasonings. Reflux is often made worse by foods such as chocolate, peppermint or spearmint that tend to relax the sphincter muscle which connects the oesophagus to the stomach.

Avoid large meals, especially late in the day. Eat smaller meals more often – perhaps five times a day – and eat slowly to help to avoid bloating and pressure. Sit down and relax at every meal. Try not to eat in the two or three hours before bed-time, and don't snack at bedtime. Sit up straight during and after meals; bending over or lying down increases pressure on the stomach and promotes reflux. Stop smoking; nicotine relaxes the sphincter muscle. You should limit your alcohol intake to the odd glass of wine or beer. Drinking cabbage juice (which contains glutamine) and also more water seems to help. Water washes the stomach acid down to the stomach where it belongs. Drinking chamomile or ginger teas between meals may bring some relief.

The use of nonprescription antacids to treat heartburn by neutralising stomach acid is questionable; the problem is not too much acid, but acid in the wrong place. However, these preparations may help to ease an attack that may have already started. If you find that they do help, follow instructions and never take them for longer than recommended. 'Proton pump inhibitors' such as omeprazole are effective drugs for acid reflux.

Infertility

EAT PLENTY OF

- A balanced diet with plenty of fruit and vegetables, lean meat, fish or poultry, wholegrain breads, cereals and grains, as well as low-fat dairy products

LIMIT

- Coffee and other sources of caffeine

AVOID

- Alcohol and smoking
- Becoming overweight or underweight

Defined as the inability to achieve a pregnancy after at least two years of trying, infertility affects up to 15 per cent of couples. Experts cannot explain why the infertility rate has almost doubled in the past 25 years, but at least three factors stand out: the growing trend for couples to delay marriage and parenthood until their most fertile years are past, the rise in sexually transmitted diseases and a puzzling drop in sperm production.

Many couples assume that infertility rests with the woman; in fact, men are just as likely to be infertile. In 40 per cent of cases, the problem lies with the male, and in 40 per cent of cases, with the female. The cause can't be identified

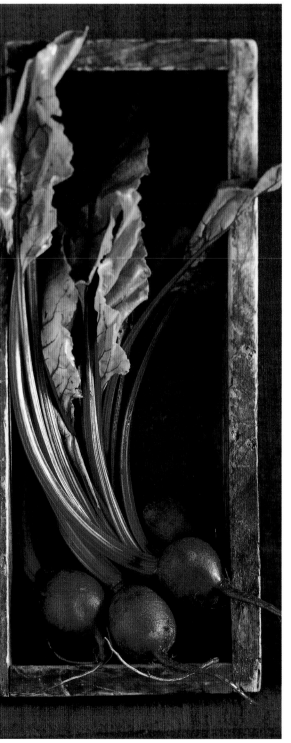

◀ **High in fibre**
Eating vegetables rich in fibre, such as beetroot, and less fatty food helps to control episodes of indigestion and heartburn caused by reflux.

in the remaining 20 per cent, or both partners may be contributing factors. While nutrition is not a leading cause of infertility, consuming a healthy diet enhances the chance of conceiving and delivering a healthy baby.

Female infertility

The leading cause of female infertility is the failure to ovulate. Ovulation may be influenced by the diet, hormonal imbalances and a variety of other factors. Women who are very thin or markedly overweight often do not ovulate because the amount of body fat is closely associated with oestrogen levels. Women who have very little body fat – professional athletes, dancers, models and chronic dieters – often stop menstruating and ovulating. Women who are obese may have abnormally elevated levels of oestrogen, which can also result in a failure to ovulate.

Conception and weight. Any woman who wants to get pregnant should try to achieve her ideal weight before conception. This should be done by eating a balanced diet; a woman who is underweight when she conceives is likely to have such problems as anaemia during pregnancy. The baby may be smaller than normal and is more at risk for health problems. Dieting during pregnancy

Did you know?

Coffee can reduce fertility in women

Researchers at Johns Hopkins University found that women who drank more than three cups of coffee a day reduced their chances of conceiving in any given month by 25 per cent. If you are trying to conceive, it is wise to cut down on the amount of coffee you drink every day.

Folic acid helps to prevent birth defects

To lessen the risk of having children with neural tube defects such as spina bifida, doctors advise all women planning on (or capable of) becoming pregnant, to take 400mcg folic acid as a supplement from about three months before conception until the twelfth week of pregnancy.

Good dietary sources of folate include fortified breakfast cereals, leafy greens, legumes, salmon, avocado and oranges.

could be dangerous to the foetus. An overweight woman should lose excess weight before trying to conceive; this also lowers her risk of developing high blood pressure or diabetes during pregnancy.

Essential nutrients. Women who take high-dose oral contraceptives are likely to experience temporary infertility until their hormonal levels return to normal and they again start to ovulate. Most oral contraceptives now used do not have adverse effects on nutrient levels, or on fertility once they are stopped. Before attempting pregnancy, a woman's diet should emphasise foods that are rich in nutrients – fruit and vegetables for vitamin C; milk for calcium; and fortified breads and cereals, lean meat, poultry and seafood for the B vitamins as well as iron, zinc and other minerals.

Alcohol and smoking are known to reduce fertility in both women and men; a recent study indicated that large quantities of coffee may have a similar effect.

Male infertility

A low sperm count is the major cause of male infertility, and for unknown reasons, men worldwide are producing fewer sperm than a few decades ago. Some scientists believe certain pesticides, which have oestrogen-like effects, may be linked

to the declining count. The use of alcohol and tobacco lower sperm production and should be avoided if there is difficulty conceiving.

Zinc. Inadequate zinc may lower male fertility; a recent study found that men who consumed 1.4mg daily produced fewer sperm and had lower levels of the male hormone testosterone than men whose daily zinc intake was 10.4mg – the zinc Reference Nutrient Intake (RNI) for adult men is 12mg.

Vitamin C. Inadequate intake of vitamin C may impair male fertility. One study correlated low levels of vitamin C with an increased tendency of sperm to clump together, a problem that all but disappeared after three weeks of taking vitamin C supplements.

Folic acid. Researchers studied a group of healthy men who had low intakes of fruit and vegetables and did not take supplements. Their study suggests that low levels of folic acid in these men were linked to decreased sperm count and decreased sperm density. The role of the vitamin is unclear, but researchers believe normalising folate levels through diet may offset diminished sperm levels. The best food sources of folic acid are dark green vegetables (such as broccoli, spinach, lettuce, peas and Brussels sprouts), avocado, salmon, oranges, liver, dry peas and beans. Other evidence suggests that vitamin B_{12} (found in all foods derived from animal products) may improve sperm count and motility, even in men who are not B_{12} deficient.

Inflammatory bowel disease

See Crohn's disease and Ulcerative colitis

Irradiation

Extending shelf-life

Food manufacturers, distributors and growers are constantly looking for ways to maintain the quality of fresh produce and extend its shelf-life. Irradiation is among the newest and most controversial of these methods to be introduced.

◀ **A symbol that irradiated foods must now bear** Advocates of irradiation emphasise that the technique can increase food supplies in many developing parts of the world, especially in the tropics, where food spoilage destroys much of the produce. Irradiation could conceivably solve chronic food shortages in these areas.

Irradiation involves exposing foods to ionising energy in the form of gamma rays from cobalt 60, or from types of X-rays, or by using an electrically generated electron beam. The electron beam and X-ray methods do not use any radioactive material.

The technology is considered desirable by some sections of the food industry as it can be used to improve shelf-life of some foods. In the UK seven categories of food may be irradiated: fruits, vegetables, cereals, bulbs and tubers, spices and condiments, poultry, fish and shellfish. Irradiation kills micro-organisms such as moulds and yeasts that cause foods such as strawberries to go bad. It can stop potatoes, onions and garlic from sprouting, and irradiation of poultry can destroy food-poisoning bacteria such as salmonella or *campylobacter*. Irradiation of meat, particularly hamburgers, can reduce the number of harmful *E. coli* bacteria. High doses of irradiation may also kill unwanted insects and pests that get into food crops such as wheat or may be present in foods imported from countries where hygiene and handling standards are lower than may be desirable.

At the highest dose approved in Britain, food is sterilised. This level of irradiation may be used in the preparation of special diets in hospital for patients with weakened immune function.

Food irradiation causes great debate. There is some concern that irradiation may result in the loss of some nutrients. Low to moderate-dose irradiation does not affect the mineral content or nutritional value of proteins, carbohydrates or saturated fats in foods. However, irradiation does cause changes to the structure, texture, appearance and taste of some foods. While some of these changes may not result in any greater changes than occur with conventional cooking methods, there is evidence that some nutrients may suffer, especially the fat-soluble vitamins A, D, E and K. There is also concern that irradiation may mean that foods that are less than fresh will still be sold.

Although it is not allowed in the UK, when animal fats are irradiated, compounds called 2-alkylcyclobutanones are formed. Some studies have shown that one of these compounds, known as 2-dodecyclobutanone (2-DCB), can cause strand breaks in DNA, which raises the prospect of cancer. Many researchers in the USA still believe that the benefits of irradiation outweigh any possible risks.

In many cases irradiated foods look and taste just like unprocessed foods. This has led to concern that customers will not be able to tell the difference.

British and EU regulations require the labelling of irradiated foods. A number of tests have been validated for the detection of irradiated foods, and regular surveys are undertaken by the Food Standards Agency. Further research into testing is taking place. For the average shopper, however, there is no reliable visual way to test if food has been irradiated.

Did you know?

Irradiation may protect people whose immune systems are compromised

Food irradiation adds an extra measure of food safety for AIDS patients and others with lowered immunity; these people are warned not to eat uncooked fruit and vegetables and to make sure that all meat, fish, eggs and other foods that may harbour disease-causing bacteria or parasites are cooked until well done. Food-borne diseases are a major hazard for those with compromised immunity. High-dose irradiation may eliminate this.

Irritable bowel syndrome

TAKE PLENTY OF

- Non-alcoholic, caffeine-free fluids
- Smaller meals
- Probiotic yoghurts which contain beneficial bacteria

LIMIT

- Alcohol
- High-fibre breakfast cereals, breads

AVOID

- Fried and other fatty foods
- All sources of caffeine
- Wind-producing foods, such as lentils and beans, if they cause a problem

Afflicting up to 20 per cent of all adults, irritable bowel syndrome (IBS) is often characterised by abnormal muscle contractions in the intestines, resulting in too little or too much fluid in the bowel.

Symptoms vary markedly from one person to another. Some people experience urgent diarrhoea. Others experience the type called spastic colon, with alternating bouts of diarrhoea and constipation, as well as abdominal pain, bloating,

People with IBS must learn to relax

It is common for stress to exacerbate irritable bowel syndrome symptoms, so make an effort to develop effective relaxation techniques, such as meditation, yoga and biofeedback. A psychotherapist or counsellor can help you to identify the stress factors in your life and develop better methods of managing them. Exercise can be very therapeutic for people with IBS because it helps to reduce stress; it can also normalise bowel function if constipation is a problem.

cramps, wind and nausea, mostly after eating. Still other symptoms may include mucus in the stool and feelings of incomplete evacuation after moving the bowels. Some people may also complain of fatigue, anxiety, headache and depression.

There are no tests for IBS, which is diagnosed by ruling out ulcerative colitis, cancer and other diseases. Although it may be aggravated by food intolerances or allergies, no specific cause has been established. It may be worsened by stress and emotional conflict and so may be a psychosomatic disorder. Various dietary factors can play a major role in exacerbating or calming IBS.

Medicine may be prescribed to quell abnormal muscle contractions and alleviate diarrhoea. But self-care, stress reduction and dietary modification are the mainstays of therapy. A recent study suggests that bacterial overgrowth in the bowel may be a cause of IBS. In one study, 78 per cent of IBS patients were found to have bacterial overgrowth in the small intestine. In 53 per cent of those who did, the overgrowth was eradicated by antibiotics and in 48 per cent of these patients, treatment eliminated the disease.

Tracking your triggers

The first step in learning to control IBS symptoms is recognising the factors that may trigger symptoms. A diary that records IBS symptoms along with stressful events and all foods and beverages ingested can help to pinpoint possible culprits. A woman should determine whether symptoms flare up during certain times of her menstrual cycle. When tracking IBS symptoms, jot down the nature and location of any pain, the frequency and consistency of stools and any related problems, such as headaches. Your diary should also note all medications taken, including supplements.

Do one simple thing

Take one or two peppermint oil capsules

Peppermint is a time-honoured remedy to calm the digestive tract. To alleviate IBS, many practitioners of natural medicine recommend taking one or two enteric-coated capsules of peppermint oil between meals. The oil should not be taken by people suffering from acid reflux disease.

Dietary modification

Because IBS differs from person to person, it's essential to develop an individualised regimen to treat your symptoms. To begin, avoid foods that your diary suggests are causing problems.

Eat several small meals a day instead of large ones. This can reduce the meal-stimulated increase in bowel contractions and diarrhoea.

Eat slowly. Eating too quickly may increase swallowed air, which promotes irritating intestinal wind. Also, poorly chewed foods can be more difficult to digest.

Drink lots of water. To maintain adequate fluid, drink at least eight glasses of water or other beverages daily, but avoid such potential bowel irritants as alcohol and caffeine.

Avoid fatty foods. Most doctors advise those with IBS against eating fried and other fatty foods because fat is the most difficult nutrient to digest. Many people find that it helps to avoid beans and other wind-producing foods.

Soluble or insoluble fibre? Choose the type of fibre you eat, according to your condition. Foods high in soluble fibre, such as oats, brans and pulses, absorb water and are helpful for bouts of diarrhoea. On the other hand, if constipation is the predominant symptom, a diet that includes ample fresh fruit and vegetables, wholegrain breads and cereals, nuts and seeds and other insoluble fibre foods is usually recommended. Insoluble fibre helps to bulk up stools and ease elimination, relieving IBS-associated constipation. If constipation is persistent, ask your doctor about taking ground psyllium seeds or a faecal softener. Avoid chronic laxative use, which can lead to problems with vitamin and nutritional deficiencies.

Avoid sugar alcohols. The sugar substitutes sorbitol, lactitol, maltitol and mannitol are used in a variety of foods and can trigger IBS symptoms in some people. For others, the lactose in milk and possibly fructose may exacerbate symptoms.

Jams and spreads

BENEFITS

- Jams and spreads contain simple sugars for quick energy

- Peanut butter provides useful amounts of protein, B vitamins and minerals

DRAWBACKS

- Jams are less nutritious than fresh fruit

- Peanut butter is high in fat and calories

- Chocolate spreads are high in sugar, fat and calories

Jams were developed in ancient times as a means of preserving fruit that would otherwise quickly spoil. When preserved, fruit resists spoilage because it lacks the water that micro-organisms need in order to grow. Surface moulds can be prevented from forming by sealing homemade marmalades and preserves with an airtight layer melted candle wax (unperfumed) or a circle of greaseproof paper dipped in brandy. Fruit boiled in sugar will gel via the interaction of fruit acids

and pectin, a soluble fibre that is drawn out of the fruit cell walls by cooking. Apples, grapes and most berries contain enough natural pectin; other fruit, such as apricots and peaches, need to have it added. Low-calorie, reduced-sugar jams are gelled with a special pectin that sets at lower acidity and with less sugar. These products are often sweetened with concentrated fruit juice and some are thickened with starches.

For nutritional value, there's no comparison between jams and fresh fruit, because most of the vitamin C and other nutrients in fruit are destroyed by intense cooking. While fruit preserves contain substantial amounts of pectin – a soluble fibre that helps to control blood cholesterol levels – this benefit is offset by their high sugar content. Simple sugars, however, make jams a source of quick energy.

Peanut butter

The high fat content of peanuts makes them easy to grind into a paste, but the oil quickly turns rancid when exposed to oxygen and light. Some commercial peanut butters are made with preservatives, stabilisers and added salt and sugar; check the label if you wish to avoid these ingredients.

In products that do not contain emulsifiers, the oil that rises to the top of the jar can be poured off to reduce the fat content. It's best to store peanut butter in a glass container in the refrigerator, where the darkness prevents the loss of B vitamins, and the cold retards oil separation. Peanut butters that don't separate may contain hydrogenated vegetable oils or emulsifiers. Hydrogenated oils contain trans fatty acids, which are bad for the heart and should be avoided.

Peanut butter can be a valuable nutritional resource for children. Two teaspoons contain about 62kcal, with 3g of protein, 4g of unsaturated fat and significant amounts of B vitamins and magnesium. Look for brands with no added sugar or salt for the best nutritional value.

J

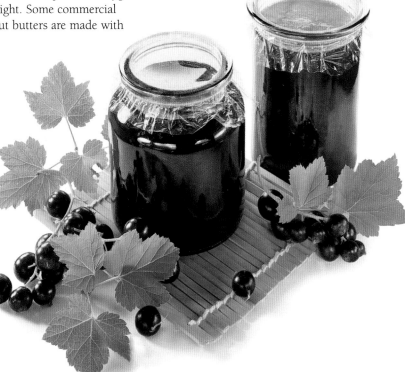

Other spreads

Lemon curds have little nutritional value and are largely sugar. Processed cheese spreads are high in saturated fat and sodium, but contribute a little protein and some calcium. Chocolate and nut spreads are high in fat, sugar and calories.

Jaundice

CONSUME

■ Fish, poultry, red meat and soya foods

■ Green cabbage and pulses for folate

■ Oats and unsweetened muesli

LIMIT

■ Fatty, spicy and sugary foods

AVOID

■ All alcoholic beverages

A yellowing of the skin and the whites of the eyes is the hallmark of jaundice. This condition typically occurs when bilirubin, a pigmented component of bile, builds up in the blood. Bilirubin is a by-product produced by the liver as it breaks down red blood cells to recycle their iron. It is mixed with bile, a digestive juice that is made by the liver, and is eventually excreted from the body in the urine or stool. Jaundice develops if the bilirubin is allowed to accumulate in the body.

There are three general types of jaundice: the most common is due to hepatitis or some other liver disorder; another, known as obstructive jaundice, usually results from gallstones or another gall-bladder disease and the least common involves an abnormality in bilirubin metabolism.

Each year many people are afflicted with liver and gall-bladder disorders, but not all of them develop jaundice. Among those who do, hepatitis – an inflammation of the liver– is the likely cause. Five major forms of viral hepatitis have been identified to date; the liver inflammation may also be due to alcohol or drug abuse, adverse reaction to a medication, as well as bacterial, parasitic or fungal infections of the liver. Some strains of viral hepatitis are highly contagious and can enter the human body through water or food that has been contaminated by human waste. Hepatitis can also be spread through blood transfusions from an infected person or by direct contact with infected body fluids or the use of contaminated syringes.

In addition to jaundice, and depending on its cause, symptoms may include fever, fatigue, nausea, vomiting, diarrhoea and loss of appetite. In a few cases, hepatitis may be serious enough to result in liver failure, coma and death.

In other forms of jaundice, the urine may be dark in colour due to increased bilirubin content, and the stools light, clay-coloured or whitish, a sign that bilirubin is not being excreted from the intestinal tract. Jaundice may also be due to Gilbert's syndrome (a disorder of bilirubin metabolism), which affects 3 to 5 per cent of the population and may be misdiagnosed as hepatitis. In Gilbert's syndrome, chronic jaundice is the only abnormality and does not signify liver disease. A few rare forms of jaundice are inherited.

Infant jaundice

It is not uncommon for a baby to develop jaundice during the first few days after birth, especially if the infant is premature. This is known as physiological jaundice, and is usually caused by a liver that is not yet fully functional. There are usually no other symptoms, and the condition typically clears up within a week, as the liver matures.

Exposing the baby to ultraviolet light hastens the process, as the light changes bilirubin to a form that is more readily excreted.

Feeding the infant soon after birth and continuing with frequent feedings helps to reduce the risk of jaundice by stimulating the intestinal tract to produce frequent stools, which increases the excretion of bilirubin. Jaundice during the first few days of life does not mean that the child will necessarily have future liver problems.

Dietary approaches

Any modification of the diet depends on the underlying cause of the jaundice. With a nutritious, well-balanced diet and rest, viral hepatitis often resolves itself – but it may take several weeks. However, many people find it difficult to eat at the very time that they need extra calories to help the liver to recover and regenerate its damaged cells. Many individuals report that their appetite decreases and their nausea increases as the day progresses, suggesting that breakfast may be the best tolerated meal of the day. Oats and unsweetened muesli will help to avoid the constipation which often accompanies jaundice.

Eat a diet high in protein. When recovering from hepatitis, a person should consume a healthy diet with sufficient protein daily, from both animal and vegetable sources. The best sources are lean meat, poultry, fish, eggs, dairy products, tofu or legumes and grain products.

If the appetite is poor, intersperse several small meals a day with a nutritious snack (such as a milk-shake or an enriched liquid drink). Fried and very fatty foods, which are difficult to digest, should be avoided; a small amount of fat is acceptable, however, to provide needed calories and add flavour. In general, the fats in dairy products

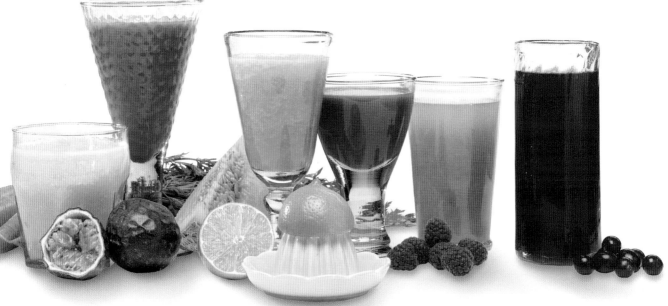

and eggs are easier to digest than those in fatty meats and fried foods. Try to avoid eating spicy foods, too.

Avoid alcohol and large quantities of sweets because they may limit the appetite for more nutritious foods. Alcohol should not be consumed, because it places added stress on an already sick liver. For some, it may be tolerated after recovery, but some liver disorders require total abstinence from alcohol for life. There is some evidence that herbal preparations based on milk thistle may help to treat liver dysfunction.

Juices

BENEFITS

■ Juicing provides a concentrated form of fruit and vegetables

DRAWBACKS

■ Juicing removes pulp and fibre

■ Can be high in calories, in quantity

By now just about everyone knows that fruit and vegetables are packed with vitamins, minerals and many other substances that protect against cancer and other diseases. Mainstream doctors and alternative practitioners alike are urging their patients to eat more fruit and vegetables, preferably raw or with minimal processing in order to preserve their nutrients. New recommendations call for at least nine servings of fruit and vegetables each day – more than the amount usually eaten in the UK.

Drink your fruit and vegetables

Fruit and vegetable juices are one way to add fruit and vegetables to your diet as well as to keep your body hydrated. They provide fluids as well as the nutrients of the fruit and vegetables they were made from. However, if you are watching your calories, drinking juice may not be your best choice. Despite the nutrition in every glass, the calories from the natural fruit sugar can add up quickly. In addition, the fibre of the fresh fruit and/or vegetable makes the whole foods more filling and satisfying than the juice. For example, a fresh orange has about 55kcal and 2.5g of fibre. A 150ml glass of fresh orange juice has about 54kcal and no fibre.

When you buy juices, choose the unsweetened varieties that do not have added sugars. Watch for words such as 'fruit drink' or 'fruit juice drink'. These drinks are not generally nutritionally equivalent to fruit juice. They tend to be higher in sugar and have varying proportions of fruit juice.

Vegetable juices tend to have less sugar than fruit juices. The only caution with canned vegetable juice is a higher salt content. Check labels carefully, and choose juices that are low in salt.

C A U T I O N

Babies need nothing but breast milk for the first six months; after the age of six months, a baby may be given diluted juice – but pure juice, not sugared squashes. Juice, while rich in some nutrients, does not have the important vitamins that breast milk or infant formula have. A baby should never drink juice instead of milk, it would be difficult to get the nutrients necessary for growth and development. And drinking juice is filling, so the baby won't want to drink milk. In addition, juice can also lead to diarrhoea, poor weight gain and tooth decay. When you do offer juice, give it in a cup or beaker, not a bottle. Undiluted juice poses a threat to the teeth of all children, because of its acid content. Offer juice only with meals and encourage your children to eat whole fruits instead of sweets.

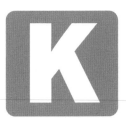

Kale

BENEFITS

- An excellent source of beta carotene and vitamin C

- A good source of folate, calcium, iron and vitamin B_6

- Contains bioflavonoids and other substances that protect against cancer

DRAWBACKS

- May cause wind in some people

A member of the cabbage family, kale looks like collard but with curly leaves. It is a hardy autumn vegetable that grows best in a cool climate; in fact, exposure to frost improves its flavour. Although the types of kale that form leafy red, yellow and purple heads are used more often for decorative purposes (both in the garden and on the table) than as a food, all varieties are edible and highly nutritious.

Like its relatives in the cabbage family, kale is an excellent source of vitamin C and beta carotene, which the human body converts to vitamin A; in fact, 80g of cooked kale contains more than a day's supply of vitamin A and well over 100 per cent of the daily requirement of vitamin C, as well as 34 per cent of the folic acid, 11 per cent of the iron and 15 per cent of the vitamin B_6 requirements. It also provides more than 2g of fibre and has only 19kcal; yet, it is filling, making kale an ideal, highly nutritious food for anyone who is weight-conscious.

In addition, kale contains more iron and calcium than almost any other vegetable; its high vitamin C content enhances the body's ability to absorb these minerals. Serving kale with a lemon dressing or in the same meal as another acidic citrus fruit further boosts absorption of the iron and calcium.

Kale is rich in bioflavonoids, carotenoids and other cancer-fighting compounds. It also contains indoles, compounds that may lessen the cancer-causing potential of oestrogen and induce the production of enzymes that protect against disease.

To prepare kale so as to preserve its rich stores of beta carotene and vitamin C, cook it quickly in minimal water; it can also be steamed, chopped and stir-fried with other vegetables or simmered until tender in broth to make a tasty soup. Kale shrinks considerably during cooking; it takes about four generous handfuls of raw greens to make a medium serving. Kale, raw or cooked, produces wind in some people.

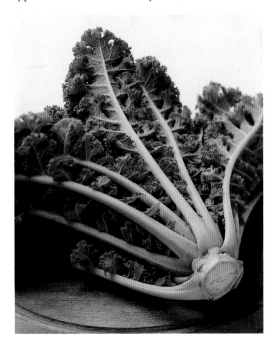

Kidney disease

CONSUME PLENTY OF

- Liquids to replace lost fluids and maintain fluid balance

- Protein according to specific needs, which may be high or low in various types of disease

LIMIT

- Salt to reduce fluid retention and prevent high blood pressure

AVOID

- Non-prescription painkillers, vitamin pills and calcium supplements, which have side effects and interactions that may cause kidney damage

Kidney disease may be either a primary condition, such as kidney stones, or a consequence of other disorders, such as hypertension, atherosclerosis or diabetes – all of which can severely damage the organs' blood vessels. Older men are susceptible to kidney infections stemming from enlargement of the prostate. Pregnant women and those with diabetes are vulnerable to infections of the urinary tract. Side effects from drugs are common and preventable causes of serious kidney disorders. For example, aspirin, paracetamol and other nonsteroidal anti-inflammatory drugs (NSAIDs) and calcium with vitamin D supplements are among the non-prescription drugs that can damage kidneys; combining aspirin and paracetamol is especially damaging. When you see your doctor, be sure to mention any non-prescription

▶ **Fluids for healthy kidneys**
Liquids are extremely important when it comes to the proper functioning of the kidneys. Water, juices and lemonade help to prevent the formation of stones.

medications or vitamin supplements you have been taking, even if only rarely.

Healthy people will stay healthy if they follow a diet that will help to prevent kidney disorders. Drink plenty of liquids to flush the urinary system and replace lost fluids, and consume a low-fat diet that emphasises starchy foods, vegetables and fruit.

Diet is crucial in treating kidney problems when they do arise. If you have a serious kidney disease, your doctor will probably refer you to a clinical dietitian for advice about changes to your diet. The allowable types and portions of foods differ, depending upon the type and severity of the kidney disorder.

Kidney stones

Kidney stones are common, and 4 to 8 per cent of adults will suffer from kidney disease at some stage in their life. The incidence is two to three times higher in men, possibly because of their failure to drink enough water to ensure adequate rehydration after sweating. About 30 to 50 per cent of those who suffer one attack will have another.

Kidney stones usually form when crystalline minerals – normally flushed away in the urine – stick together to form clumps, ranging in size from a grain of sand to coarse gravel. The cause may be gout or another metabolic problem, or it may be a structural or metabolic abnormality within the kidney. When kidney stones block any part of the urinary system, especially the ureters or bladder, they cause intense pain. Stones may pass through the system; others must be removed surgically or by sound-wave treatment (lithotripsy).

In order to prevent recurrences, it is important to determine the cause of the kidney stones. Most are formed of calcium oxalate or calcium phosphate. Less commonly, stones may form from uric acid crystals, especially in those people who suffer from gout. A fourth type, cystine stones, occurs in fairly rare metabolic diseases.

Fluids, fluids and more fluids. Regardless of the type of stone, it's essential to drink enough liquids to maintain fluid balance and flush away the minerals that accumulate to form stones. Most people with stones could reduce the risk of recurrence by increasing their water intake so that they excrete about 2 litres of urine a day.

Although most stones contain calcium, it's not a good idea to cut down on dietary calcium unless your doctor specifically orders it. Restricting calcium in the diet may actually increase the incidence of stones in some people, whereas a high-calcium diet has been shown to reduce it. Make sure you get a good intake of calcium from your food. If the body fails to get enough calcium, it will rob the bones in order to get the mineral, thus increasing the danger of osteoporosis.

Phosphorus-rich foods contribute to the formation of calcium phosphate stones. Phosphorus is found in high quality protein. The balance of phosphorus and calcium in the diet is very delicate, however, and restricting the intake of one may interfere with the other. Take advice from a doctor or dietitian when changing your intake of either essential mineral in order to maintain balanced nutrition.

Foods high in oxalate. Oxalate-rich foods include rhubarb, nuts, beetroot, tofu, chocolate, tea, berries, red currants, tangerines, wheatbran and wheatgerm, most of the dark green leafy vegetables, sweet potatoes, baked beans, lentils and beer. Many people believe that these foods must be avoided, but this is unnecessary and eliminating

● **Myth.......**
People with kidney stones should cut down on calcium-rich foods.

.......Reality ●
There is recent evidence that adequate calcium intake actually reduces the risk of calcium oxalate stones because calcium combines with oxalate in the digestive tract and prevents oxalate from being absorbed.

K

all these foods would deplete the diet of essential vitamins and minerals. A doctor or dietitian will provide a list of foods that can be eaten in moderation with little risk of causing a recurrence. People with gout should keep to a low-fat diet to reduce the risk of uric acid stones.

Kidney stones are rare in strict vegetarians. While the connection between stones and protein is not fully understood, it is known that protein increases the acidity of

Kidney transplant

Although an individual who has received a kidney transplant must follow dietary guidelines, the diet is usually less restrictive than the one followed during dialysis treatment. But because the diet is affected by medications taken to prevent rejection of the new kidney, the doctor and dietitian will continually make adjustments as recovery progresses.

In the weeks immediately following a transplant, most people are advised to eat more protein, such as eggs, low-fat meat, fish, poultry, skimmed milk and low-fat cheese. Carbohydrates are generally limited to prevent interactions with the high doses of steroids that must be taken to prevent rejection. Starchy foods are allowed, but excess sugar should be avoided. Salty foods and most processed foods should be eliminated, and no salt should be added. The doctor will provide guidelines regarding potassium-rich foods. Supplements may also be prescribed.

A moderate weight gain after receiving a kidney transplant is not unusual; however, if weight does become a problem, high-fat foods should be avoided. Between-meal snacks can include raw vegetables and fruit, and fat-free yoghurt.

urine, which probably plays a role. Many people could reduce the risk of recurrence of stones by cutting their daily protein intake to between 0.8 and 1.0g per kilogram of body weight. It's easier to reduce protein intake if you cut down on animal products. Eating a variety of foods such as rice and beans can supply the essential amino acids.

Nephritis

Inflammation of the kidney – known medically as nephritis – may result from a bacterial infection or other causes, including the side effects of drugs. Infections sometimes arise elsewhere in the body and reach the kidneys through the bloodstream, or enter the body through the urinary tract and travel up through the bladder to the kidneys. Kidney infections, like stones, require a doctor's intervention and must be treated with antibiotics. No special dietary measures are necessary; however, people with kidney infections should drink plenty of fluids. A daily glass of cranberry juice may help to prevent recurrence of urinary tract infections in susceptible people.

Kidney failure

Kidney failure may be either a temporary response to acute shock or injury or a severe long-term state necessitating drastic treatment. Acute kidney failure may be caused by severe infection, burns, diarrhoea or vomiting, poisoning (including drug effects or interactions), surgery or kidney injury.

When the problem is resolved, kidney function usually returns to normal. Chronic kidney failure may be caused by untreated hypertension, poorly controlled diabetes or an inborn condition. Severe chronic, or end-stage, kidney failure requires regular dialysis – a procedure in which a machine

removes waste products from the blood – or where possible, kidney transplantation.

Diet is extremely important in the management of kidney failure. General recommendations include restricting phosphorus, potassium, protein and salt. Fluids must be monitored. With too little, the electrolytes are out of balance; with too much, fluid retention causes oedema and electrolyte problems, and contributes to high blood pressure and even congestive heart failure. Protein must be adjusted as kidney function, dialysis or stress levels change.

Studies show that if protein is limited to about 1g per kilogram of body weight per day, the patient on dialysis will receive the essential amino acids but reduce the risk of further kidney damage. Proteins from fish, egg whites and legume and grain combinations are preferable to those in meat because they contain less saturated fat.

Kidney failure requires highly specialised and individualised medical care. No changes in diet should be made without first getting a doctor's approval. Consult regularly with a dietitian who will monitor the diet and make any necessary adjustments in the amounts of nutrients, including vitamin and mineral supplements.

Kiwi fruit

BENEFITS

- An excellent source of vitamin C
- A source of potassium and fibre
- Can be used as a meat tenderiser

On the outside a kiwi fruit looks like a fuzzy brown egg; on the inside its bright green flesh is sprinkled with a ring of small,

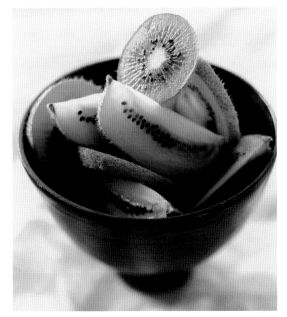

black seeds. It has a distinctive, somewhat tart flavour with overtones of both fruits and berries.

The kiwi fruit originated in China and was known as the Chinese gooseberry until New Zealand fruit growers renamed it after their national bird and began exporting it. Kiwi fruit are now also grown in Australia and have become increasingly plentiful. They are harvested while green and can be kept in cold storage for six to ten months, making them available for most of the year. Ripe kiwi fruit are eaten raw; even the skin can be consumed if it is defuzzed first.

A 75g kiwi fruit provides about 44mg of vitamin C and is rich in phytochemicals. It also provides some potassium and pectin, a soluble fibre that may help to control blood cholesterol levels. Kiwi fruit contains both lutein and zeaxanthin, antioxidants associated with eye health. It is also a perfect fast-food snack – simply cut one in half and scoop out the fruit with a spoon. A 75g serving has only 37kcal. Actinidin, an enzyme that is a natural meat tenderiser is found in kiwi fruit. The fruit can be used

as a marinade to tenderise tough meats. Rubbing the meat with a cut kiwi fruit and waiting 30 to 60 minutes before cooking will tenderise the meat without imparting any flavour from the fruit.

Actinidin will also prevent gelatine from setting and will curdle milk and cream; these effects could be prevented by poaching the fruit beforehand. However, this is not a good idea, as cooking the fruit turns it to mush.

Kohlrabi

BENEFITS

- High in vitamin C, potassium, and cancer-preventing antioxidants and bioflavonoids
- High in dietary fibre

DRAWBACKS

- May cause wind in some people

Similar to both cabbages and turnips, kohlrabi comes from the same cruciferous plant family. Because the bulb, which is the edible part of the plant, is not as rich in nutrients as the flowers or leaves, kohlrabi is not in the same nutritional league as broccoli, Brussels sprouts and kale. Still,

it is a good source of vitamin C; an 80g serving of cooked kohlrabi provides 54 per cent of the Reference Nutrient Intake (RNI) for adults, as well as 19 per cent of the folic acid and 13 per cent of the vitamin B_6 requirements. It also has 192mg of potassium, 1.6g fibre while providing only only 14kcal.

This vegetable is high in bioflavonoids, plant pigments that work with vitamin C and other antioxidants to help to prevent the cell damage that promotes cancer. Kohlrabi is also high in indoles, chemicals that may reduce the effects of oestrogen, and thus may reduce the risk of breast cancer. Isothiocyanates, another group of compounds in kohlrabi, promote the action of enzymes that may protect against colon cancer.

Kohlrabi should be harvested before it reaches full maturity; otherwise, it becomes woody. It is usually steamed until tender. People who get wind after eating other cruciferous vegetables may have the same response to kohlrabi.

K

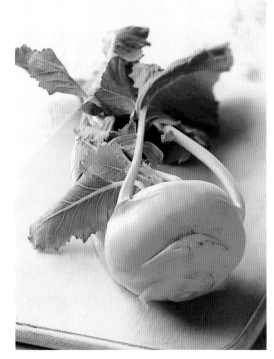

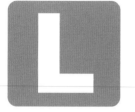

Lactose intolerance

CONSUME

- Lactose-reduced milk, soya or rice milks, lactase enzyme drops or lactase enzyme tablets if you are unable to digest milk

- Cheese, which contains little lactose, and yoghurt

AVOID

- Foods that cause any discomfort

Lactose intolerance is the inability to digest the natural sugar found in milk. It has to be broken down by an enzyme called lactase into

If you must drink milk

If you are lactose intolerant, but want to include milk products as part of your diet, here's what to do:

- Drink small amounts – try 100ml and gradually work your way up.

- Drink milk with meals – never on an empty stomach.

- The active cultures in yoghurt will help you to digest its lactose.

- Eat cheeses that contain only negligible amounts of lactose.

- Drink lactose-free milk.

- Read labels for hidden milk ingredients.

- Use enzyme drops or tablets before eating dairy products.

glucose and galactose before it can be absorbed and used by the body. If you don't have enough lactase to handle the lactose in the food you eat, you will experience a variety of unpleasant symptoms such as wind, bloating, diarrhoea and cramps after the ingestion of lactose-containing foods. This is because the unabsorbed lactose passes into the colon, where it is consumed by bacteria. The by-products of this bacterial activity is wind, which is responsible for the discomfort. The condition can be diagnosed by measuring the amount of hydrogen exhaled before and after ingesting lactose. An excessive amount of hydrogen confirms you have lactose intolerance. Except for a few inedible shrubs, milk is the only source of lactose. Once prehistoric humans were weaned, they never had lactose again; hence, they no longer needed lactase, the enzyme that breaks down milk sugar in the digestive tract.

If you are lactose-intolerant, the wisest course is to give up milk and milk products. No adult actually needs milk – it is possible to get the nutritional benefits that milk offers from other foodstuffs, such as calcium-fortified soya milk, sesame seeds, pulses and nuts.

Some lactose-intolerant adults may be able to tolerate small quantities. A lactose-intolerant child should not consume lactose at all.

Acquired intolerance

Transient or permanent lactose intolerance may follow an illness that injures the intestinal lining such as gastrointestinal illness, coeliac disease or inflammatory bowel disease. It may follow treatment with antibiotics or anti-inflammatory drugs. In most cases, the intolerance

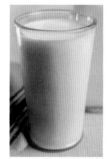

is temporary and disappears when bowel health returns to normal. In other cases, lactose intolerance is a 'threshold intolerance'. This means you can handle small amounts of lactose but increasing doses cause a problem. You need to assess how severe your symptoms are, and be prepared to stop eating foods containing dairy products if they become too severe.

Avoiding lactose

Lactose is found in all dairy products, including milk and yoghurt. Cheese contains only traces of lactose. Lactose can also be found as an ingredient or component of various food products such as confectionery, processed meats, some artificial sweeteners and even some medications. Read labels carefully and look for milk, milk solids, cream, whey, cheese flavours, curds and non-fat milk powder. If you see any of these listed on the table of ingredients, avoid the product.

Beware of milk from goats and sheep. If you are lactose-intolerant, avoid goat's and sheep milk, as well, as they also contain lactose. Check the amount of lactose in Greek-style yoghurt.

Get enzymes to help. For people with intolerance who still want dairy products, supermarkets sell lactose-reduced dairy products, and pharmacies carry enzyme drops that can be added to milk, and enzyme tablets that can be taken before eating dishes containing dairy products.

Warning: Don't confuse lactose intolerance with milk allergy, which is hypersensitivity to the proteins in dairy products. If you are allergic to milk, consuming a lactose-reduced product will not prevent a reaction.

Lamb

BENEFITS

- An excellent source of protein and B-complex vitamins
- A source of minerals, including iron, zinc and phosphorus

DRAWBACKS

- Some cuts are high in saturated fat

Lamb is a high-quality, nutritious meat, rich in minerals and the B vitamins, particularly B_{12}. Lamb is branded according to its age, which is judged by the number of teeth the animal has. Lamb meat comes from animals that are less than 12 months old and have no permanent teeth. Milk-fed lamb is eight to ten weeks old and spring lamb is three to ten months old. Mutton is from animals at least two years old while the category between lamb and mutton is known as hogget. Mutton comes from sheep older than one year, and it has a more robust taste.

Lamb is the primary meat in parts of Europe, North Africa, the Middle East and India. It has never enjoyed the same popularity in other countries. North Americans consume about 50 times more beef than lamb. Australians and New Zealanders eat more beef than lamb, but only marginally. In the UK, lamb is popular and features often in the traditional diets of Afro-Caribbeans and Muslims. Fears that scrapie, the sheep equivalent of BSE could cross from cattle to sheep have so far proved unfounded. The Food Standards Authority advises that there is no need to avoid lamb.

Lamb comes in a variety of cuts including legs, shoulder, chops, cutlets, mince, shank and spareribs. Although some cuts are slightly higher in fat, lamb is not marbled like beef. Since much of its fat is on the outside of the meat, it can be trimmed before cooking. The meat is tender, because it is the relatively little-used muscle of young animals. A 100g portion of lean roast leg of lamb contains about 190kcal, with about 30g of protein and about 9g of fat.

Lamb is a rich source of protein, B-complex vitamins, as well as some iron, phosphorus, potassium and calcium. Because it is easily digested and almost never associated with food allergies, it is a good protein food for people of all ages.

Lamb is a source of conjugated linoleic acid (CLA), a group of fatty acids that occur naturally in meat and milk products from ruminant animals. Animal studies have found that CLA improved cholesterol profiles and delayed the development of atherosclerosis. In addition, CLA may have anti-carcinogenic properties. Although it is premature to draw definitive conclusions about the protective benefits of CLAs, there is growing interest and research in this area.

Leeks

BENEFITS

- Low in calories, with some potassium, iron, folate and fibre

DRAWBACKS

- May cause flatulence

Leeks are closely related to onions and they are distant cousins of asparagus. All three are members of the lily family. Although the entire leek is edible, most people prefer to eat only the white, fleshy base and tender inner leaves and to discard the bitter dark green leaf tops.

Leeks probably originated in warm regions of Asia or the Mediterranean, but they are now cultivated in temperate to cool climates. Leeks are the national symbol of Wales.

Low in calories, leeks provide vitamins, minerals and fibre. An 80g serving of cooked leeks contains only 17kcal with 1.5g of fibre and 120mg of potassium. It supplies 14 per cent of the Reference Nutrient Intake (RNI) of vitamin C and 16 per cent of the RNI for folic acid, as well as useful amounts of iron.

Like all vegetables in the onion group, leeks may have a protective effect against stomach cancer, and like onions, leeks may help to lower cholesterol. On a more negative note, they can cause flatulence.

Leeks are useful in a range of dishes where their mild oniony flavour is desired. You can boil and sieve them with potatoes for a chilled vichyssoise soup; braise them in fat-free stock to serve hot; or use them as a basis in vegetable soups and casseroles. TThey can be added to rice dishes or pasta.

In traditional medicine, leeks were used to treat a variety of ailments including sore throats, gout and kidney stones. Because of their potassium content, they are also an effective diuretic.

L

Lemons

BENEFITS

- An excellent source of vitamin C
- May help to relieve rheumatism

DRAWBACKS

- The peel contains an irritating oil

Ideal for flavouring everything from fish to vegetables to tea, lemons are perhaps the most widely used of all citrus fruits. Sweetened, diluted and chilled, fresh lemon juice is an old-fashioned summer thirst quencher. It's also an excellent source of vitamin C; the juice from one medium lemon (75ml) has about 27mg of vitamin C, which is well over 50 per cent of the Reference Nutrient Intake (RNI) for adult women. To get the all the juice out of a lemon, put it in warm water or in the microwave for 30-40 seconds before squeezing.

Many recipes call for fresh lemon zest, which is the grated outer peel. The zest is rich in an antioxidant chemical called rutin, which may help to strengthen the walls of veins and capillaries. Because lemons are often sprayed with fungicides to retard mould growth and pesticides to kill insects, wash them thoroughly before grating the peel. Select lemons that have not been waxed (wax may seal in fungicides). Lemon peels contain limonene, an oil that can irritate the skin in susceptible people. Limonene is being studied for its anti-tumour activity and may prove useful against breast cancer.

Favourite lemon home remedies

A tablespoon of lemon juice in a cup of honey-sweetened hot water is a popular sore throat remedy.

Sipping unsweetened diluted lemon juice or sucking a lemon slice can stimulate saliva flow in people who have a dry mouth. This should be done in moderation, however, since the high acidity of plain lemon can damage tooth enamel.

Lettuce and other salad greens

BENEFITS

- Low in calories
- Some varieties provide beta carotene, folate, vitamin C and potassium

DRAWBACKS

- Often eaten with large amounts of oily or high-fat creamy dressings

A green salad is often part of a healthy dinner, and although many vegetables may be used in it, lettuce is by far the most common. It is one of the most popular vegetables sold in supermarkets because health-conscious people are eating more salads these days, and also so many lettuces and other fresh salad greens are available all year-round, thanks to modern refrigeration and swift transport links.

People watching their weight are especially partial to salads – they are low in calories yet filling, since they provide fibre. But a large bowl of salad greens that has only 14kcal can quickly become more fattening than a steak if it's drowned in a high-fat dressing. There are, however, many tasty low-fat alternatives – herb vinegar mixed with a little olive oil, a sprinkle of herbs and lemon juice or some low-fat yoghurt combined with a little garlic, chopped parsley and lemon juice.

Good nutrition

Some types of lettuce and other salad greens contain beta carotene, folate, vitamin C, potassium and iron, but the amounts vary greatly from one variety to another. Beta carotene works against degenerative diseases, and folate is very good for pregnant women. In general, salad vegetables with dark green or other deeply coloured leaves have more beta carotene and vitamin C than the paler varieties. Cos lettuce, for example, has five times as much vitamin C and more beta carotene and folate than iceberg lettuce.

Such salad greens as curly endive, lamb's lettuce, rocket and watercress are all more nutritious than lettuce; many people also find them more flavoursome, and they are readily available in restaurants and supermarkets. Some, such as rocket, curly endive, mizuna and watercress, are slightly bitter, and provide an interesting flavour and texture contrast when they are added to a salad of lettuce and other types of greens.

Rocket, a member of the same plant family as broccoli, cabbage and other cruciferous vegetables, has a tangy, peppery flavour when grown during the cool spring and autumn months, and a stronger, mustard-like taste if harvested during summer. This is one of the most nutritious of all salad greens: a 100g serving has more calcium than most other salad greens and is a source of vitamin C, beta carotene, iron and folate – all for only about 12kcal. Watercress, another cruciferous vegetable, is also a nutritional winner: 25g contains a mere 6kcal yet it provides 16mg of vitamin C and useful amounts of beta carotene, iron, folic acid and vitamin B_6.

Deeply coloured lettuces and greens are also high in bioflavonoids, plant pigments

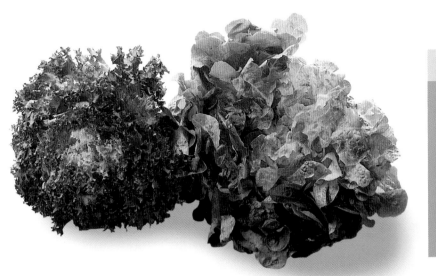

Do one simple thing

Toss your salad greens with oil

Make your salad with a variety of salad greens rich in beta carotene, such as watercress, curly endive and rocket, and a little flavoured vinegar, lemon juice and olive oil. Oil enhances the absorption of carotenoid, which may help in preventing some types of cancer and vision-loss.

known to work with vitamin C and other antioxidants to prevent cancer-causing cell damage. Lettuce and other greens can be combined with a broad spectrum of raw fruit or vegetables, cold pasta or chunks of chicken or tuna to make a low-calorie, highly nutritious main dish. Baby spinach is often used as a salad green; although cooking makes some of its nutrients a bit easier to absorb, a spinach salad still provides good amounts of beta carotene, folate, vitamin C and some calcium.

What is the best way to wash your lettuce?

This was investigated by spraying lettuce with bacteria and storing it overnight at 40°C, then washing by one of three methods:

1 The lettuce was cored and washed in a sink of water, and left to air dry;

2 It was cored and washed intact under running tap water, and left to air dry;

3 The leaves were separated and then washed in a sink full of tap water and dried in a spinner.

The third method was the best.

Another recommended method is to wash lettuce leaves in – or spray them with – vinegar, leave them for 5 minutes to kill germs, and then rinse thoroughly with running tap water.

Types of salad greens

There are dozens of different varieties of lettuce; some of the more widely available are listed below. Make your salads with a variety of greens to elevate your fibre intake and increase your antioxidant levels.

Butterhead lettuce forms soft, loosely packed heads of tender, mildly flavoured leaves.

Cos lettuce has long, crisp, dark green leaves that form a loose head. Also called romaine, it is used to make Caesar and similar salads.

Curly endive has a somewhat bitter taste. It is nutritious but not widely used because of its assertive flavour.

Iceberg lettuce, a crisp, tightly packed head lettuce, is the most widely consumed variety of lettuce. It is nutritious, but provides lower levels of vitamins than some other varieties of lettuce and greens.

Lamb's lettuce has small, delicate leaves. It is also called corn salad or mache and is most often found in gourmet shops.

Lollo rosso has green leaves with a distinct reddish tinge round their frilly edges. They have a mild flavour and make a good garnish.

Radicchio is an Italian chicory that looks like a small cabbage with firm, reddish-purple leaves. It has a crisp texture and a bitter flavour.

Rocket resembles dandelion leaves and has a peppery flavour.

Watercress grows in streambeds; A member of the cruciferous family, it has a strong, sometimes hot flavour, and is believed to be protective against some cancers.

Limes

BENEFITS

■ An excellent source of vitamin C

■ Can be used to flavour and tenderise meat, poultry and fish

DRAWBACKS

■ Peel contains psoralens, which increase sun sensitivity

In the mid 1700s James Lind, a Scottish naval surgeon, discovered that drinking the juice of limes and lemons prevented scurvy, the scourge of sailors on long voyages. Soon British ships carried ample stores of the fruit, earning their sailors the nickname 'limey'. It was later learned that vitamin C deficiency causes scurvy, and that limes are very high in this essential nutrient.

The juice of one medium lime (50ml) has 19mg of vitamin C. Limes are high in bioflavonoids and other antioxidants, which may help to protect against cancer and other diseases. Limonene, found mainly in the zest of lemons and limes, may help to reduce cancer risk.

Like lemons, limes are useful as flavouring agents. They are widely used in Thai cooking. They can also tenderise and heighten the flavours of other foods, especially fish and poultry. Lime juice can also be used as a salt substitute for meat and fish dishes. A sprinkling of lime juice over a fruit salad prevents discoloration.

Lime peel contains psoralens, chemicals that can make the skin sensitive to the sun; thus, care should be taken to minimise skin contact with lime peels. It may be advisable to peel limes before squeezing their juice into food.

Linseed (or flax)

BENEFITS

- A good source of fibre and alpha-linolenic acid
- Contain lignans

DRAWBACKS

- The omega-3 fats in linseed oil oxidise rapidly; oxidised fats generate free radicals

Linseed, also known as flax in some countries, is a tiny seed packed with a variety of components that can play an important role in your diet. They are a great source of soluble fibre, they can help to lower cholesterol levels and consequently lower heart disease risk. Studies at the University of Toronto showed that 25g to 50g of linseeds a day helped to lower blood cholesterol significantly. The insoluble fibre in linseeds is good for preventing constipation.

Linseeds are a rich source of alpha linolenic acid (ALA), one of the omega-3s. ALA is an essential fatty acid, also thought to be a 'heart healthy' fat. Because your body can not manufacture this fatty acid, you must consume it in foods. Omega-3 fatty acids help to reduce the thickness of blood so the heart doesn't have to work as hard to push the blood through the blood vessels. They also lessen the 'stickiness' of blood platelets, cutting their tendency to form clots.

Linseeds may protect against some cancers; they contain lignans, which convert in the body to compounds that are similar to the body's own oestrogen but have much weaker activity. They can occupy oestrogen receptors in cells and block the effects of more powerful oestrogens. That is why numerous studies are currently looking at the role linseeds may play in lowering the risk of hormone-linked cancers, such as of the breast

CAUTION

Once extracted from the seeds, linseed oil oxidises rapidly, making it ideal for its traditional use in oiling cricket bats and in varnishes and paints. But for human consumption, it is important to avoid oxidised fats as they increase production of free radicals which can damage tissues. Unless you are sure the oil is freshly pressed and has been kept refrigerated since pressing, it is best avoided. The natural coating on the seeds themselves protects the oil from oxidation.

or colon. Animal studies have already shown that linseeds can reduce tumour size and can even influence the incidence of tumour development. Human studies are limited, but one study showed that the tumour growth in breast-cancer patients was reduced when they were given muffins containing 25g of ground linseeds daily.

Linseeds contain no gluten, are very inexpensive and have a pleasant nutty flavour. There is no recommended daily amount, but many studies use 1 to 2 tablespoons of linseeds daily.

Many of the whole linseeds you eat will pass straight through you. However, some are gradually broken down by intestinal bacteria and release their ALA. If you prefer to use ground linseeds, grind them in a food processor as close as possible to when you will be consuming them. Any ground seeds not used should be kept in the fridge or freezer in an opaque airtight box.

Linseed oil provides omega-3 fatty acids but not the fibre and the lignans of the seeds. Linseed oil should be kept in the fridge and has a limited shelf life; check its freshness before purchase. It breaks down with heat so is not a good choice for cooking.

Here are some pleasant ways to get linseeds into your diet:
- Add them to cereal, muffin batters, breads, pancake mixes and biscuits.
- Stir ground linseeds into yoghurt or smoothies, juice or stewed fruit.
- Sprinkle on salads for a pleasant, nutty flavour.
- Add to casseroles, meatballs or meat loaf.
- Make a pesto sauce with fresh basil, garlic, ground linseeds, linseed oil and freshly grated Parmesan cheese.
- Sprinkle linseeds over steamed vegetables just before serving.

Liver

See Offal

Liver disorders

EAT PLENTY OF

- Oily fish, as well as walnuts, beans, whole grains, linseeds and rapeseed oil for omega-3 fatty acids

- Fresh fruit and vegetables for vitamins, minerals and phytochemicals

- Small meals and snacks, if they are more appealing than large meals

AVOID

- Alcohol in all forms

The liver, located in the upper right abdomen and protected by the ribs, performs thousands of vital chemical and metabolic functions – including the storage of fat-soluble vitamins, iron and other minerals and glycogen for future needs. It manufactures cholesterol, amino acids and other essential compounds, removes waste substances from the blood, detoxifies alcohol and environmental chemicals and metabolises most medications.

Amazingly, our bodies can still function when only a quarter of the liver is healthy enough to operate. Unlike most other organs, even after severe damage, the liver can regenerate itself by growing new cells. When severely diseased or subjected to excessive abuse, however, the liver will fail – often with fatal results.

Liver diseases are common, but experts feel that many cases could be prevented by careful attention to diet and hygiene. The most common disorders are hepatitis (usually caused by a virus spread by sewage contamination or by direct contact with infected body fluids),

cirrhosis and liver cancer. The risk of liver cancer is higher in those people who have cirrhosis or who have had certain types of viral hepatitis; but more often, the liver is the site of secondary (metastatic) cancers spread from other organs.

Symptoms are often not felt until the disease is advanced. The most recognised symptom of liver disease is jaundice, the yellowing of the skin and the whites of the eyes, caused by a build-up of bile pigments (bilirubin) in the skin.

People with liver disease may be deficient in the water-soluble vitamins, such as folate, niacin and thiamin, as well as the fat-soluble vitamins A and D. Lack of vitamins is most common among those with alcohol dependency, who may often substitute alcohol for food. Even when food intake is maintained, alcohol places undue demands on the liver, which must give precedence to detoxifying it over its other metabolic functions. Liver disease is also linked with problems in metabolising carbohydrates.

Food for the liver

A diet that is low in fats, alcohol and sugars is the key to maintaining a healthy liver. Cut down on tea and coffee and avoid spicy foods as they place a strain on the liver.

Eat small, frequent meals. The diet of a person recovering from a liver disorder should place the least possible burden on the organ; they should not eat fatty foods that are hard to digest. They often have a poor appetite and find it easier to eat frequent, nutritious snacks rather than large meals.

Eat foods rich in fatty acids. Omega-3 fatty acids seem to facilitate the processing of fats in the liver; a diet that is rich in these nutrients lowers the rate at which the liver manufactures triglycerides, which is beneficial for people with

circulatory and heart problems. These fatty acids are found in salmon and other oily fish, walnuts, beans, whole grains, linseeds and rape seed oil.

Get lots of protein. Including sufficient protein in the diet is important. Studies have shown that people with liver disease need at least 0.8g of protein per kilogram of body weight per day, but the recommended amount is 1.2–1.5g per kilogram. There is also some evidence to support the use of vegetable protein foods such as those found in soya, peas and legumes, especially for people who develop mental confusion, a condition called hepatic encephalopathy. A good supply of carbohydrates is also needed to meet the body's energy needs.

Consume plenty of vitamin D. Liver disease may cause a thinning of the bones (osteoporosis) if the body's stores of vitamin D, which helps the body absorb calcium, are depleted; such cases may require the use of calcium and vitamin D supplements. For the most part, however, vitamins and minerals should be provided adequately within the diet; supplements can upset the nutritional balance and, in the case of excessive iron, can cause severe liver damage.

Absolutely no alcohol. Alcohol should be avoided until complete recovery; in some cases, however, it must be eliminated for life. For protection against liver disease, adults should follow the advice on safe limits: no more that 14-21 units a week for women, and no more than 21-28 units a week for men.

Lobster

See Shellfish

L

'Low-carb' diets

Do they work?

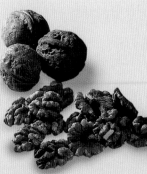

A few years ago, low-carbohydrate diets were all the rage. Chances are, you or someone you know got swept up in the excitement. Atkins, South Beach, The Zone, Protein Power. . . there is a long list to choose from. But did they work? What are the long-term health consequences of these diets?

HOW LOW-CARBOHYDRATE DIETS WORK

Proponents of these diets believe that carbohydrates stimulate the production of insulin, the hormone responsible for transporting glucose into the cells, where it is used for energy, with excess amounts being stored as fat. The theory is that since protein-rich foods do not cause the same rise in insulin levels, substituting them for carbohydrate foods promotes the use of stored fat for energy, resulting in weight loss.

The diets range from extreme to more moderate. Some of the more extreme, like the Dr Atkins or the South Beach diet, recommend a carbohydrate level of 20g or 30g per day during their initial stages. Health authorities recommend a minimum of 130g of carbohydrate per day, with most people eating well over 200g per day. More moderate diets, like The Zone, suggest carbo-hydrates represent 40 per cent of energy (the current recommendation ranges from 45 to 55 per cent), balanced with protein and fat at every meal.

Many low-carbohydrate diets allow unlimited amounts of meat, poultry, fish and eggs, some non-starchy vegetables, nuts, seeds, oils and other fats. Some allow small amounts of fruit, dairy and whole grains. Processed carbohydrates, like breads, pasta, cereals and sugary foods, are restricted.

We don't yet fully understand the implications of low-carbohydrate diets, but we are beginning to get a better picture of the pros and cons of this weight-loss approach.

SHORT-TERM BENEFITS

There's good evidence that in the first six months, low-carbohydrate diets can result in more rapid weight loss than conventional low-calorie, low-fat diets. Some studies show that those on low-carbohydrate diets may lose up to twice as much as those on conventional diets.

Low-carbohydrate diets can initially be easier to follow because the higher levels of protein and fat suppress appetite and keep dieters feeling full longer.

Compared to conventional diets, low-carbohydrate diets, in the short term, may have a more beneficial effect on both HDL cholesterol (the 'good' cholesterol) and triglyceride levels. Both factors are important for cardiovascular health. In one six-month study, people who were on a low-carbohydrate diet saw their 'bad' LDL cholesterol drop and their HDL increase slightly. Those on a low-fat diet showed a similar reduction in total cholesterol, but some of the loss came from a drop in HDL cholesterol. Later research has countered this (see panel, right).

LONG-TERM DISADVANTAGES

The early weight-loss effect of low-carbohydrate diets decreases over time. After a year, there is no significant difference in weight loss using a low-carbohydrate diet versus a conventional approach with restricted calories and fat.

Many of the stricter low-carbohydrate diets put the body into ketosis, which is the accumulation in the blood of ketones, by-products of fat metabolism. Ketosis causes nausea, dehydration, dizziness, fatigue and bad breath. The longer term effects of chronic ketosis on health are unknown.

Constipation is often a side effect of many low-carbohydrate diets, because of their low-fibre, high-fat profiles.

Lack of variety, can make the diet difficult to stick with in the longer term, as well as a potential for inadequate intake of important vitamins and minerals.

There are no studies on the long-term effects of these diets. Effects of high fat and protein intakes on bone health, cancer rates and cardiovascular and kidney function are unknown.

Recent research highlights

- Four controlled studies have shown that during the first 6 months, low-carbohydrate diets result in greater weight loss than conventional low-calorie, low-fat diets. However, this gap decreases with time and the difference in weight loss after 12 months is no longer significant.

- There are no studies assessing the long-term health consequences (particularly kidney health, bone health and cardiovascular function) of a high-protein, high-fat diet.

- In the short term, low-carbohydrate diets have a stronger positive impact on HDL cholesterol levels and triglyceride levels than conventional diets. There is no difference in the effect on total cholesterol and LDL cholesterol levels between conventional and low-carbohydrate diets.

- Many low-carbohydrate diets are also calorie-restricted, either because the programme restricts them or because dieters are choosing to eat less food. The weight loss on these diets is probably from simply eating less.

- Findings are hard to assess in studies of low-carbohydrate diets because of high dropout rates by participants.

- A recently published 12-month study reported that 30 per cent of those on a low-carbohydrate diet experienced a rise in LDL cholesterol levels (unlike in previous studies), 91 per cent had gastro-intestinal problems (mostly constipation), 60 per cent reported headaches. Bad breath, muscle weakness and cramps were common.

Low-carbohydrate diets allow far less than the recommended servings of fruit and vegetables associated with good health. In addition, scientific research has linked excessive meat consumption to colon and prostate cancer, and high protein intake with calcium loss from bones.

Did you know?

Low-carbohydrate diets deny that all calories are created equal

Proponents believe that there is something about a low-carbohydrate, high-protein diet that allows you to eat more calories than someone on a low-calorie, low-fat diet, while you lose more weight. This strikes at the heart of one of the dietary establishment's long-revered beliefs that a calorie is a calorie. Studies also show that those following low-carbohydrate, high-protein diets actually consume just over 1400kcal a day – much the same as is recommended in conventional weight-loss diets.

BOTTOM LINE

There is convincing evidence of the short-term effectiveness of low-carbohydrate diets. But over longer periods of time, it has been found that these diets lose their advantage over low-calorie, low-fat diet approaches. In addition, significant concerns over long-term health effects remain.

Whatever your weight-loss goals, remember that good health is an important goal too. A healthy, well-balanced diet is strongly linked to a decreased incidence of many diseases.

L

Lupus

CONSUME PLENTY OF

- Fruit and vegetables such as grapefruit, broccoli, cabbage and Brussels sprouts for antioxidants and bioflavonoids
- Dairy products and fortified soya and rice beverages for calcium
- Foods rich in essential fatty acids such as oily fish, nuts, walnuts and linseeds

LIMIT

- Fats, especially animal fats

AVOID

- Alfalfa in all forms
- Celery, parsnips, parsley, lemons, limes and figs if you are sun sensitive

Also known as systemic lupus erythematosus (or SLE), lupus is a chronic auto-immune disease. Arthritic joint pain, skin rashes, debilitating fatigue and dry mouth are the most common symptoms. It can also damage organs throughout the body, particularly the kidneys. Lupus strikes about nine times as many women as men. Often a mild disease, lupus can be serious and even life threatening for some.

Lupus is believed to be caused by a genetic predisposition, triggered by factors such as a virus; it may be worsened by other factors, such as sun exposure, infection, stress and some foods and drugs.

Lupus is such a variable disease that there is no one treatment regimen that helps everyone. The patient and doctor may have to try different approaches to find one that seems to work.

Therapy often calls for a non-steroidal anti-inflammatory drug (NSAID) to try to suppress inflammation, as well as hydroxy-chloroquine (a drug long used to fight malaria), which can increase resistance to sun exposure and help to prevent lupus rashes and joint pain. For more severe cases, steroids or other immuno-suppressive drugs may be prescribed.

Harmful foods

Alfalfa in any form. Even herbal supplements containing alfalfa worsen lupus symptoms; other legumes may have a similar effect.

Mushrooms and some smoked foods. These may also cause problems for lupus sufferers.

Foods containing psoralens. If you are one of the majority of lupus patients whose disease is worsened by exposure to the sun or unshielded fluorescent light, avoid foods containing psoralens, such as celery, parsnips, parsley, lemons and limes, which heighten photosensitivity.

High-protein, high-fat foods. Many lupus patients note an improvement after they decrease the consumption of fatty high-protein foods, especially animal products. A vegetarian diet that allows eggs, skimmed milk and other low-fat dairy products may be suggested.

Helpful foods

Wholegrain cereals, vegetables and fruit. They are high in the anti-oxidant vitamins and minerals: vitamins C, beta carotene, zinc and selenium. They are beneficial not only for lupus itself but also protect against heart disease. People with lupus tend to have high blood cholesterol levels, which may be worsened by steroid medications.

> ## C A U T I O N
>
> If you are taking cyclosporin, a powerful immune system suppressor, do not have grapefruit or grapefruit juice; although they are generally recommended for most lupus patients, they greatly increase the body's ability to absorb cyclosporin, leading to severe toxicity.

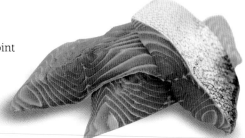

▲ Salmon for vitamin D
Fish, such as salmon, is an important dietary component for sufferers of lupus, as it is a good source of vitamin D. Exposure to the sun, the usual source of vitamin D, is not recommended for those with lupus.

Some studies have shown that lupus is associated with an increased level of oxidised blood fats and lower levels of circulating vitamin E; preliminary studies found that vitamin E may slow the progress of lupus. Vitamin E is found in nuts, seeds, oils and wheatgerm.

Eat cruciferous vegetables, bioflavonoids and oily fish. Broccoli and other cruciferous vegetables contain indoles that alter the metabolism of oestrogen in a way that may have a positive impact on lupus. Fresh citrus fruit, especially grapefruit, is high in bioflavonoids that seem to help lupus patients. Because most lupus patients need to avoid exposure to the sun, their diet must provide adequate vitamin D. Good sources are fortified soya beverages, salmon, herrings, margarine and butter. It has been found that fish oils have anti-inflammatory effects and may help to relieve joint pain, soreness and stiffness associated with lupus.

Drugs and diet

If you take aspirin or other NSAIDs, take them with meals. If you are taking corticosteroids, cut back on salt; it increases water retention and contributes to high blood pressure. Steroids also increase the risk of osteoporosis, so eat calcium-rich dairy products, canned sardines or salmon (with their bones) and dark green leafy vegetables.

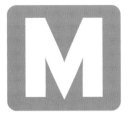

Mandarins

BENEFITS

- A good source of vitamin C, beta carotene and potassium
- Contain pectin, a soluble fibre that helps to control blood cholesterol

DRAWBACKS

- Oils in peel may irritate the skin of some people

These sweet citrus fruits with loose-fitting skins originated in China, but they are now grown in many parts of the world. The name 'mandarin' originated from the Chinese Imperial court. One variety that flourished in Tangiers in Morocco, came to be known as tangerines – the name most commonly used in Europe.

Mandarins have also been crossed with other citrus fruits to produce different varieties, including tangelos.

Mandarins are very popular with children as they are easy to peel.

Like oranges, mandarins and tangelos are an excellent source of vitamin C. Just one mandarin or tangelo provides about 100 per cent of the Reference Nutrient Intake (RNI) of this important antioxidant vitamin. Tangelos also provide small quantities of beta carotene, which the body converts to vitamin A, and both mandarins and tangelos have some folate as well as 160mg of potassium, and only about 40kcal.

They are also high in pectin, a soluble fibre that helps to lower blood cholesterol, and contains tangeretin, a flavonoid linked in experimental studies to reduced growth of tumour cells.

Like other citrus fruit, mandarin skin contains oils that can cause an itchy rash. However, because mandarins are so easy to peel, this can usually be avoided.

Types of mandarin

As a result of global marketing, mandarins are available in the UK for most of the year. Good-quality tangerines with be firm to slightly soft, heavy for their size and pebbly skinned with no deep grooves. You may find some of these varieties in your supermarket:

Clementine. This variety was first developed in Mediterranean countries (it is sometimes called an Algerian mandarin). The fruit is small, sweet and juicy, but can be difficult to peel as the tight-fitting skin breaks easily.

Ellendale. A cross between a mandarin and a sweet orange, this variety has deep orange-coloured skin that is very easy to peel. The sweet, richly flavoured flesh is bright orange.

Honey murcott. This variety has a greener, thinner skin than other mandarins, but the flesh is more orange and the flavour is outstandingly sweet.

Imperial. An early season mandarin with smooth glossy skin and sweet orange flesh.

Tangelo. A cross between a tangerine and a grapefruit, the tangelo looks like an orange with a pear-shaped neck. Its taste is tangier than a mandarin and is sweeter than a grapefruit.

Mangoes

BENEFITS

- An excellent source of beta carotene and vitamin C, and a good source of vitamin E
- Low in calories, high in fibre

Mangoes used to be regarded as a somewhat exotic fruit in the UK; Native to India and southern Africa, but they are now widely grown throughout the tropics.

Mangoes are considered a comfort food in many parts of the world. They contain an enzyme with digestive properties similar to papain found in papayas – which also makes them a very good tenderising agent for meat.

Nutritional value

Like other orange or deep yellow fruit, mangoes are high in beta carotene, which the body converts to vitamin A. Mangoes are also high in vitamin C which, along with vitamin A is an antioxidant. One medium-sized 150g mango has

M

about 86kcal and 56mg vitamin C, which is more than 100 per cent of the Reference Nitrient Intake (RNI). It also provides 4g of fibre, 1.58mg of vitamin E and a good amount of vitamin B$_6$; mangoes are also high in pectin, a soluble fibre that is important in controlling blood cholesterol.

However, mangoes are also quite high in sugar: a medium-sized mango is about 14 per cent sugar. As they are fairly acidic, they may contribute towards dental decay if eaten very often.

There are hundreds of different varieties of mango, ranging in size from 100g to more than 1.5kg.

Mangoes are usually picked while still somewhat green, but if possible, the skin should be turning yellow, becoming more orange or red as the fruit ripens.

When buying a mango, look for one with flesh that yields slightly when you press it gently. It should also have an orange or reddish skin. Large dark spots on the skin may mean that the flesh is bruised. (If the skin is completely green, the fruit may be useful for some Asian dishes that call for green mango.) Smell before buying. A flowery fragrance indicates that the mango is ripe and at the peak of its flavour. If you place an unripe mango in a

How to eat a mango

Some mango lovers advise eating the ripe fruit in the bath, where you can enjoy it without worrying about the juice running down your chin and onto your clothes. Here's a more practical approach. Make two vertical cuts – one on each side of the seed – and use a sharp paring knife to remove one half of the fruit from the large seed. You can then score the flesh into a crisscross, diamond pattern, making it easy to eat. Then repeat the process with the other half of the fruit.

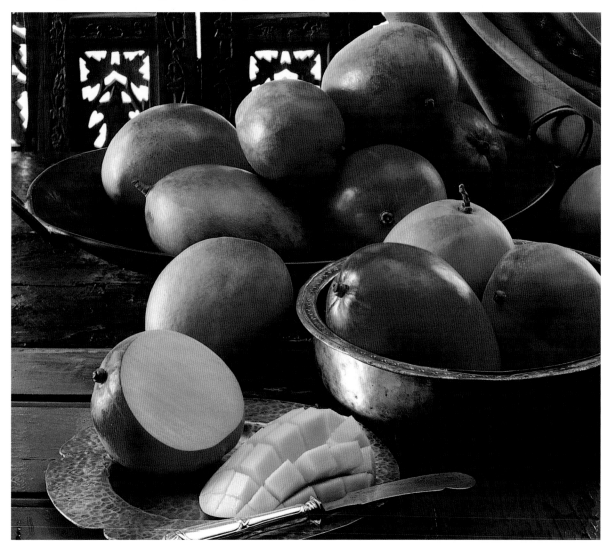

paper bag in a cool location, it will ripen in two or three days. (Do not put it in a sunny spot, as this can spoil the flavour.) Ripe mangoes should be eaten as soon as possible. They make a delicious addition to a tossed mixed salad.

Margarine

See Butter and margarine

Mayonnaise

BENEFITS

■ A source of vitamin E, depending upon the type of oil used

DRAWBACKS

■ High in fat, cholesterol and calories

■ Raw eggs may pose a salmonella risk in fresh mayonnaise

The rich flavour and creamy texture of mayonnaise accounts for its wide popularity in fast foods and salad dressings. There are several ways to make mayonnaise, but all involve the same basic ingredients – eggs and vegetable oil, as well as vinegar or lemon juice – whipped together to form a semi-solid spread. Egg yolks act as the emulsifiers that allow the oil and vinegar or lemon juice to blend. Mustard, salt, pepper, sugar and a number of other seasonings may be added. Some mayonnaises are good sources of vitamin E, yielding about 20 per cent of the adult Reference Nutrient Intake (RNI) in 1 tablespoon. The precise amount varies, however,

Allergy alert
Many commercial brands of mayonnaise and salad dressing have fillers made of gluten, which should be avoided by anyone with coeliac disease.

according to the type of oil used; those made with sunflower, cotton-seed and safflower oils are highest in this antioxidant nutrient. (The labels of commercial mayonnaise do not often specify the type of oil used.) The eggs do contribute protein and some minerals, but the amounts are negligible considering the number of calories per serving. A tablespoon of mayonnaise provides about 10g of fat and about 100kcal, depending on the type, which is roughly the same amount in a tablespoon of butter or margarine. Exact values vary and reduced-fat varieties are available, so check the nutrition information panel for commercial varieties of mayonnaise.

Homemade for quality – but take care
You can make your own mayonnaise at home. Most recipes call for olive oil – largely monounsaturated fat – although polyunsaturated oils, such as corn or safflower, can be used instead for a lighter flavour. Fresh mayonnaise should be used within two or three days. Even then, it could become a source of food poisoning if allowed to stand at room temperature for more than an hour. Commercial mayonnaise is safer, because its high vinegar content and antioxidant preservatives discourage the growth of disease-causing organisms.

Raw eggs used in homemade mayonnaise can be a potential source of salmonella, unless they are obtained from a reliable source.

'Light' varieties
Reduced-fat mayonnaise-type salad dressings contain less fat and fewer calories than ordinary mayonnaise. Although similar in texture and appearance, these salad dressings have a more acidic flavour, which can be tempered by adding a small amount of yoghurt.

Five ways to cut calories

SIMPLE WAYS TO REDUCE THE FAT

1 If you really don't like a snack made without mayonnaise, halve the amount that you use. And remember that some moist fillings used in sandwich bars, such as tuna salad, are made with mayonnaise.

2 Try mustard or chutney in a sandwich instead of mayonnaise for fewer calories (only about 7kcal per level teaspoon) and no fat.

3 Salad dressings made with mayonnaise are packed with calories and fat. Lemon juice livens up a fresh salad and adds neither fat nor calories. Low-fat yoghurt dressings with herbs are also healthier alternatives.

4 When you must have the luxury of mayonnaise, temper the damage by mixing it half and half with low-fat natural yoghurt.

5 Replace half the amount of mayonnaise with low-fat cottage cheese, whipped in a blender for a creamy consistency.

Low-fat and cholesterol-free mayonnaise and low-fat mayonnaise substitutes are available. The low-fat versions substitute air, water, starches and other fillers for some of the oil. Some contain a lot of sugar, so check the ingredient list, and some may contain gluten, so if you have coeliac disease, check for this, too.

Make your own, to be safe
A homemade recipe for mayonnaise uses tofu, egg whites, lemon juice, salt, mustard and a little bit of olive oil. Or you can make an imitation mayonnaise with natural yoghurt mixed with lemon juice and herbs to use in coleslaw.

Medicine-food interactions

The hidden dangers

In the body, drugs share the same route of absorption and metabolism as nutrients. This creates the potential for interactions, sometimes with dangerous consequences.

WHEN FOOD AFFECTS MEDICINE

The most common problem is when foods interfere with absorption, making a drug less effective. Calcium, for example, can bind to the antibiotic tetracycline, interfering with its absorption. Nutrients or other components of food can also interfere with a drug's metabolism, or how it is broken down in the body. Foods can also affect the elimination of drugs from the body. So some drugs should not be taken with food, while others must be taken with food to prevent stomach irritation.

WHEN MEDICINE AFFECTS FOODS

Some drugs interfere with the absorption of nutrients. For example, some cholesterol-lowering medications reduce the absorption of fat-soluble vitamins. Others affect the body's use or elimination of nutrients. For example, diuretics, which can cause a depletion of potassium, and lead to a deficiency.

DANGEROUS INTERACTIONS

The following are some of the more serious interactions that can occur between food and medicine:

MAO inhibitors and foods containing tyramine: Mixing monoamine oxidase (MAO) inhibitors – a class of medications used to treat depression – with foods high in tyramine produces one of the most dramatic and dangerous food-drug interactions. Symptoms include a rapid rise in blood pressure, severe headache, collapse and even death. Foods high in tyramine include aged cheese, chicken liver, some red wines, yeast extracts, processed meats, dried or pickled fish, legumes, soy sauce and beer.

Grapefruit and pomegranate: These juices contain a compound that can increase the absorption of some drugs, which can result in receiving a larger dose than was intended. Drugs that are affected may include AIDS medications, cholesterol-lowering 'statins', calcium channel blockers, antihypertension drugs, oral contraceptives and cyclosporin, an immune system suppressant. It is wise to consult your doctor, if you are taking any of these medications, before drinking either grapefruit or pomegranate juice. Compounds in the juice can stay in the blood for 24 hours, so there may be effects even if the medicine is not taken with the juice.

Foods high in vitamin K: Vitamin K is essential for clotting blood. Foods high in vitamin K, such as kale, spinach, Brussels sprouts, broccoli and other leafy greens, can interfere with anti-coagulants or blood thinners.

Alcohol: Alcohol can slow down the body's metabolism, so medications stay active longer than they should. Ask your doctor or pharmacist if your medication is safe with alcohol as some combinations can be fatal. To be safe, try to avoid it when taking non-prescription medications.

Did you know?

High blood pressure drugs deplete potassium

Many antihypertensive drugs deplete the body's potassium, although ACE inhibitors increase it. If your potassium level is low, eating bananas may help, but in most cases, you are better having your potasium levels monitored by your doctor who will probably prescribe a potassium supplement.

Six tips for taking medicines safely

1 Always carry a list of your medications and doses.

2 When your doctor prescribes a new medicine, mention any other drugs you are taking. This includes non-prescription drugs and vitamin supplements.

3 If you have any side effects from a medication, contact your doctor or pharmacist immediately.

4 It is usually best to take prescription medications with a full glass of water, sitting or standing, not lying down. Take them with water, not soft drinks or grapefruit or pomegranate juice.

5 Don't mix your medications with food or drink unless instructed to by your doctor or pharmacist.

6 Always read and follow any directions that come with your medication.

Foods and drugs that don't mix

Before taking any medication, always read the package instructions and ask your doctor or pharmacist about any dietary precautions. In some cases, drugs alter nutritional needs; in other instances, foods can interfere with the way a medicine works. The table below shows how particular foods can interact with some of the more commonly used drugs.

DRUGS	EFFECTS AND PRECAUTIONS
ANTIBIOTICS	
Cephalosporins, penicillin	Take on an empty stomach to speed absorption of the drugs.
Ciprofloxacin	Avoid dairy products, caffeine and supplements, which contain calcium, iron or zinc, for 2 hours before and after taking the medication.
Erythromycin	Don't take with fruit juice or wine, which decrease the drug's effectiveness.
Sulphonamides	Increase the risk of vitamin B_{12} deficiency.
Tetracycline	Dairy products decrease its efficacy. Lowers vitamin C absorption. Take 1 hour before or 2 hours after eating.
ANTICOAGULANTS	
Warfarin	Foods high in vitamin K can reduce the drug's effectiveness. Do not increase or decrease the usual intake of broccoli, spinach, kale, Brussels sprouts or cabbage.
ANTICONVULSANTS	
Phenytoin, phenobarbital	Increase the risk of anaemia and nerve problems due to a deficiency of folate and other B vitamins.
ANTIDEPRESSANTS	
Fluoxetine	Reduces appetite and can lead to excessive weight loss.
Lithium	A low-salt diet increases the risk of lithium toxicity; excessive salt reduces drug's efficacy.
MAO inhibitors	Foods high in tyramine (aged cheeses, processed meats, legumes, wine, beer, among others) can bring on a hypertensive crisis.
Tricyclics	Many foods, especially legumes, meat, fish and foods high in vitamin C, reduce absorption of the drugs
ANTIHYPERTENSIVES, HEART MEDICATIONS	
ACE inhibitors	Take on an empty stomach to improve the absorption of the drugs.
Alpha blockers	Take with liquid or food to avoid an excessive drop in blood pressure.
Antiarrhythmic drugs	Avoid caffeine, which increases the risk of an irregular heartbeat.
Beta blockers	Take on an empty stomach; food, especially meat, increases the drugs' effects and can cause dizziness and low blood pressure.
Digitalis	Avoid taking with milk and high-fibre foods such as oatmeal, which reduce absorption. Increases potassium loss. Avoid black liquorice which lowers potassium.
Diuretics	Increase the risk of potassium deficiency.
Potassium-sparing diuretics	Unless a doctor advises otherwise, don't take diuretics with potassium supplements or salt substitutes, which can cause potassium overload.
Thiazide diuretics	Increase the reaction of MSG. Stick to a low salt diet and increase potassium intake.

DRUGS	EFFECTS AND PRECAUTIONS
ASTHMA DRUGS, DECONGESTANTS	
Pseudo-ephedrine	When prescribed for colds, avoid caffeine, which increases feelings of anxiety and nervousness.
Theophylline	Char-grilled foods and a high-protein diet reduce absorption. Caffeine increases the risk of drug toxicity.
CHOLESTEROL-LOWERING DRUGS	
Colestyramine	Increases the excretion of folate and vitamins A, D, E and K.
Gemfibrozil	Avoid fatty foods, which decrease the drug's efficacy in lowering cholesterol.
HEARTBURN AND ULCER MEDICATIONS	
Antacids	Interfere with the absorption of many minerals; for maximum benefit, take medication 1 hour after eating.
Cimetidine, famotidine, sucralfate	Avoid high-protein foods, caffeine and other items that may increase stomach acidity.
HORMONE PREPARATIONS	
Oral contraceptives and HRT preparations	Sodium increases fluid retention. Avoid salt and use fewer processed foods that contain sodium. Drugs reduce the absorption of folate, vitamin B_6 and zinc; increase intake of foods high in these nutrients. The oestrogen in HRT reacts with caffeine to increase the risk of Parkinson's disease.
Steroids	Sodium increases fluid retention. Increase intake of foods high in calcium, vitamin K, potassium and protein to avoid deficiencies.
Thyroid drugs	Iodine-rich foods and turnips lower the drugs' efficacy.
LAXATIVES	
Mineral oils	Can cause a deficiency of vitamins A, D, E and K.
PAINKILLERS	
Aspirin and stronger non-steroidal anti-inflammatory drugs	Always take with food to lower the risk of gastro-intestinal irritation; avoid taking with alcohol, which increases the risk of bleeding. Frequent use of these drugs lowers the absorption of folate and vitamin C.
Codeine	Increase fibre and water intake to help to avoid constipation.
SLEEPING PILLS, TRANQUILLISERS	
Benzodiazepines	Never take with alcohol. Caffeine increases anxiety and reduces the drugs' efficacy.

M

Melons

BENEFITS

- Low in calories

- Orange varieties are high in beta carotene

- Most are good sources of vitamin C and potassium

- Some are high in pectin, a soluble fibre that helps to control blood cholesterol levels

There are many types of melon; among them cantaloupe, galia, honeydew, charentais and the traditional watermelon. Although mostly water, melons are very nutritious, providing beta carotene, which the body converts to vitamin A, vitamin C, potassium and other minerals.

Cantaloupe and other deeply coloured varieties are high in beta carotene; a large slice (200g) of cantaloupe provides 52mg of vitamin C, more than the Reference Nutrient Intake (RNI), 420g of vitamin B_6, more than 3,530mcg of beta carotene, 380mg of potassium and only 38kcal. Honeydews are also low in calories, high in vitamin C and a good source of

Did you know?

Watermelon may help to prevent prostate cancer

Watermelon is a good source of lycopene, an antioxidant linked with a lower rate of prostate cancer.

potassium. A 200g slice of water-melon contains about 62kcal, 16mg of vitamin C and just a little less potassium than the others.

Many melon varieties are high in bioflavonoids, carotenoids and other plant pigments that may help to protect against cardiovascular

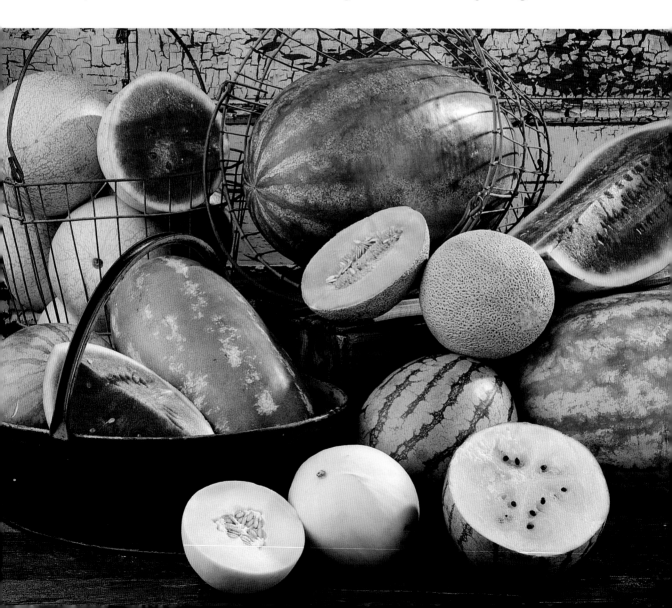

disease, cancer and other diseases. Because melons are made mostly of water, they may stimulate the kidneys to work more efficiently. Although melon flesh is not high in insoluble fibre, it does contain pectin, a type of soluble fibre that may help to keep blood cholesterol levels in check.

How to buy a melon

Because melons do not contain starch that converts to sugar, they don't continue to ripen after they are picked from the vine; therefore, melons that are harvested before they are fully ripe never achieve their peak flavour.

In order to select a vine-ripened melon, check the stem area for a smooth, slightly sunken scar; this indicates that the melon was ripe and easily pulled from its vine. In contrast, if part of the stem still adheres to the scar, the melon was picked while it was still green and not fully ripe.

When purchasing melons, don't be shy about sniffing the fruit to see if it is fully ripe; a ripe melon will have a deep, intense fragrance.

A ripe watermelon should rattle when you shake it, because the seeds loosen as the fruit matures; thumping the melon should produce a slightly hollow sound. Watermelons come in several colours, but in all instances the rind should be firm and smooth, with a yellowish undertone.

To best preserve nutrient content, buy melons whole (some stores offer halves or quarters). Certain nutrients, especially vitamin C, are diminished by exposure to the air.

◀ **Cool and refreshing − and packed with nutrients**
Melons contain pectin, a type of soluble fibre that may help to keep blood cholesterol levels in check. They are also low in calories.

Memory loss

EAT

■ Breakfast every day

■ Lots of fruit and vegetables for vitamin C, beta carotene and flavonoids

■ Include some vegetable oils, nuts and wheatgerm for vitamin E

Mild lapses in memory are common with age and simple forgetfulness is usually relatively benign. Profound memory loss is a universal symptom of dementia or Alzheimer's disease. Benign age-related memory loss may result from shrinkage of the brain's nerves, diminished production of brain chemicals or restricted blood flow to brain tissue. Genetic factors, head injuries, viruses, obesity and cardiovascular disease may, however, contribute to Alzheimer's disease.

Exercise and a healthy diet help to preserve brain longevity and sustain memory. Protective brain nutrients include carbohydrates and B vitamins, which help to ensure healthy nerve transmission and enough neurotransmitters.

Eat breakfast. Eating breakfast can do wonders for your memory, according to researchers from the University of Toronto. A study of healthy men and women, aged 61 to 79, showed that taking in calories from either protein, carbohydrates or fat boosted their performance on memory tests. Previous research has shown that carbohydrates can fuel memory-based performance, perhaps because of the rise in blood sugar they provide. The rise in blood sugar could then increase glucose supply to the brain. But this study showed that any food, regardless of source, can help. While it appears that any breakfast is better than no breakfast, the researchers think that carbohydrates still generally give longer term benefits to memory.

Coffee may give a memory boost

That afternoon coffee break may do more than you think to get you through the day, especially if you are an older adult. Researchers at the University of Arizona found that memory in older people is often at its best in the morning and declines in the afternoon. When half the seniors in their study drank 350ml of decaffeinated coffee both morning and afternoon, their memory performance showed a significant decline from the morning to the afternoon. The group that drank regular coffee, however, maintained their morning performance levels throughout the afternoon as well.

Get plenty of carotenoids and vitamin C. There is some evidence that high levels of beta carotene and other carotenoids and vitamin C are associated with superior memory performance in people 65 or older. Researchers believe these anti-oxidants may delay brain ageing and enhance mental longevity and fitness by combating free radicals in the brain. Experimental research suggests that flavonoids in blueberries may slow age-related decline in mental function.

Consume lots of vitamin E. Other research is looking at the link between blood levels of vitamin E and memory function in the elderly. In one large study, more than 4,000 people performed tests designed to assess their ability to remember facts. Those classified as having poor memory were more likely than others to have low blood levels of vitamin E. Another study showed an association between past intake of vitamin E and mental acuity in old age, and other studies have found vitamin E helpful in slowing the progression of Alzheimer's disease.

Iron may also be important for memory. Research suggests that depressed levels of iron can impair memory function. Studies have

M

shown that when children have an iron deficiency, they score better on tests of memory when this deficiency is corrected.

Try ginkgo biloba. Current research indicates that ginkgo biloba extracts may have a limited effect on improving memory. As with other herbal products, the lack of standardisation is a concern, as is the possibility that labels may not reflect contents accurately.

Investigate sage oil. Recently, researchers at the UK's Northumbria and Newcastle universities followed up on the recommendation of some old-time herbalists to improve memory with sage oil by giving it to a group of 44 adults in a placebo-controlled study. People who took the sage oil performed much better on their memory performance tests.

One more supplement. Phosphatidylserine, a naturally occurring compound in the brain that maintains cell membrane fluidity, is available as a supplement, extracted from soya. Limited evidence suggests that it may be of some help in cognitive function but more studies are needed.

Menopause

EAT PLENTY OF

- Dairy produce for calcium
- Fresh fruit and vegetables for vitamins, minerals and bioflavonoids
- Soya and linseed products for phytostrogens and omega-3 fatty acids
- Oily fish for vitamin D and omega-3s

LIMIT

- Alcohol and caffeine

Menopause is defined as the end of a woman's monthly menstrual periods. This process usually begins at around

45 to 50 years of age, as a result of a progressive decline in levels of the hormone oestrogen, and concludes around the age of 55. The start of this time is called perimenopause and the period after menopause is called postmenopause.

Menopause used to be viewed as the beginning of old age. Today a majority of women in developed countries will live more than a third of their lives after menopause.

During menopause, fluctuations in oestrogen levels can cause hot flushes, night sweats, insomnia, vaginal dryness, weight gain and difficulty in concentrating. While some women experience few or no symptoms of menopause, others experience severe symptoms that cause them extreme discomfort.

Menopause can also affect a woman's life expectancy and quality of life. Before menopause a woman's hormones protect her from the risk of heart disease, but with the onset of menopause that protection is lost. From about 55 years of age onwards, women die of heart disease at about the same rate as men. In addition, the gradual loss of bone mass that most women experience from the age of 30 onwards is drastically accelerated at menopause. Bone loss results in part from the lack of oestrogen as well as from inefficient absorption of calcium. A woman may lose 10 to 20 per cent of her bone mass in the decade following menopause, with a slower but still significant loss thereafter. This bone

thinning, or osteoporosis, increases the risk of fractures, which can lead to disability and pain.

Hormone replacement therapy (HRT)

In the past, many women have chosen to counteract the effects of oestrogen loss with hormone replacement therapy, a combination of oestrogen and progesterone prescribed by their doctors. HRT was designed to treat symptoms of menopause, but medical experts also believed that it provided some protection against chronic diseases. However, recent findings of a major US study on HRT, showing that the risks of taking HRT appear to outweigh the benefits, have caused many women, and their doctors, to rethink this strategy.

The Women's Health Initiative Study, which included more than 16,000 women, concluded that, although HRT is effective in relieving symptoms of menopause, its long-term use increases a post-menopausal woman's risk of breast cancer, heart disease, stroke and blood clots. A combined therapy of oestrogen and progestorone also seems to increase the risk of dementia after the age of 65. As a result of these findings, experts are now recommending that HRT be

▶ **Helpful linseeds**
Linseeds are packed with omega-3 fatty acids.

Do one simple thing

Try linseeds to reduce hot flushes

Eat 1 to 2 tablespoons of linseeds a day. These pleasant, versatile seeds contain omega-3 fats, which help against heart disease. They also contain a type of phyto-oestrogen called lignans, which may help to reduce hot flushes. Try adding the seeds to cereal or yoghurt for a tasty snack.

Four important nutrients for menopause

1 Vitamin E. Considered useful in alleviating hot flushes and thought to offer some heart protection although a recent study showed that 400 IU of vitamin E taken twice daily reduced hot flushes only slightly more than the placebo. Include foods such as nuts and seeds, egg yolk and wheatgerm that contain vitamin E. Women with diabetes should check with their doctor first.

2 Calcium. To help to prevent the development of osteoporosis. Good sources are milk and milk products, sardines, almonds, broccoli and calcium-enriched soya milk. To absorb calcium, the body needs vitamin D, which can be made by the skin after exposure to the sun; dietary sources of this vitamin include butter and margarine, eggs and oily fish.

3 Magnesium. Works with calcium to maintain bone density. Found in whole grains, milk and milk products, tofu, nuts and seeds and legumes.

4 Phyto-oestrogens. May help to alleviate hot flushes. May also protect against heart disease and osteoporosis. Foods rich in phyto-oestrogens include soya foods, linseeds and legumes.

used in the lowest possible dose, for the shortest period of time, when symptoms of menopause are so severe that they are interfering with quality of life.

To treat milder symptoms, and to avoid development of chronic disease, women are encouraged to adopt a healthy lifestyle and to try other approaches, which can include dietary changes, exercise and herbal remedies.

Diet

It may require a little more effort than simply swallowing a pill but a healthy diet can help to ease menopause symptoms and reduce the risk of chronic disease. Here are some helpful dietary strategies:

Eat foods known to reduce menopausal symptoms. Follow a diet that is high in whole grains, fruit and vegetables and low in saturated fats. It will provide you with plenty of fibre, vitamins and minerals, phyto-oestrogens and bioflavonoids, all important for long-term health and to help minimise menopausal symptoms.

Watch out for trigger foods. These are foods that can worsen symptoms like hot flushes, insomnia and mood swings. Some common culprits are coffee, tea, chocolate, colas, alcohol and spicy foods.

Include soya foods. Some studies have shown that soya foods not only help to protect against heart disease, but they also can help to ease hot flushes. Soya foods contain isoflavones, which have a weak oestrogenic effect in the body. They come in many shapes and sizes, including tofu, soya beans, soya beverages, soya nuts and soya protein. While soya foods may be safe enough, the safety and efficacy of isoflavone supplements have not been thoroughly demonstrated.

Exercise regularly

Regular exercise may help to lessen mood swings and hot flushes. At least 30 minutes of exercise, four to five times a week, is recommended.

Herbal products

Long before hormone replacement therapy, women often sought relief for their menopausal complaints with herbal remedies. Some of the more popular ones – for which there is some evidence of efficacy – are listed below. The evidence, however, is not compelling and the amounts of these substances found in commercial preparations is not standardised, which makes it difficult to assess results. Always check with your doctor before you start taking any of these herbal preparations.

Black cohosh (*Cimicifuga racemosa*). A number of studies have shown that black cohosh can help many unpleasant symptoms of menopause, including irritability, poor concentration, insomnia and depression, but it has been linked to liver disease.

Chasteberry (*Vitex agnus-cactus*). This herb has been useful in the management of fluid retention, hot flushes, anxiety and depression.

St John's wort (*Hypericum perforatum*). St John's wort has been shown to be effective in managing some mild to moderate cases of depression. It may interact with several prescription medicines, so check with your phramacist.

Red clover (*Trifolium pratense*). Extracts of red clover are marketed to help with menopausal symptoms. Chemical analysis does indeed show the presence of oestrogenic compounds, but two studies found no difference between red clover

M

and a placebo for treating such menopausal symptoms as hot flushes and vaginal dryness over a period of 12 weeks. Still, many women claim that their symptoms are alleviated by red clover preparations.

Menstrual problems

LIMIT

- Alcohol and caffeinated drinks

AVOID

- Highly salted foods, which promote fluid retention and bloating

Most women in their reproductive years recognise the mild cramps or slight twinge in the lower back as the normal effects of menstruation. These effects are not symptoms of any sickness and do not usually interfere with normal activities. Many women, however, experience discomfort and even temporary disability from the severe cramps and nausea that can precede their periods, sometimes lasting several days. Some others have to deal with irregular, sparse or even excessive bleeding that can make it difficult to plan and enjoy activities.

Premenstrual syndrome

More than 150 symptoms – notably, bloating, irritability, food cravings, breast tenderness, headache and constipation – have been linked with premenstrual syndrome (PMS), which is often attributed to hormonal changes during the latter half of the menstrual cycle. For 10 per cent of the women who suffer from PMS, these symptoms can cause serious social problems, disrupting work and family activities and even putting the sufferer at risk through anger.

Eat foods with a low Glycaemic Index. No food can prevent PMS, but certain substances in food may offer relief from some symptoms. Doctors advise a balanced diet combined with exercise. Women should eat regular, moderate meals, spaced through the day, based on a combination of whole grains, legumes, vegetables and fruit. Slowly digested carbohydrates may help by increasing production of serotonin, a brain chemical that regulates mood. Foods with a lower glycaemic index are best because they raise blood sugar levels more slowly, helping to control appetite and possibly cravings. Fats, highly refined foods and caffeinated drinks should be avoided and sodium intake should be reduced. Alcohol has been found to trigger or worsen many symptoms and so should be avoided in the days before menstrual periods.

Get more calcium. Calcium may help to reduce mood disturbances, cramping and bloating resulting from PMS. Some researchers believe PMS symptoms may be the result of low calcium levels, the symptoms of which are very like the symptoms of PMS. Best calcium sources include dairy products, fortified soya or rice beverages, canned salmon or sardines and leafy greens. Women with PMS may have low magnesium levels, which may predispose them to PMS-induced headaches and depression. Foods rich in magnesium include sunflower seeds, nuts, lentils and legumes, tofu, soya beans, figs and green vegetables. Some research suggests that foods rich in vitamin B_6 may be useful. The vitamin B_6 may help to stimulate production of serotonin and reduce anxiety and depression caused by PMS. Best food sources are wheatgerm, red meats, pork, chicken, fish, wholegrain cereals, bananas, peanuts, avocados and potatoes.

A caution about vitamin B_6. If you take supplements, do not exceed 50mg per day. Excess has been associated with nerve damage.

Watch those food cravings. Many women crave sweets – in particular, chocolate – just before their period starts. An occasional piece of chocolate won't do much harm, but eating large amounts of sugary foods only adds empty calories and can worsen the craving for sweets by disrupting normal blood sugar levels. It's much better to satisfy such cravings with healthy carbohydrates, such as fresh fruit, wholegrain bread or fresh vegetables, which are metabolised at a slower rate than sweets. These snacks are also packed with fibre, which helps to prevent the constipation that some women experience as part of PMS.

Don't neglect exercise. Women who exercise regularly are less likely to suffer from PMS. The difference may be related to the levels of endorphins, which are released at an increased rate during exercise. Endorphins are chemicals in the brain that are natural mood elevators. They can increase the sense of well-being and help the body to deal with stress.

Try evening primrose oil. This oil, available in capsules and in liquid form, contains an essential fatty acid called gamma linolenic acid (GLA). This fatty acid may help to block the inflammatory prostaglandins that contribute to cramps and breast tenderness.

Painful periods

Menstrual cramps (dysmenorrhoea) are most common among young women who have never been pregnant. In most cases there is no underlying health problem, and symptoms often ease somewhat after pregnancy, or with the onset of use of oral contraceptives.

Herbal teas may help. Raspberry leaf tea contains a substance that is thought to relax the uterus and ease cramping. Chamomile tea also has antispasmodic action and may help. Drink the tea while relaxing in a warm bath or lying down with a heating pad over your abdomen to relieve muscle cramps and tension.

Take an anti-inflammatory. Prostaglandins, hormone-like substances that cause uterine contractions, play a part in causing menstrual cramps, but the precise mechanism is unknown. Aspirin, ibuprofen and other nonsteroidal anti-inflammatory drugs (NSAIDs) can block prostaglandin production and alleviate menstrual cramps. Use these drugs with care, because they can cause stomach irritation and bleeding problems.

In some instances, painful periods are related to other conditions, such as fibroid tumours (benign uterine growths) or endometriosis (the growth of uterine tissue outside the uterus). These conditions all require the attention of a gynaecologist.

Heavy periods

Menstrual bleeding tends to be heavy and irregular at the beginning and end of a woman's reproductive years. Heavy periods, caused by hormonal fluctuations, often occur in the months following the first period (known as menarche) and in the year or two preceding menopause.

Eat lots of iron-rich foods. A healthy adult woman needs 14.8mg of iron daily. However, excessive blood flow may result in a greater loss of iron, with a risk of anaemia; extra iron may be necessary. Good sources are red meat, tofu, beans, pulses, fortified breakfast cereals, leafy green vegetables and dried fruit. To help the body to better absorb iron, a food rich in vitamin C should be eaten at the same meal.

A woman who has persistently heavy or irregular periods should see her doctor to determine if she has a problem requiring treatment or, if she is approaching middle age, to obtain information about dealing with her menopause.

Missed periods

The most likely reason for a missed period is pregnancy. However, the cause may be hormonal imbalances related to obesity or diabetes, thyroid disease, a change in contraceptive pills or an eating disorder such as anorexia nervosa. Women involved in high-level athletic training are prone to menstrual problems, because they lack the critical amount of body fat to maintain adequate oestrogen levels. A meal plan can provide the nutrition essential to maintain top athletic performance while guarding against excess weight. A woman who is not having regular menstrual periods should see a doctor for a thorough check-up.

Migraines and other headaches

LIMIT

■ Coffee, tea, colas and other beverages containing caffeine

AVOID

■ Alcohol, especially red wine, port, champagne and beer

■ Any food shown to trigger your attacks

■ Skipping meals

Headaches afflict about 70 per cent of adults at least occasionally, often seriously enough for many to seek medical relief. Most headaches are transient and due to tension or a temporary condition, such as a cold or the flu, but some reflect a serious underlying problem. Recurrent headaches warrant medical attention. When you see your doctor, bring a detailed written description of your headaches: their severity, ranging from mild to incapacitating; their frequency; their duration; the exact areas affected by the pain; and any related symptoms you've noticed, such as nausea.

Migraine headaches

Most migraine sufferers usually experience a one-sided, severe, throbbing or pulsating headache, often accompanied by nausea or vomiting and sensitivity to light and sound. Migraines are also called vascular headaches, because they usually involve spasm of the arteries of the head, resulting in a pulsating pain. The headaches may last from a few hours to several days.

About 10 per cent of migraine sufferers experience a warning aura before the headache starts; this early symptom involves a visual disturbance, such as partial or temporary loss of sight or flashes of light and colour. An aura may also cause tingling on one side of the face or body or a disturbance in the sense of smell. Even those who don't experience an aura may have warning signs in the few hours leading up to a migraine, such as feeling cold, craving a specific food, mood changes, a sudden burst of energy or frequent yawning.

Migraines affect about 15 per cent of women and about 6 per cent of men, and are most common in the 25 to 34 age group, but some start in childhood. Doctors think that dietary, hormonal, emotional and environmental triggers may cause blood vessels in the brain to constrict and then relax. The distorted blood vessels prompt nerve endings to send out pain signals.

M

The food-migraine link

Many foods, additives and other dietary components can cause migraines, but the triggers vary greatly from one person to another. The following list covers the more common ones.

- Aged cheeses, Brie, Camembert and Swiss cheeses.
- Breads containing dried fruit, crumpets and muffins.
- Fermented foods, including pickles, soy sauce and miso.
- Some legumes, especially dried beans, lentils and soya products.
- Nuts, seeds, peanut butter and muesli bars.
- Chocolate and cocoa.
- Offal and meats that are salted, dried, cured, smoked or contain nitrites.
- Sardines, anchovies and pickled herring.
- Many fruits, including avocados, bananas, citrus fruit, figs, grapes, pawpaws, passionfruit, plantains, pineapples, raspberries and red plums.
- Alcohol, especially red wine.
- Chicken livers, bacon, ham and pâté.
- Seasonings and flavour enhancers, especially artificial sweeteners, stock cubes and fish sauce.
- Sulphites used as preservatives in wine and dried fruit.
- Monosodium glutamate (MSG).

Try relaxation techniques. In addition to using relaxation techniques, some doctors suggest taking a course in biofeedback to learn how to raise the temperature of your hands, thereby diverting some of the blood flow from the head to another part of the body. This technique can be used at the start of an attack.

Medications. For acute attacks, a simple analgesic such as aspirin, paracetamol or a nonsteroidal anti-inflammatory drug (NSAID) may also help, but can cause gastrointestinal problems. NSAID products available include ibuprofen and naproxen. Products combining paracetamol with codeine may also give relief, although they usually cause constipation. An anti-emetic (metoclopramide or domperidone) may be needed to stop vomiting. Specific anti-migraine drugs such as sumaptriptan (Imigran) may be used.

Sumatriptan is a serotonin antagonist available as an oral medication, a nasal spray or injection. It may not be effective if taken during the aura phase. Migraine headaches are thought to be due to some blood vessels widening, and sumatriptan aims to normalise these blood vessels.

If there are more than two attacks a month, they are increasing in frequency, causing severe disability or you cannot tolerate the drugs used in acute attacks, doctors may prescribe pizotifen (Sanomigran) which is an antihistamine and serotonin antagonist; beta blockers (such as propranolol); topiramate (Topamax) which is an anti-epileptic drug used only under supervision; amitriptyline (which is as yet unlicensed); or

sodium valproate (an anti-epilepic drug, also unlicensed as yet). In addition, high-dose riboflavin (400mg) has been tested for preventing migraine, but the initial results from one small study have not been duplicated in placebo-controlled trials. Coenzyme Q_{10} looks more promising, but more studies are required. Magnesium is also being examined for its anti-migraine affects.

Known migraine triggers

The triggers that can set off a migraine vary widely from one person to another. A number of the following triggers can be avoided entirely; others can be minimised.

Environmental triggers. These include glare, bright lights, loud noises, strong odours, cigarette smoke and changes in temperature, weather or altitude.

Hormonal triggers. Experienced by women and are usually related to the menstrual cycle; they can also be caused by the use of oestrogen supplements or high-oestrogen oral contraceptives.

Activity triggers. These include irregular or no exercise, inadequate or excessive sleep, eyestrain and motion sickness.

Do one simple thing

Try herbal migraine relief

Take one or two capsules of freeze-dried feverfew daily to reduce headache episodes. Recent research shows that regular feverfew dosing may decrease the frequency and intensity of migraine headaches and their nausea. Start slowly, because feverfew can produce allergic reactions in some people. If you have no side effects, you can continue this regimen indefinitely. It cannot, however, stop an attack that has already started.

Emotional triggers. These tend to be the negative ones, such as anger, resentment, depression, fatigue, anxiety and stress.

Dietary triggers. These may be the easiest to control. Keep a food diary, note what foods seem to prompt symptoms, and then seek help from a dietitian. Eat regular meals, because hunger or low blood sugar can trigger a headache.

The caffeine in coffee and other beverages – as well as in many non-prescription analgesic drugs – can play a dual role in migraines. Regular and excessive ingestion can add to the frequency of the headaches.

On the other hand, once you are completely off caffeine, you may be able to use it to abort an impending attack, because it constricts dilated blood vessels. At the first sign of an aura or a pain, drink a cup of strong coffee, take two aspirin and lie down in a dark, quiet room. The episode may pass within an hour.

Cluster headaches

The most incapacitating of all vascular headaches, this type lasts from 15 minutes to 3 hours and typically occurs in clusters, coming and going repeatedly over several days or weeks and then going away for months or even years. Often starting during sleep, they cause excruciating, stabbing pain on one side of the head, usually behind or around one eye. Red, watering eyes, swollen or drooping eyelids, runny nose and facial sweating are typical symptoms, too.

Cluster headaches are far more common in men than in women, especially among those who are heavy smokers and frequent alcohol users. Eliminating these habits may banish the headaches. In addition, keeping a diary of food and lifestyle factors may reveal that some of the factors known to trigger migraines can also prompt cluster headaches.

Tension headaches and other types

Tension headaches are the most common type and are caused by muscle contractions or an imbalance of natural chemicals in the brain. The pain causes a bandlike pressure around the head and there may be a sense of tightness in the head, neck and shoulder muscles. They often begin in the afternoon or evening and produce a steady pain.

Prevention is the best approach; relaxation techniques, such as biofeedback, massage, meditation and visualisation, work for many people and can abort an attack.

Another recommendation is to eliminate from the diet all foods and drugs that contain caffeine, which can increase tension and anxiety, contributing to headaches.

Headaches also may be due to sinusitis, an inflammation of the lining of the sinus cavities, causing a deep, dull ache around the eyes and sometimes in the forehead and ears. A good diagnostic clue is that the pain worsens when you bend over.

Rebound headaches can result from overuse of nonprescription analgesics, prescription medications, sedatives and caffeine (which is a common ingredient in such drugs), resulting in a vicious cycle of growing tolerance and increasing dependence. These tend to be mild to moderate headaches. Although you may have to go through a painful week or more to withdraw from dependence on these drugs, you will feel better in the long run.

Dental problems, too, can cause very severe one-sided headaches that may feel just like migraines, especially if a tooth is abscessed.

The many other factors that can cause headaches include squinting for long periods in bright sunlight, eyestrain, hunger, excessive alcohol consumption and too little or too much sleep.

Milk and milk products

BENEFITS

- An excellent source of calcium

- A good source of vitamins A and D (full-cream milk only) and B_{12}, riboflavin, phosphorus, zinc and magnesium

- Dairy products, including low-fat varieties, are high in protein

DRAWBACKS

- Whole milk and cream are high in fat

- Some people cannot digest milk sugar

- Milk protein can trigger allergic reactions in susceptible children

- Unpasteurised milk is a relatively common cause of food poisoning

Milk is an excellent source of dietary calcium, a mineral needed to build healthy bones and teeth and to maintain many of the basic functions of the human body. Calcium helps to prevent osteoporosis, and recent

Did you know?

You may be able to lose weight by drinking milk instead of soft drinks

A 2003 study indicated that dairy products may play a role in weight loss. A group of 323 girls in Hawaii lost both weight and abdominal girth when they consumed just 1.5 servings of dairy foods daily. One cup of milk or a small piece of cheese resulted in 0.9mm less abdominal fat and a decrease of as much as 1kg of body weight.

This may not be as controversial as it sounds, for there is a growing body of evidence that small amounts of low-fat dairy products as part of a calorie-controlled diet can lead to better loss of weight, overall. One reason may be that people who drink milk in place of soft drinks might also eat less junk food and have a healthier lifestyle.

The milk controversy

There is a debate regarding the most popular source of dietary calcium – dairy products – and how much we should consume. Some believe that two servings of dairy produce per day will help to prevent osteoporosis. Others believe that our need for dairy foods is greatly overstated and that too much dairy may actually cause harm. What is clear is that an adequate intake of dietary calcium is necessary to reduce the risk of osteoporosis, and milk is a convenient source. Milk is also a good source of protein and riboflavin. Also, getting calcium in dairy products has been shown to have benefits beyond the health of your bones. It may lower the risk of high blood pressure as well as colon cancer. Semi-skimmed milk is recommended for everyone over the age of two (skimmed for dieters).

studies indicate that it may also protect against high blood pressure and colon cancer. Milk also provides high-quality protein, vitamins and other minerals. Three servings a day of milk or other dairy foods are now recommended. One serving is 200ml of milk, 150g of yoghurt or two slices (30g) of cheese.

Milk has two solid components: fat, including fat-soluble vitamins; and non-fat solids, which have carbohydrates, water-soluble vitamins and minerals and proteins. Casein, a protein found only in milk, makes up 82 per cent of the total protein.

Fat-soluble vitamins are lost when cream is skimmed off whole milk; but in the UK, low-fat milk is sometimes fortified with vitamins A and D and calcium. Powdered milk is fortified with vitamin D. Homogenised milk is pressure-treated to break up the fat globules and disperse them evenly.

Types of fresh milk that are readily available include whole milk (3.9 per cent fat), semi-skimmed (1.6 per cent fat) and skimmed (with 0.1 per cent fat). UHT (ultra-high temperature) milk is processed at high temperatures so it can be kept without refrigeration for long periods.

Asians, Afro-Caribbeans and some Westerners lack the enzyme that is needed to digest milk sugar (lactose) and are lactose-intolerant. The answer is to look for lactose-free milk or limit oneself to small amounts of regular milk. In general, lactose-reduced milks taste sweeter than traditional milks. Cow's milk can be allergenic in children so wait for at least a year before introducing it mixed with cereal or in cooking.

Pasteurisation

Almost all milk that is sold in the UK is pasteurised by heating to kill off harmful bacteria. Claims that raw milk is superior to pasteurised milk are not valid. Disease-causing organisms can find their way into unpasteurised milk because of contamination from the cow, its human handlers or from the milking and processing equipment. In the pasteurisation process, milk is heated hot enough and just long enough to kill most micro-organisms without compromising the taste or the nutritional content of the milk.

Most health regulatory bodies urge pregnant women, and people with weakened immune systems, to avoid raw-milk cheeses as harmful bacteria may have survived the cheese-making process.

Storage

When buying milk, note the 'use by' date on the carton. Look for milk dated several days in the future (very often, placed at the back of the chest). Even pasteurised milk contains bacteria and will quickly spoil unless refrigerated. Place milk

towards the back of the refrigerator, where it is colder than in the door. A temperature just above freezing is ideal; however, milk should not be frozen. Milk is very sensitive to light, which rapidly breaks down the riboflavin and causes unpleasant changes in taste.

Cardboard containers preserve their content better than clear plastic or glass; milk stored in bottles should be kept in the dark.

Omega-3 in dairy foods

It is now possible to buy full-cream and semi-skimmed milks (and other dairy products) that have been enhanced by the addition of omega-3 fatty acids. Two 250ml glasses of full-cream milk can supply 50 per cent of the Reference Nutrient Intake (RNI) of omega-3s, and the same amount of semi-skimmed provides up to 30 per cent of the RNI.

Goat's milk

Although it has a more pungent taste than cow's milk, goat's milk is a pleasant alternative to soya or rice-based milk substitutes. It has similar quantities of protein, fat and lactose to cow's milk, but much less vitamin B_{12}. Goat's milk is no better tolerated by people with lactose intolerance or milk allergies than cow's milk.

Chocolate milk

Made from milk with added sugar and cocoa powder, most brands of chocolate milk contain about 1 per cent fat. The amount of sugar in chocolate milk is about the same as is contained in unsweetened orange juice but protective factors in milk reduce the dental hazards inherent in acidic beverages.

▶ **The many faces of milk**
Whether as a drink, yoghurt or one of the many varieties of cheese, milk packs a powerful nutritional punch.

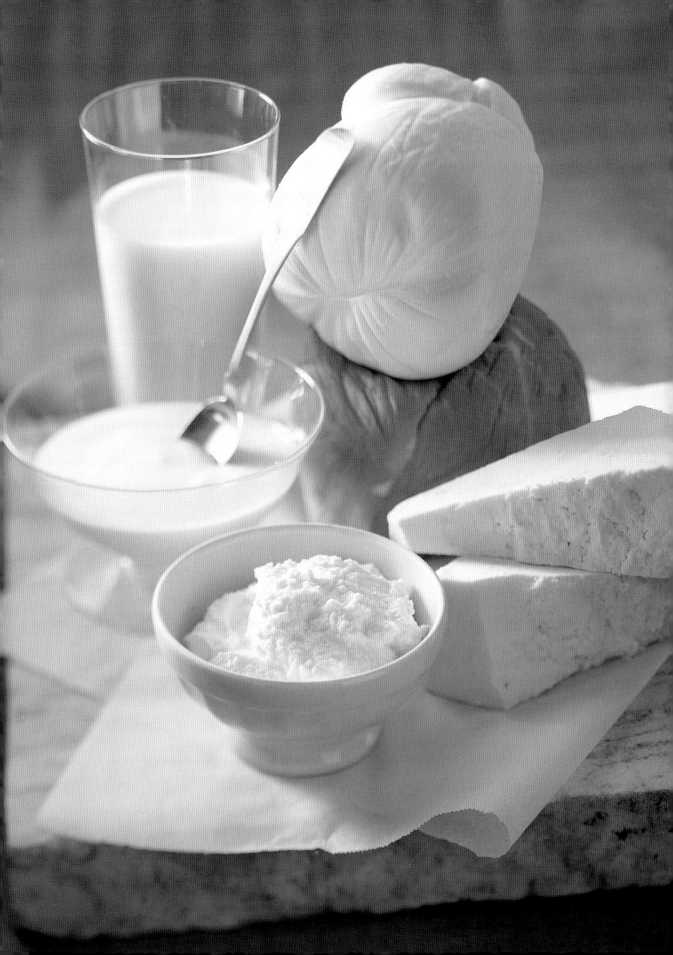

Minerals

All you need to know

Minerals are essential nutrients that your body needs in small amounts in order to work properly. They constitute about 4 per cent of your body weight and perform a variety of functions: they are essential to the architecture of bones and teeth; they are important constituents of body fluids, helping enzymes to work; and they facilitate nerve transmission.

Minerals are generally classified according to daily dietary requirement and fall into two categories: essential minerals (of which the body requires more than 100mg a day) and trace minerals, also called trace elements, of which the body requires less than 100mg a day. Essential minerals include calcium, iron, magnesium, phosporus, potassium, sodium and sulphur. Whether iron belongs in this group is controversial as the Reference Nutrient Intake (RNI) for iron varies with age and sex, but it is usually less than 100mg a day. Some food experts include chloride as an essential mineral, too. Trace elements include boron, cobalt, copper, chromium, fluoride, iodine, manganese, molybdenum, selenium, silicon and zinc.

All these minerals are vital to health and since the body is unable to make them on its own, they must be provided from food.

Other minerals are sometimes listed as trace elements: these include aluminium, arsenic, cadmium, mercury, nickel and vanadium, but there is little evidence that they are of nutritional value, and may even be considered pollutants as they are toxic, even at low levels. However, small doses of arsenic have been shown to send some forms of cancer into remission and may also help to thin the blood.

A varied and balanced diet provides all the essential minerals; supplements are generally not recommended, because many are highly toxic if taken in large amounts. There are a few exceptions – such as during pregnancy, when extra iron may be needed. Also, the mineral content of foods varies according to the composition of the soil where the plants are grown or animals are grazed. Therefore, people may need dietary supplements in areas where the soil is deficient in a particular mineral.

A number of factors influence the body's ability to absorb and metabolise minerals. In general, the body is more efficient in absorbing a mineral during periods of increased need; thus, a person who is anaemic will absorb more iron from the diet than an individual who has a normal reserve of the mineral. Unprocessed bran may bind with some minerals to reduce absorption; in contrast, vitamin C increases the uptake of iron and some other minerals. Most high-fibre foods, on the other hand, provide more minerals than they bind.

THE ESSENTIAL MINERALS

Minerals make up about 4 per cent of normal body weight; most of this comes from the essential minerals that are stored in the bones. But minerals also circulate in the blood.

CALCIUM. The most abundant mineral in the body, calcium weighs in at roughly 1,000g to 1,300g in the typical adult male, compared to 750g with 900g for women. Because calcium is essential for building and maintaining strong bones and teeth, it's not surprising that these structures hold 99 per cent of the body's calcium. This mineral also ensures proper nerve and muscle function as it moves in and out of bone tissue and circulates through the body. Calcium helps to prevent osteoporosis, regulate blood pressure and may reduce the risk of colon cancer.

Milk products are convenient sources of calcium; but they may not be tolerated by people with lactose intolerance. Even in those who are not affected, it is wise to limit dairy intake of these foods. Fortunately, the mineral is also found in fortified soya and rice beverages, canned sardines and salmon (if the bones are eaten), tofu (soya bean curd), broccoli and a variety of other vegetables and fruits. In general, the

▶ Bone builders
Minerals are necessary for proper muscle and nerve function, and for building bones.

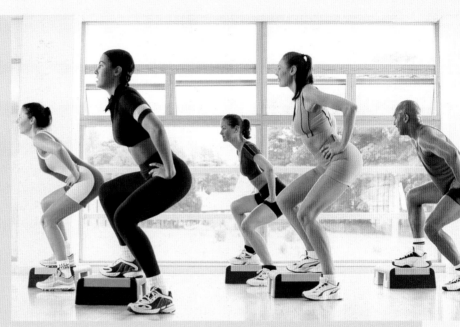

calcium in milk or soft bones is easier to absorb than that in plant foods. Both vitamin D and lactose-containing foods enhance calcium absorption. Phytates found in cereals and oxalates found in vegetables such as spinach and beetroot can interfere with absorption. In the UK, white and brown (but not wholemeal) flour is fortified with calcium, so bread products are a good source of the mineral.

Calcium deficiency can cause rickets in children and a disorder characterised by brittle, porous bones (osteoporosis) in adults. In some cases, calcium deficiency is due to a lack of vitamin D, which the body requires to absorb the mineral. The deficiency may also be a result of physical inactivity, especially complete bed rest, which increases calcium loss.

IRON. The body has only 3g to 5g of iron, 75 per cent of which is in haemoglobin, the pigment in red blood cells that carries oxygen. Iron-deficiency anaemia is the most common nutritional deficiency in developed countries. There are two types of iron: haem is found in red meat, pork, lamb, poultry, fish and other seafood; non-haem is also found in animal products, including eggs, as well as in vegetables, fruit, juices, grains and fortified cereals. About 20 to 30 per cent of haem iron is absorbed; lesser amounts of non-haem iron are absorbed, depending upon need and other dietary factors. Consuming non-haem iron with vitamin C or meat, fish or poultry increases its absorption; bran and the tannins in tea and red wine reduce its absorption. As the body breaks down old red blood cells, it recycles most of their iron.

A healthy adult man loses about 1mg of iron per day; compared with 1.5mg per day in a woman who is still menstruating. Those most likely to develop an iron deficiency are teenagers, menstruating women, pregnant women, preschool children, some athletes and people on restricted diets.

MAGNESIUM. The body contains only about 28g of magnesium, 60 per cent of which is stored in the bones; the rest circulates in the blood or is stored in muscle tissue. Magnesium is essential to build bones and is needed for proper muscle function, energy metabolism, to transmit nerve impulses and to make genetic material and protein.

Magnesium is found in green leafy vegetables, nuts, whole grains, beans and milk.

A deficiency of magnesium is rare. The RNI for magnesium is 300mg for men; 270mg for women, with an extra 50mg needed during lactation. Reserves can be depleted, however, by alcoholism, prolonged diarrhoea, liver or kidney disease, severe diabetes and a poor diet.

PHOSPHORUS. The second most plentiful mineral in the body, phosphorus works in conjunction with calcium and fluoride to give

(continued on page 259)

Do one simple thing

Watch your iron intake

Researchers continue to debate the potential risk of ingesting too much iron. Studies have shown that people with very high levels of iron in their blood are at increased risk of heart problems. In one study healthy men were given high doses of iron and then had their blood flow measured. Researchers found that the normal blood vessel dilation was reduced by as much as a third. Doctors recommend iron supplements only in cases of known deficiency. Consult your GP before taking iron supplements, as excess iron is harmful for those with haemochromatosis – a genetic disorder affecting 1 in 400 people that causes too much dietary iron to be absorbed.

M

All about minerals

MINERAL	BEST FOOD SOURCES	ROLE IN HEALTH
ESSENTIAL MINERALS		
Calcium	Milk and milk products; fortified soya and rice beverages; canned sardines and salmon (including bones); dark green vegetables; some types of tofu.	Builds strong bones and teeth; vital to muscle and nerve function, blood clotting and metabolism; helps to regulate blood pressure.
Magnesium	Leafy green vegetables; legumes and wholegrain cereals and breads; meats, poultry, fish and eggs; nuts, milk.	Stimulates bone growth; necessary for muscle function and metabolism.
Phosphorus	Meat, poultry, fish, egg yolks, legumes, dairy products.	Helps to maintain strong bones and teeth; component of some enzymes; essential for proper metabolism.
Potassium	Avocados, bananas, citrus and dried fruit; legumes and many vegetables; wholegrain products.	Along with sodium, helps to maintain fluid balance; promotes proper metabolism and muscle function.
Sodium	Dairy products, meat, seafood, salt, seasonings, most processed foods.	With potassium, regulates the body's fluid balance; promotes proper muscle function. Excess sodium is a major health problem.
Sulphur	Protein from animal and vegetable sources	Component of two essential amino acids which help to form many proteins in the body. Present in every cell.
Chloride	Seafood, milk, eggs, meat, also a component of salt.	Maintains proper body chemistry. Used to make digestive juices.
TRACE MINERALS		
Chromium	Brewer's yeast, wholegrain products, liver, cheese, chicken, mushrooms, molasses.	Works with insulin to metabolise glucose.
Copper	Liver, shellfish, legumes, nuts, prunes.	Promotes iron absorption; essential to red blood cells, connective tissue, nerve fibres and skin pigment. Component of several enzymes.
Fluoride	Fluoridated water; tea.	Helps to maintain strong bones and teeth.
Iodine	Iodised salt, seafood, foods grown in iodine-rich soil.	Necessary to make thyroid hormones.
Iron	Liver, meat, seafood, tofu, eggs, legumes, fortified cereals, dried fruit, whole grains, leafy greens, nuts and seeds.	Needed to produce haemoglobin, which transports oxygen throughout the body.
Manganese	Tea, nuts, legumes, bran, leafy greens, whole grains, egg yolks.	Component of many enzymes needed for metabolism; necessary for bone and tendon formation.
Molybdenum	Liver and other offal; dark green leafy vegetables; wholegrain products, legumes, nuts.	Component of enzymes needed for metabolism; instrumental in iron storage.
Selenium	Brazil nuts, poultry, seafood, wholegrain products, onions, garlic, mushrooms, nuts, brown rice, offal.	Antioxidant that works with vitamin E to protect cell membranes from oxidative damage.
Zinc	Oysters, meat, yoghurt, milk, eggs, wheatgerm, nuts.	Instrumental in metabolic action of enzymes; essential for growth and reproduction; supports immune function.

The table presents current Reference Nutrient Intakes (RNIs). The RNIs are set to meet the known needs of practically all healthy people Source: Department of Hea

(continued from page 257)

DAILY REFERENCE NUTRIENT INTAKE (RNI) FOR ADULTS OVER 19	
MALES	FEMALES
700mg 19-50+ years	700mg 19-50+ years
300mg	270mg
550mg	550mg
3,500mg	3,500mg
1,600mg	1,600mg
Not set	Not set
2,500mg	2,500mg
Not set; safe intake 25mcg	Not set; safe intake 25mcg
1.2mg	1.2mg
Not set	Not set
140mcg	140mcg
8.7mg	14.8mg 19-50 years 8.7mg 50+
Not set; safe intake 1.4mg	Not set; safe intake 1.4mg
Not set; safe intake 50-400mcg	Not set; safe intake 50-400mcg
75mcg	60mcg
9.5mg	7mcg

bones and teeth their strength and hardness. On average, phosphorus makes up 1 per cent of normal body weight; 85 per cent of this is in the bones, and the remainder is found in soft tissue. Phosphorus is essential for many metabolic processes and the storage and release of energy. It is also essential for the activation of the B-complex vitamins and many enzymes. Foods that are high in calcium also tend to be high in phosphorus; other good sources include meat, fish, eggs and nuts. A deficiency of phosphorus would be very rare.

POTASSIUM. Along with sodium, potassium helps to regulate the body's balance of fluids. Potassium is essential for many metabolic processes; it is also instrumental in the transmission of nerve impulses, proper muscle function and maintaining normal blood pressure. Most plant foods contribute varying amounts of potassium; especially rich sources include dried fruit, bananas, tomatoes, citrus fruits, avocados, potatoes, milk and melons.

Prolonged diarrhoea, vomiting or the use of diuretics to treat high blood pressure can lead to a potassium deficiency; typical symptoms include an irregular heartbeat, muscle weakness and irritability. Caution is necessary when taking potassium supplements, however; an overdose can cause nausea, diarrhoea and serious cardiac arrhythmias that can result in sudden death.

SODIUM. Table salt is composed of sodium and chloride, and the terms salt and sodium are often confused. Sodium is found in all body fluids and is largely responsible for determining the body's total water content. Like potassium, sodium ions help to regulate nerves and muscles. These two electrolytes are responsible for maintaining the fluid balance inside and outside the body cells. Sodium maintains the acid–base balance, sends nerve impulses and helps

M

muscle contraction. Lack of sodium is very rare; overconsumption is much more common. Salt intake is linked to high blood pressure; it can also cause swollen ankles and fingers and other signs of a build-up of body fluids. Sodium occurs naturally in many foods but most of what we consume has been added in processing or food preparation. Added salt is rarely required.

SULPHUR. Most sulphur in the body is obtained as part of the protein intake as well as in three of the B vitamins. An inorganic form of the mineral – sulphites – used to preserve the colour of dried fruits, can trigger asthma attacks. In its pure form, sulphur acts as an anti-fungal and antibacterial agent.

CHLORIDE. A component of table salt, chloride is needed for nerve conduction and to make hydro-chloric acid, which the stomach uses in order to digest food. Almost all diets supply adequate chloride; deficiencies are rare but they may occur during periods of excessive sweating or prolonged vomiting or diarrhoea.

THE TRACE MINERALS

Only very small, or trace, amounts of the following minerals are required in order to meet normal body requirements.

COPPER. A component of many enzymes, copper is essential for making red blood cells, skin pigment, connective tissue and nerve fibres; copper also stimulates the body's absorption of iron. Excessive zinc has been shown to reduce the body's ability to absorb and store copper. A copper deficiency may result in anaemia, deterioration of the heart muscle, inelastic blood vessels, various skeletal defects, nerve degenera-tion, abnormalities of the skin and hair as well as infertility. Liver is the richest source of copper, but the

Myth.......
Chromium supplements build muscle and burn fat.

.......Reality
Short-term use of low doses of chromium are generally harmless, but chromium can affect insulin in the blood and cause the blood sugar level to go too low. Possible side effects of chromium include weight gain, headache, insomnia and other sleep problems, skin irritation and mood changes. High doses can cause severe side effects: for example, diabetics who use chromium may develop kidney problems. Other possible effects include vomiting, diarrhoea, bleeding into the gastrointestinal tract and the worsening of any behavioural or psychiatric problems.

mineral is also found in seafood, legumes, nuts and seeds, prunes and barley. Be careful of using unlined copper pans in cooking. This can result in copper toxicity. Excessive copper in the system can cause severe liver disease and mental deterioration; some metabolic disorders can cause a build-up of copper in the liver and other tissues. People who suffer from Wilson's disease, for example, must take medication in order to eliminate the copper from their body.

CHROMIUM. Insulin and chromium appear to act together to metabolise glucose, the body's major fuel. Brewer's yeast is very high in chromium; other good sources include wheatgerm, wholegrain products, liver, cheese, chicken, mushrooms, peas and molasses. Chromium supplements do not prevent the onset of diabetes and may exacerbate it once it is present.

FLUORIDE. Best known for preventing cavities and other dental disorders, fluoride is also needed to maintain strong bones. Fluoride occurs naturally in some areas; in fact, it was in these regions that the relationship between decreased incidence of tooth decay and fluoride was first noted. Some groups oppose adding fluoride to drinking water. The prevailing scientific opinion, however, is that fluoridating drinking water at current levels is an appropriate health measure and has significantly reduced the incidence of cavities.

IODINE. This mineral has only one known function in humans: it is necessary to make thyroid hormones. An iodine deficiency can result in a goitre; in severe cases, it can lead to hypothyroidism. A baby born to a woman with a severe iodine deficiency may develop cretinism, a type of mental retardation. Seafood, kelp, milk and vegetables grown in iodine-rich soil are good sources of the mineral. Iodised salt is advisable in areas where the soil lacks iodine.

MANGANESE. A component of numerous enzymes, manganese is important for metabolism and is needed to build bones and tendons. Manganese deficiency is unknown in humans, largely because most plant foods contain small amounts. Legumes, nuts, seeds, peas, leafy greens, whole grains, egg yolks and some fruits are good sources.

MOLYBDENUM. Another component of many enzymes, molybdenum helps to regulate iron storage and is instrumental in the production of uric acid. A deficiency of this mineral almost never occurs.

SELENIUM. This very important antioxidant interacts with vitamin E to prevent the free radicals produced during oxygen metabolism from damaging body fat and other tissues. Research is looking at its role in lowering the risk of lung, prostate, stomach and colorectal cancers.

Foods high in selenium include Brazil nuts, some meats and fish, seafood, wholegrain products, oats and brown rice. Plant foods, especially wheat, provide much of the selenium in the diet. Intakes have fallen in the UK with the decline in the use of selenium-rich North-American hard wheats. European wheat has a lowel level. Recommended RNIs are 60mg a day for women and 57mg for men; current intakes average 39mg a day. Selenium toxicity can occur and there have been cases among people taking high doses. Symptoms include nausea, diarrhoea, fatigue, skin and nerve damage and the loss of hair and nails.

ZINC. An essential component of many enzymes, zinc is necessary for some metabolic processes, normal growth and sexual development and proper immune system function. It is also needed to make genetic materials and for proper wound healing. Deficiencies result in increased susceptibility to infection, fatigue, appetite loss, balding and impaired taste. Zinc is found in many foods; especially good sources are red meats, oysters and other seafood, eggs, milk, yoghurt, wheatgerm and nuts. The phytates in some wholegrain products, however, may bind with the zinc they contain and prevent its absorption.

Limit zinc supplements to no more than 25mg a day; excessive amounts can be toxic and can depress the immune system, increasing the susceptibility to infection. Taking large doses of supplementary zinc can interfere with your body's absorption of copper, can reduce HDL cholesterol and impair red blood cell formation.

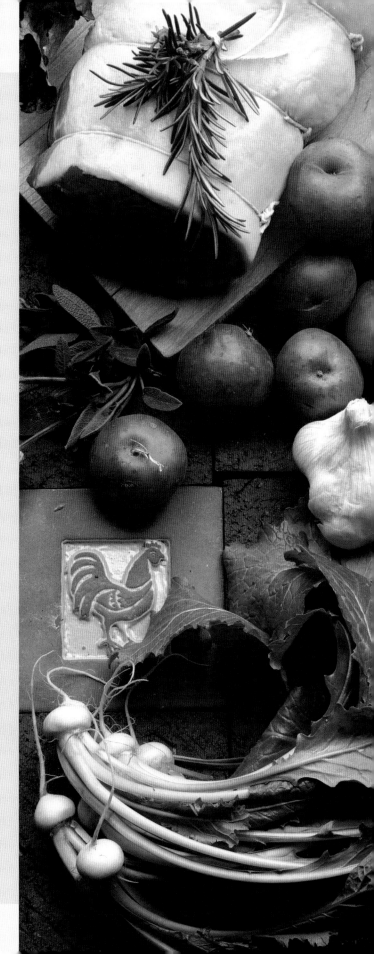

Mononucleosis

See Glandular fever

Mood and diet

CONSUME

- Small meals or snacks throughout the day; do not skip meals
- Foods rich in B vitamins, omega-3 fats and low-GI carbohydrates

AVOID

- Caffeine, alcohol and sugary foods

Everyday foods can affect people's moods quite profoundly. The link between mood and food is complex: nutritional deficiencies, food intolerance and the level of glucose (blood sugar) in the bloodstream can all have an effect. Deficiencies of some of the B vitamins, for example, can result in memory loss and low mood.

Vegetarians and vegans may have vitamin B deficiency and should boost their intake of B vitamins with beans, brown rice, soya products, wholegrain cereals and yeast extract.

'Stressors' and 'supporters'. A survey backed by the mental health charity, Mind, found that eating the right foods could have a profoundly beneficial effect on the moods of the people in the survey. Many foods fell into the category of a stressor – a food that lowered the mood and created negative feelings. The most common foods were sugar, caffeine, alcohol, foods containing wheat, foods with additives in them, dairy products and saturated fats.

Foods that fell into the category of supporters – that had a beneficial effect – were water, vegetables, fruit, oil-rich fish, nuts and seeds, wholegrain foods, fibre, protein and organic foods. Many of the people who took part in the survey said that they felt better when they avoided stressor foods and ate more supporter foods. This bears out the received wisdom that good-quality food has a beneficial effect on the whole person.

The effect of serotonin. The amino acid tryptophan, found in complete proteins, such as meat, milk and eggs, is used by the brain to produce serotonin. This neuro-transmitter not only regulates sleep, but may also play a role in relieving certain types of depression. It has also been claimed that meals rich in carbohydrates can increase the levels of serotonin in the brain. A typical effect of serotonin is the drowsiness that follows a sugary snack or a high-carbohydrate lunch.

Selenium's benefits. Selenium is a mineral which is now thought to have an effect on mood; a low intake of selenium is linked with a greater incidence of depression and low mood. Wheat products provide selenium and intakes have fallen in the UK now that selenium-rich North American hard wheats are no longer imported. European-grown wheat has a lower level of selenium. It is possible to buy bread that has been made with selnium-rich Canadian wheat.

Caffeine. The best-known mood-altering dietary item is caffeine, the stimulant found in coffee, tea, colas and chocolate. While a cup of coffee may be a welcome eye-opener, too much caffeine can cause palpitations, anxiety and sleeplessness.

Limit alcohol. Alcohol is a depressant that slows down certain processes, including respiration, which decreases the supply of oxygen to the central nervous system. Alcohol can actually cause

◀ **A calming meal**
A capsicum stuffed with rice and pine nuts provides the amino acids and carbohydrates used to make soothing brain chemicals.

depression and interfere with sleep, which can cause irritability, anxiety and depression.

Don't skip meals. Eating small amounts of food frequently can keep energy levels and mood more constant. Skipping meals can have a negative effect on mood and energy.

Moods and junk food. There is growing evidence that removing junk food from the diet of various groups of people has a remarkably positive effect. Prisoners whose diet was improved showed a marked improvement in their moods, attitudes and behaviour. Improving the diet in school canteens may prove equally positive. Eating more salads may help, as lettuce is known to have a calming effect.

Comfort food. Chocolate appears to give an instant lift to the spirits and act as an antidepressant, giving the famous 'chocolate high'; the caffeine in it increases alertness.

Mouth ulcers

CONSUME PLENTY OF

- Lean meat, legumes, fortified cereals, dried fruit and other high-iron foods

- Dark green leafy vegetables, wheat germ and legumes for folate

- Animal products for vitamin B_{12}

AVOID

- Salty, spicy and acidic foods, or any other food that worsens symptoms

- Alcohol and very hot beverages

Mouth ulcers with bright red inflamed borders can occur singly or in clusters; they may be aphthous ulcers. Other types of ulcer can be caused by a trauma, such as a jagged tooth, or more serious disorders. Simple aphthous ulcers tend to be acutely painful for the

Do one simple thing

Chew an antacid tablet to relieve the pain

Any non-prescription antacid tablet will do. Or you could hold the tablet on the mouth ulcer and let it dissolve. It will ease pain by neutralising the acids that eat into the ulcer. A damp tea bag will have the same effect.

first few days, last for a week or two and then heal without consequence. Larger ulcers may take months to heal and be accompanied by fatigue, fever and swollen lymph nodes.

Although the cause of mouth ulcers is unknown, doctors believe that an abnormal immune response or a viral infection may be the problem. Stress or local trauma, such as from ill-fitting dentures, may precipitate an attack.

In some cases, mouth ulcers may be a symptom of an allergic reaction to foods, anaemia, coeliac disease, Crohn's disease, cancer or lupus.

A warm salt water wash is one of the best treatments. Your pharmacist will be able to advise on an over-the-counter treatment. For recurrent or severe ulcers, your dentist may prescribe a protective paste to speed the healing.

Mouth ulcers and nutrition

Deficiencies of iron, vitamin B_{12} and folate have been associated with an increased risk of mouth ulcers; mashed potato made with milk will supply B vitamins and should not aggravate the mouth.

During attacks, avoid any food or beverage that may irritate the sores. The most common offenders are hot drinks, alcohol, salty or spicy foods and anything acidic.

Try a diet of bland soft foods. If painful ulcers interfere with eating, try sipping liquid or puréed foods through a straw.

Multiple sclerosis

CONSUME PLENTY OF

- Fibre-rich foods to prevent constipation

- Cranberry juice to ward off cystitis

- Puréed foods to ease swallowing

LIMIT

- Caffeine to avoid bladder irritation

AVOID

- Foods that could cause choking

A chronic, often disabling disease of the central nervous system that mostly strikes people between the ages of 20 and 40, multiple sclerosis (MS) is characterised by the gradual destruction of the myelin sheaths that insulate the nerve fibres, thus robbing nerves of the ability to transmit impulses. Although the symptoms vary depending on where in the brain and spinal cord myelin is destroyed, most people suffer abnormal fatigue, impaired vision, slurred speech, loss of balance and muscle co-ordination, difficulty chewing and swallowing, tremors, bladder and bowel problems and, in severe cases, paralysis.

MS and nutrition

A low-saturated-fat, high-fibre diet that has fruit, vegetables and whole grains can be helpful in managing MS by providing energy and nutrients to maintain and repair tissues, to fight infections and to keep the risk of constipation low.

The Swank diet. Some MS support groups advocate the Swank diet (named after the professor who proposed it in 1950), which eliminates most animal fats. There have been some impressive results from it, but it is not easy to stick to. Several studies have found that essential omega-3 polyunsaturated

M

fats found in seafood and omega-6 fats from vegetable oils and walnuts may be beneficial in treating MS. More studies are under way.

Some more controversial diets that have been proposed for treating MS may lead to unbalanced or poor nutrition. Among them are liquid diets, crash diets that can lead to potassium deficiency, raw food diets, diets that restrict intake of pectin and fructose and gluten-free or no-dairy-food regimens. None of these has been proved effective.

Vitamin B$_{12}$. A deficiency in this vitamin mimics the symptoms of MS, and as it is needed to maintain myelin, there is a possible link. But tests with vitamin B$_{12}$ supplements. have shown no significant benefits.

Antioxidants. Some scientists believe that free radical damage can promote the progression of MS. Antioxidants are believed to counter the effect of these free radicals, so it is prudent to include antioxidant-rich foods in your daily diet. These include fruit and vegetables for vitamin C, beta carotene and many nonvitamin antioxidants; vegetable oils, nuts and seeds for vitamin E; and whole grains, nuts and seafood for selenium.

Vitamin D. Some studies suggest that vitamin D may prevent the progression of the disease or may play other protective roles.

People with MS are also at risk of osteoporosis, and vitamin D plays an important role in lowering this risk. Good food sources include sardines, salmon, herrings, butter and margarine. Studies also show benefits from sunlight. In societies where more milk is drunk, there seems to be a greater incidence of MS; this may be linked to lactose.

The main role of diet in MS is to help people to control symptoms, such as fatigue, constipation, urinary tract infections and problems with eating. A balance

---

Women can cut their risk of MS by 40 per cent with vitamin D

Women are twice as likely as men to develop multiple sclerosis, and they can reduce their risk by 40 per cent simply by consuming a daily dose of vitamin D of about 400 IU or 10mcg – or so a recent Harvard University study shows.

Researchers found that the risk of developing MS was lower with a high vitamin D intake from supplements or from food. Sunlight is also an important source of vitamin D for protection against MS.

---

between healthy diet, exercise and rest can help to minimise fatigue. Eating more frequent but smaller meals helps to provide a constant source of energy.

Managing complications

Watch your weight. It is especially important to maintain a suitable height/weight ratio. Excess weight can add to mobility problems and strain the respiratory and circulatory systems. Skin becomes irritated and breaks down more easily in overweight, relatively inactive people. Being underweight is to be avoided, because it may decrease resistance to infection and increase the risk of developing pressure sores and other skin ulcers.

Fluid intake. Urinary tract infections are often a problem for people with MS, particularly when they have to undergo frequent catheterisations. Drinking cranberry juice increases urinary acidity and may create an environment hostile to bacteria. If urinary incontinence is a problem, people with MS should avoid caffeinated drinks, such as coffee, tea and colas. Caffeine has a diuretic effect and irritates the bladder.

Fibre intake. Constipation is aggravated by an inadequate fluid intake. Plenty of water and fibre-rich

---

foods, such as fruit, vegetables and wholegrain products, encourage good bowel function. Prunes and bran cereal are good breakfast choices.

Avoid problem foods. Some people with MS have problems with bowel incontinence, which may be worsened by diet. Try eliminating coffee, alcohol and spicy foods from the diet for a few days; then reintroduce them one at a time to see if the problem recurs. Because nicotine can stimulate the bowel, it is important not to smoke.

Be careful with food textures. Reduce problems with chewing and swallowing. For example, substitute smoothies, yoghurt, fruit and vegetable purées, thick soups and milky desserts for firm or dry dishes. Serve chopped spinach in place of salad, or diced, stewed fruit instead of a fresh apple or pear. Use a blender or food processor and serve smaller but more frequent meals. Your doctor may recommend a speech therapist for advice about positioning food in the mouth or changing breathing patterns to relieve swallowing difficulties.

Muscle cramps

CONSUME PLENTY OF

- Water to maintain the circulation and help to flush lactic acid and other waste products from the muscles

- Low-fat dairy products for calcium to regulate muscle contractions

- Potassium-rich foods, such as bananas, citrus fruit, dried fruit, tomato juice, cantaloupe, courgettes, potatoes, milk and avocado

- Carbohydrates, such as rice, legumes and pasta, for energy

- Fortified wholegrain cereals for iron and wholegrain breads for B-complex vitamins needed for energy conversion

■ Caffeine in coffee, tea and cola, which can decrease the circulation to muscles

■ Highly salted foods, which can cause fluid retention

■ Smoking, which restricts the blood supply to the muscles

Cramps are painful spasms that mainly affect muscles in the legs and feet. A cramp generally lasts a few minutes and then ends on its own, although massage and stretching can hasten the process, and certain foods may help to prevent its recurrence.

The human body is made up of about 600 groups of muscles, which constitute 40 per cent of an average person's weight. Each muscle is made up of many thousands of long fibres bound together with connective tissue. The bundled fibres can shrink or lengthen, allowing muscles to contract or relax.

How muscles get energy

Most of the fuel necessary for muscular activity comes from glucose, the end-product of carbohydrate metabolism, which is stored as glycogen in the liver and muscles.

Vitamins. The vitamins in the B group are crucial to the process by which energy is derived from carbohydrates, proteins and fats. In fact, our need for thiamin is directly related to the amount of energy we expend.

Minerals. We need iron to form haemoglobin, the blood pigment that supplies muscles with oxygen for energy conversion. Also critically important to muscle function are sodium, potassium and chloride; these minerals are known as electrolytes, because their

electrically charged particles (ions) relay nerve impulses from the brain to the muscles, instructing them when to contract and relax. Calcium is the trigger for muscle contraction. And to come full circle, potassium is stored in the muscles with glycogen and – like glycogen – it is rapidly depleted whenever the muscles undergo a vigorous workout.

When muscles burn glycogen for energy, lactic acid forms as a waste product and remains in the muscle tissue until circulating blood clears it away. During periods of intense exercise, a build-up of lactic acid can cause severe muscle pain. The pain, which is similar to muscle cramps, dissipates with rest, which allows the blood to remove the extra lactic acid.

The correct fluid balance is important in muscle function. The spasms of true cramps may be caused by an inadequate supply of blood to the muscle, overstretching, or an injury. If the fluid volume is too low, the electrolyte balance is thrown off kilter, the kidneys respond by conserving sodium at a high rate, fluid is retained in the tissues and there is not enough circulating fluid to flush out waste products and keep the muscle contraction mechanism working smoothly. There should be enough water to keep electrolytes in

the proper concentration for relaying impulses from the nerves to the muscles, but not too much water, which dilutes the blood and lowers the electrolyte concentration.

Electrolyte depletion is not often a problem, because these minerals are amply supplied by a properly balanced diet. Although the electrolytes are excreted in sweat, the amounts lost are very small, even with heavy perspiration during vigorous activity. The exception is potassium, which is drawn out of body stores along with glycogen.

Managing muscle cramps

People who may suffer from leg cramps include athletes, who deplete their glycogen reserves through intense activity and lose potassium and salt in heavy perspiration; those being treated for hypertension with beta-blocking drugs or diuretics, which increase the amount of potassium excreted in the urine; and women in the later months of pregnancy, who lose larger amounts of potassium in the urine.

Eat lots of high-potassium foods. A daily serving of a high-potassium food – for example,

▶ **Cramp control**
Certain foods are claimed to help to reduce muscle cramps, including yoghurt, pasta, bananas, tomato juice, milk, water, oranges and wholegrain bread.

M

some dried fruit; a glass of tomato juice, citrus juice or milk; a slice of melon, an orange or a banana – can help to banish leg cramps and prevent their recurrence. Caffeine and nicotine constrict blood vessels, decreasing the circulation to the muscles and contributing to cramps. If cramps are a problem and you smoke, make every effort to quit; also switch to decaffeinated beverages.

People confined to bed rest or chair rest for extended periods often suffer leg cramps. Apart from dietary measures, the best remedy is regular exercise to tone the muscles and improve the circulation. Try curling and uncurling the toes a dozen times in quick succession; or straighten the leg, bend the foot upwards, and then extend it and point the toes a dozen times in quick succession. Repeat these exercises throughout the day.

Occasional cramps that abate within a few minutes are no cause for concern. Frequent or prolonged cramps or spasms accompanied by other symptoms, particularly in older adults, should be evaluated by a doctor. Quinine can sometimes bring relief from muscle cramps, but the amount in tonic water is insufficient.

Restless legs

Some people are awakened during the night by a jerking of their leg muscles; others suffer an aching, uneasy sensation that doctors call 'restless legs syndrome'.

Some medications that affect the nervous system may cause these conditions; often, they occur with no apparent cause. A dietitian may detect iron, folate or magnesium deficiencies and recommend adding iron-rich foods to the diet or taking supplements. In some cases, drugs may help; getting out of bed and walking or frequently changing positions may give some relief.

Mushrooms and truffles

BENEFITS

- Fat-free and very low in calories
- Useful source of copper and some B vitamins
- Some are rich in plant chemicals, which may boost immune function

DRAWBACKS

- Wild mushrooms may be poisonous
- Truffles are expensive

All types of mushrooms, as well as truffles, are classified as fungi. They are primitive plants that cannot obtain energy through photosynthesis and therefore draw their nutrients from humus, the partially decomposed tissues of more complex vegetation. Many varieties of fungi live symbiotically with trees. The fungus draws sugars from the tree roots, while at the same time supplying the tree with minerals, such as phosphorus, which it gets from the soil more efficiently than the tree can.

Mushrooms and truffles have another unique feature. Their cell walls are made of chitin, the same material that forms the external skeleton of insects. By contrast, higher plants' cell walls are made of cellulose, which we value not as a

Did you know?

Mushrooms grow like magic

If not picked, a white button mushroom will double in size every 24 hours. First it becomes a closed cup mushroom, then the cup opens to show the brown gills. If left undisturbed, it grows on to become a large flat mushroom with open gills. As the mushroom increases in size, its flavour increases.

Truffles: an expensive delicacy

Defying all attempts to cultivate them, truffles grow underground among the roots of certain trees such as oaks or beeches. Their pervasive, earthy scent is due to the hormone androstenol – which some claim is identical to the one secreted in the saliva of male pigs. Trained sows are more efficient than dogs at rooting up the prized fungus in the truffle-growing regions of France and Italy.

nutrient (we can't digest cellulose) but as fibre that promotes the elimination of digestive waste.

Used in every age and culture as food, mushrooms have also served as medicines and as stimulants or hallucinogens. Evidence that Stone Age humans used dried mushrooms as tinder was provided by 5,000-year-old Oetzi, the Iceman, whose body was discovered in the Tyrolean Alps.

Many varieties

The common white mushroom, *Agaricus bisporus*, was first cultivated by the French more than 300 years ago in abandoned gypsum quarries near Paris. Today, mushrooms are cultivated on beds of manure, straw and soil in buildings controlled for temperature and humidity. Only recently has it become possible to cultivate a number of other species on a commercial scale and a wide range of mushrooms is now offered by many supermarkets, including brown varieties such as portobellos, the delicate brown or grey oyster, orange chanterelles, the chewy shiitakes with their dark brown caps and white gills, the crisp white enokis with their long, thin stems and tiny caps and the ominously black but perfectly safe trumpets of death. Although cultivated, many varieties, especially the popular portabello mushroom, manage to preserve much of the rich, earthy flavour of field mushrooms.

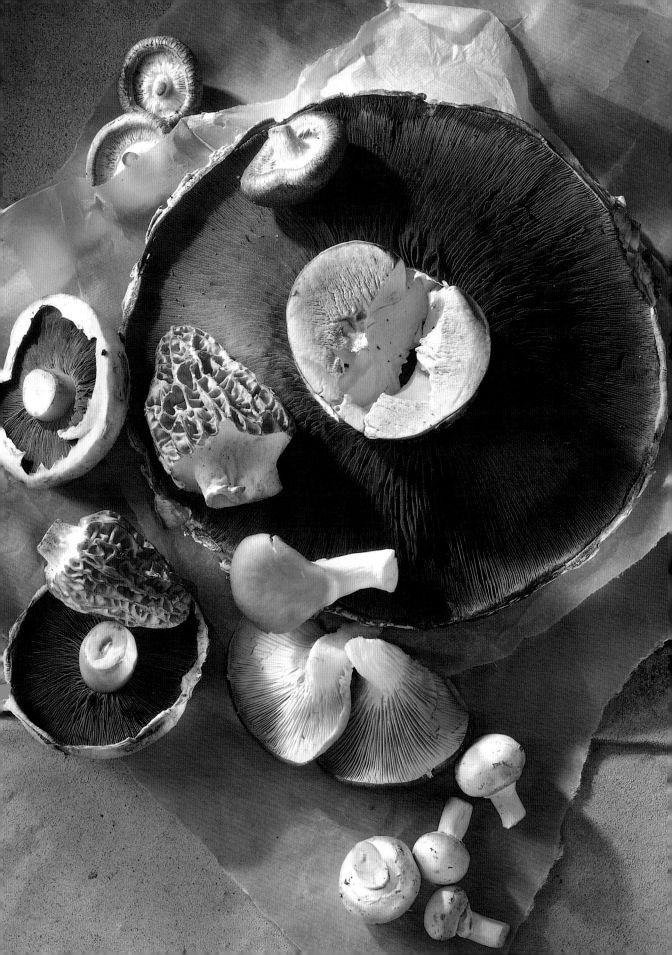

Mushroom advice

- When buying mushrooms, look for firm buttons with no bruises. All mushrooms are hand picked, but bruise easily. Handle them carefully.
- Flavour develops as the mushrooms grow, so the largest of any variety have the most flavour.
- Don't store mushrooms in cling wrap or plastic. Place them in paper or cloth bags and store in the vegetable crisper of the refrigerator.
- Five days should be the maximum storage time in the refrigerator.
- Wipe mushrooms just before using them, but do not peel them or remove the stalks. The nutrition of mushrooms is just under the skin and will be lost by peeling. Just slice, quarter or chop with the skins intact.
- Cook mushrooms quickly. If using them in a slow-cooking dish such as a casserole, add the mushrooms for the last 20 minutes.

With its firm, meaty texture, the portabello is especially suitable for barbecuing and can take the place of meat in a meal. Many other mushroom varieties, including cèpes and tree-ears, are available dried.

Their concentrated glutamic acid – a naturally occurring form of monosodium glutamate (MSG) – makes mushrooms natural flavour enhancers in many dishes.

Warning: Many common species of wild mushroom produce toxins that are quickly lethal whether eaten raw or cooked. Because there is no feature that readily distinguishes dangerous mushrooms, and inedible varieties often closely resemble edible ones, never gather or eat wild mushrooms unless a mushroom expert has identified them as safe.

Nutritional value

A good substitute for meat in many recipes, mushrooms can be cooked with grains to make a meatless 'meat' loaf. They are also appetising and nutritious on their own. Extremely low in calories (100g contains only 13kcal), mushrooms are virtually fat-free and a valuable source of dietary fibre. The same amount of mushrooms provide 30 per cent of the Reference Nutrient Intake (RNI) of copper and useful amounts of the B vitamins such as B_2, niacin, B_6 and folate. Fourteen button mushrooms, or 4 heaped tablespoons of sliced mushrooms will count as one of the fruit and vegetable portions we are should eat every day.

Mushrooms are a long-time staple of many Asian diets, and Japanese scientists have taken the lead in investigating their possible health benefits. Japanese studies have shown that certain mushrooms may favourably influence the immune system, with potential benefits in fighting cancer, infections and such auto-immune diseases as lupus and rheumatoid arthritis. This effect may be related to the high content of glutamic acid, an amino acid that seems to be instrumental in fighting infections, among other immune functions. Shiitake mushrooms contain lentinan, a phytochemical that may help to boost immune activity, as well as eritadenine, which may help to lower cholesterol by promoting cholesterol excretion. Other compounds in shiitakes are being studied for their role in lowering heart disease and cancer risk as well as high blood pressure. All mushrooms contain good amounts of potassium, which can have a positive effect in lowering blood pressure. In addition, tree-ear mushrooms, used in many Chinese dishes, inhibit blood clotting and are thought to lower cholesterol. This may prove valuable in treating some heart diseases.

Researchers at Beckman Research Institute in California have early laboratory findings that suggest substances in the common white mushroom (*Agaricus bisporus*) slow an enzyme used in the production of oestrogen, which may promote cancer in postmenopausal women. More tests are still needed.

Toxins

Mushrooms contain toxins that are reduced by cooking – but they still give off poisonous fumes. The common white button mushroom contains trace amounts of the carcinogen agaritine, but cooking decreases the effect. Scientists have found that most naturally occurring carcinogens cause cancer only when long-term, high doses are taken and that they pose no risk to humans.

Truffles

These gourmet fungi, essential to haute cuisine for their unique flavour, have defied all attempts at commercial cultivation. They grow underground, usually around beech trees, and are sniffed out by trained pigs or dogs. The black or Périgord truffle and the white or Italian truffle are outstanding varieties. They are eaten in such small quantities, however, that their nutritional value if negligible.

CAUTION

Some wild mushrooms, although safe to eat on their own, can be deadly when consumed with alcohol.

M

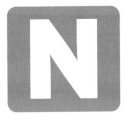

Nail problems

CONSUME PLENTY OF

- Lean meat, poultry and fish for iron and high-quality protein
- Citrus fruit for vitamin C
- Dark green leafy vegetables, whole-grain products, legumes and fruit juices for folate and other B vitamins

AVOID

- Overuse of nail polish removers and other harsh chemicals

Many nail problems stem from abuse – from picking and biting to the overuse of nail polish removers, glues and other harmful chemicals. In rare cases, however, unhealthy nails reflect a nutritional deficiency or an underlying medical problem.

Normally, nails grow about 3mm a month, although illness, age and even cold weather slow the rate of growth. Nails are composed of keratin, the same hard protein that forms the outer layer of skin (the epidermis) and hair. The visible portion, called the nail plate, rests over the tips of the fingers and toes and grows out of the lunula, the pale half-moon at its base. The cuticle acts as a protective seal between skin and nail. Only the lunula is living tissue; the rest is made of dead cells.

Even though nails are mostly dead tissue, they are an important indicator of a person's state of health; this is the reason a doctor carefully examines them for clues to many diseases. Soft, spoon-shaped nails that curve upwards, for example, point to iron-deficiency anaemia. Rounded, club-shaped nails indicate either impaired circulation or a lung disorder; thickened, discoloured nails may be due to a fungal infection; psoriasis can cause pitting; and horizontal ridges may indicate a systemic infection or debilitating illness.

Healthy nails are strong and smooth, with a pinkish cast. Just like hair, they need moisture for flexibility; without it, they become yellowish and break or chip easily. Nails require a steady supply of oxygen and other nutrients to remain healthy. But because the body efficiently delivers nutrients to where the need is greatest, and as the nails are not vital organs, they are one of the first parts to be neglected if there is greater demand elsewhere in the body.

Many of the nail problems that reflect diseases and nutritional deficiencies disappear when the underlying condition is corrected. In order to make keratin, the

Nail conditioners

Brittle and splitting nails are often caused by excessive dryness, which increases with age and is exacerbated by exposure to detergents and other chemicals. Soaking the fingers in water, then applying a moisturising hand cream or a special nail conditioner can restore lost moisture and prevent further loss. Application of nail hardeners may also help to seal in moisture and provide a protective hard surface over the nails. Dermatologists generally recommend protein hardeners or products that contain nylon rather than ones made with formaldehyde, which causes adverse reactions in some people.

● **Myth.......**
Gelatine, calcium or zinc supplements aid nail health.

.......Reality ●
These nutritional supplements, promoted as nail builders, healers and hardeners, have little if anything to do with nail health. In reality, gelatine is an incomplete protein and lacks the amino acids to give nails strength. Nails contain very little calcium, so taking supplements will not enhance their growth or strength. And the same is true of zinc. In the past, the white spots that sometimes develop in nails have been attributed to a zinc deficiency. Those spots, however, are usually caused by an injury, and taking zinc will not get rid of them.

body needs high-quality protein from lean meat, poultry, fish, seafood and other animal products; a combination of grain products and legumes will also supply complete protein.

You may need iron-rich foods. A more common nutrition-related problem involves iron-deficiency or other anaemias, in which the blood does not deliver adequate nutrients to the nails. Increasing the consumption of iron-rich foods – lean meat, poultry, fish, seafood, dried apricots and enriched cereals – may be enough to cure mild iron-deficiency anaemia. A doctor should be consulted, however, to determine whether the anaemia is due to other nutritional deficiencies or to chronic hidden bleeding. (Never self-treat with iron supplements; they can lead to toxicity and many other serious problems.) Vitamin C helps the body to absorb iron from plant sources; so a balanced diet should include citrus fruit and a variety of other fresh fruit and vegetables.

Try folate. Some types of anaemia that affect the nails are caused by a deficiency of folate, an essential B vitamin. Whole

N

grains, legumes, dark green leafy vegetables, peas, nuts and orange juice are good sources of folate and other important B vitamins.

▶ **Succulent sweetness**
Nectarines continue to ripen after they are picked, so choose firm fruits when you buy.

Nectarines

BENEFITS

■ A good source of vitamin C

■ Provide some potassium

■ Contain pectin, a soluble fibre

Sweeter and more nutritious than peaches, their genetic cousin, nectarines were named after the Greek god Nekter; their juice was later called the drink of the gods. This juicy fruit, which is often described as being like a peach without the fuzz, is available with white or yellow flesh. One medium-sized nectarine (about 150g) has 60kcal and provides 56mg vitamin C, which is more than 100 per cent of the Reference Nutrient Intake (RNI) and 250mg of potassium. The yellow-fleshed nectarines also have small amounts of beta carotene.

The flesh of nectarines is rich in antioxidants – especially carotenoids – that help to protect against cancer and other diseases by reducing the cellular damage that occurs when the body burns carbohydrates, fats or proteins. Nectarines are also contain pectin, a soluble fibre that may help to control blood cholesterol levels. The skins contribute insoluble fibre, which helps to prevent constipation.

Cutting or peeling a nectarine releases an enzyme that causes a darkening of the flesh. The fruit may look a little less appetising, but the browning doesn't alter its flavour or nutritional value. This discolouring process can be slowed by dipping the fruit in a little lemon or lime juice.

Selecting the best

Buy fruit that is moderately firm but brightly coloured. The fruit is ready to eat when the flesh yields to gentle pressure and has a sweet, fruity fragrance. Reject nectarines that are hard or have a greenish skin. These were obviously harvested too early, and even though they will soften, they will never achieve peak sweetness and flavour.

Neuralgia

EAT PLENTY OF

■ Lean meat, poultry, eggs and low-fat dairy products for vitamin B_{12}, and breads and wholegrain cereals for thiamin; also eat spinach, potatoes and melons for vitamin B_6

■ Vegetable oils, nuts, seeds, avocado, wheatgerm and wholegrain foods for vitamin E

AVOID

■ Alcohol in all forms

Neuralgia is an umbrella term for any type of throbbing pain that extends along the course of one or more of the peripheral nerves. Neuralgia is classified by both the part of the body affected and the cause. In some cases, doctors can't find a cause; in others, the cause is an infection or underlying disease, such as arthritis, diabetes or syphilis. Tumours, both cancerous and benign, can cause neuralgia, as do structural problems in which nerves become compressed or pinched. Sciatica, the throbbing pain that can extend from the lower back and buttocks to the feet, is one of the most common examples. Various medications, as well as toxins, can also produce neuralgia.

Keep up vitamin B_6 levels. The long-term use of hydralazine (a powerful antihypertensive) or isoniazid (used in the treatment of tuberculosis) can result in vitamin B_6 deficiency, manifested by sensory loss and neuralgia. Anyone taking these drugs should follow a diet that provides extra B_6; good sources include lean meat, poultry, fish, spinach, sweet and white potatoes, watermelon, bananas and prunes. **Warning**: Self-treating with high doses can damage sensory nerves.

Don't neglect vitamin B_{12}. A deficiency of vitamin B_{12}, found only in animal-based products, can lead to degeneration of the spinal cord and widespread neuralgia, as well as pernicious anaemia. Most B_{12} deficiencies are due to a lack of intrinsic factor, a substance made by the stomach that is necessary to absorb the vitamin. A strict vegetarian diet can also result in vitamin B$_{12}$ deficiency. However, if you suspect you need any of the B vitamins, take a vitamin B complex supplement.

In rare cases, malabsorption problems resulting in low vitamin E levels can cause a type of neuralgia. Doctors usually give supplements of 30mg to 100mg a day; good dietary sources include nuts, seeds, wheatgerm, vegetable oils, eggs, poultry and seafood.

Nuts and seeds

BENEFITS

- Rich in minerals such as potassium, calcium, iron, magnesium and zinc

- Many are good sources of vitamin E, folate, niacin and other B vitamins

- A good source of protein and essential fats

DRAWBACKS

- High in calories

- Nut and seed oils can turn rancid

- Peanuts may trigger allergic reactions

- May cause choking in small children and people with swallowing problems

- Moulds in peanuts and other nuts may produce cancer-causing aflatoxins

Nuts and seeds are the embryos of various trees, bushes and other plants. They are packed with all the nutrients needed to grow an entire new plant and have been valued for their nutritional content since prehistoric times.

Coconuts are the world's leading nut crop, followed by peanuts, which are actually legumes but often classified and consumed as nuts. Nuts of all kinds are highly nutritious and research has linked nut consumption with a variety of health benefits.

Nutritional value

Most nuts and seeds are a rich source of vitamins, especially folate, B vitamins and vitamin E; minerals such as iron, calcium, magnesium, manganese, phosphorus, selenium, zinc and potassium; fibre; essential fatty acids; plant compounds such as flavonoids; as well as plant sterols.

Certain nuts are higher in certain nutrients. A 50g serving of almonds, hazelnuts, peanuts, pine nuts or pistachios provides more than 340mg of potassium – about the same as a banana.

A 30g serving of almonds provides over 70 per cent of the Reference Nutrient Intake (RNI) of vitamin E and a similar serving of hazelnuts has slightly more. Nuts and seeds are one of the best food sources of vitamin E, an important antioxidant that enhances the immune system, protects cell membranes, and helps to make red blood cells.

A 50g serving of cashews contains 3mg of iron; pine nuts or pistachios have 2mg. Pumpkin, sesame seeds and linseeds are also good sources. A 50g portion of almonds has 120mg of calcium in it, making it a useful source of calcium, particularly for people who are on dairy-free diets.

Most nuts and seeds also contain magnesium, phosphorus and zinc, as well as B vitamins such as niacin, thiamin and folate; 50g of sunflower seeds contains 100 per cent of the RNI for thiamin, and just 30g of peanuts contains 33mcg of folate – 17 per cent of the RNI – along with useful amounts of potassium, zinc, magnesium, copper and selenium. Peanuts also contain resveratrol (the beneficial substance found in red wine) as well as other antioxidants.

Brazil nuts are high in the anti-oxidant selenium. Just three nuts provides 100 per cent of the RNI for this mineral.

Walnuts are especially rich in ellagic acid, an antioxidant that may inhibit the growth of cancer cells. Walnuts are also rich in omega-3 fatty acids. In one study men and women with high cholesterol levels

N

added walnuts to a healthy Mediterranean diet. Their LDL cholesterol and heart disease risk both dropped.

Hazelnuts are rich in vitamin E, fibre and copper and contain iron, zinc and potassium. Just 30g of sunflower seed kernels contains more than 100 per cent of the RNI of vitamin E. Sunflower seeds are also rich in selenium, copper, fibre, iron and zinc.

Most nuts provide good amounts of protein. With the exception of peanuts, however, they lack lysine, an essential amino acid necessary to make a complete protein. This amino acid can easily be obtained by combining nuts with beans and pulses in the same meal. Nuts can provide a good source of protein in a vegetarian diet.

Peanuts, in particular, provide an inexpensive source of protein and are rich in monounsaturated fats.

Finally, most nuts and seeds are a good source of dietary fibre. With most nuts, a 50g serving provides about 4g to 5g of fibre.

Facts about nuts

- Peanuts are legumes, not nuts, and they grow underground – hence their other name, ground nuts.

- Gathered from trees in the Amazon basin, Brazil nuts are rarely cultivated.

- There are two varieties of almond – the edible type is sweet; the inedible, or bitter, almond contains a form of cyanide.

- Pistachios have a light brown shell and pale green flesh.

- Weight for weight, both pumpkin and sesame seeds have more iron than lamb's liver does.

- Betel nuts are frequently chewed by many Asians despite the probability that they contain a carcinogen and are likely to be responsible for numerous cases of oral cancer.

Health benefits

Researchers have been investigating the potential health benefits of nuts, such as their cholesterol-lowering effects, their association with a lower risk of stroke and their role in weight management.

Their healthy qualities may be attributed to their fatty acid profile along with their protein, fibre, vitamin E and magnesium content.

Nuts also contain plant sterols that can lower cholesterol and may offer some protection against cancer.

Several large studies have found that a regular intake of nuts protects against heart disease.

The Nurses' Health Study found that women who ate more than 140g of nuts per week had a 35 per cent lower risk of heart attack and death from heart disease compared with those who never ate nuts or ate them less than once a month.

The Physician's Health Study found that men who ate nuts two or three times per week had a 47 per cent reduced risk of sudden death from cardiac arrest compared with those who rarely or never ate nuts.

And several studies show that almonds and other nuts significantly lowered levels of LDL cholesterol in those who already had elevated cholesterol levels.

The issue of fats

Nuts and seeds tend to have a high fat content but, with the exception of coconuts and palm nuts, the fats are mostly mono or poly-unsaturated. These are considered to be heart-friendly fats, especially when they replace saturated fats. In most research, nuts and seeds have had the best effect when used as a substitute for, not an addition to, highly saturated fats. However, being high in fat, nuts are also extremely calorific and should therefore be eaten in moderation.

For example, macadamia nuts have more than 748kcal per 100g; pecans are a close second. Other nuts and seeds contain from 595kcal to 666kcal per 100g. Peanuts contain around 560kcal per 100g. Chestnuts are the exception; 100g contains only 170kcal.

Store nuts in their shells in cool, dry conditions, because they are prone to contamination with moulds. Imported nuts with a trace of mould on the shell or kernel may be contaminated with poisonous substances called mycotoxins.

Mouldy nuts from tropical countries are especially dangerous if they contain highly carcinogenic mycotoxins, called aflatoxins, which may cause liver cancer. Peanurts are particularly prone to this form of contamination and, even though those imported into Britain are routinely checked for these moulds, it is safest to eat only peanuts that are sold in packets. Never eat the peanuts sold for use in bird food.

Refrigerate or freeze shelled nuts; their oil quickly turns rancid. They can be taken out and used as you need them, and won't take long to thaw at room temperature.

Other problems

Some nuts, especially peanuts provoke allergic reactions in many people. Symptoms range from a tingling sensation in the mouth to hives and, in extreme cases, to anaphylaxis, a life-threatening emergency. But because the different varieties are not closely related, a person who is allergic to walnuts, for example, may be able to eat another type of nut or seed.

Warning: Choking deaths are often traced to nuts. Young children and those who have difficulty in chewing and swallowing should not be given nuts at all, even if they are finely chopped.

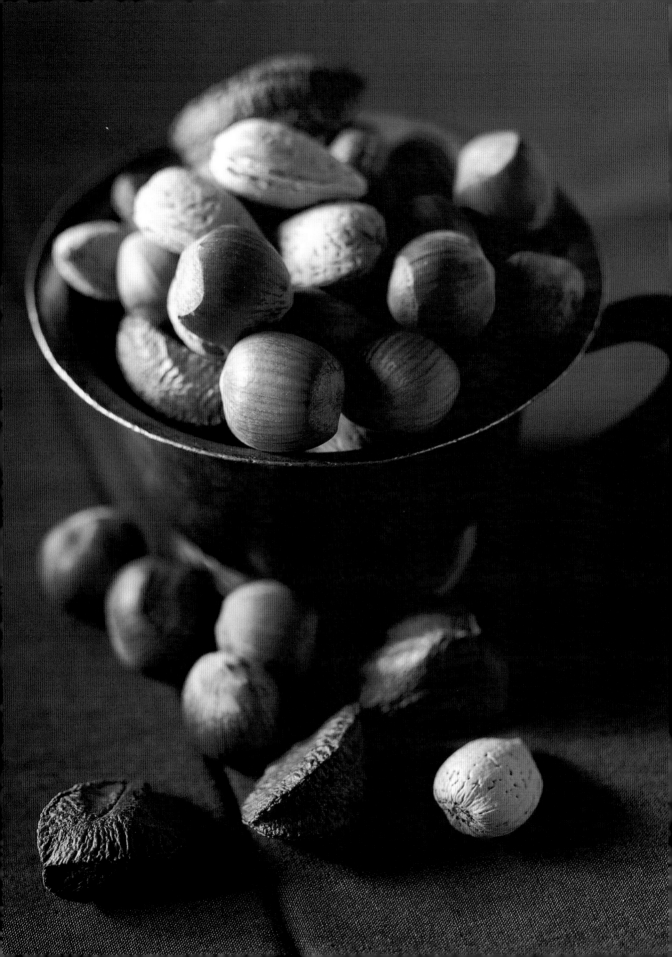

Oats

BENEFITS

■ An excellent source of soluble fibre

■ A source of iron, manganese, zinc and vitamin E, thiamin, niacin, riboflavin, folate and other B vitamins

Rolled oats and other wholegrain oat products such as oat bran and oat flakes are a tasty, convenient, versatile and economical source of nutrients and phytochemicals. Commonly used as a breakfast cereal and in baking, oats can be added to many dishes, including burgers and fish cakes, and can be used to thicken soups and sauces, to add a lighter texture to stuffing, or as a topping for fruit crumble. Oats have good effects on cholesterol, blood pressure, blood sugar and gastrointestinal health.

On a weight for weight basis, oats contain a higher concentration of protein, fat, manganese, thiamin, folacin and vitamin E than other unfortified whole grains. Oats also contain polyphenols and saponins, powerful antioxidants with disease-fighting properties.

Health benefits

Oat bran is high in beta-glucan, a soluble fibre that can help to lower blood cholesterol levels, possibly reducing the risk of heart attacks. To reduce blood cholesterol by roughly 5 per cent and lower heart attack risk by about 10 per cent, a person needs to eat 3g of beta-glucan a day – the amount found in 100g of oats. The inclusion of oats as a part of a diet low in saturated fats, and as part of a healthy lifestyle, can help to reduce blood cholesterol. Some studies have shown that oats not only lower LDL cholesterol but may also boost levels of the protective HDL cholesterol.

Regular consumption of rolled oats may reduce the risk of heart disease in women in other ways than through cholesterol reduction. The Nurses' Health Study found that those who ate oats five or more times per week had a heart disease risk reduction of 29 per cent. The authors suggest that there is more to this effect than just the soluble fibre: antioxidants may also play a role. Oats contain a unique blend of antioxidants, including the avenanthramides that prevent LDL cholesterol (the 'bad' cholesterol) from being converted into the oxidised form that damages arteries. And Yale University researchers have found that eating a large bowl of oatmeal may counter the harmful reduction in blood flow that may happen after eating a high-fat meal.

Oats take a long time to digest and therefore keep you feeling full longer. It is thought that both the protein and fibre in oats contribute to this effect. In one study that compared rolled oats with a sugared flaked cereal for breakfast, the researchers found that subjects who ate oats at breakfast consumed a third fewer calories for lunch, thus helping with weight management.

Oats can also help to reduce blood pressure. A study in Minnesota looked at a group of people who were taking medication for high blood pressure. Half of them were asked to eat about 5g of soluble fibre a day in the form of one and a half cups of oatmeal and an oat-based snack, while the other half ate cereals and snacks with little soluble fibre. The people who were eating the oats showed a significant reduction in blood pressure.

Oats also have been shown to reduce both blood sugar and insulin levels, an important asset in controlling diabetes. Human studies confirm that oat-soluble fibre reduces after-meal blood sugar and insulin in both healthy people and people with diabetes.

Although there is a very small amount of gluten in oats, many people with coeliac disease find that oats don't cause the same problems that other gluten-containing foods do. Current advice is to introduce small amounts into the diet to see if there is any adverse reaction; limit the amount to no more than 50g a day. Children and severe sufferers of coelic disease should discuss it with a doctor before eating oats.

There are many varieties of oats:
• Rolled oats are minimally processed – only the outer hull is removed. They are very nutritious but they are chewy and must be soaked before cooking.

- In the UK, rolled oats are also called oatmeal, rolled oatmeal or old-fashioned oats. They are steamed, rolled and flaked so that they cook quickly.
- Instant oats consist of very thin, precooked oat flakes that need only to be mixed with a hot liquid. They often have salt and flavourings added.

Obesity

EAT MODERATE AMOUNTS OF

- Healthy carbohydrates, such as wholegrain pasta, potatoes, unrefined rice, legumes and wholegrain products for energy, vitamins and fibre
- Fresh vegetables and fruit for vitamins and minerals
- Fish, skinless poultry and lean meat for high-quality protein and minerals

AVOID

- High-calorie items, such as sweets, chocolate, pastries, fatty meats, sweet fizzy drinks, alcohol and potato crisps

Obesity is the most common nutritional disorder in the Western world. In the UK, 44 per cent of adults are overweight and by 2010, one in three will be obese. The number of obese and overweight children has risen to 22 per cent and the incidence of Type 2 diabetes in children (normally seen only in overweight adults) is increasing.

Many experts believe that it is not just the amount of fat but also its distribution that is a key factor in the risk to health. For example, excess abdominal fat has been linked to other, more serious health problems, including heart disease, stroke and Type 2 diabetes, than has fat in the hips and thighs. This is because the liver converts more of the abdominal fat into forms that circulate in the bloodstream.

Few people are truly 'fat and happy'; obesity can have devastating effects on health. Because slimness is highly valued in our culture, people who are overweight often have a poor self-image and are subjected to discrimination.

Obesity can also cause physical problems such as shortness of breath, skin chafing and difficulty moving around, making it hard to enjoy a normal life. Obese people have an increased risk of coronary heart disease, high blood pressure, stroke, diabetes, gallstones and certain types of cancer. Other health consequences include damage to the weight-bearing joints. This leads to osteoarthritis and disability, which perpetuate the vicious circle by restricting movement, leading to further weight gain. Obesity is frustrating and often difficult to overcome. Newspaper and magazine articles and advertisements attest to the constant demand for safe, sure and rapid weight loss.

Causes of obesity

If we eat more than we need, the surplus food is converted into, and stored as, fat.

Watch empty calories. No foods need to be totally forbidden, but empty calories in alcohol, sweetened fizzy drinks, sugary desserts and high-fat, high-salt snack foods should be avoided. Weight loss is its own reward. As weight is shed, the urge to lose more will grow and the desire for fatty, sugary foods will gradually fade.

Eating too much food and exercising too little are the key factors. One theory holds that each person has a biological set point for his or her 'ideal' weight, and that the body adjusts its metabolism to maintain this set point whenever the person eats more or less than is expended. This set-point theory may be valid; nevertheless, research

Assessing body weight

The most widely accepted methods to assess weight and body fat are body mass index (BMI) and waist circumference.

BODY MASS INDEX

To calculate your BMI (metric):

1. Measure your weight in kilograms (kg).
2. Measure your height in metres and square it.
3. Divide your weight in kilograms by your height in metres squared. **BMI = kg/m²**

To calculate your BMI (imperial):

1. Measure your weight in pounds (lb).
2. Measure your height in inches and square it.
3. Divide your weight in pounds by your height in inches squared and multiply by 703. **BMI = lb/in² x 703**

BMI CATEGORIES

- Underweight = less than 18.5
- Normal weight = 18.5 to 24.9
- Overweight = 25 to 29.9
- Obesity = 30 or greater

WAIST CIRCUMFERENCE

An accumulation of fat around the abdomen is closely related to increased health risk. Measure midway between your lower rib and the top of your hip bone (about level with your navel).

Men with waist measurements of 94cm (37in) are at increased risk. When their measurements go up to 102cm (40in) they are in the high risk category. For women, increased risk starts when the waist measures 80cm (32 in) and becomes high risk when the waist measurement goes up to 88cm (35in).

Did you know?

Obesity is linked to cancer risk

Women who gain 20kg or more after the age of 18 are twice as likely to develop breast cancer after the menopause than those who remain approximately the same weight.

shows that we can reset our set point through gradual weight loss and increased physical activity.

Set a good example. Obesity often seems to run in families, but probably not because it is in the genes, but because it is in the lifestyle: parents who overeat, themselves, encourage overeating in their children. It is true that fat cells are laid down in childhood and are likely to remain for a lifetime. They may grow larger or smaller to accommodate fat stores, but the number usually remains the same. That's why a person who was obese as a child may always store fat more readily than a person who started life thin.

Because metabolism slows with age, some put on weight as they approach middle age. Older people also may be less active; in either case, calorie needs decline with age, and a person's food intake should be scaled back accordingly.

Controlling obesity

The biggest challenge is not losing weight but keeping it off. Most dieters regain all the weight they've lost within one to five years. The only successful route to permanent weight loss is a combination of exercise and diet.

However, anyone who is 20 per cent or more above their ideal weight should see a doctor before embarking on any exercise plan or diet. Very low-calorie diets or fad diets usually lead to the yo-yo

phenomenon, in which people lose weight, then quickly regain all they've lost and a lot more. The additional weight is often even harder to shed.

Limit calories. A diet providing about 1,400kcal a day for a woman and 1,800kcal for a man is a reasonable approach. Combined with a moderate exercise programme, it should allow a loss of 0.5kg (about a pound) a week. Since the aim is to find a diet you can live with in order to keep weight off permanently, it's better to shed weight gradually by eating moderate amounts of lean meat and other high-protein foods, pasta and other healthy carbohydrates and ample vegetables and fruit. Low-fat dairy products supply calcium and other nutrients.

For any weight-loss programme to be successful, a combination of healthy eating and regular exercise is essential.

Offal

BENEFITS

- Good source of protein and potassium
- Liver and kidneys are excellent sources of vitamin B_{12}, folate, niacin and iron

DRAWBACKS

- Most offal is high in cholesterol
- Liver may harbour toxins
- High levels of vitamin A may be dangerous during pregnancy

Any edible parts of an animal, apart from the flesh, are classed as offal. Since the BSE scare of the 1990s, the British government has banned the sale of these types of offal for human consumption: the brain, spinal cord, thymus gland (sweet-breads), spleen and intestines of

cattle over six months of age. However, tripe (stomach) still appears regularly on the menus of some restaurants. Pâtés and popular luncheon meats, such as liverwurst, are often made from offal.

Liver

Because the liver is a storehouse for vitamin A, iron and many other nutrients, it follows that it is also a highly nutritious meat source. A 120g serving of lamb's liver provides up to 30 times the Reference Nutrient Intake (RNI) of vitamin A, five times the RNI for B_6, 50 times the RNI of vitamin B_{12} and more than 100 per cent of the RNIs for folate and copper and 50 per cent of the RNI for iron. Unlike other meats it contains vitamin C.

The 235kcal contained in a 100g serving of liver and its cholesterol content of approximately 400mg are its two drawbacks. However, an occasional serving of liver in an otherwise low-fat, low-cholesterol diet is probably not harmful.

When buying liver, you will find calves' liver has a softer texture and is more delicate than that of sheep or pigs. Chicken liver is delicate, too, and is used mostly in paté.

One of the liver's main functions is to metabolise and detoxify various chemical compounds. Thus, the liver may harbour residues of antiiotics and other drugs fed to meat animals, as well as environmental toxins. For this reason, some doctors advise against eating liver on a regular basis.

Liver is one of the richest dietary sources of vitamin A, which is needed for healthy skin and resistance to infection. However, when one consumes more vitamin A than is needed, the excess is stored in the body. In time a build-up of vitamin A can result in liver damage, fatigue and other problems. Studies show, for example, that consuming five to ten times the RNI of vitamin A before and during early pregnancy can increase the risk of birth defects. Normally, it's difficult, if not impossible, to consume toxic amounts of vitamin A from an ordinary diet. But because liver is so high in this nutrient, anyone who regularly consumes it several times a week may develop a toxicity. So it is advisable for women who hope to become pregnant, or who are pregnant, to avoid eating liver.

However, liver is a valuable food for anyone who is suffering from iron-deficiency anaemia, but its high cholesterol count should not be overlooked – it should not be eaten more than once a week.

Other offal

Next in popularity to liver, comes kidneys. But there are other, highly nutritious forms of offal which can add useful amounts of nutrients to the diet.

- Kidneys are low in fat and high in protein. They provide large amounts of vitamin B_{12}, riboflavin and iron, and useful amounts of B_6, folate, niacin and vitamin C.
- Heart is also high in vitamin B_{12}, iron and potassium; in addition, it provides high-quality protein and less fat and cholesterol than other offal does.

- Tongue is high in fat, but contains useful amounts of iron and the B vitamins, especially B_{12}.
- Tripe provides high-quality protein and small amounts of some minerals and vitamins.

Oils

BENEFITS

- Provide essential fatty acids needed for hormone production
- Make possible the absorption of fat-soluble vitamins A, D, E and K
- Improve texture and flavour of food

DRAWBACKS

- High in calories
- Saturated types may raise blood cholesterol levels

Throughout history, various plant oils have served as an essential source of concentrated energy and nutrients during times of need. Before refrigeration was invented, preserving foods with oil was critical to survival.

Today, even with a limitless supply of healthy foods, oils are an important diet component. They add an appetising flavour, aroma, texture and appearance to foods, and because they take longer to digest than the other main food groups, they satisfy hunger for longer.

Oils and fats belong to the lipid family and differ only in their melting points. Oils are liquid at room temperature; fats are solid. Some fats contain fatty acids, which are needed in moderate amounts for several essential body functions. All fats and oils have a practically identical calorie content: 99kcal in 15ml or per level tablespoon. They provide a concentrated source of energy and fatty acids that are essential to build and maintain cell walls. Fats are also necessary to make growth and sex hormones and prostaglandins (the hormone-like substances that regulate many body processes), as well as to absorb and use fat-soluble vitamins A, D, E and K. Vegetable oils contain no cholesterol; it is found only in animal products.

Among the oldest crops for oil are olives – which have been grown for both oil and fruit in the Mediterranean for at least 6,000 years – and sesame, grown from Africa to India. Coconut palms and oil palms flourished untended in the tropics, where foragers gathered the nuts to extract oils. As techniques for extracting and preserving oils have improved, many more plants have been introduced to cultivation. Currently, the main oil crops are coconut, corn, cottonseed, olive, palm, peanut, rapeseed, soya bean and sunflower.

The oils are concentrated in seeds or fruit, which are broken down by pressing or grinding. For some oils the tissues are further treated with solvents and heat to remove the last of the oil. Most oils are refined by by soaking parent seed or fruit in a lye solution, followed by centrifugation and filtration to remove undesirable solids and steam deodorisation; some go through 'winterisation' to remove substances that crystallise and make the oil cloudy when it is chilled, such as in the refrigerator.

Health profile

Oils contain varying amounts of saturated, monounsaturated and polyunsaturated fatty acids. Saturated fats tend to raise levels of artery-clogging LDL cholesterol. Fats that are polyunsaturated and monounsaturated tend to lower LDL cholesterol, especially when they replace saturated fats in the diet.

O

CAUTION

If you like to make flavoured oils by adding herbs, garlic or other ingredients, keep them refrigerated, and use them or throw them out after two days. Oil can support the growth of the bacterium that causes botulism, which is potentially fatal. Commercially prepared flavoured oils usually contain additives that prevent bacteria from growing.

People who are concerned about cholesterol are encouraged to avoid most saturated fats and replace them with mono and polyunsaturates. The saturated fatty acids mostly responsible for raising cholesterol are myristic, lauric and palmitic acids. Coconut, cottonseed, palm and palm kernel oils contain high levels of these damaging fatty acids. Palm, palm kernel and coconut oils, like animal fats, are solid at room temperature and are saturated. The best all-purpose dietary oils are corn, olive, groundnut, safflower, rapeseed, soya bean and sunflower oils, which contain mainly mono- and/or polyunsaturated fats with very low levels of saturated fats.

Oils used to make margarines and shortenings are often processed by hydrogenation to give them a solid consistency and increase their shelf life. The process of hydrogenation creates trans fatty acids, which raise detrimental LDL cholesterol levels and lower HDL levels. Many spreads are now made with minimal trans fatty acids and are better for cholesterol watchers than butter. (Some contain plant sterols or stanols which actively help to lower raised cholesterol levels.)

About 15 to 20 per cent of the fat in margarine is saturated; both of these products have much less than the 60 per cent saturated fat content of butter.

◄ **Flavoured oils**
Oils now available include: sesame, olive, virgin olive, cold-pressed extra virgin olive, groundnut, walnut, sunflower, hazelnut, garlic, chilli oil and more.

Do one simple thing

Use oil instead of butter on your bread

Dip your bread in olive oil instead of using butter. If you dip lightly, you'll consume fewer calories – and very little saturated fat.

Using oils

Monitor your oil consumption by buying single-source oils, such as pure rapeseed or olive, rather than blended oils. Read labels: a blended oil often has an overwhelming proportion of the cheapest and probably least healthy oil listed on the label, with only a token amount of the more expensive, better quality oil. Check labels, too, for the oil content of processed commercial foods, especially baked goods. If a label states 'Contains one or more of the following oils: corn, safflower or coconut', the product is probably made mainly with coconut oil because it's the least expensive of the three listed oils.

Oils add a distinctive flavour and texture to salads and sauces. Along with margarines, they can replace dairy fats in many baking recipes. Virtually no oils are needed in the preparation of foods for grilling, barbecuing and roasting. When frying, you can keep oil absorption low by making sure the oil is at the correct temperature before you add raw foods. Fry at high temperatures where possible, in order to seal food quickly and minimise the amount of oil soaked up. Coating food in crumbs will increase the amount of oil absorbed. Before serving fried foods, drain off any excess oil on a paper towel.

Omega-3 fatty acids

Fish oils contain omega-3 fatty acids, which protect against heart disease and may help people with certain inflammatory conditions such as rheumatoid arthritis. The full benefit of the oils can be obtained from eating at least one serving of oil-rich fish a week. Similar fatty acids are also found in several plant oils, including rapeseed, linseed and walnut. However, scientist are not certain that these plant omega-3s offer the same health benefits as those found in fish oils.

Fish oil supplements should be taken with care. High doses have been known to cause nausea and diarrhoea. Because fish oils have a blood-thinning effect, supplements are not advised for anyone who is taking blood-thinning medications such as heparin or warfarin.

Also, it is best to avoid fish liver oil supplements, which are concentrated sources of vitamins A and D. These supplements can be toxic when taken in large amounts over a long period of time.

Mineral oils

Oils that have been extracted from petroleum and other forms of non-digestible hydrocarbons are sometimes used as laxatives, particularly by people who are trying to lose weight rapidly by purging. This is a dangerous practice that interferes with the absorption of many nutrients, especially fat-soluble vitamins. It may also cause embarrassing bowel leakage.

Okra

BENEFITS

- A good source of vitamin C and fibre

- Good source of folate, and contains some iron, calcium and magnesium

- Low in fat and calories

- Often used as a thickener in soups and stews

DRAWBACKS

- Glutinous consistency is displeasing to some people

A relative of the hibiscus, okra was brought to the Americas from Africa in the 1600s. It is sometimes known as 'ladies' fingers'. The dark green pods are the main ingredient in spicy Creole stews or gumbos.

Okra is now widely available in almost all supermarkets and green-grocers in the UK. Choose small, young pods that snap crisply when broken in half. Dull or dry-looking okra should be avoided. Don't wash them until just before you cook them; the moisture will make them slimy. Store untrimmed, uncut okra in a paper bag in the refrigerator.

This low-calorie vegetable is high in folate; 80g of boiled okra has 22kcal and provides about 20 per cent of the Reference Nutrient Intake (RNI) of folate and 30 per cent of the RNI for vitamin C. They also contain the phyto-chemicals lutein and zeaxanthin which may help to reduce the risk of age-related macular degeneration. Sixteen okra, when cooked, weigh

▼ **Powerful pods**
Use okra to thicken your soup; it could lower your cholesterol.

O

about 80g and make up one of the five to seven recommended daily portions of vegetables.

Okra's thickening properties and unique flavour make it a wonderful addition to stews and soups. As it cooks, it releases sticky juices that thicken any liquid to which it is added. This is due in part to the soluble fibres, including pectin, which may help to lower blood cholesterol levels by cutting bile absorption in the intestine and forcing the liver to use circulating cholesterol to make more bile.

Those who are put off by its gummy consistency should try steaming or blanching the pods until they are just tender. Don't slice the okra before cooking – less juice will be released if the inner capsule remains intact. Prepare okra along with an acidic vegetable, such as tomatoes, to reduce its gelatinous consistency. Some people prefer eating okra raw with dips, as part of a fresh vegetable tray or in a salad.

Olives and olive oil

BENEFITS

■ High in monounsaturated fats, which benefit blood cholesterol levels

■ High in vitamin E and antioxidants

DRAWBACKS

■ Some varieties of olives are high in sodium

The all-purpose crop of the Mediterranean area, olives are indispensable in the preparation of traditional Mediterranean dishes. Once a staple product for cooking, lighting, cosmetics and high-quality soap, olive oil is now used most often in salad dressings and as a

cooking oil – which is high in monounsaturated fatty acids, that may raise levels of the beneficial HDL cholesterol, and very low in saturates. Olives and their oil are thought to contribute to the low rate of heart disease in Mediterranean countries.

Raw olives are so unpalatable that they have to be treated to remove bitterness by being pickled in brine made from a lye solution or dry-salt cured. This means they can be high in sodium, which may raise blood pressure in some people.

Three commercial methods of processing are the Spanish method, which ferments unripe green olives; the American method, which soaks half-ripe olives in an iron solution to achieve a black colour; and the Greek method, which preserves the fully ripe, almost black fruit.

A serving of ten olives contains between 30 and 40 calories and provides some vitamin E.

Olive oil

The primary source of fat in the healthy Mediterranean diet, olive oil is rich in unique disease-fighting phytochemicals, vitamin E and monounsaturated fat, which all help to prevent cholesterol from being deposited in the arteries. The antioxidant phytochemicals hydroxytyrosol and oleuropein may work together, according to

laboratory studies, to help to protect against breast cancer, high blood pressure, infection-causing bacteria and heart disease. Lignans, present in extra virgin olive oil (achieved through pressing the olives only once), may protect against cancer by suppressing early cancer changes in cells. Olive oil contains 99kcal per tablespoon.

The classification of olive oil is the same worldwide and is governed by the International Olive Oil Council. Its acidity, which can be affected by the quality of the olives as well as harvesting and pressing techniques, determines the oil's classification and whether any refining is needed. Minimally processed oil, such as extra-virgin or cold-pressed oil, has the best flavour and the highest content of antioxidants.

Virgin olive oil is the oily juice pressed from the olive. It is unrefined. The term virgin refers to oils that are slightly more acidic than extra-virgin ones; they must contain no more than 3g of free oleic acid per 100g.

Extra virgin olive oil is the least acidic and has a maximum acid level of 1g of free oleic acid per 100g of oil. It is highly regarded as it offers the widest variety of flavours and aromas with a 'fruity' flavour. The flavour differences are due to the regions of cultivation, the climate, the variety of olive and the manner in which the olives are harvested.

Extra light and light olive oils are the most refined. They are no lower in calories or fat and lack the taste and many of the benefits of the other olive oils.

To preserve flavour, store olive oil in an airtight container in the refrigerator or other dark, cool place. Refrigerated olive oil will solidify, so you will have to let it reach room temperature before it is pourable.

▼ **Green or ripe?**
Green olives are unripe; dark olives are fully ripe.

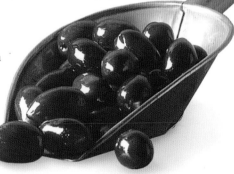

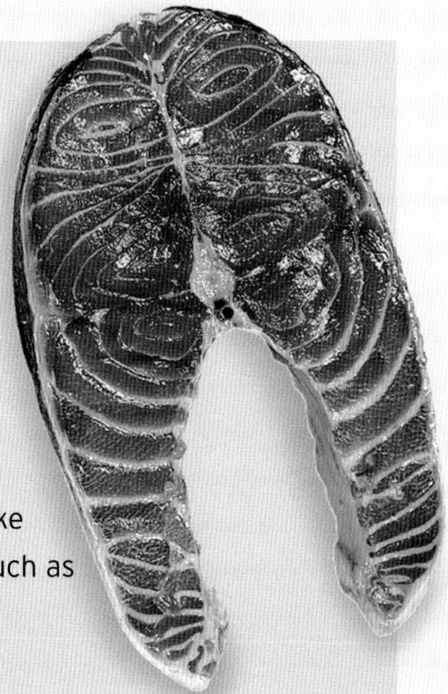

Omega-3s and omega-6s

Essential fatty acids

Omega-3 and omega-6 fatty acids are called essential fatty acids because they are needed for human health but the body can't make them itself. So we need to get them from the foods that we eat, such as oil-rich fish, nuts and seeds and plant oils.

Essential fatty acids are used to manufacture and repair cell membranes and to produce prostaglandins, which affect the whole body. It is important to maintain a good balance of omega-3s and omega-6s in the diet as these two substances work together to promote health. Omega-3 fatty acids help to reduce inflammation and most omega-6 fatty acids tend to promote inflammation. So an imbalance of these essential fatty acids contributes to the development of disease. The balance of omega-3s and omega-6s in our diet has changed dramatically over the past 100 years or so. The two families share a common metabolic pathway and many nutritionists are concerned that a high intake of omega-6s compared with the intake of omega-3s may affect the metabolism of omega-3s, with unfavourable health results. Currently the British diet provides these fatty acids in a ratio of about 7:1 in favour of omega-6s; most experts believe the optimal ratio is 4:1. So we need to pay attention to good food sources of omega-3s. (The Mediterranean diet has a much better balance between them, perhaps because there is less use of those oils and margarines that are high in omega-6s.)

DIFFERENT TYPES

The three best known types of omega-3 fatty acids are alpha-linolenic acid (ALA), eicosapentaenoic acid (EPA) and docosahexaenoic acid (DHA). The body has enzymes that can convert ALA to EPA and DHA, the two types of omega-3 fatty acids readily used by the body. You get the EPA and DHA directly and more efficiently from eating oil-rich fish, most of which are found in cold waters.

EPA and DHA are found in fish such as salmon, swordfish, trout, fresh tuna, mackerel, herring and sardines. ALA, on the other hand, is found mainly in linseeds and walnuts, with smaller amounts in dark green leafy vegetables.

HEALTH BENEFITS

Scientists originally made the connection between omega-3s and health while studying the Inuit people of Greenland. They found that as a group, the Inuit suffered far less from certain diseases, such as heart disease, rheumatoid arthritis and psoriasis than other populations. Yet the Inuit diet was high in fat from eating whale, seal and salmon. Researchers found that these foods were rich in omega-3 fatty acids, providing real disease-fighting benefits. Similar findings came from Japanese studies, too.

Best food sources of omega-3 fatty acids in fish

The omega-3 content of fish varies, but these are the best sources. Figures are given for a 100g edible portion of fish.

- Salmon: 3.0g
- Sprat: 2.4g
- Huss: 2.5g
- Pilchard/sardine: 2.2g
- Herring/mackerel: 2.0g
- Tuna: 1.6g
- Crab/rainbow trout: 1.2g

O

Omega-6 fatty acids may help to relieve premenstrual and menopausal symptoms. One, gamma linolenic acid (GLA), is extracted from the evening primrose and has been used as a treatment for fibrocystic breast disease and aching joints.

CAUTION

Because fish oil can reduce the time it takes blood to clot, you should use supplements only under your doctor's supervision, especially if you are also taking a blood-thinning medication such as warfarin.

lower triglycerides and raise HDL. ALA may not be as effective for people with diabetes as they may lack the ability to efficiently convert ALA to the more usable EPA or DHA.

Researchers are continuing to explore the benefits of these essential fatty acids. The evidence is strongest for heart disease and related concerns, but there are now a wide range of other possible therapeutic uses.

HEART DISEASE

Evidence suggests that EPA and DHA found in fish help to reduce risk factors for heart disease, including high blood pressure and high levels of triglycerides. Research has also shown that these fatty acids can inhibit the development of plaque and blood clots that lead to strokes, reduce cardiac arrhythmias and offer protection from sudden cardiac death. Studies of heart-attack survivors have found that daily omega-3 supplements can reduce the risk of death, subsequent heart attacks and stroke. The Food Standards Agency suggests that we should eat at least two portions of fish a week, of which one should be oily fish.

DIABETES

People with diabetes often have high triglyceride and low HDL levels. Omega-3 fatty acids from fish oil (EPA or DHA) can help to

◀ **The power of greens**

Dark green leafy vegetables are a source of alpha-linolenic acid (ALA), an omega-3 fatty acid that may help to protect us from developing heart disease.

ARTHRITIS

Several studies have concluded that omega-3 supplements can reduce tenderness in joints, decrease morning stiffness and allow a reduction in the amount of medication needed to relieve the pain experienced by people suffering with rheumatoid arthritis.

DEPRESSION

People deficient in omega-3s in their diet may be at increased risk for depression. These fatty acids are important components of nerve cell membranes. They help nerve cells to communicate with each other, maintaining good mental health.

ATTENTION DEFICIT HYPERACTIVITY DISORDER (ADHD)

Children with ADHD may have low levels of essential fatty acids. Research has shown that those with lower levels of omega-3 fatty acids demonstrate more learning and behavioural problems than those with normal levels. There are no well-controlled studies that look at the effect of omega-3 fatty acid supplements on these symptoms, but a diet high in these fats remains a reasonable approach.

BREAST CANCER

The balance between omega-3 and omega-6 fatty acids appears to be an important factor in the development and growth of breast cancer. More research is needed, however, before we can understand this relationship. Researchers have speculated that omega-3s in combination with other nutrients such as vitamin C, vitamin E and selenium may prove to have value in the prevention and treatment of breast cancer.

Onions

BENEFITS

- Spring onion tops are a good source of vitamin C and beta carotene
- May lower raised blood cholesterol and reduce the risk of heart disease
- Reduce the ability of the blood to clot
- Mild antibacterial effect may help prevent superficial infections
- Sulphur compounds may block carcinogens
- Used as a decongestant in traditional medicine

DRAWBACKS

- Can cause bloating and flatulence
- Raw onions taint breath

Folklore is filled with fascinating facts about the onion – among them that Alexander the Great fed huge quantities to his troops to strengthen them for battle. The Egyptian tomb paintings abound with onions; in fact, they are depicted more often than any other plant. Early Hebrew writings reveal that it was one of the foods that the Jews longed for after their flight from Egypt. And throughout history, healers have accorded onions near-magical powers to cure everything from baldness to infections.

Onions are members of the allium plant family, which includes garlic, leeks and shallots. There are scores of different varieties of onion, with new ones constantly emerging. In general, however, onions are divided into two categories: spring onions, which have a mild flavour and

---

Better raw than cooked

Cooking onions at a high heat significantly reduces the benefits of diallyl sulphide – a cancer-protective phytochemical they contain.

---

whose green tops and bulbs are eaten; and globe onions, which have a more pungent flavour and dry outer skins that are discarded. Shallots possess features of onions and garlic, but are milder.

With so many sizes, shapes and flavours, and so many varieties of spring and other onions available year-round, choosing an onion can be tricky. Spring onions and larger white onions should have crisp, dark green tops and firm white bottoms. Although they will keep for a few days in the refrigerator, they should be used before they begin to soften.

Other types of onion should be firm, with crackly, dry skin. Reject any that feel soft, have black spots (indicating mould) or have green sprouts showing at the top (these are well past their prime). They should have a mild odour – a strong, oniony smell points to decay. Onions should be stored in a cool, dry place away from direct light, which can give them a bitter taste. Preferably in open baskets where circulating air will keep them fresh. They should not be stored near potatoes, which give off moisture and a gas that causes onions to spoil more quickly.

Red onions have a mild, rather sweet flavour, which makes them a favourite for salads and sandwiches. Stronger white and yellow varieties are ideal for cooking, because they become milder and sweeter upon heating and they also impart a pleasant flavour to other foods. There are a number of new sweet varieties of yellow onions, which are often named for the areas where they were originally developed.

The many uses of onions

Cooked or uncooked, onions are extremely versatile and have many culinary uses: sliced raw in salads and sandwiches; cooked into stews,

---

Lung cancer protection

A study published in the *Journal of the National Cancer Institute* reported on the significant correlation between the high intake of dietary flavonoids and a reduced risk of lung cancer. Food sources of the flavonoids that offer the best protection include onions, as well as apples and grapefruit.

---

soups and omelettes; and baked, boiled, sautéed or fried and served as a side dish. Spring onions can be included in a raw vegetable tray, chopped into salads or dressings, or braised and served hot. Build a light meal around a bowl of French onion soup. In order to reduce the calorie content, use a defatted broth stock and just a sprinkling of low-fat cheese.

Health benefits

Cooks value onions more for the flavour they impart to other foods than for their nutritional content. Although onions are not high on the nutritional scale, spring onions are a useful source of vitamin C and their green tops provide some beta carotene.

Recent research has verified some of the centuries-old beliefs about onions. For example, folk healers have long recommended onions as a heart tonic; researchers have now documented that adenosine, a substance in onions, hinders clot formation, which may help to prevent heart attacks. Studies also indicate that onions may protect against the artery-clogging damage of cholesterol by raising the levels of the protective high-density lipoproteins (HDLs). This means that they may offer some protection against heart attack and stroke. Still other studies suggest that eating ample amounts of onions may help to prevent high blood pressure. Sulphur compounds in onions can

O

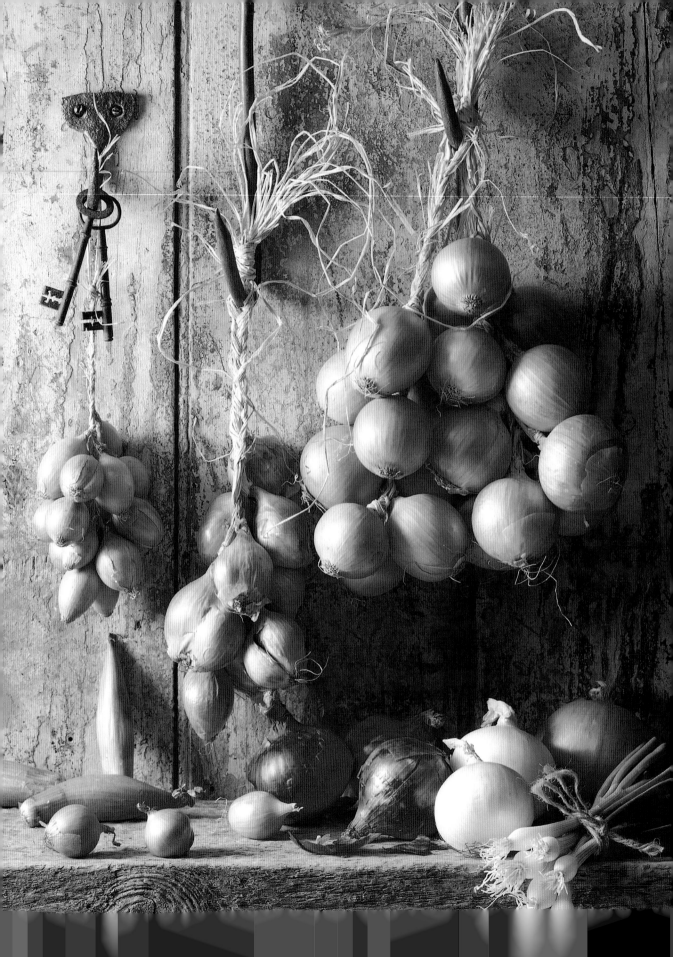

leave an unpleasant odour on the breath and hands, but they also block the cancer-causing potential of some carcinogens. In addition, onions contain substances that have a mild antibacterial effect, which may validate the old folk remedy of rubbing a raw onion on a cut to prevent infection.

Cutting an onion allows its sulphur compounds to combine with enzymes and release volatile molecules that react with moisture in the eyes to form sulphuric acid. Tearing is a natural reaction of the eyes to eliminate the irritant. This effect may help to clear congested nasal passages during a cold.

A syrup made from onions and honey is an old cough remedy. But eating raw onions can cause bloating and flatulence in some people, and may trigger migraines in others.

Oranges

BENEFITS

■ An excellent source of vitamin C

■ A good source of folate and potassium

DRAWBACKS

■ May produce allergic reactions in some susceptible people

One of our most popular fruits, oranges are usually associated with vitamin C, and with good reason. One medium-sized orange (150g) provides 80mg, twice the Reference Nutrient Intake (RNI) for women. As an antioxidant, vitamin C protects against cell damage by the free radicals produced when oxygen is used by the human body, and it may reduce the risk of certain cancers, heart attacks, strokes and other diseases. Oranges also contain rutin, hesperidin and other bioflavonoids – plant pigments that may help to prevent or retard

Do one simple thing

Eat the pithy part

Eat the orange with some of the pith (the spongy white layer between the zest and the pulp). A good amount of the fruit's fibre and antioxidant plant chemicals are found there, although it may cause flatulence.

tumour growth. Beta-cryptoxanthin is a carotenoid in oranges and mandarins that may help to prevent colon cancer. Nobiletin, a flavonoid found in the flesh of oranges, may have anti-inflammatory actions and tangeretin, the flavonoid found in tangerines, has been linked in experimental studies to a reduced growth of tumour cells. They also have smaller amounts of other vitamins and minerals including thiamin, folate and potassium.

Oranges are low in calories (one medium orange contains about 56kcal). They are a low GI food, serving very well as hunger busters, which makes them ideal for people with diabetes, and great for every-one wanting longer-lasting energy. An additional benefit is that the membranes between the segments of the fresh fruit provide a good amount of pectin, a soluble dietary fibre that may help to control blood cholesterol levels.

Fresh oranges are a delicious snack or dessert and a delightful ingredient in salads and some meat dishes. A small glass (150ml) of freshly squeezed juice has 54kcal and 59mg of vitamin C; it counts as one of the recommended servings of fresh fruit we should have daily. Commercial orange juice is popular but tastes different to fresh juice. This is partly because it is often made from juice concentrates and these

may contain oils from the orange skin. Most orange juice concentrate is imported from Brazil. High consumption can add many calories with a 500ml bottle having 180kcal. Those watching their weight should restrict consumption to half a cup.

The peel of the orange is dried to make candied orange peel or flavourings. Caution is needed, however, because the peel may be treated with sulphites, which can trigger serious allergic reactions in susceptible people. Also, orange peels contain limonene, an oil that is a common allergen. Many people who are allergic to commercial orange juice, which becomes infused with limonene during processing, find they can tolerate peeled oranges.

Types of orange

The following are the most common types of orange.

- Valencias, the most commonly grown variety, are used for both eating and juicing.
- Blood oranges are sweet, deep red oranges originating in Italy.
- Navel oranges are sweet and seedless; they are the second most common type.
- Sevilles are sour oranges that are used mostly for marmalades.

O

Organic foods

Are they worth the cost?

If you are concerned about pesticide residues in foods today, you can turn to organic products – but don't assume that they will be nutritionally superior.

Only a decade or so ago, organic foods were found only in health-food shops or at farmers' markets. Today supermarkets stock organic fruit and vegetables, meats, milk, poultry, cereals, eggs and honey. Organic wines, yoghurt, cream and cheeses are also available. However, only 3 to 4 per cent of the produce bought in Britain is organic, and about 70 to 75 per cent of organic food is imported.

Major retailers promote organic foods, but consumers are often reluctant to pay more for inferior-looking fruit and vegetables. Nevertheless, sales have tripled in the last decade or so, and the market is worth an estimated £1 billion annually. Part of the problem is also that the country has only about a fifth of the farmland needed to meet the growing demand for locally grown organic foods.

THE MEANING OF 'ORGANIC'

Organic food is produced by farmers who grow, handle and process crops without synthetic fertilisers, pesticides or herbicides, or artificial ingredients. Organic food is not irradiated and does not contain genetically engineered ingredients. Organic meat, poultry, eggs and dairy products come from animals that are given no antibiotics or growth hormones.

Organic food crops can, however, be grown with pesticides – just not synthetic ones. One popular organic pesticide is *Bacillus thuringiensis*, a naturally occurring soil bacterium that is toxic to the larvae of several species of insects but harmless to wildlife and people. Not all of these organic pesticides are harmless, however – some can cause allergic reactions, for example. Naturally occurring copper compounds can also be used in organic agriculture, even though they are potentially toxic in large quantities.

Organic foods can also be contaminated with synthetic agricultural chemicals carried by the wind from other fields, or that persist in the soil. However, in these cases, the pesticide levels are much lower than in conventional foods.

The notion of organically farmed produce appeals to a public which became increasingly anxious about pesticides and additives used in intensive farming.

Keeping pests at bay while you grow your own

There are many ways of keeping your own, home-grown fruits and vegetables healthy, while maintaining an organic, pesticide-free environment for them:

- Plant aromatic summer savory to protect runner beans, fragrant buckwheat to keep pests off broad beans, or pot marigolds to prevent whitefly in your greenhouse.

- Surround your garden with a thick hedge to attract birds and put out food for them in winter to encourage them to visit your garden; they will eat slugs and insects.

- Dig a pond which will encourage frogs and toads; they will also help to keep down the slug population.

- If all else fails with slugs, sink a jam jar into the bed and pour a little beer into it; slugs will die a blissful death.

- Leave a pile of logs in a corner, to shelter beetles which will prey on pests.

- A patch of nettles will attract ladybirds, which feed on any aphids that may appear.

- Fine mesh placed over susceptible plants will keep away carrot fly, cabbage root fly and cabbage white butterflies without affecting growth.

- A mulching material made of natural bark or wood chippings suppresses weeds and has nutrients that benefit the soil.

- Use an organic fertiliser; it keeps bacteria in the soil healthy, promoting healthy plant growth.

The British government is giving support to organic farming, not only to meet consumer demand, but also because it recognises that it is a more environmentally friendly form of agriculture.

IS ORGANIC FOOD MORE NUTRITIOUS?

Some studies suggest there is a difference in nutritional value, but they are far from conclusive. One study published in the January 2003 *Journal of Agricultural and Food Chemistry* found that frozen organic corn had 52 per cent more vitamin C than conventional corn. An August 2002 Italian study in the same journal found that organic peaches and pears have higher levels of health-protective polyphenols, and slightly more vitamin C (8 per cent). Another found that organic soup had more salicylic acid – an anti-inflammatory compound found in food – than non-organic soup. Even if the differences shown in these studies are real, they are small. You'd get a lot more vitamin C eating an extra orange than in eating organic corn for dinner.

The label 'organic' is not meant to be a nutrition claim. Nor does it mean that the food is any less likely to be contaminated with pathogens that cause food-borne illness: organic chickens can be contaminated with salmonella and other food-borne pathogens, just like conventional chickens. Nor is it safer to eat raw organic eggs than raw conventional eggs.

THE SAFETY FACTOR

Is organic food safer to eat than conventionally produced food? Synthetic pesticides, herbicides, fungicides, insecticides and other agricultural chemicals can certainly have adverse health effects on the farm workers who use them. But the evidence is not conclusive about their effect on consumer health. Unfortunately, for consumers, what needs to be determined is the effect of lower levels of intake over a lifetime, which is more difficult for researchers to establish.

There may be a greater benefit in shielding children from pesticide residues since their bodies are smaller and they eat a less varied diet. In a University of Washington study, Seattle preschoolers whose

What's best to buy?

Since organic food is often more expensive, it makes sense to shop selectively. One way to save money is to buy organic produce only for those foods where the non-organic forms have been documented to have the highest pesticide residues. Although there is no evidence that fruits and vegetables with higher residues pose a hazard, selecting the organic versions of these is a logical place to start:

- Choose these organic fruits: peaches, nectarines, apples, grapes, pears, cherries, raspberries and strawberries.
- Choose the following organic vegetables: green beans, spinach, peppers, celery and potatoes.
- Consider organic meat. While most people worry about fruit and vegetables, animals actually accumulate more residues, especially in their fat. Cattle raised to produce organic beef have not had hormone implants in their ear, a practice that occurs in many other cattle.
- Choose organic poultry and eggs as the hens will not have been given routine antibiotics as growth promotants.
- Choose organic wheat products, including cereals. These have not been treated with fumigants during storage.

families ate primarily organic foods had much lower urine levels of organophosphate pesticides. While the researchers found that children who ate conventional foods were more likely to be exposed to these pesticides at levels above those recommended by the United States government, such guidelines have a wide margin of safety. So there's no clear evidence that there is a risk to eating conventional food, or a benefit to eating organic ones.

Research is also being carried out to determine if there is a link between the decline in male fertility and the increasing use of agro-chemicals over the past 50 years. There is a claim that men who eat organic foods have higher sperm counts than those who don't.

THE BOTTOM LINE

Scientists are concerned that modern agricultural methods and our liberal use of pesticides are upsetting the delicate ecological balance and creating major problems. There are also many questions being raised about the link between pesticide use and cancer rates. Thanks to the increasing availability of organic foods, consumers who are concerned about chemical residues and can afford the extra cost, can now purchase organic alternatives.

Osteoporosis

GET PLENTY OF

- Low-fat milk, yoghurt, canned fish with bones and other foods rich in calcium

- Foods rich in vitamin D, such as oily fish and eggs

- Expose skin to sunlight for 10 to 15 minutes each day

- Weight-bearing exercise

LIMIT

- Foods rich in phytic acid, such as wheat bran, brown rice and nuts

- Foods containing oxalic acid such as spinach, rhubarb and chocolate

- Coffee, tea and other drinks containing caffeine, and alcohol

AVOID

- Smoking

Throughout life, our bones are in a state of constant renewal. While some cells eat away at the existing bone, releasing calcium into the bloodstream, other cells are forming new bone and depositing calcium into it. In young, healthy people, there is equal activity between the two types of cell, but with age, we lose more calcium than is put back and the bones become weak and extremely porous. Fractures can occur with little or no pressure; this condition is called osteoporosis. Lack of oestrogen appears to be its key contributing factor, but a decline of androgens – the male hormones – is also involved, coupled with an inadequate intake of calcium and vitamin D.

Throughout childhood, bones grow in length and density. In adolescence bones build density and finish growing in length (ages 11 to 14). Peak bone mass is usually reached in your 20s. The denser your bones, the lower the risk of osteoporosis later. Once peak bone mass is achieved, you can't improve it; it's determined by genetics and nutrition.

Both men and women begin to lose some mass with increasing age. In women, the loss is greatly accelerated with the decline in oestrogen production at menopause. Osteoporosis affects both women and men, but women of Northern European and Asian ancestry have the highest risk. Women of African and Mediterranean descent are less affected, perhaps because they tend to have more bone mass and get the sun needed to make vitamin D.

Although exercise can help the bones at any age, an excessive level of athletic training in adolescent girls could rob their body of the fat they need to produce and store oestrogen. Highly trained teenage athletes and ballet dancers may have menstrual irregularities and are more at risk for developing early, severe osteoporosis. Anorexic girls who lose their normal layer of fat are at high risk as well.

Smoking greatly increases the risk of severe osteoporosis. Women who smoke have lower levels of oestrogen at all ages, and may enter menopause up to five years earlier than nonsmokers. Nicotine is known to interfere with the body's ability to use calcium.

Women whose ovaries are surgically removed have an abrupt stop to oestrogen production rather than a gradual decline. They may suffer more severe osteoporosis than those who have normal menopause. Kidney diseases and the use of steroid drugs also are risk factors.

Prevention

Osteoporosis prevention should begin in childhood, with a healthy diet and regular exercise. Plenty of calcium, the building block of bone, and vitamin D are needed. The recommendations for calcium are 550mg a day for 7-10 year old girls and boys; 1,000mg a day for boys 11-18 and 800mg a day for girls 11-18; and 700mg a day for men and women from 19 onwards.

Calcium. Foods rich in calcium include milk and dairy products, nuts, fortified soya and rice drinks, dried beans and peas, tofu, canned fish eaten with the bones, dark green leafy vegetables. The darker the greens, the more calcium they contain. Spinach is the exception: it is high in oxalic acid, which inhibits the absorption of calcium.

Skimmed milk gives more calcium, volume for volume, than whole milk. Fat-reduced cheese, yoghurt, and lactose-free milk are excellent calcium sources for people who have a lactose intolerance. Strict vegetarians can get calcium from fortified soya and rice drinks, tofu, beans, lentils, nuts and green vegetables. In fact, we all need plenty of fruit and vegetables: studies indicate that they help in protection against osteoporosis.

Did you know?

Strong bones are developed in adolescence

Adolescence is the critical window for developing strong bones to last a lifetime. One recent study found that women over 50 who had drunk less than a glass of milk a day as girls had significantly lower bone density and twice the risk of fractures compared with those who drank a glass or more. The difference existed no matter how much milk the women drank as adults or how much calcium they took.

If your GP recommends a calcium supplement, check how much elemental calcium is in each pill. Calcium citrate is easily absorbed; calcium carbonate is less well absorbed, but satisfactory, although it occasionally causes constipation, bloating and wind. Calcium gluconate is well absorbed but may infrequently cause diarrhoea. Taking supplements along with meals helps absorption. Bone meal and dolomite supplements are not recommended; they may be contaminated with heavy metals.

Vitamin D. Just as important as calcium is vitamin D; the body needs it in order to absorb calcium. It has always been assumed that most people make enough vitamin D within the body from the action of sunlight on the skin. Studies now show vitamin D deficiency in elderly people in nursing homes and also in women and children where cultural or religious beliefs mean the skin is covered. Vitamin D can also be obtained from oily fish, egg yolks, butter and margarine.

Vitamin K. New research suggests that vitamin K may help to increase bone density and also reduce fracture rates. Both the Nurses' Health Study and the Framingham Heart Study found that people who consume the most vitamin K have a lower risk of hip fractures than those who consume less. Friendly bacteria that live in your intestine help to make a large percentage of the vitamin K you need, and the rest can be found in leafy green vegetables, green peas, broccoli, spinach, Brussels sprouts, cos lettuce, cabbage, kale and liver. There is some in egg yolks, dairy products and plant oils.

Soya. Studies suggest that soya may play a role in prevention of osteoporosis as it contains isoflavones, a type of plant oestrogen that may help to conserve bone mass, particularly during perimenopause and menopause.

Linseeds/flaxseeds. A study of postmenopausal women suggests that linseeds, which are high in lignans, may retain bone mass, elevate antioxidant status and help to prevent urinary loss of calcium.

Vitamin C. Studies have linked higher intakes of vitamin C with higher bone density. Vitamin C also helps to form the connective tissue that holds bones together. Some of the best food sources are fruit and vegetables, especially citrus fruit, berries, melons and peppers.

Phosphorus. Also essential to bone formation, it is found in most foods that contain calcium as well as meat, poultry and eggs.

Regular weight-bearing exercise. Walking, jogging, aerobics, tennis and dancing are all excellent in helping to maintain bones. They improve the circulation, bringing vitamins and minerals to the bones and strengthening them for old age.

What to avoid
Evidence indicates that the following should be avoided.

Sodium. It also can cause the kidneys to excrete calcium. Cut down on salt used in cooking and at the table; also, cut back on processed and canned foods.

Caffeine. Drinking lots of coffee, tea or colas increases the amount of calcium you excrete.

High levels of dietary protein. This too can cause calcium to be excreted. Eating more plant proteins in place of animal proteins is a strategy to keep your protein intake more moderate.

Medications can affect the levels of calcium in the body. Antacids containing aluminium can promote calcium excretion. Calcium is also lost during long-term use of other drugs, including certain antibiotics, diuretics and steroids.

● **Myth.......**
Black cohosh, red clover and chasteberry can help to combat osteoporosis.

.......Reality ●
While many women try these herbal remedies to relieve menopausal symptoms, there is no evidence that black cohosh, red clover or chasteberry have any effect on calcium metabolism related to bone loss.

Beyond diet
Many doctors recommend a baseline bone density scan for women when menstrual periods become irregular. Depending on the results, the doctor may recommend calcium and vitamin D supplements.

Medical treatment
For women, hormone replacement therapy (HRT), to replace oestrogen lost at menopause, is an option used where other treatments have failed. HRT does decrease bone loss and is useful if started early in the menopause, but bone loss will resume when the HRT stops. However, it is not considered appropriate for the long-term treatment of osteoporosis.

Newer, non-hormonal drugs offer men and women an alternative. These include bisphosphonates, such as alendronate. They decrease bone loss and shift the balance towards the formation of healthy tissue. Calcitonin, a hormonal preparation taken by injection or as a nasal spray, works in a similar fashion.

Yet another new medication is raloxifene (Evista), which helps to prevent osteoporosis by modulating the body's oestrogen receptors. This drug, while not a hormone, offers many of the same benefits as oestrogen without increasing the risk of breast and uterine cancers.

O

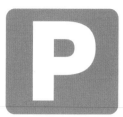

Papaya

BENEFITS

- An excellent source of vitamin C

- High in beta carotene

- An extract is used to tenderise meat

DRAWBACKS

- Can cause dermatitis in some people

Papaya is known as 'paw paw' in some countries. They are simply different varieties of the same fruit, which is native to tropical America. There is also a dwarf Philippine variety of the fruit that has red-flesh and is popular in Asian countries.

The green skin of the papaya fruit generally turns yellow or orange as the fruit ripens, although the skin on some varieties remains greenish even when ripe.

Fruit from female plants tend to be globular or oval while those from hermaphrodite plants are usually long and narrow.

Like most yellow-orange fruit, papayas are high in vitamin C and beta carotene, the plant form of vitamin A. A medium-sized papaya (150g) supplies more than twice the adult Reference Nutrient Intake (RNI) of vitamin C and almost 30 per cent of the RNI of vitamin A, but with only 54kcal.

Some varieties of papaya contain papain, an enzyme that is similar to the digestive juice pepsin. Because this enzyme breaks down protein, papain extract from papayas is marketed as a meat tenderiser.

It has also been used medically to treat ruptured spinal disks, but this treatment has fallen out of favour in most places. Topical ointments containing papain are sometimes applied to promote the shedding of dead tissue. Papain causes the dermatitis that some people experience when handling papayas; this irritation is not necessarily an allergic reaction.

Usually eaten raw, the fruit should be washed, split open and the black seeds scooped out. These seeds are normally thrown away, but they can be dried and used like peppercorns.

Unripe green papaya is used in Thai and other Asian dishes. A few pieces of papaya added to a stew tenderises the meat, while its pectin serves as a natural thickener.

◀ **The seeds of a papaya are edible too** Rinse papaya seeds and add to a salad for a nutty and slightly peppery taste.

Parkinson's disease

CONSUME PLENTY OF

- Fresh vegetables, fruit and fibre-rich wholegrain products

- Fluids to promote good digestion

- Soft or puréed foods to ease swallowing, if required

LIMIT

- High-protein foods if taking levodopa

AVOID

- Excessive weight gain

About 120,000 people in the UK are afflicted with Parkinson's disease, a chronic and progressive nerve disorder that causes uncontrollable shaking or tremors, a fixed staring expression, muscle rigidity, stooped posture and an abnormal gait. The disease varies from one person to another; some people develop speech problems and difficulty swallowing, while others suffer progressive dementia. Parkinson's affects men and women equally and is most common over the age of 55. Every year, 10,000 new patients are diagnosed.

Parkinson's disease is caused by a decrease in the brain's production of dopamine, which is an essential chemical that transports signals from one brain cell to another in order to produce smooth, coordinated muscle movements. The symptoms of Parkinson's disease are due to the progressive destruction of a part of the brain, the *sustantia nigra* where cells make dopamine and another chemical, acetylcholine, which control the movement of the body. When the level of dopamine falls to 80 per cent, the balance between the two chemicals is upset and messages from the brain to some parts of the body are interrupted or travel very slowly. Some studies have shown a higher incidence of Parkinson's among agricultural workers suggesting that the use of pesticides may be linked to the disease.

Parkinson's grows progressively worse over time, which is why it is called a 'degenerative disorder'.

There is no way to screen for Parkinson's before the symptoms occur, and there is no cure for the disease, but various medications, especially levodopa, can reduce symptoms and slow the progression. Some preliminary research indicates that the dietary supplement coenzyme Q_{10} may be beneficial. Physiotherapy and speech therapy also have been found to be helpful. There are also surgical treatments, such as the new and very successful deep brain stimulation (DBS) that has been pioneered in France.

The role of diet

Although there are no nutritional treatments for Parkinson's disease, diet can help to increase the effectiveness of treatment with levodopa and manage the problems that occur, such as constipation and difficulty in eating.

Make treatment more effective. To be its most effective, levodopa should be absorbed from the small intestine as soon as possible after it is taken. Some doctors advise taking the drug 20 to 30 minutes before meals, but if this provokes nausea, it can be taken with a carbohydrate snack, such as fruit or bread. Protein delays the absorption of some medications, so levodopa should not be taken with high-protein foods. Some reports say that taking the whole day's protein allowance in the evening is less likely to create problems.

A proper diet helps to control other symptoms. Constipation can be minimised by consuming ample fresh fruit and vegetables, whole-grain cereals and breads and other high-fibre foods, as well as drinking six to eight glasses of water or other fluids daily.

Exercise promotes healthy bowel function and is advised for anyone with Parkinson's disease, because it preserves muscle tone and strength.

It is also important to try to avoid becoming overweight, as this makes mobility even more difficult.

Problem solving

Patients with advanced Parkinson's often have trouble chewing and swallowing food, because the tongue and facial muscles may be affected. There are ways to relieve the worst of these sysmptoms.

Excessive drooling and shaky hands. These are common problems. Medications can help to reduce drooling, and meals should centre on foods that are easy to chew and swallow. These include cooked cereals or well-moistened dry cereals, poached or scrambled eggs, soups, mashed potatoes, rice, pasta, tender chicken or turkey, well-cooked boneless fish, puréed or mashed vegetables and fruit, custard, yoghurt and juices. If eating is tiring, try smaller but more frequent meals.

Avoiding choking. Sit up straight and tilt your head slightly forward when swallowing. Take small bites, chew thoroughly and swallow everything before taking another bite. Concentrate on moving food backwards in your mouth with your tongue, and swallow again if you feel that food did not go down completely.

Sip a little liquid between bites to help wash food down. If you do cough or choke, lean forward and tuck your chin down while coughing.

Stay independent. Try to do as much for yourself as you can, but know when to accept help. Getting over-tired worsens the symptoms

Parsnips

BENEFITS

- A useful source of vitamin C, vitamin E and folate
- High in carbohydrate and fibre
- A source of potassium

Parsnips have a sweet, nutty flavour that goes well with other vegetables in soups or stews. Excellent roasted, they can also be served instead of potatoes or other starchy foods. This winter root vegetable tastes best after the first frost; exposure to cold begins to convert its starch into sugar. Parsnips are a nutritious food. An 80g portion has 53kcal, 4g fibre, 280mg of potassium, 33mcg of folate and 8mg of vitamin C.

When buying parsnips, reject any that are soft and shrunken. If the tops are still attached, cut them off before storing so they don't draw moisture and nutrition from the roots. They can be kept for a few weeks in the fridge.

Pasta

BENEFITS

- A useful source of protein, B vitamins and dietary fibre
- Low in fat and sodium
- Versatile and inexpensive

DRAWBACKS

- Often topped with high-fat sauces

Introduced to the UK by the Italians, pasta has become a staple in many homes. It is a healthy food product made from durum wheat, which is the most nutritious type of wheat. Pasta has a good level of nutrients, including protein and fibre, and it is digested and broken down to blood glucose slowly, giving all types of pasta a low Glycaemic Index (GI). Some diet books claim that pasta made from white flour has a high GI, but data published by reliable researchers shows that pasta has a low-to-medium GI. A medium portion of cooked pasta contains 230kcal, 7g of protein and 2g of dietary fibre. Wholegrain pasta contains about two and a half times the fibre of white pasta, and a diet rich in whole grains has been shown to lower the risk of diabetes and heart disease, as well as several forms of cancer.

Some supermarkets also carry pastas made from corn, rice, buckwheat and other types of flour as well as varieties flavoured with spinach and tomato, which have a little more nutrition. Egg pasta has only relatively small quantities of egg. Although the vegetables and pepper powders added to some pasta add flavour, they add very little else.

Healthy pasta sauces

Pasta dishes can be transformed by the addition of sauces. Traditional ingredients include olive oil, garlic, onions, mushrooms, tomatoes and fresh basil. Many classic sauces, such as four cheeses, pesto and bolognaise, are high in fat and calories. The following are ideas for creating tasty, healthy dishes.

- Toss pasta with fresh, diced tomatoes and herbs.
- Use half of the oil, cheese and nuts in a pesto recipe, while increasing the basil and garlic. Add white wine or lemon juice if the sauce is too dry.
- Purée cooked vegetables in a blender or food processor, simmer them with herbs and spices and toss with spaghetti or another pasta.
- When making a cream sauce, substitute low-fat milk or evaporated skimmed milk for the cream.
- Toss a pasta salad with a dressing made from non-fat yoghurt instead of soured cream or mayonnaise.
- Combine pasta with beans, lentils or other legumes to create a high-protein vegetarian meal.
- Instead of a buttery cheese sauce, toss pasta with a broth and sprinkle it lightly with grated Parmesan or pecorino cheese.
- Add vegetables instead of meat to a light tomato sauce.

The calorie question

Pasta itself is not especially high in calories. A 230g portion of cooked pasta contains about 230kcal. In southern Italy, where pasta is served almost daily, it is usually served with a tomato-based sauce and a small amount of highly flavoured finely grated hard cheese. Such a meal, based on the same amount of cooked pasta, would contribute around 380kcal and 6g of fat. Add a green salad to complete the meal and the total energy content would not be excessive. But if your pasta is accompanied by a cream-based sauce and sprinkled liberally with cheese, the energy content of the meal could easily reach around 700kcal with the fat content at around 40g. Pasta itself isn't

▼ **A medley of pastas**
Not all pastas are equal. Egg noodles contain a little extra protein; white pastas contribute some nutrients; but wholegrain pastas add considerably more dietary fibre.

Did you know?

Pasta is a 'mood food'

The brain uses the chemical serotonin to make us feel good. When you eat carbohydrates such as pasta, there's an increase in blood sugar and serotonin levels. The good feelings may last for several hours. Eating protein with the pasta, however, can negate the effect, while wholegrain pastas, which take longer to break down, prolong it.

fattening – it is its accompaniments that are. There are also ways that you can cut the calories, even with something that seems inherently fatty, such as a lasagne. By using a small quantity of very lean meat and adding vegetables such as mushrooms, tomatoes, aubergine and grated courgette to the sauce and substituting low-fat ricotta cheese for the usual rich cheese sauce, you can cut the energy level from 700kcal to around 500kcal.

Nutrition

Pastas are a useful source of iron (about 1.2mg in a **230g** serving) and B vitamins. Although the protein in pasta (about 8-10g in the same sized serving) lacks some essential amino acids, these can easily be obtained from a light sprinkling of Parmesan cheese as a topping (21kcal per level teaspoon). Egg noodles provide complete protein, and contain only an insignificant increase in fat.

A versatile food

Pasta is most nutritious when it is used as a 'vehicle' for healthy foods such as vegetables and fish.

For lunch, toss some cooked pasta with vegetables, tuna or thinly sliced chicken. Sauté or stir-fry fresh vegetables and toss them with pasta to make an entrée, a side dish or a main course. For a special occasion, try topping linguine or angel hair

pasta with a seafood medley of clams, mussels, prawns and scallops. Remember, when cooking pasta, adding salt to the water is optional and there is no need to add oil to stop pasta from sticking. Simply give the pasta a quick stir when you add it to the water and keep an eye on it as it cooks.

Tortellini, bow-shaped farfalle and fusilli are a just few of the interestingly shaped and colourful pastas that are ideal as beginner foods for toddlers. For a change, spaghetti and tagliatelli can replace noodles in stir-fries.

Do one simple thing

Measure the portion you put on your plate

The easiest way to keep your portion size under control is to weigh out the dry pasta before cooking. You should allow 75-100g of dry pasta for each person. This will equate to 230kcal per serving.

Peaches

BENEFITS

■ A good source of vitamin C, beta carotene (yellow-fleshed varieties only), with useful amounts of potassium

■ A good source of dietary fibre

DRAWBACKS

■ May provoke allergic reactions in susceptible people

Nutritious and versatile, peaches can be enjoyed fresh, added to fruit salads or cooked with meat and poultry dishes. They can also be baked, grilled, flambéed or poached to create pies, crumbles and other desserts ideas.

While there are hundreds of varieties, peaches are usually classified into one of two categories: freestone, with a loose, easily removed stone, or clingstone, in which the stone is firmly embedded in the fruit. Freestones are usually much bigger than clingstones, with a more delicate flesh that bruises easily. They are mostly sold fresh, and will usually be white-fleshed.

Clingstones are very often bright yellow. The fruit has to be peeled before it is used for canning, stewing or making peach jam. The stones are removed after cooking.

Fresh peaches are a low-calorie source of vitamin C. They contain fibre, especially pectin, a soluble fibre that may help in lowering high blood cholesterol. A medium-sized peach contains only 35kcal and, if eaten unpeeled, provides more than three quarters of the daily requirement for vitamin C.

Canned peaches lose more than 80 per cent of their vitamin C and, if in syrup, are higher in calories than the fresh variety; for example, 110g of peaches canned in heavy syrup has 61kcal, as opposed to 43kcal in juice-packed brands – so always look for fruit in juice.

Volume for volume, dried peaches contain the most calories, because it takes about 3kg to produce just 500g of the dried fruit. Ten dried peach halves (about 120g) provide

Peach-picking tips

● Look for yellow or creamy peaches with a rosy blush on their cheeks. Avoid peaches with green undertones – they were picked too early.

● Select peaches with unwrinkled skin and no bruises.

● Sniff the stem end of the peach. You should be able to smell the peachy fragrance.

● Watch out for peaches with tan circles. It's an early sign of decay.

262kcal; on the plus side, they are also a more concentrated source of various essential nutrients. Those ten halves provide 1,300mg of potassium and 8mg of iron. After eating dried peaches, brush your teeth to remove their sticky residue; it can create dental problems if it is left for any length of time.

Dried peaches often contain sulphites, a preservative that is known to produce an allergic reaction in susceptible people.

Peaches may produce an allergic reaction in people who react to such related fruit as apricots, plums and cherries, as well as almonds. They also contain salicylates, which may provoke a reaction in aspirin-sensitive people.

▼ Cooked peaches for dessert
Baked halves of yellow-fleshed peaches, stuffed with redcurrant jelly and crumbled digestive biscuits make a delicious dessert.

Many of the peaches on sale in British supermarkets are imported, which means they can be on sale at almost any time of year.

Keep in mind that peaches do not increase in sweetness after picking, so when choosing fruit avoid those that are rock hard. A peach should feel heavy, indicating that it is juicy, and it should have a sweet odour. The skin should be smooth and have a warm yellow or reddish colour. Avoid any peaches that are bruised or look 'tired'.

In terms of texture, it is best to choose relatively soft peaches if they are to be eaten straightaway. If you buy firm peaches, placing them in a paper bag at room temperature will hasten the ripening process. Unless they are going to be eaten within the day, store ripe peaches in the refrigerator; they will keep for three to five days.

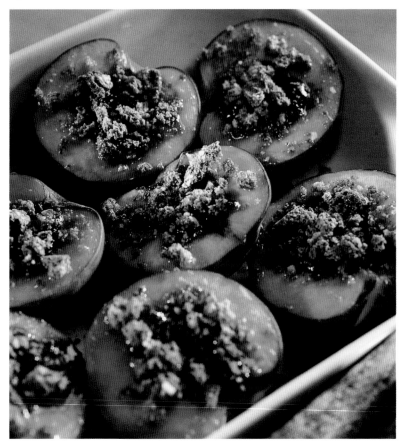

Pears

BENEFITS

- A good source of dietary fibre
- Good ource of vitamin C

DRAWBACKS

- Dried pears often contain sulphites, which provoke asthma attacks or allergic reactions in susceptible people

Called the 'butter fruit' by many Europeans in reference to its smooth texture, a pear makes an ideal snack, dessert or even a sweet or spicy side dish. Pears are a delicious treat when served fresh, but they can also be baked, sautéed or poached in red wine with spices, to make superb desserts.

One medium-sized pear has about 60kcal – most of which are in the form of natural fruit sugar – and provides 75 per cent of the Reference Nutrient Intake (RNI) for vitamin C and about 3.3g of fibre. The fibre in pears includes pectin, a soluble fibre that helps to control blood cholesterol levels and cellulose, an insoluble fibre that promotes normal bowel function.

Dried pears provide a more concentrated form of calories and nutrients than fresh pears; however, their high sugar content and sticky texture may promote tooth decay. Dried pears may also contain sulphites, which can provoke asthma or an allergic response in susceptible individuals.

Canned pears lose most of their vitamin C due to the combined effect of peeling and heating. They are also higher in calories, especially if they are packed in heavy syrup.

Varieties of pear

There are many varieties of pear grown throughout the world but those seen most often for sale in the UK include: Gold Williams (also

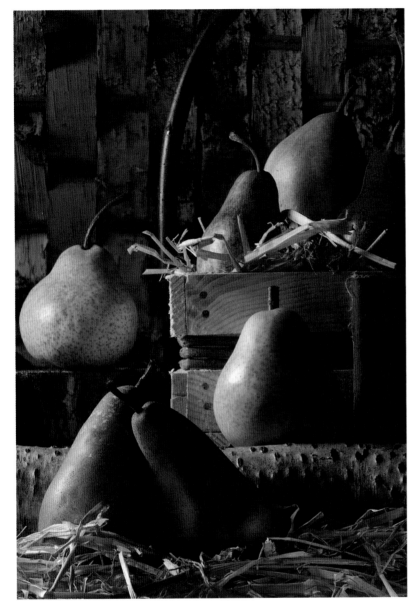

- Split peas are high in purines, which can precipitate a flare-up of gout symptoms in people with this disorder

Throughout history the pea has been a plant of significance. It is mentioned in the Bible, and dried peas have even been found in Egyptian tombs. In more recent times pea plants provided data for Gregor Johann Mendel, the founder of modern genetics.

Peas are classified as legumes, and as such, they form a complete protein when combined with grains. Fresh or frozen peas are handier than dried, because they do not require as long a cooking time as dried and can even be eaten raw. (There is no truth to the notion that eating three dried peas a day lowers blood cholesterol.)

Besides being high in protein, fresh green peas are a good source of pectin and other soluble fibres, which help to control blood cholesterol levels. The pods are high in insoluble fibre, which helps to prevent constipation. Green peas are lower in calories and fat than other high-protein foods; an 80g serving contains about 60kcal and 5g of protein. It also provides about a quarter of the vitamin C and a third of the thiamin and 10 per cent of the iron and folate required daily, as well as 2.2mg of zinc.

Peas contain lutein, a plant chemical that is linked to lowered risk of macular degeneration, the leading cause of loss of vision in older adults.

The younger green peas are, the sweeter and more tender they are; very young peas can be eaten in their pods. Once picked, green peas should be eaten or refrigerated, because their sugar quickly converts to starch. After shelling, green peas can be eaten raw or cooked. To minimise the loss of vitamins, peas

known as Bartlett), a medium-sized pear with a green skin that becomes yellow as the pear ripens; there is a Red Williams, too, which is very intensely coloured.

Juicy Conference pears have a distinctive bronze-coloured skin with a rough texture. Their long, sleek shape contrasts with the rotund shape of the crisp, juicy, yellow-green Packham. Comice are large, with a gentle red blush to the skin. Imported pears offer many lesser-known varieties.

Peas, sugar snaps and mangetout

BENEFITS

- A source of vitamin C, folate, thiamin, niacin and beta carotene

- High in pectin and other types of fibre

- Provide protein, iron, zinc and some potassium

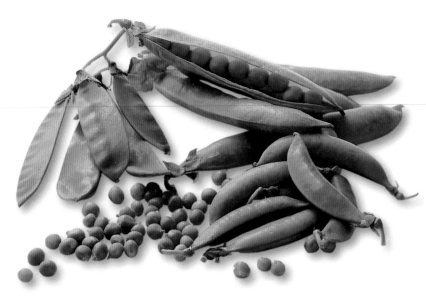

should be cooked in as little water as possible until just tender. Cooking some of the pods together with the peas or with soup stock adds flavour and nutrition; discard the pods before serving.

Peas are also sold frozen or canned. Of the two, frozen peas are nutritionally better than canned, which have fewer nutrients, added salt and less colour and flavour. To cook frozen peas, drop them into boiling water, and by the time the water has come to the boil again, they will be cooked.

Sugar snap or snow peas are often used in stir-fried dishes and salads and are widely available. Their flat pods are edible because these peas have been bred with a particular type of fibre. They contain slightly less protein than green peas. They are, however, higher in vitamin C (80g of raw sugar snap peas supplies about 26mg, which is more than 50 per cent of the RNI for women). In addition, they have less iron. Eaten in their fibrous pods,an 80g serving of sugar snap peas has about 27kcal.

Like other legumes, dried peas are high in purines, which can precipitate an attack of gout in people with this disease and so should be carefully avoided.

Peppers

BENEFITS

■ An excellent low-calorie source of beta carotene and vitamin C

Peppers, which are also known as sweet peppers, are related to chillies, or hot peppers. Both are native to the Western Hemisphere and were named by Spanish explorers who confused them with the unrelated peppercorn.

The four-lobed peppers are the most common of the sweet varieties. Depending on the degree of ripeness, peppers range in colour from green to yellow to red. Those picked while green will not become red, because they ripen only on the vine. Peppers grow sweeter as they ripen, which is the reason red ones are sweeter than yellow ones, which, in turn, are sweeter than green ones.

Other varieties may be orange or purple-brown. Related vegetables include banana peppers, which derive their name from their yellow colour and elongated shape; hot chillies and orange-red pimentos, which are heart shaped.

Peppers of all colours can cause indigestion in susceptible people. Cooking them does not reduce the risk of a disgestive disturbance.

Nutritional value

One 125g pepper contains only 40kcal and the vitamin content varies according to colour. Weight for weight, peppers are a better source of vitamin C than citrus fruit. One medium green pepper provides more than 300 per cent of the adult RNI for vitamin C, and red peppers provide 400 per cent. A green pepper supplies less beta carotene than a red pepper. In addition, all peppers supply both vitamin B_6 and folate.

Deeply coloured peppers are high in bioflavonoids, plant pigments that may help to prevent cancer; phenolic acids, which inhibit the formation of cancer-causing nitrosamines; and plant sterols, precursors of vitamin D that are believed to protect against cancer. Peppers also supply lutein and zeaxanthin, antioxidants linked to a reduced risk of macular degeneration, the leading cause of vision loss in older adults.

Peppers can be stir-fried, roasted, stuffed and baked, or served raw in a salad, or along with other vegetables and a delicious low-fat dip. Steaming, stir-frying and other fast cooking methods do not greatly lower their nutritional value.

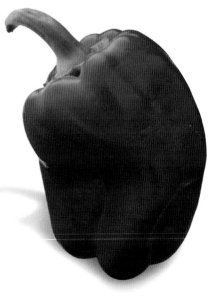

Pesticides and pollutants

How safe are our foods?

Pesticides help to assure an abundant food supply, but there is some concern that their overuse may adversely affect human health and the environment. Eating a variety of foods helps to minimise exposure. Certain foods, especially colourful fruit and vegetables, may boost the body's ability to detoxify potentially toxic compounds.

The productivity of modern agriculture depends to a large degree on a wide array of complex compounds synthesised by the agricultural chemicals industry. These include fertilisers and pesticides applied to crops, antibiotics and hormones given to livestock and additives included in animal feed. The system provides an abundance of food at a very low cost.

Inevitably, though, most crops retain traces of pesticides – they also accumulate in farmed meat to a somewhat greater degree. Potentially harmful chemicals can enter the food supply during growing, processing and packing. Environmental pollutants – heavy metals such as mercury, persistent toxic compounds such as PCBs and dioxins – in the air, water and soil may also make their way into the food supply.

A tiny trace is not necessarily harmful. The risk to your health is likely to depend not only on the toxicity of a substance, but also on the extent and type of exposure you receive. As the famed alchemist Paracelsus stated in the 16th century, 'Only the dose makes the poison'.

Workers exposed to pesticides during their manufacture and farmers who use them face much higher risks than people who eat foods with trace residues of the same chemicals. In the same way, pesticides that are harmful in large doses in animal tests may pose little danger to human health when consumed in tiny amounts as part of a varied and balanced diet. However, some toxic compounds persist for years in the environment,

and they can become more and more concentrated as they move up the food chain, making certain foods a risk to human health.

ARE PESTICIDES SAFE?

It's like asking if medicines are safe. It depends on which one, in what dose, how and by whom it is taken and for what reason. Two aspirin may take an adult's headache away but may result in a child getting a disease called Reye's syndrome – and the full contents of a bottle can kill just about anyone. So it is with pesticides. It depends on how they are

Antibiotics in the food supply

Sometimes a substance that's added to food affects human health, but only indirectly. That's the case with antibiotics given to beef cattle, pigs, poultry and other livestock. There is little, if any, direct effect on the people who eat the meat from these animals. But the widespread use of these antibiotics – many of which are very similar to the ones used to treat human illness – may be helping to weaken some of medicine's strongest weapons.

Agricultural scientists discovered that when healthy animals are given very small (subtherapeutic) doses of antibiotics, they often grew faster and fatter and were able to fight off the infections that inevitably pass from one animal to another in closely confined conditions. Unfortunately, if the subtherapeutic doses fail to kill all the bacteria and create resistant organisms that are then eaten in undercooked meat, the result is food poisoning that's hard to treat. The UK has banned antibiotic growth promoters; they are now only used to treat actual disease, with the theoretical risk that use of antibiotics may increase as animals succumb to infection.

Mercury in the food chain

Mercury, a heavy metal that enters the atmosphere primarily from coal-burning electric utilities, becomes more toxic when bacteria in lakes and oceans convert it into methylmercury, which fish then absorb into their fat tissues. The bigger a predatory fish – like swordfish – the more methylmercury it's likely to harbour.

Methylmercury is particularly toxic to pregnant women, breastfeeding mothers and young children up to six years of age. Even low-level exposure can affect the developing brain and have neurological and behavioural effects. In Europe, levels of mercury found in sea fish are carefully monitored and limits are set. Freshwater fish are equally scrupulously checked for mercury that may have escaped from industrial and medical waste and entered the water system.

Seafood is nutritious – a low saturated-fat source of high quality protein, rich in heart-healthy omega-3 fatty acids – so public health experts are eager to determine the level of mercury in seafood that can be safely consumed.

used. After all, pesticides are designed to kill their targets, whether insects, weeds or fungi. The best we can do is to evaluate the risks and the benefits of each substance and make appropriate judgments.

Because high doses of certain pesticides have been linked to health problems in animals, it is not surprising that many people are concerned that residues of them in foods we eat could cause birth defects, neurological diseases and even cancer. Several agricultural pesticides are indeed classified as 'possible' or 'suspected' human carcinogens. Because there is no known threshold for carcinogens scientists believe that the greater the overall residue taken in, the higher the possible risk of developing cancer.

Fortunately, food surveys find that many people actually have very low overall exposure to pesticide residues. And the level of that exposure has been declining in the last few years and will likely decline further. One reason is that newer pesticides tend to break down more quickly in the environment, often before food crops are harvested. And new agricultural approaches such as integrated pest management (IPM) can reduce pesticide use even more. IPM refers to the appropriate use of insect traps, crop rotation, natural insect predators and the more specific use of pesticides when needed to control pests. The small but growing market for organically grown foods also, by definition lowers the use of synthetic pesticides.

PROTECTING INFANTS, CHILDREN AND WOMEN

Certain groups of people may be more susceptible to pesticide residues in food. Infants and children, in particular, tend to consume larger amounts of single foods such as rice cereal or bananas, and they take in more food per body weight than adults – after all, their bodies are small and they're growing rapidly. A child who eats potatoes could become, in theory, sick from pesticide residues, even if the level was safe for adults. Scientists admit there are many gaps in our knowledge of how pesticides affect the growth, development and health of children.

Another population group about which too little is known is pregnant and breastfeeding women. When women breastfeed their infants, studies show, they pass along small amounts of potentially toxic compounds such as PCBs (polychlorinated biphenyls) to their infants, although scientists emphasise that the many benefits of breastfeeding far outweigh any potential risks.

There is also concern that certain pesticides that mimic the major female hormone oestrogen can disrupt endocrine systems, damaging reproductive health. Some critics of the pesticides believe these so-called oestrogen disruptors are behind a worldwide drop in sperm production. Other experts contend that the amounts in food are minute and safe.

Just as the effects of pesticides may be greater in infants, pregnant or breastfeeding women, so any potential adverse effects of antibiotic and hormone residues would be greater in these groups. Antibiotics are no longer used as growth promoters and there is a limit to the amount of copper and zinc that can be used for this purpose. Hormone implants to promote growth in cattle have also been banned in the EU since 1988. There was disagreement over the safety of these compounds. Regulatory authorities in the United States insisted that the hormones given to beef cattle were only what the animal already produced and were safe. However, despite protests, imported US beef does not contain hormones. The ban on the use of hormones in the EU arises from the difficulty in establishing safe levels of growth hormone residues. There is also concern over whether antibiotics given to animals can affect the humans who eat their meat, creating organisms that are resistant to normal antibiotic treatments.

If you wish to avoid all these problems, buy organically grown vegetables, fruit and cereals and organic meat, poultry and eggs. All are available now in supermarkets and at the increasing number of farmers' markets in the UK.

HOW PESTICIDES ARE REGULATED

In the UK, all agricultural or veterinary chemical products must be assessed and registered before they can be sold. The Pesticides Safety Directorate measures, monitors and assesses residues in food to ensure protection of public health and safety for people and animals, and also for the environment. They also evaluate whether the products work effectively and monitor the market for compliance.

More than 60 per cent of the foods monitored by the PSD are found to be free of residues, and limits are placed on foods found to have more than the Maximum Residue Level (MRL). MRLs are set for a wide range of food products and ensure that no more than a limited (and presumed safe) amount of residue is present in each. The safety limit is based on a number of factors, including the character of the pesticide, the level of residue in a particular food, the amount of that food people are likely to consume at a single meal or over a longer period and the bodyweight of the consumer. The short and long-term effects are then estimated.

In the UK, the committee that monitors residues in foodstuffs is the Pesticide Residues Committee (PRC). It targets foodstuffs which may be at high risk and can enforce the offending suppliers to adhere to the agreed guidelines. Foods are screened for residues of many heavy metals (antimony, arsenic, cadmium, copper, lead, mercury, selenium, tin and zinc). Heavy metals are found, in very small amounts, in many foods; most are there through environmental sources such as pollution from leaded petrol and industrial leakages and emissions. Other exposure to heavy metals can occur through occupational risks and inhalation. At present, there are no established maximum limits for heavy metals in foodstuffs, but they are under review.

Heavy metal levels in fish are watched carefully and EU controls on the acceptable levels of lead, cadmium and mercury in fish have been tightened. Shark, swordfish and giant tuna, in particular, have given the most cause for concern and new limits have been set. Because of the danger of mercury content, pregnant women are advised to limit their tuna consumption to no more that four cans or two fresh tuna steaks a week. Large freshwater fish, such as pike, may also contain harmful levels of mercury. Anglers should check with their local water authority before eating the fish they catch.

Breads, biscuits, cereals, coffee, nuts and chocolate are also tested for aflatoxins and related substances that are known carcinogens that develop in certain moulds in foods. Meats, dairy products, eggs and infant formulas are also tested to see if they contain some antibiotic residues.

Each food in the survey is chemically analysed to measure the levels of pesticide residues, contaminants and other substances and this data is then related to food consumption data.

While there are obviously many checks in place, pesticides present some difficulties. In some cases, health consequences of pesticide residues have only become apparent years after use and even when a product such as DDT is discontinued, residues remain in the environment and the food chain for many years. We also have little knowledge of the cumulative effect of the many pesticides to which we are exposed.

P

WHAT YOU CAN DO TO LOWER YOUR RISK

Eating a well-balanced diet rich in fruit and vegetables protects against possible risks from agricultural residues. It's true that the fruit and vegetables themselves may contain small quantities of pesticide residues, but scientists agree that the protection offered by the healthy compounds in these foods greatly outweighs the risks posed by the residues. And for those contaminants we can't avoid, our bodies are remarkably well equipped with preventive mechanisms to detoxify them. Here are five ways to minimise your risk:

1 Eat a wide variety of foods. Doing so helps to protect you from overeating any one type of food that may have high levels of pollutants or pesticides.

2 Trim the animal fat. Whether a contaminant is harmful or not depends on how long it lingers in the body or the environment. A substance that resists chemical or biological breakdown accumulates as it is ingested by one species after another, steadily building up as the food chain progresses from small, weak species to the large and dominant. The highest levels of pollutants, therefore, are ingested by large animals. Many of these persistent pollutants are stored in an animal's fat, which is why choosing lower-fat foods and trimming fat from meat can help to reduce the amount of pollutants you consume.

3 Buy organically grown foods and wash non-organic fruit and vegetables well to remove traces of pesticides. Organic meats and chicken are also produced without the use of antibiotic growth promoters.

4 Eat fruit and vegetables, whole grains, nuts and seeds. They're rich in the fibre and antioxidants that may help to protect the body from carcinogens.

5 Eat your broccoli – and cauliflower, cabbage, watercress and Brussels sprouts. They contain compounds that release isothiocyanates, which stimulate the liver to produce enzymes that can detoxify carcinogens before they cause harm. Phenolic compounds (in apples and other fruit) and bioflavonoids (high in citrus fruit) protect in similar ways.

Other elements of a healthy diet may help to counter any carcinogenic pesticide residues. Sulphur compounds in onions and garlic may have cancer-protective activities – they bind to carcinogens, neutralising them. And calcium, abundant in dairy products as well as in dark green leafy vegetables, may help to guard against colon cancer.

A low-fat diet that provides ample vegetables and fruit will be naturally rich in detoxifying compounds. But many other factors, such as heredity, lifestyle and exposure to environmental pollutants, affect your susceptibility to disease. Our food supply has low and declining levels of pesticide residues, but there are always risks, and a healthy lifestyle is the best protection.

Did you know?

Fish from the Baltic Sea are affected by pollutants

Swedish researchers have found that fishermen exposed to high levels of organochlorine pollutants (such as dioxin, DDT and PCBs – all now banned) from eating fish from the Baltic Sea, have a higher proportion of the male Y chromosomes in their sperm. An egg fertilised by a Y chromosome sperm will produce a male baby, but whether this higher proportion of Ys will produce more male babies is not yet known. The quality of their sperm was also affected by the pollutants.

P

Pickles and other condiments

BENEFITS

- Sauerkraut is a good source of vitamin C, iron, potassium and other nutrients

- Pickles are low in calories

DRAWBACKS

- Most pickles and condiments are extremely high in sodium

- Sweet pickles, tomato sauce and chutneys are high in sugar

- In large amounts, pickled foods may increase the risk of cancer

Pickling was a traditional way to store food over winter. Long before vitamin C and other nutrients were identified, sauerkraut – pickled cabbage – was used to prevent scurvy during long sea voyages.

In pickling, food is preserved by saturating it with acid, which prevents most micro-organisms from growing. Although minerals are usually retained in the process, many vitamins are lost – the exception to this is sauerkraut.

There are two basic methods of pickling: soaking or cooking the food in a vinegar-based solution; and brining, a fermentation process. In the first method, vegetables are presoaked in brine to draw off moisture that would dilute the vinegar. They are then sealed in jars to mature, usually with pickling spices. This method is used for sweet and sour pickles. Chutney and tomato sauce are cooked, pulped variations on the basic pickle. Bacteria rarely grow in them but moulds and yeasts may flourish on imperfectly sealed surfaces. Fermented pickles, such as dill pickles, are vegetables that are immersed in a brine that is strong enough to inhibit the growth of unwanted bacteria but mild enough to nourish several species that produce lactic acid. This and other compounds contribute to the characteristic flavour. (Dill pickles are also flavoured with dill seeds.) Bacteria are not added to the brine; they are attracted to the mixture from the surrounding air. Fermented pickles are more difficult to make than vinegar pickles because, given the wrong temperature or salt concentration, hostile bacteria will thrive and make them unpalatable.

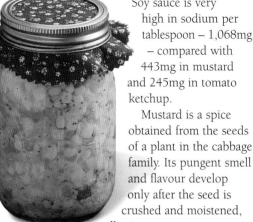

Sauerkraut

One of the few pickled dishes served as a vegetable, sauerkraut has only 9kcal in a 100g serving. It provides 10mg of vitamin C, 1.2mg of iron and small amounts of the B vitamins, calcium, fibre and potassium. Sauerkraut is high in sodium (590mg per 100g), and the salt content may be increased by the foods often served with it, such as smoked sausages.

Tomato and other sauces

Most tomato sauce is made from tomatoes, although apples, pears, mangoes and other soft fruit can be used. The huge variety of barbecue sauces are variants on the basic tomato sauce recipe of tomatoes, brown sugar, vinegar, salt, pepper and spices. These sauces have a negligible nutritional value, although tomato sauce does contain some of the antioxidant lycopene which is valuable for prostate gland health. The high salt content in most sauces may be harmful to people with high blood pressure or on a low-salt diet.

Soy sauce is very high in sodium per tablespoon – 1,068mg – compared with 443mg in mustard and 245mg in tomato ketchup.

Mustard is a spice obtained from the seeds of a plant in the cabbage family. Its pungent smell and flavour develop only after the seed is crushed and moistened, allowing enzymes to react with isothiocyanates to form mustard oils. Most mustards are sold premixed, and many specialty varieties, which are mixed with white-wine or herb-flavoured vinegars, are marketed both as fine pastes and as coarser blends that contain unground seeds. The addition of turmeric gives some types their brilliant yellow colour and extra tanginess. In making prepared mustard, the dry powder is usually blended with wheat flour to improve its mixing qualities; people with coeliac disease, who are gluten sensitive, should look for mustards that don't contain wheat.

Cancer risk

A diet that is high in pickled or salt-cured foods and condiments has been linked to an increased risk of stomach and oesophageal cancers. This is thought to stem from their high levels of nitrates, which are converted to cancer-causing nitrosamines during digestion. Nitrates are often used in the pickling solution to impart flavour and prevent the growth of unwanted micro-organisms. Vitamins A and C, beta carotene, and other antioxidants are thought to inhibit the cancer-causing potential of nitrosamines; eating ample fresh vegetables and fruit may counteract any risk from pickled foods.

P

Pineapples

BENEFITS

- A good source of vitamin C, with useful amounts of dietary fibre and manganese

DRAWBACKS

- May cause dermatitis in individuals sensitive to bromelain, an enzyme in pineapples

Native to South America, pineapples are now grown in tropical areas worldwide. The majority of the crop is reserved for canning and juicing; the rest goes on the market as fresh fruit. Although pineapples are available year round, their peak season takes place during the summer months.

The sweet and tangy flavour makes fresh pineapple a delicious choice; it can be added to fruit salads, or barbecued or baked with seafood, ham, poultry or other meats. As pineapple is cooked, its texture softens due to the breakdown of cellulose, a type of fibre in its walls.

Healing properties

Fresh pineapple contains bromelain, an enzyme that is similar to papain in papayas that dissolves proteins. Consequently, fresh pineapple is a natural tenderiser for meat and poultry when it is added to stews or marinades. If pineapple is to be used in a jelly or a dessert combined with gelatine, however, it is better to use the canned fruit or boil it beforehand to deactivate the bromelain; otherwise, the gelatine (a form of protein) will not set properly and will become soupy.

Bromelain is an anti-inflammatory enzyme, and preliminary research suggests that it may reduce the risk of blood clots, thereby lowering the risk for heart attack and stroke. This is difficult to explain, since bromelain is a protein and such proteins are readily broken down in the digestive tract. Topically applied, bromelain may help to control tissue swelling and the inflammation associated with arthritis, strains and sprains, but it can also irritate the skin of susceptible people.

An 80g portion of fresh pineapple chunks contains 33kcal and provides a quarter of the daily requirement of vitamin C. Pineapple is high in soluble fibre, which helps to control high blood cholesterol. Pineapple is a good source of ferulic acid, a plant chemical that may help to prevent the formation of cancer-causing substances.

Canning does not significantly lower pineapple's vitamin C; 80g of canned fruit, regardless of whether it is juice or syrup, retains 10mg of vitamin C. However, canning heats the fruit enough to destroy its bromelain, so such products can be used to make jellied desserts. Pineapple is often canned in syrup, which adds calories. Juice-packed chunks contain 38kcal per 80g, compared with 51kcal in the same amount packed in heavy syrup.

After picking, a pineapple will not ripen further. When buying a pineapple, look for one that exudes a fragrant odour and has light or deep yellow flesh. Brown patches indicate spoilage. If you are buying the fruit whole, make sure that it seems dense and heavy for its size and that the leaves are green. Small, yellow-fleshed pineapples are usually sweeter than larger fruit with paler flesh.

Pizza

See Fast food

Did you know?

Pineapple contains an anti-inflammatory enzyme

Pineapple contains bromelain, may help to control the inflammation associated with arthritis and many other conditions. Research suggests that bromelain's anti-inflammatory property may also reduce blood clots, which may lower the risk of heart attack and stroke.

Plums and prunes

BENEFITS

- A useful source of vitamin C, potassium, iron and fibre

- Prunes help to relieve constipation

DRAWBACKS

- May cause allergic reactions in susceptible people

- Prunes may lead to tooth decay

Plums are a nutritious, low-calorie food, whether eaten fresh, cooked or canned. One medium (50g) fresh plum contains only 20kcal and is a good source of such dietary fibres as cellulose and pectin. It also supplies useful amounts of several nutrients, including 2mg of vitamin C and 132mg of potassium. Canned plums contain comparable amounts of riboflavin and potassium but are significantly lower in vitamin C (one canned plum provides only 1mg). Fruit canned in heavy syrup is higher in calories than fresh – for example, one canned plum packed in a sugary syrup yields 40kcal.

Plums contain anthocyanins, the reddish blue pigments that lend them their intense colour. These antioxidant pigments may help to protect against cancer and heart disease by mopping up free radicals, unstable molecules that damage cells.

Fresh plums do not ripen after they have been picked; so when buying, look for brightly coloured fruit that yields slightly to the touch. Colour, which varies from one variety to another – and there are more than 2,000 varieties – may not be a good indicator of ripeness. Over-ripe plums tend to be soft, with a bruised or discoloured skin, and they are sometimes leaky. Firm plums can be stored for a day or two at room temperature to soften. Plums may produce an allergic reaction in individuals allergic to apricots, almonds, peaches and cherries, which come from the same family. Similarly, people who are allergic to aspirin may also have problems after eating plums.

Prunes

Although all prunes are plums, not all plums are prunes. Prunes are the dried fruit from a few particular species of plum trees whose fruit has firm flesh and is naturally high in sugar and acidity. These traits allow the fruit to dry without fermenting if the stone is left in.

Like all dried fruit, prunes contain very little water and are a more concentrated source of energy and nutrients than their fresh fruit counterparts. They are also higher in calories and natural fruit sugar (80g of stewed prunes contain 72kcal and five dried, pitted prunes contain approximately 70kcal), and they leave a sticky residue on the teeth that can cause cavities. On the plus side, prunes are rich in fibre: five prunes contain 3g of fibre as well as good amounts of iron and potassium.

Prunes are popular as a remedy for treating constipation. This effect can be attributed to prunes' high dietary fibre content; they also contain dihydroxyphenylisatin, a natural laxative.

Unlike other types of juice, prune juice retains many of the fruit's nutrients because it is made by pulverising prunes and dissolving them in hot water. A glass (150ml) of prune juice contains 2g of dietary fibre and 315mg of potassium. But it contains more calories than other fruit juices, about 86kcal per 150ml portion. Prune juice is naturally high in sugar, so needs no additional sweeteners. It is not as good a source of fibre as whole prunes but, as it contains the same natural laxative, it can help to relieve constipation.

Pomegranates

BENEFITS

- Good source of vitamin C, potassium

- Rich in plant chemicals

DRAWBACKS

- May interact with some medication

The word 'pomegranate' is Old French for 'seeded apple', a fitting name for this apple-sized fruit filled with jewel-like clusters of red seeds. There are many types cultivated around the world.

Pomegranates have a leathery, deep red to purplish rind. The interior is bursting with hundreds of tiny, edible seeds packed into compartments called arils and separated by bitter, cream-coloured membranes. The fruit can be eaten out of hand by deeply scoring vertically and then breaking it apart. The clusters of juice sacs are then lifted out and eaten.

Pomegranate is often consumed as juice and can be juiced in several ways. The sacs can be removed and put through a basket press or the juice can be extracted by reaming the halved fruit on an ordinary juice squeezer. Another approach is to soften the fruit by hand and then make a cut in the stem end and place it over a glass to let the juice run out, squeezing the fruit from time to time. One pomegranate yields about 75ml of juice. The juice can be used to make jellies, sorbets or sauces, as well as to flavour cakes and baked apples. Pomegranate molasses is available in Middle Eastern food shops and some delicatessens. It is excellent served with chicken or lamb. Pomegranates

P

▶ **Pomegranate seeds**

Both the seeds and the fleshy seed covering of this fruit are edible.

...are a good source of potassium: one medium pomegranate has about 360mg, more than in most oranges, as well as 50 per cent of the RNI for vitamin C.

Pomegranates and their juice are rich in anthocyanins and ellagic acid, both of which have antioxidant properties. The juice has two to three times the antioxidant capacity of equal amounts of red wine or green tea, and anthocyanins make an important contribution to the pomegranate's antioxidant power. Drinking little pomegranate juice daily may improve cardiovascular health by significantly reducing oxidation of LDL cholesterol.

Warning: Pomegranate juice can have severe reactions if taken with certain medicines, such as those used to lower cholesterol levels. It appears to increase the blood levels of many medications.

Pork

BENEFITS

■ Fresh, lean pork is a good source of high-quality protein, B vitamins and zinc

DRAWBACKS

■ Ham, bacon and other cured pork products are high in salt and may also be high in fat

■ Risk of trichinosis if undercooked

Thrifty cooks used to boast that when it came to pigs, they could use everything but the squeal. A pig yields not only chops and other cuts of fresh meat, but cured or processed products, such as ham and bacon as well as skin for gelatine.

Globally, pork continues to be the world's most eaten meat, with consumption continuing to grow. The latest data shows that of the world's meat consumption, 41 per cent is pork (versus 29 per cent poultry and 25 per cent beef). Over the past 20 years, the volume of pork consumption has increased by 73 per cent worldwide.

Surprisingly, pork is one of the leanest meats; it is the products made from it that can be high in fat. Trimmed, lean pork is close to skinless poultry in its calorie and fat content. A 100g serving of lean roast pork has 185 calories and 7 per cent fat, compared with 150 calories and 5 per cent fat in the same amount of chicken.

Pork supplies substantial amounts of high-quality protein and the B vitamins thiamin, riboflavin, niacin, B_6 and B_{12}; it provides 100 per cent of the Reference Nutrient Intake (RNI) of thiamin, niacin and B_{12}. Lean pork provides minerals such as potassium, magnesium, iron and zinc. About half the iron in pork is haem iron, the most readily absorbed and digested type of dietary iron. The tenderloin, loin chops and centre-cut leg are the most lean. Pork cooked to an internal temperature of 70°C will remain moist and tender.

Once the visible fat is removed, pork also has less saturated fat than other meats. The problems occur with processed pork products where the fat is incorporated into the product, as occurs with bacon, some types of ham and luncheon meats that are made from reconstituted

meat, salami and smoked sausages. Pork sausages are also high in fat and all processed pork products are high in sodium. Two rashers of lean grilled bacon, for instance, contain 10-14g of fat, with 40 per cent from saturated fat and 144kcal.

Bacon also contains nitrates, which can lead to the formation of carcinogenic nitrosamines. Another health problem is the possibility that undercooked pork can transmit tapeworm eggs, trichinosis or other parasites. Always check that pork is thoroughly cooked and that juices run clear, before serving it.

Potatoes

BENEFITS

■ A good source of vitamins C and B_6, and potassium and other minerals

■ An inexpensive, filling and nutritious starchy food

■ A source of fibre

DRAWBACKS

■ Green and sprouted potatoes may contain solanine, a potentially toxic substance

Potatoes are native to the Andes Mountains and were first cultivated by Peruvian Indians at least 4,000 years ago. Spanish explorers introduced potatoes to Europe in the 1500s, where they became a staple food source for the poor. Potatoes are now cultivated worldwide; in fact, they are the world's largest and most economically important vegetable crop. In the UK, potatoes are a major part of the diet – recent figures revealed that the average Briton will eat 100kg of potatoes a year – often in processed forms that are high in fat and salt.

There are many varieties of potato. They are members of the nightshade family, and are related to peppers and tomatoes. Surprisingly, yams and sweet potatoes do not belong to the potato family.

Potatoes are very nutritious and relatively low in calories. When eaten with the skin, they are high in complex carbohydrates and fibre; a 150g baked potato (with the skin) provides 25mg of vitamin C, which is more than 50 per cent of the adult Reference Nutrient Intake (RNI) for women, along with 100 per cent of the RNI for vitamin B_6, 1,130mg of potassium, good amounts of folate and thiamin and a moderate amount of iron. The skins are rich in chlorogenic acid, a phytochemical that has anti-cancer properties.

Potatoes have a relatively high Glycaemic Index (GI), which may be an issue for people with diabetes.

However, since potatoes are rarely eaten on their own, their GI may be less important. Combining potatoes with meat, fish, chicken or green peas will reduce their glycaemic effect. Waxy potatoes (the type that don't mash well) have a lower GI than floury potatoes that mash easily. New potatoes are digested more slowly than mature white potatoes or red potatoes.

Many people think potatoes are fattening, but this is true only when they are fried or served with butter, margarine, soured cream or rich sauces. A 200g baked or boiled potato has about 140kcal, a small amount of protein and 0.5g fat. The same potato turned into potato chips has around 378kcal and up to 15g of fat. One-half cup of mashed potatoes with milk and butter or margarine provides about 182kcal, and 7.5g fat. In addition, French fries and other processed potatoes are almost always high in salt.

When preparing potatoes, it is best not to remove the skin because some of the fibre and many of the phytochemicals are in the skin or just near the surface; instead, scrub potatoes under water with a vegetable brush. If you do peel them, try to remove as thin a layer as possible. Once sliced or peeled, raw potatoes will discolour when exposed to oxygen, so cook them

Why potatoes sometimes turn black

Potatoes contain small amounts of iron from the soil, in an ionic form known as ferrous iron. When a potato is cut, or cooked, the ferrous ion reacts with oxygen and converts to a form called ferric iron. The ferric iron-chlorogenic acid complex is black. This can often be seen as harmless blue-black spots in cooked potatoes.

immediately or place them in water with vinegar or lemon juice added. Baking, steaming or microwaving preserves the maximum amount of nutrients. Pierce a potato's skin with a fork before baking or microwaving to avoid having it burst. It is preferable to steam potatoes, but if you boil them, leave the skin on, use as little water as possible and cook in a covered pot. Some nutrients, particularly vitamin C, are lost during boiling. To salvage some lost nutrients, add the potato water to soups or stews.

When shopping, look for potatoes with few eyes and no black spots. Avoid potatoes with a green tint to the skin, and remove any sprouts; they will taste bitter and may contain solanine, a toxic substance that can cause diarrhoea, cramps, migraine or drowsiness. Store potatoes in a dark, cool place, but not in the refrigerator.

P

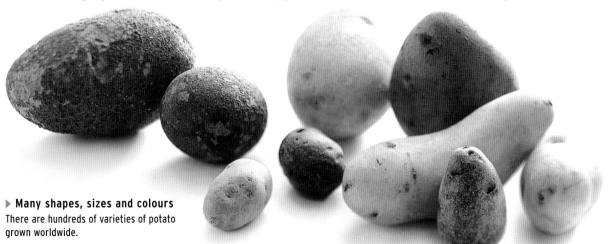

▶ **Many shapes, sizes and colours**
There are hundreds of varieties of potato grown worldwide.

Did you know?

A 'new' potato is not just a small potato

A 'new' potato is one dug before the plant's foliage has died down. It has a soft skin that can be rubbed off, a waxy texture and more intense flavour.

Temperatures below 7°C convert the starch to sugar, giving the potato a strange taste. Don't store potatoes and onions together; the acids in onions aid the decomposition of potatoes, and vice versa.

Poultry

BENEFITS

■ An excellent source of protein

■ A good source of the B vitamins and several minerals

DRAWBACKS

■ Susceptible to bacterial contamination

■ Skin is high in fat

Higher in protein and lower in saturated fat than red meats, poultry – including chicken, turkey, duck, goose, guinea fowl, pigeon, pheasant and quail – is an excellent source of high-quality protein, with all the essential amino acids, as well as some copper, iron, phosphorus, potassium and zinc.

All poultry has a similar range of nutrients; the main difference, apart from flavour, is in the fat content. A 100g portion of roasted, skinless light turkey is the lowest in calories and fat, with 153kcal, 2g of fat and 33g of protein, compared with 195kcal, 10.5g of fat and 25g of protein in a comparable portion of skinless roasted duck. A 100g serving of roasted chicken breast without skin has 153kcal, 3.6g of fat and 30.2g of protein compared with

the same serving with skin at 216kcal, 22g of protein and 14g of fat. Most poultry fat is under the skin; removing the skin before eating the meat greatly reduces fat content. The fattiness of a duck can be reduced by pricking the skin all over before roasting it to allow the fat to drain off. You can roast, grill or barbecue poultry with the skin on to preserve moisture, but it's best to remove it before eating.

Poultry meat is a good source of many B vitamins. Duck and dark-meat turkey are good sources of haem iron, the most absorbable form of this important mineral. A 100g serving of cooked skinless chicken breast supplies 12mg of niacin, almost 100 per cent of the Reference Nutrient Intake (RNI). Duck and turkey are also excellent sources of niacin, which is vital for energy metabolism, healthy skin and healthy digestive and nervous systems. Dark turkey is quite high in selenium. A 100g serving contains 17mcg, which is 25 per cent of the RNI. Poultry contains tryptophan, an essential amino acid that may help to ease depression and insomnia. Though all poultry has vitamin B_6, light-meat chicken and turkey are the best sources with

Poultry fat content

	GRAMS OF TOTAL FAT PER 100G (ROAST MEAT, NO SKIN)
■ Chicken	3.6
■ Duck	10.5
■ Goose	22
■ Partridge	2
■ Pheasant	4
■ Pigeon	2
■ Turkey	2

Did you know?

Dark meat has more fat

Lovers of the dark meat from a turkey should know that the legs and thighs contain more iron but also slightly more fat than the breast meat. While a 100g portion of roasted breast (without skin) contains about 2g of fat, the same amount of dark meat without the skin contains about 4g of fat.

100g providing 0.5mg or more than half of the RNI. Turkey, duck and dark-meat chicken also provide generous amounts of zinc.

Dark poultry meat comes from muscles that get more exercise. That's why the drumsticks have darker meat than the breast, and why game birds, which spend much of their life on the wing, often have dark breast meat.

Poultry safety

Because most poultry is sold with its skin on, it is susceptible to spoilage from bacteria that remain on the skin and in the cavity after processing. Kept at the average 4°C fridge temperature, chicken skin becomes slimy in about six days, indicating a 10,000-fold increase in bacteria. Don't keep poultry for more than two to three days. All raw poultry should be washed under running water. Wash your hands often during preparation, and scrub knives and chopping boards in hot, soapy water.

Poultry is properly cooked when the leg joints move easily and the juices run clear if the thigh is pierced with a knife. The best way to judge readiness is to use a meat thermometer. Put the thermometer into the breast of a whole chicken, thigh of a whole turkey or into the thickest part of cut-up poultry. Stuffing cooked inside poultry or cooked separately should reach 75°C before being served.

Stuffed poultry should be cooked at 190°C (375°F, Gas mark 5); for birds under 4kg allow 20 minutes per kilogram plus 70 minutes. For birds heavier than 4kg, allow 20 minutes a kilogram plus an extra

90 minutes. Never stuff the body cavity of a turkey; stuff the neck pouch only. Use leftovers within a day or two, or freeze them.

Pregnancy

CONSUME PLENTY OF

- Lean meat, poultry, fish, dried beans, lentils and eggs for protein and iron
- Milk and dairy products, canned sardines and salmon (with bones included) and other high-calcium foods
- Citrus fruit, dark green vegetables, legumes, whole grains and fortified cereals for folate

LIMIT

- High-fat foods
- Sugary desserts and confectionery
- Coffee and other caffeinated drinks

AVOID

- Drinking alcohol and/or smoking

  Liver and fish liver oil supplements high in vitamin A
- All drugs unless prescribed by a doctor

At no other time in a woman's life is good nutrition more essential than during pregnancy. While the need for calories increases by only a small amount, if at all, the need for some nutrients more than doubles, and a woman needs to plan her diet carefully to meet these needs. She should work with her doctor or other health professional providing prenatal care to design an eating programme that supplies the best nutrition for her and her baby.

A woman planning a pregnancy should also evaluate her eating habits. Even before trying to conceive, she should eat well to achieve ideal nutritional status as well as a healthy weight. Women who are too thin often have difficulty conceiving and then have low-birth-weight babies, while those who are overweight have a greater risk of gestational diabetes and giving birth to an oversized baby. Infants who are either too small or too large at birth often suffer serious problems, including respiratory disorders and an increased risk for diabetes, high blood pressure and obesity later in life.

Pregnancy is also the time to abstain from alcohol or limit consumption to one or two units of alcohol, once or twice a week, because alcohol causes the most harm to a foetus during the first few weeks of a pregnancy, and the woman may not know that she has conceived. Studies show that women who have more than one or two drinks a day tend to have undersized babies. A greater danger is incurred by heavy drinkers during early pregnancy; these women have a high risk of giving birth to a baby with foetal alcohol syndrome, a constellation of congenital defects that may include mental deficiency, facial and heart malformations, an undersized head and retarded growth.

The use of vitamin supplements also should be evaluated. High doses of vitamin A should be stopped several months before attempting pregnancy, because large stores of the vitamin can cause severe birth defects. Women who are planning a pregnancy should take a daily 400mcg folic acid supplement from the time they stop using contraception until the twelfth week of pregnancy.

Nutritional guidance

The recommended gain for a woman of average weight having an average pregnancy is about 10kg-15kg. Underweight women may need to gain as much as 12kg-18kg, and women who are overweight may be advised to gain no more than 7kg–11kg. An obese woman should not try to lose weight in pregnancy; to do so exposes her baby to numerous hazards.

The pattern of weight gain is just as important as the amount gained. It is normal for most women to gain no weight during the first trimester. After that, a healthy woman at ideal weight before conceiving should gain an average of up to 0.5kg a week; underweight women should gain slightly more each week; overweight women should gain weight more slowly. Losing the weight after the birth is important: studies show

P

Food cravings

From pickles to ice cream, stories abound about the food cravings of pregnant women. The cravings are certainly real, but they rarely reflect any true nutritional problem. The one exception is craving ice, which may be a sign of iron-deficiency anaemia. Some women, however, inexplicably develop pica, a craving for bizarre, inedible substances, such as clay, soil, paint, coffee grounds and laundry starch. Some studies have linked such cravings to iron deficiency, even though in reality, eating soil, clay or starch lowers iron absorption.

that failing to shift pregnancy fat can lead to problems in subsequent pregnancies. However, crash diets after birth are very dangerous, too.

Most women need to add about 190–260kcal to their daily diet to support normal foetal growth, especially during the last two trimesters. This is a relatively small amount, despite the saying about 'eating for two'. A woman who doubles what she normally eats will certainly gain excessive weight during her pregnancy. Appropriate foods that add sufficient extra calories include 200ml skimmed milk plus two pieces of fruit; or an egg and two slices of toast. Pregnant women need at least three portions of dairy foods a day.

Protein. A pregnant woman needs to consume an extra 5g of protein daily – the amount found in 125ml of skimmed milk or 25g of cooked meat. Some studies suggest that excessive protein may be detrimental to the baby, causing delayed growth or premature birth. When selecting protein-rich foods, include lean meats, poultry and fish, which are also good sources of B vitamins and iron and other trace

▶ **Eating for two**
Being pregnant should not mean eating double portions; however, a healthy balance of nutritious food will help the baby to get off to a good start.

minerals. Other foods high in protein include eggs, cheese, nuts, seeds, grains and legumes.

Lacto-ovo vegetarians can obtain protein from milk and eggs as well as from legumes, nuts and seeds; vegans, who eat only plant foods, should consult an accredited dietitian on how to plan an adequate diet.

Vitamin supplements. Experts agree that women should take 400mcg of folic acid supplements from when they stop contraception until the twelfth week of pregnancy, as well as 10mcg of vitamin D daily. Many doctors believe that a diet that includes a variety of foods in the right amounts will meet most needs, but others prescribe multivitamins as added insurance against deficiencies.

Calcium. A pregnant woman needs 700mg of calcium a day. Because many women do not get enough calcium, it's a good idea to increase consumption of calcium-rich foods before becoming pregnant. This is especially important for women under 30, whose bones are still increasing in density. Low-fat milk and dairy products are the best dietary sources of calcium; other good sources include fortified soya and rice drinks, tofu, canned sardines and salmon with the bones included, nuts and seeds and leafy green vegetables. 200ml milk has 246mg of calcium – which is more than a third of the recommended 700mg. A 30g portion of Cheddar cheese contains 222mg and a 150g pot of yoghurt contains about 290mg.

If you're not a milk drinker, you can get about the same amount of calcium from 200ml of fortified soya or rice drink, 500g of baked beans, 100g of canned salmon, with the bones, 90g sardines or 100g almonds. Calcium is also present in bok choy, and other Asian greens. If you take calcium supplements, have them with meals to aid absorption and reduce intestinal upsets.

Coping with morning sickness

Despite its name, morning sickness can occur at any time of the day, but it usually disappears after the first three months of pregnancy. In order to ease the nausea and vomiting, try these strategies:

- Eat dry cereal, biscuits or dry toast before you get out of bed.
- Avoid greasy foods or anything that increases nausea.
- Instead of three big meals, eat several small meals during the day.
- To quell nausea, sip ginger ale or suck a piece of fresh or preserved ginger.
- Try an acupressure bracelet, such as those used to prevent motion sickness.
- Have someone else prepare food if cooking odours provoke nausea.

Iron. A woman's iron requirement doesn't change during pregnancy; there is no need to take extra iron.

Folic acid. Adequate folic acid, or folate, can help to prevent birth defects involving the brain and spinal cord, such as spina bifida – a condition in which the spine does not form normally. It is estimated that 50 to 70 per cent of such defects could be prevented if all women of child-bearing age took folic acid. The Reference Nutrient Intake (RNI) calls for 200mcg of folic acid for women who are not pregnant; this increases to 400mcg during pregnancy and then changes to 350mcg during breastfeeding.

Because the most critical period for folate consumption is during the first four to six weeks of pregnancy, when the foetal central nervous system is being formed, women planning to become pregnant are generally advised by their doctors to take a supplement while trying to conceive. Good dietary sources include green leafy vegetables, oranges, lentils, peas, beans, liver, asparagus, avocado and salmon.

Sodium. In the past, pregnant women were routinely advised to cut down on salt because it was thought to increase the risk of toxaemia, a potentially life-threatening condition. There is no evidence, however, that salt restriction prevents or alleviates toxaemia. It is, however, still a very good idea to limit salt for other health reasons, including avoiding high blood pressure.

Artificial sweeteners. Controversy has swirled around the use of artificial sweeteners. Extensive studies on aspartame suggest that it is safe to use during pregnancy, unless the woman has phenylketonuria (PKU). Saccharin can cross the placenta, but there is no proof that it harms the foetus. Acesulfame-K and sucralose pass through the digestive tract and are excreted unchanged, and no toxic effect has been shown. Most experts believe that sweeteners used in moderation are not harmful during pregnancy.

Caffeine. A recent study found an increased risk of spontaneous abortion and low birth weight in pregnant women who consumed more than 150mg of caffeine per day. There is some evidence to suggest that high levels of caffeine may delay conception. And yet other studies have failed to find any association between caffeine consumption and birth defects or premature birth.

Since adverse effects on pregnancy outcomes have been linked to high caffeine intake, it would be wise to limit caffeine intake to 300mg per day. Each of the following contains about 300mg of caffeine: three mugs of instant coffee (100mg each); four cups of instant coffee (75mg each); three cups of brewed coffee (100mg each); six cups of tea (50mg each); eight cans of cola (up to 40mg each); four cans of 'energy' drink (up to 80mg each) or eight bars of plain chocolate weighing 50g each (50mg each). The caffeine in milk chocolate is about half that of plain chocolate.

Remember that caffeine is also found in some cold and flu remedies, so check with your doctor or pharmacist before taking any.

Alcohol. If you are pregnant, it is wise to avoid alcohol altogether, but if you really want to have a drink, limit it to one or two units, once or twice a week.

A unit is half a pint of standard strength beer, lager or cider; or a pub measure of spirits. A glass of wine is about 2 units and 'alcopops' are about 1.5 units.

Fish. Mercury is a widely found pollutant which can show up in deep sea fish. Pregnant women and

CAUTION

Food safety is important during pregnancy. Foods contaminated by *Listeria monocytogenes*, bacteria which are widespread in our environment, can cause listeriosis, which is especially dangerous for pregnant women and may cause abortion.

To prevent listeriosis, take the following steps: avoid delicatessen meats unless they are reheated until steaming hot; avoid soft cheeses such as Brie and Camembert, blue-veined cheeses and fresh cheeses such as ricotta (hard cheese, semi-soft cheeses such as mozzarella, and pasteurised processed cheese slices can be safely consumed); avoid pâté or meat spreads, smoked seafood unless it is an ingredient in a cooked dish; do not drink raw or unpasteurised milk or eat foods that contain unpasteurised milk. Avoid rare and undercooked meats and raw fish such as sushi.

To avoid salmonella, avoid foods with uncooked eggs in them and cheeses made from unpasteurised milk. In addition, make sure that all ready meals are thoroughly heated.

Avoid raw shellfish because it may contain harmful bacteria and viruses that could cause food poisoning.

women who may become pregnant should avoid eating any shark, swordfish or marlin. In addition, limit the amount of tuna you eat to no more than two tuna steaks (weighing 140g cooked or 170g raw) or four medium-sized cans (with a drained weight of about 140g) of tuna a week. This is because, at high levels, mercury can harm a baby's developing nervous system.

Most fish is very good for your health and the development of your baby, and it is important to have at least two portions of fish a week, with one being an oily fish. If you do eat fish, limit your intake of oily fish (salmon, mackerel, sardines, pilchards and fresh trout) to no more than two portions a week.

P

Probiotics

Beneficial bacteria

The term probiotic means 'for life'. Probiotics are organisms
that live in the intestinal tract and contribute to its health;
they are commonly referred to as the 'friendly', 'beneficial' or 'good' bacteria,
that act against 'bad' bacteria to maintain a balance and help to fight disease.

Probiotic organisms are found in live
yoghurts and sometimes in supplement
form. To be effective, probiotics must reach
the colon in sufficiently large numbers by resisting
the effects of digestion such as gastric juices in
the stomach and bile in the small intestine. On
reaching the colon, probiotic organisms must be
able to reproduce themselves to establish a viable
part of the flora. In order to maintain the friendly
Bifidus bacteria as a viable part of the colonic
flora, regular 'topping-up' with daily consumption
of new supplies of probiotic organisms is required.

Probiotics have a number of ways of working,
including affecting inflammatory processes,
secreting compounds that regulate cell function
and protecting the intestine against invasive 'bad'
bacteria. They may also inhibit the growth of
disease-causing bacteria by preventing their
attachment to the intestine and by producing
substances that suppress their growth.

Probiotic bacteria naturally living in our gut
perform a number of important functions
including the digestion of food and manufacture of
certain vitamins. Some experts believe they play a
vital role in helping to strengthen the immune
system and helping to reduce blood cholesterol
levels. They also help to keep our intestines
healthy by crowding out and preventing the
growth of unfriendly bacteria.

Unfortunately the delicate balance of good
and bad bacteria in the gut can be upset easily,
allowing unfriendly bacteria to gain the upper
hand. Several factors including stress, poor diet,
illness and prescription drugs such as antibiotics
can upset this balance. An imbalance of bacteria
in the gut bacteria, a condition doctors call,
dysbiosis, has been linked with several health
problems, including constipation, diarrhoea,
irritable bowel syndrome, inflammatory bowel
disease, gastroenteritis, colon cancer, thrush,
candidasis, food allergies and ME.

Prebiotics are non-digestible carbohydrates,
such as fructosoligosaccharides (FOS), that
selectively stimulate the growth of the friendly
Bifidus bacteria in the large bowel. Certain foods
including banana, chicory, garlic, onion, artichoke,
and asparagus are naturally rich in FOS and some
probiotic drinks have FOS added; FOS can also be
found in supplements.

The science of probiotics is an exciting field
and while the research looks promising, more
research is still needed.

- Probiotics in the form of fermented dairy
products and foods such as sauerkraut have
been consumed in some parts of the world for
literally thousands of years
- Different types and brands of probiotic contain
different species of bacteria. Each probiotic
strain is unique and can have varying effects.
A probiotic that claims it is helpful for one
thing may not be effective for another. If you
decide to take a probiotic in tablet form it's
important to buy a reputable brand. In one
study carried out it was discovered that many
brands of probiotic supplement didn't contain
the bacteria they say they did.
- Probiotic bacteria from probiotic drinks and
supplements cannot live in the gut so they
need to be consumed on a regular basis.
Probiotic bacteria in yoghurts and drinks foods
only have a shelf life of a few weeks so itis
important to use them before their 'use by' date.

Prostate problems

CONSUME PLENTY OF

- Tomatoes and tomato products, red grapefruit and watermelons for lycopene

- Nuts, seafood, fish, bread, wheat bran, wheatgerm, oats and brown rice for selenium

- Vegetable oils, nuts and seeds and wheatgerm for vitamin E

- Fruit, vegetables and whole grains for antioxidants

- Pomegranate juice

- Fluids to flush the bladder

LIMIT

- Fatty foods

AVOID

- Alcohol, caffeine, spicy foods and other substances that could irritate the urinary tract

- Excessive weight gain

The prostate, a golf-ball-size gland located just below the bladder, is the source of many male urinary problems, including cancer, benign enlargement and inflammation (prostatitis). Urinary tract infections, lifestyle habits and a high-fat diet may predispose a man to some of these problems.

As men age, the prostate tends to enlarge, a condition called benign prostatic hypertrophy (BPH). About a third of all men over 50 will experience this non-cancerous enlargement that can cause severe obstruction of urinary flow. The condition occurs more often as men age, but especially between the ages of 60 and 70. By the time they over 80, about four out of every five men in the UK are treated for prostate enlargement each year.

Consult a doctor if you suspect enlargement, because it may indicate the presence of a malignant growth. Prostate cancer is the second most common cancer in men, after testicular cancer, and is likely to effect 1 in every 11 elderly men in the UK. If treated in an early stage, it is highly curable. Prostate cancers usually occur in older men and are generally slow growing. Until regular screening becomes commonplace, older men should talk to their GPs if they suffer any urinary problems such as difficulty in urinating, a weak or intermittent flow of urine, increased frequency of urination and even occasional incontinence.

The role of diet

Diet may play a role in maintaining prostate health, and may help to ward off cancer.

Lycopene. A recent study of nearly 48,000 men found that this substance, found in tomatoes, tomato products, red grapefruit and watermelons appears to reduce the risk of prostate cancer, endorsing recommendations to increase consumption of fruit and vegetables, which are high in other antioxidants and bioflavonoid pigments that protect against various cancers. Cooking appears to release more of the lycopene in tomatoes, so tomato-based pasta sauces and homemade tomato soups may be especially beneficial. Lycopene is fat soluble so is better absorbed when eaten with a little fat.

Vitamin E. It is known to reduce inflammation and may protect against prostate cancer. Men, especially smokers, appear to be at increased risk. Good sources include wheatgerm, vegetable oils, nuts and seeds and whole grains.

Selenium. It may protect against prostate and colorectal cancers. This antioxidant is found in nuts,

especially Brazil nuts, seafood, some meats, fish, wheat bran, wheatgerm, oats and brown rice.

Isoflavones. Soya products can help to prevent enlargement of the prostate, may help to protect against prostate cancer and may slow the growth of tumours. This effect is attributed to isoflavones – plant chemicals that help to lower a male hormone that stimulates the overgrowth of prostate tissue.

Eat lots of cruciferous vegetables and omega-3s. Fish and vegetable oils high in omega-3 fats seem to reduce the risk of prostate cancer. A diet high in saturated animal fats has been linked to an increased incidence. Vegetables from the cruciferous family such as broccoli, cabbage and cauliflower contain isothiocyanates, which are phytochemicals that appear to be protective. Whole grains offer fibre, selenium, vitamin E and phytochemicals, all of which play a role in the prevention of cancer.

Pomegranate juice helps. Drink 250ml of pomegranate juice daily – it can slow the progress of prostate cancer, and even act to prevent it.

Drink plenty of fluids. Anyone with an enlarged prostate should drink plenty of water and other nonalcoholic fluids and reduce intake of caffeine.

P

Protein

A body-building nutrient

Protein is the quintessential nutrient that every cell in the human body requires for growth or repair. Also, the antibodies that protect us from disease, the enzymes needed for digestion and metabolism, as well as hormones such as insulin, are all proteins.

Every cell in the body needs protein; it is needed for the growth and repair of everything from muscles and bones to hair and fingernails. Cholesterol travels through the bloodstream attached to lipoproteins (fat-carrying proteins). Connective tissue made from protein forms the matrix of bones; chromoproteins are a combination of protein and pigments that form haemoglobin; keratin, still another type of protein, is used by the body to make hair and nails. The neurotransmitters that deliver messages to the brain are made from amino acids derived from dietary protein.

With so many essential functions, you might assume that protein should make up the bulk of the diet, but this is not the case. In an ideal balanced diet, only 12 to 15 per cent of daily calories should come from protein. Healthy male adults only need about 55g of protein every day which could come from a 180g portion of lean roast chicken or about 225g of steamed trout. An average woman needs about 45g a day and a child needs about 28g a day. Most Westerners eat far more than that – about 100g a day.

AMINO ACIDS

Proteins are exceedingly complex and diverse structures built of amino acids that are linked together into long chains by peptide bonds. There are many thousands of different proteins, but they all have a backbone of carbon atoms interlaced with nitrogen atoms. Various groupings of atoms can be attached to this backbone.

The human body requires 20 different amino acids to build all the proteins it needs. Of these, 11 can be made in the body, but the other nine, referred to as essential amino acids, must come from the diet. Just as the various letters in the alphabet are joined to make words, so too are amino acids arranged in an almost infinite number of different ways to form the more than 50,000 different proteins in the body. Proteins are made up of hundreds of amino acids. DNA (deoxyribonucleic acid), the genetic material that is found in the nucleus of each body cell, provides the blueprint for how amino acids are arranged to form individual proteins.

DIETARY PROTEIN

The body is constantly building protein from amino acids, some of which are recycled from the body tissue that is being rebuilt. Even so, a certain amount of protein is lost through normal wear and tear and must be replaced from the diet. But to use this protein, the body must first break it down into its individual amino acids and then reassemble them according to instructions found in the body's genetic code.

With the exception of oils and pure sugar, all foods contain at least some protein, but its quality varies according to the variety of amino acids it provides. Animal protein (apart from gelatine) provides all nine essential amino acids in the proportions required by the body and is therefore referred to as

Did you know?

High-protein meals are a pick-me-up

Most of the 35 or so neurotransmitters that tell the brain to make us feel high, low, sleepy or alert are made from amino acids that come from dietary protein. A high-protein meal provides tyrosine and can increase levels of noradrenaline that stimulate the brain. On the other hand, a high-carbohydrate meal provides the brain with tryptophan and has a calming effect.

complete, or high-quality, protein. In contrast, plant proteins (with the exception of soya, which is almost as complete as animal food) lack one or more of the essential amino acids. Because not all plant foods lack the same amino acids, the body can build a complete protein if these foods are combined in such a way that they complement each other. For example, grains are high in the essential amino acid methionine, but they lack lysine. This essential amino acid is plentiful in dried beans and other legumes, which are deficient in methionine. By combining a grain with a legume, you can obtain the complete range of amino acids. Such combinations can occur at adjacent meals, if desired.

Interestingly, low-meat ethnic diets all have dishes that provide complementary proteins: the beans and corn tortillas of Mexico; the rice and dahl of India; the tofu, rice and vegetable combinations in Asian cuisine; and the chickpeas and bulghur wheat in Middle Eastern dishes. Strict vegetarian diets can supply ample protein by combining complementary grains and legumes. However, if an essential amino acid is missing, usually from starvation, the body breaks down lean tissue to get it.

Moderate cooking makes protein easier to digest because heat breaks down some of the bonds that join amino acids together. Overcooking, however, can cement some amino acids together, making the protein more difficult to digest and to break down into individual amino acids.

In the stomach, long chains of amino acids are broken into shorter chains called polypeptides. Digestion continues in the small intestine, where pancreatic and other enzymes complete the process. The individual amino acids are absorbed into the bloodstream and transported to the liver, where some are used to make lipoproteins and new enzymes. Others are returned to the bloodstream, which carries them to cells.

Because amino acids are not stored as such, those that are not used in a relatively short time are returned to the liver, where the nitrogen is removed and passed on to the kidneys to be excreted as urea. The remaining protein molecules are usually converted to glucose for energy.

HIGH-PROTEIN WEIGHT-LOSS DIETS

High-protein, low-carbohydrate diets are very popular. While people do lose weight on these diets, there is concern about the effects of high protein and high fat intakes on kidney function, bone health, cardiovascular function and cancer rates. A diet that is high in protein may be low in fruit and whole grains and consequently low in the numerous beneficial compounds that these foods provide.

Although nutrition experts have concerns about the use of very high protein diets, emerging research suggests that increasing protein slightly, so that protein provides around 20 per cent of total energy, may have a beneficial effect in terms of weight management because higher protein foods seem to be more satisfying and create a sense of fullness.

EXCESSIVE PROTEIN

The typical Western diet provides more protein than the human body needs. This does not pose a serious threat for healthy persons, but too much protein adds to the workload of the kidneys and liver. Thus, people with diseases affecting these organs may be put on a low-protein diet. Don't undertake a diet of this sort without medical supervision.

CAUTION

Purified protein and amino acid powders or pills are often promoted as high-energy, muscle-bulking supplements for athletes and body-builders, as well as weight-loss aids for dieters. There is no evidence that athletes benefit from high protein intakes. A balanced diet provides all the needed protein; any excess is just excreted. Taking individual amino acid supplements can have some unforeseen consequences. Studies have also shown that amino acid supplements can upset normal protein synthesis, setting the stage for nutritional imbalances. Some researchers also maintain that taking protein supplements increases calcium excretion and may increase the risk of osteoporosis. Excessive intake of dietary protein may also cause the same problem.

P

Prunes

See Plums and prunes

Psoriasis

EAT PLENTY OF

■ Fruits and vegetables for antioxidants

■ Oily fish for omega-3 fatty acids

CUT DOWN ON

■ Offal and alcohol

No creams or lotions will solve skin problems unless you eat to provide your skin with the nutrients it needs for repair and renewal. Psoriasis – a chronic condition which tends to run in families – affects one person in 50 in Britain and the United States. It is characterised by scaly pink patches, commonly appearing on the elbows, knees, shins and scalp; fingernails and toenails are also often affected.

Although there is as yet no cure for the disease, a combination of a healthy diet and prescribed skin ointments enables most sufferers to keep their symptoms under control.

Many people with psoriasis find that their symptoms improve after they have been in the sun. Moderately severe psoriasis may be treated with PUVA (the combination of a light-sensitive psoralen drug and exposure to longwave ultra-violet light). Recent research has found that sufferers do not metabolise vitamin D, and a patient may be prescribed an ointment containing synthetic vitamin D analogues.

Psoriasis can be either helped or exacerbated by food choices. Oily fish – such as mackerel and trout – have been shown to relieve some symptoms of psoriasis and should form a regular part of the diet. As well as vitamin D they contain omega-3 fatty acids which have an anti-inflammatory effect, as do the antioxidants in fruit and vegetables.

Many people find that simply cutting out certain foods results in a marked improvement. Examples of foods which may be worth excluding are dairy produce, animal fats, meat and spices. Cut out offal because this contains an essential fatty acid called arachidonic acid, which the body converts to pro-inflammatory prostaglandins, which will irritate the condition. However, it is wise to consult a nutritionist before eliminating too many foods from the diet.

Reducing alcohol intake may also be beneficial, since it is a vasodilator – it widens blood vessels and increases the blood flow to the skin – which causes the skin to become reddened and warm, exacerbating the itching and flaking of psoriasis.

Pumpkins

BENEFITS

■ A rich source of beta carotene and vitamin C

■ A good low-calorie source of potassium

■ High in fibre

■ The seeds are a good source of protein, iron, zinc, B vitamins, vitamin E and fibre

Like all orange-pigmented vegetables, pumpkins are rich in beta carotene – this is what gives them their bright orange colour. Beta carotene is used by the body to make vitamin A. Pumpkins also contain calcium, iron, folate and vitamin C.

Pumpkins are naturally low in salt and fat, and3 tablespoons of cooked pumpkin will provide one of your daily portions of vegetables.

An 80g serving of cooked pumpkin contains just 10kcal, making it an ideal accompaniment to a meal.

They are popular for baking and can also be used in pumpkin soup, pumpkin pies or sliced and cooked on the barbecue. Try baking chunks of pumpkin with the skin on and then remove the skin after cooking. Slices of pumpkin, sprayed with olive oil and cooked for a few minutes in a hot pan, are also delicious with pasta or cooled for use in a salad.

Pumpkin seeds, known as pepitas, are a good source of protein. Just 30g of pumpkin seeds provides 7g of protein – similar to an equal serving of peanuts – as well as 3mg of iron (20 per cent of the adult RNI). They are high in unsaturated vegetable oil, a source of vitamin E, and are an excellent source of zinc, with 30g of seeds providing almost a third of the RNI for zinc. They also provide fibre. Pumpkin seeds are easy to prepare: scoop out the seeds, wash them and let dry, then bake them on an oiled baking sheet at 120°C for an hour. Add them to muesli, toss them into a salad or nibble them as a healthy snack.

Because pumpkins have hard shells, they are ideal for storing. Pumpkins last about a month in a cool, dry place.

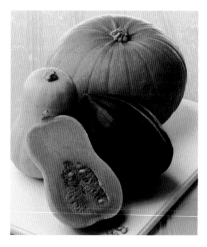

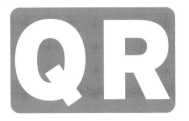

Quince

BENEFITS

- An excellent source of vitamin C, and also provides potassium
- High in pectin, a soluble fibre

DRAWBACKS

- Often cooked with large amounts of sugar to offset tartness
- Seeds contain a cyanide compound

A member of the same rose family as apples and pears, the quince has an acidic tartness and is unsuitable to eat raw. Cooking cuts the acids, and the fruit takes on a mellow flavour similar to that of an apple, with the texture of a pear.

Quinces are high in vitamin C; a medium (250g) provides more than 40mg, or 100 per cent of the adult Reference Nutrient Intake (RNI). The same sized quince provides 500mg of potassium and good amounts of fibre.

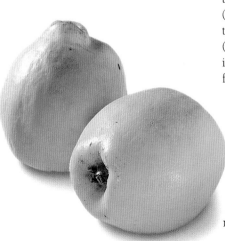

There are about 50kcal in a medium-sized quince; it is also high in pectin, a soluble fibre that helps to control levels of blood cholesterol. Because pectin forms a semi-solid gel when cooked, quinces are ideal for making jams and jellies.

Quinces may be round or even pear-shaped. Look for fruit that is firm, with pale yellow skin covered with fuzz; reject any fruit that is irregularly shaped or bruised. Poaching and baking are the most nutritious methods of preparing the fruit. Don't be misled by the tartness of raw quince; the fruit becomes sweeter as it cooks. Long, slow cooking also changes the colour of the flesh from yellow to pink or red.

Quinoa

BENEFITS

- An excellent source of iron, magnesium, potassium, zinc and other minerals
- A good source of B-complex vitamins
- High in protein

DRAWBACKS

- Not widely available and more expensive than most grains

Although it is often classified as a grain, quinoa actually belongs to the same plant family as spinach (*Chenopodiaceae*). Although the tops of the green leafy quinoa plant (pronounced 'keen-wah') are edible, it is the seeds that are served most frequently.

For more than 5,000 years, quinoa has been the staple food of peoples of the Andes, where it is one of the few crops that grows well in the dry mountainous climate and poor soil. Peru and Bolivia are the top growers of quinoa in the world, producing more than 50 per cent.

A nutrient powerhouse

The tiny quinoa seeds are packed with important nutrients; 100g (dry weight) of quinoa provides about 9mg of iron, more than any unfortified grain product. The same amount of quinoa also contributes large amounts of several other essential minerals, including 210mg of magnesium, 740mg of potassium and 3.3mg of zinc, as well as numerous B vitamins, especially B_6, folate, niacin and thiamin.

Most of the 155kcal in a medium portion of cooked quinoa (about 50g dry weight) come from complex carbohydrates. However, it also provides 13g of protein, which is of a higher quality than similar products because it provides lysine, an amino acid missing in corn, wheat and other grains. This makes it an unusually complete food for humans. Quinoa is a good source of saponins, the phytochemicals that help to prevent cancer and heart disease.

It is gluten-free (which makes it an excellent food for coeliac sufferers), easy to digest and is a good source of dietary fibre. The UN has dubbed it a 'superfood'.

Quinoa cooks quickly into a fluffy, delicately flavoured grainlike dish that lends itself to many uses. It can be served as a substitute for rice, potatoes and other starchy foods; combined with vegetables, poultry or seafood to make a pilaf; and added to soups and stews.

Q

Radishes

BENEFITS

- A useful source of vitamin C

- Low in fat and calories and high in fibre

DRAWBACKS

- Can produce wind in some people

- Salicylate content may provoke an allergic reaction in people sensitive to aspirin

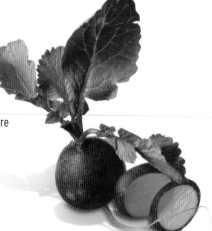

A member of the cruciferous family, the radish is closely related to kale, cabbage, turnips and cauliflower. Not especially high in nutrients other than vitamin C, radishes are tasty, as well as low in calories, making them ideal for snacking and as a spicy addition to salads, soups and Asian dishes.

Apart from their vitamin C, radishes also contain some iron, potassium and folate. Five medium raw red radishes (40g) provide 7mg of vitamin C and they contain only 5kcal. They also supply sulphurous compounds that may protect the body against cancer.

Like other cruciferous vegetables, radishes can cause bloating and wind in some people. Also, radishes contain salicylates – compounds similar to the active ingredient in aspirin; many people sensitive to aspirin may suffer an allergic reaction to radishes.

Radishes are available during spring and autumn – spring radishes having a milder flavour. The long white daikon radish is also best then. Radish leaves are a rich source of vitamin C, beta carotene and a good source of iron and calcium. Use them in stir-fries.

When selecting red globe radishes, avoid the larger ones if possible, as they may be pithy. A bright colour indicates freshness. If there are leaves on the stems, make sure they are green and crisp.

Regardless of which variety of radish you are buying, the vegetables should feel solid and have an unblemished surface.

Unless the radishes are going to be served the same day, you should remove any leaves and tops; the radishes will stay fresh longer without the tops. Store radishes in a plastic bag in the refrigerator.

Raisins

See Grapes

Raspberries

BENEFITS

- An excellent source of vitamin C

- A source of folate and contain useful amounts of iron and potassium

- Provide bioflavonoids, which may protect against cancer

- High in fibre

DRAWBACKS

- Contain a natural salicylate, which can cause an allergic reaction in aspirin-sensitive people

These fragile berries are available for a good part of the year in the UK and are usually quite expensive. Raspberries are low in calories and a rich source of vitamin C. An 80g serving of raspberries contains 20kcal and 26mg of vitamin C (more than half the Reference Nutrient Intake, or RNI). It also provides 26mcg of folate, 136mg of potassium and some iron. The vitamin C content increases the iron's absorption.

There are 2g of fibre in 80g of fresh raspberries. The seeds in raspberries provide insoluble fibre that helps to prevent constipation. The fruit is also high in pectin, a form of soluble fibre that helps to control levels of blood cholesterol. In addition, raspberries contain anthocyanins, antioxidant plant pigments that have been shown to prevent cancer and heart disease as well as ellagic acid, another cancer-fighting substance, which is not destroyed by cooking.

Raspberries spoil faster than most berries because of their delicate structure and hollow core. Once picked, they should be eaten as soon as possible. Freezing, however, will preserve them for up to a year. When thawed from frozen, they lose much of their firmness and are best used in hot desserts.

Berries often produce allergic reactions, and raspberries are no exception. Those who are sensitive to aspirin may also react to raspberries, which contain a natural salicylate, similar to the major ingredient in aspirin.

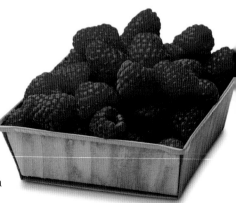

Frozen raspberries have nothing added and are frozen soon after picking, which retains their nutrients. Canned raspberries in light syrup have less vitamin C than fresh berries, with 80g providing 6mg; the sugar syrup increases the calories to 70kcal.

Raspberry vinegar and raspberry leaf tea are other traditional uses for these berries. To make raspberry vinegar, steep 500g of raspberries in a litre of wine vinegar for about two weeks, then strain. It is used as a gargle for sore throats and may be added to cough mixture.

The tea may offer some relief from period pains if taken for some days before the onset of the period, and is beneficial during the last three months of pregnancy. Its mild astringent action may be useful as a mouthwash. It is also suitable to treat mild digestive problems such as both diarrhoea and constipation.

Respiratory disorders

CONSUME PLENTY OF

- Non-alcoholic fluids
- Fresh fruit and vegetables for beta carotene, vitamin C and other antioxidants
- Lean meat, oysters, yoghurt and wholegrain products for zinc
- Live yoghurt for probiotics
- Oil-rich fish for omega-3 fats

LIMIT

- Foods that cause bloating and wind

AVOID

- Smoking, passive smoking and other air pollutants
- Alcohol

Respiratory infection is one of the most common reasons for a visit to the doctor. Respiratory disorders range from colds and flu, which are usually minor infections, to chronic diseases, such as asthma and bronchitis, which are much more problematic. Any condition that affects the passage of air to and from the lungs should always be taken seriously. The onset of respiratory symptoms is sufficient cause for you to see your doctor. The following are some of the more common respiratory disorders.

Bronchitis

Difficulty breathing, a relentless cough and production of thick mucus, or phlegm, are the main symptoms of bronchitis – an inflammation of the bronchi, or branching tubes, that carry air to and from the lungs. There may also be a low-grade fever and a burning sensation in the chest. Acute bronchitis, often a complication of a severe cold, flu or other infection of the upper respiratory tract, may require antibiotic treatment, but it usually goes away in a week or two.

Chronic bronchitis is a very serious problem that develops when the bronchial tubes are irritated over a long period of time. Cigarette smoking is the most common cause, although exposure to air pollution and occupational dusts and chemicals may also be involved. The tubes become thickened, a mucus-producing cough is present almost all of the time and air flow to the lungs is often greatly impaired. This creates an ideal breeding ground for infection and sets the stage for progressive lung damage.

Emphysema

Also known as chronic obstructive pulmonary disease (COPD), emphysema afflicts many smokers. It takes years to develop, and is

Do one simple thing

Try aromatherapy to relieve symptoms

A soothing way to relieve lung problems is to inhale the steam from a bowl of hot water that contains a few drops of highly concentrated essential oils. A combination of eucalyptus, thyme, tea-tree and lavender oils is often recommended to ease bronchitis. Eucalyptus oil is particularly good for relieving the feeling of congestion and may be helpful to people with emphysema. Peppermint oil may also be added to hot water to relieve bronchial symptoms.

often a consequence of smoking or chronic bronchitis. As the disease worsens, the air sacs (alveoli), lose their elasticity and fill with stale air, leading to an increased shortness of breath and a distended chest.

Pneumonia

There are many different types of pneumonia, but the symptoms generally include a cough with a great deal of sputum, fever, chills and chest pain. Pneumonia's causes include viruses, bacteria, fungi, parasites and exposure of lung tissue to toxic substances. AIDS patients often develop *Pneumocystis carinii*, a rare type that strikes people with weakened immunity. One common bacterial type, pneumococcal pneumonia, can be prevented by a vaccine, which is recommended for everyone over 65 and for anyone over the age of two who has a chronic disease that may increase the risk of pneumonia.

Helpful foods

A nutritious and well-balanced diet can help to prevent or reduce the severity of bronchitis, pneumonia and other lung infections because people who are in good health are more likely to be able to fight off the underlying causes.

Did you know?

A diet rich in fruit and vegetables improves lung health

There is extensive evidence from studies over the past 10 to 15 years that a diet rich in fruit and vegetables is beneficial to lung health. The most compelling evidence is linked to fruit high in vitamin C, which is associated with improved lung function in the general population of adults and children. One study looked at the relationship between diet and self-reported wheezing, doctor-diagnosed asthma and lung function in 2,633 adults. They found that eating five or more apples a week or at least three tomatoes a week was most strongly associated with increased lung function. Another study of more than 40,000 people found that those who ate the highest intake of vegetables had a much lower risk of bronchitis than those who ate the least.

Fluids. During any respiratory infection, adequate fluid intake is especially important because it helps to thin mucus and make breathing easier. Doctors generally recommend that their patients drink at least six to eight glasses of non-alcoholic fluids a day. Chicken broth and other warm fluids are comforting, but cold fluids are also beneficial.

Antioxidants. These help to protect lung tissue from the cellular damage caused by free radicals, unstable molecules that are released when the body uses oxygen. Important antioxidants are the vitamins A, C, folate and beta carotene, which the human body converts into vitamin A.

Vitamins A and C. They are also necessary to build and repair epithelial tissues, which line the lungs, bronchi and other parts of the respiratory system; the tissues act as a barrier against bacteria. In addition, these vitamins are essential to building an immunity against lung disease. A balanced diet that provides ample fresh fruit and vegetables, particularly those that are yellow, orange and dark green, will provide reasonable amounts of vitamins A and C.

Zinc. Important for boosting immunity, especially against upper respiratory infections, zinc is found in many foods, especially lean meat, oysters, yoghurt and wholegrain products. While zinc helps your immune system, excess can do the opposite. Consuming more than 40mg per day can depress your immune system, making you more susceptible to infection.

Eating approaches

People with emphysema generally feel better if they eat smaller, more frequent meals. Consuming too much at one time can increase the volume in the stomach and crowd the already distended lungs. Cut down on fried and other fatty foods. Fats remain in the stomach longer because they require more time to digest; thus, the stomach may crowd the lungs longer than when filled with other foods. Anything that causes wind and bloating should also be avoided; common offenders include beans and other legumes, cabbage, Brussels sprouts, broccoli and onions. The volume of food in the stomach can be reduced by taking liquids an hour before eating and an hour afterwards, rather than with your meals.

Some of the medications used to treat respiratory disorders can cause a loss of appetite. Ask your doctor about taking medicines straight after eating. Make your meals enticing and try not to rush; have small servings and eat slowly.

Asthmatics, in particular, should avoid any food that triggers any level of wheezing. There is also some evidence that junk foods can increase the risk of asthma.

Lifestyle habits

Smoking is by far the leading cause of chronic respiratory disorders, including chronic bronchitis, emphysema and lung cancer. If you smoke, make every effort to stop. Also try to avoid secondhand smoke and air pollutants. If your job exposes you to harmful dusts or chemical gases, be sure to wear the proper protective masks.

Alcohol lowers immunity and should be avoided during any infection. Because emphysema and chronic bronchitis predispose a person to develop lung infections, it's a good idea to abstain from all alcoholic beverages.

Rhubarb

BENEFITS

■ Contains vitamin C, potassium and fibre

DRAWBACKS

■ Usually prepared with substantial amounts of sugar or other sweeteners

■ Contains oxalic acid, which inhibits absorption of its calcium and iron

■ Leaves are poisonous

■ May aggravate joint problems in sufferers from arthritis and gout

Although it is thought of as a fruit, rhubarb is, in fact a vegetable. A 100g portion of fresh diced rhubarb yields a mere 7kcal and provides 6mg of vitamin C, as well as 290mg of potassium. The same amount also contains more than 93mg of calcium; however, rhubarb is not considered a good source of this mineral, since it also contains oxalic acid, which blocks the absorption of its calcium. Fortunately, rhubarb does not block calcium absorption from other dietary sources.

Only the rhubarb stalks are eaten – the leaves are poisonous. Because raw rhubarb stalks are stringy in texture and tart in flavour, most people eat them cooked with sugar or honey, thus inflating the calorie count to 72kcal. To avoid extra calories, cook it with sweet fruit, such as strawberries or apples, or use an artificial sweetener.

A favourite pie or crumble filling, rhubarb can also be preserved, or it can be stewed to make a compote or sauces to complement poultry.

When cooked and sweetened, rhubarb will turn pinkish brown in colour. It should not be prepared in aluminium or cast iron pots, which will interact with the acid in the vegetable and darken both the pot and the rhubarb. Do not eat the leaves: they are highly poisonous.

Rice

BENEFITS

- Provides complex or starchy carbohydrate and some B vitamins.

- Makes a complete protein, combined with beans and other legumes.

- Gluten-free and suitable for people with coeliac disease.

- Easy to digest; useful in restoring bowel function after a bout of diarrhoea.

- Rarely, if ever, causes food allergies.

For thousands of years, rice has been the staple food for more than half the world's population for whom it provides both energy and protein. With over 60,000 different types of rice grown throughout the world, there is a type of rice for every kind of dish.

Like barley and oats, rice grows in a protective husk that has to be removed if the grain is to be used as food. (Wheat and corn require less processing.) Vitamins and minerals are lost with the bran and germ that are removed in milling to make

white rice. In populations that subsist on white rice, thiamin deficiency is common. White rice also has a high GI.

Brown rice – intact kernels that retain their bran layers – is somewhat more nutritious than white rice, but it also contains phytic acid, a substance that interferes with the absorption of iron and calcium.

Since it is a refined carbohydrate, white rice is digested quickly, elevates blood sugar levels and provides energy, but with less nutritional value and fibre content than brown rice. The Glycaemic Index (GI) is an indication of how rapidly the carbohydrate in a food is converted to blood glucose compared with an equal quantity of straight glucose. Basmati rice and brown rice have a lower GI than regular short or long-grain rice.

When other foods, such as meat, are consumed with rice, the overall GI falls, as the presence of protein or fat in a meal will slow down the digestion of the entire meal. Most types of rice should be cooked in twice their volume of water, which will be completely absorbed by the grain and will preserve the nutritional content.

Popular types of rice

Rice is classified according to its size. There are long-grain varieties and short-grain, whole grain and easy-cook. (Easy-cook rice is pre-cooked, then dried so that it takes only about 5 minutes to cook.)

Long-grained white rice is still one of the most popular varieties. It has a delicate flavour and is milled to remove the outer layers of the husk and bran. Brown long-grain rice has a stronger flavour and retains the bran layer after minimal milling. This means brown rice contains more vitamins, minerals and fibre than white, and is therefore more nutritious.

Arborio. A medium-grain absorbent rice, cooking to a creamy mass. It is used in Italian risottos because it remains firm at the centre when cooked. It absorbs a larger quantity of stock during cooking.

Basmati. A long-grain, aromatic rice, native to India and Pakistan and used in Indian dishes. When cooked, the grain swells only lengthways. Basmati grains stay dry and separate and are especially suitable for pilafs. It has been described as the prince of rice.

Glutinous. A sticky rice, popular in the Far East. Almost round in shape, it has a slightly sweet flavour.

Jasmine is an aromatic rice with origins in Thailand. It has a soft, moist texture and grains that cling together. It is a fragrant rice that is widely used in Chinese cooking.

Koshihikari is a white rice that has a soft sticky texture and a slightly glossy appearance when cooked. It is used for making sushi, nori rolls and other Japanese dishes.

Pudding rice. A short-grain rice that, as its name suggests, is used for rice pudding. The grains are starchy and tend to clump together.

Some facts about rice

- Although popular worldwide, 90 per cent of all rice is still grown and consumed in Asia.

- The outer, most nutritious parts of the rice kernel are removed and fed to livestock when rice is milled.

- Rice bran oil is a rich source of some plant sterols that are effective in lowering blood cholesterol levels. The active compound is known as gamma-oryzanol. Rice bran oil is also fed to racehorses to increase their muscle mass.

- Rice originated in southern Asia about 6,500 years ago, but it did not reach Britain until the 16th century, when it was imported from Spain.

- Most of the rice eaten in Britain comes from Carolina in the USA.

R

Wild rice. This is not a true rice – it it is the seeds of a North American wild aquatic grass, found in the Great Lakes region. It is also native to some parts of Japan and China. Once gathered by hand in the wild by Chippewa Indians, wild rice is now cultivated commercially and harvested by machine. Wild rice contains more protein than true rice does and is richer in lysine, the amino acid lacking in most grains. The 'grains' are long, slim and black; they swell and burst when cooked. They are rich in the B vitamins (except for B_{12}.) Wild rice is often served mixed with Basmati rice.

Nutritional value

Ninety per cent of the calories in rice come from carbohydrates. A medium portion (180g) of boiled white rice contains about 248kcal, while the same amount of boiled brown rice has 255kcal.

Brown rice is significantly higher in fibre, with 1.4g per portion compared with 0.01g in the same volume of white rice. Brown rice also contains more selenium, magnesium and manganese.

The protein content of cooked rice, about 3-4g in a 180g portion, is less than that of other cereals, but the amino acid balance is superior to that of other grains. Rice contains only a trace of fat and virtually no sodium.

As with potatoes, it's what you eat with or on your rice that adds the calories and makes it fattening. Try adding cooked or raw diced vegetables, chopped herbs or even orange segments to a tasty dish.

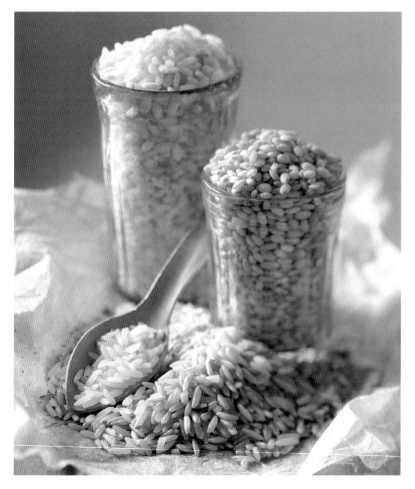

Did you know?

Sake is actually a type of beer

Rice wine, or sake, is a kind of beer that is fermented with a mould that secretes starch-digesting enzymes as it grows on rice. Sake's alcohol content is high. Unlike Western beers, which are drunk chilled, sake is still, or flat, and is served hot.

Health benefits

Rice pudding made with low-fat milk and flavoured with cinnamon is a soothing, easy-to-digest dish for convalescents. It is also a favourite with children, especially if served with a blob of low-sugar jam or preserved fruit.

Several studies have shown that rice bran helps to reduce cholesterol and may reduce the risk of bowel cancer. Some studies also show that brown rice helps to regulate glucose metabolism in people with diabetes.

As an unrefined complex carbohydrate, it provides a slower, steady supply of glucose, with a less rapid rise than occurs after eating sugars or refined white rice.

Along with lamb and a few other foods, rice rarely, if ever, provokes an allergic reaction. It is this quality that makes rice ideal as the basis of the strict elimination diet that doctors sometimes used to identify food allergens.

Rice is a true staple in menu planning. Risotto, which is made with fat-free stock and with plenty of vegetables, and pilaf, based on fat-free stock, chopped nuts and dried fruit, are economical, nutritious, low-fat meals.

Rice is an ingredient of hot and cold breakfast cereals, an excellent base for salads and a natural companion to fish, meats, vegetables and cheese. Rice bran can also add bulk to baked goods and fibre to processed cereals.

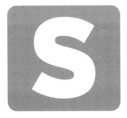

SAD (seasonal affective disorder)

TAKE PLENTY OF

- Complex carbohydrates, such as pasta, wholemeal bread, pulses, vegetables and brown rice

AVOID

- Alcohol, which can worsen depression
- Excessive intake of sweets, biscuits and cakes

People who always feel abnormally depressed and lethargic during the gloomy winter months – and whose symptoms subside in spring – may be suffering from Seasonal Affective Disorder, or SAD. This depressive condition is due to the chemical effects of light deprivation on the brain. It afflicts mainly women living in northern climates and increases the incidence of depression and suicide during the long, dark winters. SAD was not officially designated an illness until 1987, although in the 1920s doctors routinely sent depressed patients off to have a holiday in the sun during the winter months.

Light therapy

The majority of SAD sufferers feel better after one or two weeks of light therapy. This involves extra exposure to natural sunlight or high-intensity bright white light (between 5 and 20 times brighter than ordinary room lighting) for periods of half-an-hour to several hours each day. This treatment is most effective first thing in the morning, and seems to work better than the anti-depressant drugs that are sometimes prescribed for SAD.

Food cravings, especially for sugary carbohydrates, are often associated with the disorder – a starchy 'fix' makes SAD victims feel better for a while. Scientists in Switzerland have suggested that eating sweet things might trigger the release of the same mood-altering chemicals as sunlight or bright white light. Once light therapy is initiated, the craving for sugary foods may drop.

If you have SAD, try to satisfy any carbohydrate cravings by eating pasta with light sauces, beans and pulses, fresh vegetables and bread instead of high-fat, high-sugar sweets, biscuits and cakes, and try to avoid alcohol, as it can worsen depression. Standardised extracts of the herb St John's wort have proved helpful to SAD sufferers. Try to do more outdoor activities, and if you work in an office, having your desk near a window might help.

Salad dressing

BENEFITS

- A good source of vitamin E
- Oil in a salad dressing assists the absorption of some of the carotenoids found in tomatoes and salad greens

DRAWBACKS

- Cheese, creamy and oil dressings, as well as mayonnaise, are high in fat
- Additives can cause allergic or adverse reactions in susceptible people

Various dressings give flavour to lettuce and other greens; they are even more important in potato and bean salads because they help to hold the ingredients together. The olive, corn, rapeseed and other vegetable oils used in most salad dressings provide vitamin E, and because their fats are unsaturated, they do not tend to raise blood cholesterol levels. But traditional salad dressings also add lots of calories, and those made with eggs or soured cream contain saturated fats and cholesterol. Fortunately, there is an increasing number of low-fat alternatives, although these are not necessarily low in calories.

> **Don't overdress your salad**
>
> A salad that's drenched in dressing is high in unnecessary calories and becomes soggy quickly, because vinegar wilts lettuce and other greens. Use a very light sprinkling of oil to coat the greens, and mix the other ingredients – such as raw vegetables or artichoke hearts – with a small amount of vinegar. Then toss the two together just before serving.
>
> Mixed dressings are high in fat and calories, so should be used sparingly; a tablespoon of oil-based dressing has 70kcal and 7g of fat; a level tablespoon of mayonnaise has 109kcal and 12g of fat; a tablespoon of reduced calorie dressing has 43kcal and 4g of fat.

The classic vinaigrette dressing is a mixture of vinegar and oil – about two parts oil to one part vinegar – but you can reduce the amount of oil if you mix it with a wine, rice or mild balsamic vinegar. Another option is to dilute it with wine, lemon or lime or juice. You can also reduce the amount of oil by selecting one with an assertive flavour, such as walnut or extra virgin olive oil.

Using oil in salad dressings has some nutritional advantages. Some of the carotenoids found in green, orange and red vegetables are absorbed much better in the presence of fat, so adding a little olive oil dressing to a salad can

S

increase the absorption of alpha and beta carotene and lycopene, the valuable carotenoid in tomatoes.

For a creamy texture without the saturated fat, add fat-free yoghurt to the vinaigrette dressing.

Blue cheese dressings rank near the top in fat and calories. Try blending equal amounts of low-fat cottage cheese and yoghurt with a little vinegar to make a creamy dressing; then crumble in a small amount of blue cheese for flavour.

If a recipe calls for a mayonnaise dressing, start with a low-fat type. Then blend the mayonnaise with an equal part of low-fat yoghurt.

Safety issues

Commercial salad dressings are pasteurised to kill micro-organisms, and their high vinegar content discourages the growth of new ones. However, commercial dressings often contain wheat or corn starches, soya and perhaps eggs. Anyone with food allergies, coeliac disease and other food intolerances should check the labels carefully or stick to homemade.

Salt and sodium

BENEFITS

- Sodium helps to maintain fluid balance, regulate blood pressure and transmit nerve impulses
- Salt is a useful food preservative

DRAWBACKS

- Sodium promotes fluid retention and may contribute to high blood pressure

While the terms are often used interchangeably, salt and sodium are not the same. Sodium is an element that joins with chlorine to form sodium chloride, or table salt. Sodium occurs naturally in most foods, and salt is the most common source of sodium in the diet. Sodium works to maintain the body's acid-alkaline balance and helps to maintain the body's fluid balance as well as controlling nerve function and muscle movement.

The amount of sodium the body needs daily is far less than the amount that is usually consumed. Circumstances and climate will dictate the amount needed, but in general, the body needs a minimum of 1.6g of sodium a day, which will be found in 4g of salt, to maintain health. One level teaspoon of salt weighs 5g. In the UK, the average adult eats about 9g a day (about 2 level teaspoons). The World Health Organization recommends only 6g salt (2.4g sodium) a day.

Sodium is naturally present in some foods but most is added during processing or cooking. Salty foods, such as potato crisps and salted crackers, are easy to identify, but hidden sodium has to be tracked down on package labels. Cereals, processed meats like ham, canned soups, canned vegetables, prepackaged meals and commercial baked goods are usually high in sodium. Sodium is also found in monosodium glutamate (MSG); garlic salt or other seasoned salts; sea salt; meat tenderisers; condiments such as tomato sauce; soy sauce; chilli sauce and steak sauce; in soups, cured or smoked foods; olives and pickles. The more processed a food is, the higher its sodium content is likely to be.

The connection between blood pressure and salt

People with high blood pressure are typically advised to cut back on salt, because sodium affects the kidneys' ability to rid the body of wastes and fluid. When the body's sodium level is low, the kidneys retrieve the chemical from the urine and return it to the circulating blood. Some individuals, however, conserve sodium, which may predispose them to high blood pressure. As the kidneys retain more salt than

Five ways to cut salt

1 Use spices that don't contain sodium, like fresh herbs, garlic powder or fresh garlic, onion flakes (instead of onion salt), coriander, dry mustard, lemon, mint, cumin, chilli, curry, rosemary, thyme, basil, bay leaves, ginger, hot peppers, pepper, chives and parsley.

2 Make your own salad dressing rather than using the bottled ones. Use flavoured vinegars instead of salt for extra taste.

3 Eat more fresh or frozen fruit and vegetables. If you use canned vegetables, choose those with no added salt. Use fresh potatoes rather than instant and fresh cucumber instead of pickles. Add spices and herbs instead of salt to the water when you cook vegetables.

4 Eat fresh fish instead of smoked, canned or dried varieties, choose sliced roast beef or chicken instead of corned silverside, salami or other processed meat.

5 Re-educate your taste buds. Taste food before adding salt. Cook from scratch instead of packages. Do not add salt when cooking pasta or rice.

necessary, they excrete less urine so that fluid is available to maintain the sodium at the correct concentration. As a result, the heart is forced to pump harder to keep this extra fluid in circulation, and the blood pressure increases to maintain the blood flow. Restricting salt intake can correct this form of high blood pressure.

Studies have shown that as salt in the diet is increased, blood pressure goes up. Populations with low salt intake have lower blood pressure. The Yanomami Indians of Brazil add no salt to their food and hypertension is unknown.

By contrast, there are ten million adults suffering from high blood pressure in the UK, where salty snacks and processed foods are a way of life. Whether a reduced-salt diet lowers blood pressure in people who do not have high pressure to start with is not critical. Eating fewer salty processed foods automatically leads to a healthier diet, and limiting salt intake can cause no harm.

Health authorities are now convinced that by cutting back on salt from childhood onwards, the high proportion of the population with high blood pressure could be greatly reduced. This would ease the burden of costs and side effects associated with drugs used to reduce hypertension.

A large study known as DASH (Dietary Approaches to Stop Hypertension) found that keeping salt intake low had even more benefits for blood pressure than the initial DASH approach which decreased saturated fat and increased fruit, vegetables and low-fat dairy products.

Some people are more salt-sensitive than others, and they will see the biggest benefits from cutting back on salt. However, a low salt diet begun early in life appears to benefit almost everyone.

The increase in blood volume that occurs during pregnancy increases the body's need for salt temporarily, but the amount required is normally supplied in a varied, balanced diet. Pregnant women should prepare meals with only a little salt and not add salt to food at the table.

Reducing salt intake

Preparing most dishes from scratch and avoiding processed foods is the most important way to cut down on salt intake. Supermarkets and food stores now stock a growing variety of 'no added salt' versions of processed foods. All food labels now list the amount of sodium in a 'serving'; but if the serving specified on the label is much smaller than what you eat, your sodium intake could be much higher. Also check the label for coded terms, such as brine, stock, corned, cured, pickled, soy sauce and teriyaki sauce, that indicate other high-sodium ingredients have been added.

For many people, adding salt to food at the table is a reflex response to seeing the salt shaker; remove the shaker and you may not miss the salt. The amount of salt and other sodium-containing seasonings in most recipes can be cut by half or even more without a noticeable change in taste. Herbs and spices, fresh garlic or lemon juice are healthy alternatives. Adding these ingredients shortly before serving keeps flavours from being lost during prolonged cooking.

Pickles and condiments, such as mustard, tomato sauce, dressings and sauces, are high in sodium. When eating in restaurants, ask for dressings and sauces to be served on the side. In restaurants ask that food be prepared without salt.

Using a home water softener may add a lot of sodium to your water; do not drink this water or use it to mix baby foods.

● **Myth.......**
Sea salt is a healthier product than table salt.
.......Reality ●
There are no documented health advantages to sea salt, and the sodium content is similar.

Warning: Most commercial salt substitutes contain potassium. These may be dangerous for people with kidney disorders or those taking potassium-sparing diuretics or supplements. Check with your doctor before using a salt substitute, especially if you're taking a diuretic or potassium supplement.

Non-prescription medications may contain sodium. If you are on a sodium-restricted diet, it is advisable to check with your doctor or pharmacist before using medicines such as antacids, painkillers or laxatives.

Sauces and gravies

BENEFITS

- Used sparingly, sauces complement flavours and enhance appearance

- Salsa-style garnishes supply fibre and antioxidant vitamins, provided they are carefully prepared

- Pasta sauces based on fresh vegetables and olive oil are good sources of vitamins, fibre and unsaturated fat

DRAWBACKS

- Traditional sauces made from butter, flour, cream and egg yolks are very high in fat, saturated fat and cholesterol

- Asian-style sauces are high in salt and should be avoided by people on low-sodium diets

When an 18th-century Italian compared England with France, he wrote: 'England has 60 religions and one sauce, whereas France has 60 sauces and one religion'. Like so many exaggerations, this one had a grain of truth. French cuisine has always been renowned for its sauces, while British cuisine still has a weakness for gravy. Italian cooks are famous for vegetable-based sauces that are often enlivened with fresh herbs.

Whatever the type of cuisine – French, Italian, Asian, Indian or Mexican – there's an international medley of delicious and exciting sauces available that can transform an ordinary dish.

The word *sauce*, like *salsa*, comes from the root-word meaning 'salty'. Early sauces were heavily salted and spiced to preserve food and mask the flavours of any tainted meats. Sauces today are added to enhance or complement the flavours of foods.

Fresh-made sauces are limitless in variety and taste, from a world-renowned chef's classic concoctions to the home cook's on-the-spot invention. Commercially prepared sauces, such as barbecue sauces and hot pepper sauces, are made to patented formulas of ingredients.

Traditional sauce-making techniques are based on five main methods: the reduction of stock; a mixture of cooked vegetables mixed or blended to a pulp; a roux, in which similar quantities of fat and flour are cooked together, blended with milk or other liquid to a thick, velvety consistency and then flavoured; hot egg-based sauces (such as hollandaise), in which egg yolks and butter are blended into an emulsion with concentrated wine or vinegar and seasonings; and cold sauces (such as mayonnaise), where oil is blended into an emulsion with egg yolks and vinegar or lemon juice.

These traditional sauces generally contain only moderate amounts of vitamins A and D from their milk, cream, butter and egg yolk components. Considering the small portions in which they are meant to be served, however, the vitamin quotient is negligible and is far outweighed by the negative impact of saturated fats and calories. Two tablespoons of a homemade white sauce contain about 75kcal; the addition of grated cheese to make a mornay sauce typically increases the calorie count to 120kcal.

Sauces made from commercial mixes are somewhat lower in calories than homemade ones, but are often high in sodium, and supply few nutrients.

The trend away from flour-based sauces got its first big push from the health-conscious nouvelle cuisine that emerged in the 1970s. Professional chefs and home cooks began to spurn flour thickeners and butter enrichment in favour of the pure, intense flavours obtained by concentrating fat-free stocks and vegetable purées. While traditional sauces were typically laden with saturated fat and cholesterol, the new garnishes manage to add flavour in a low-fat, low-calorie form.

Salsa

Fresh salsas are mixtures of finely chopped vegetables or fruit, highly seasoned with garlic, spring onions, citrus juice and fresh herbs, such as coriander and basil. In contrast to the traditional sauces, salsa that has been made at home from fresh fruit or vegetables is virtually fat-free if made without oil. It is also high in fibre, very low in calories and rich in such antioxidants as vitamin C and beta carotene.

Commercial salsas, however, are usually modified vinegar pickles that have been cooked and thickened with starch.

What a difference a sauce makes

Choose your sauces carefully if you are trying to be health conscious. Here's what happens to the same half cup of steamed broccoli when you add different sauces.

	kcal
80g steamed broccoli	19
add 100ml white sauce	+151
add 100ml cheese sauce	+250
add 1 tbsp salad dressing	+70
add 100ml hollandaise sauce	+700

Pasta sauces

Some pasta sauces, such as Alfredo, are made with cream, butter, egg yolk and cheese, and are very high in fat and cholesterol. They should be used only sparingly, and those people with high cholesterol levels should avoid them altogether.

The variety of low-fat pasta sauces is limited only by a cook's imagination and the ingredients available. Excellent sauces can be made with fresh tomatoes chopped with herbs and garlic and blended with other ingredients. All tomato-based sauces provide some fibre, beta carotene, vitamin C, lycopene (which protects against prostate problems) and a small amount of unsaturated fat.

Gravies

Gravy is variations on the roux. Flour is cooked in fat drippings from roasted meat, then blended with a liquid to make a sauce. Packet gravies are also available. Two tablespoons of beef or mushroom gravy made from a dry mix contain about 11-17kcal.

Individuals on low-sodium diets should avoid commercial gravies, which are extremely high in salt. Gravies have substantial amounts of fat and only a negligible amount of nutrition. Although they add flavour and moisture to a meal, they should be used sparingly.

Asian sauces

Many of the sauces used in Asian cooking are extremely high in sodium. Those most familiar are soya; teriyaki; fish or oyster sauce (*nuoc mam* or *nam pla*); hoisin and other bean-based sauces; and stir-fry sauce (a mixture of other sauces). Some of these may be thickened with wheat gluten and should be avoided by people with coeliac disease. A teaspoon of soy sauce contains the 1068mg of sodium – the equalvalent of 2.7g of salt.

Traditional gravy

Here's how to make a gravy for the Christmas turkey, that has a reduced fat and calorie content and improved nutritional quality. It uses a stock-based method.

Brown the turkey giblets and trimmings in a hot oven or under the grill, drain off the fat, and simmer the browned scraps with vegetables and herbs (an unpeeled onion stuck with a clove, a celery stalk, carrot, leek and turnip; thyme, parsley stems, pepper-corns and a bay leaf) to make a rich stock. Drain the stock, discard the vegetables, then chill the stock.

This will make it easier to remove the congealed fat from the surface and greatly reduce the fat content. Next, concentrate or reduce the skimmed stock by boiling it down to a half or third of its volume.

When the turkey is done, drain the fat from the roasting pan and pour in the hot stock to dissolve the clinging browned bits of meat. Boil the liquid to blend the flavours together, season and serve hot with the turkey.

Bottled sauces

Most brands of tomato ketchup and brown sauce are high in salt and sugar. But tomato ketchup is a rich source of lycopene which may help to protect against cancer, particularly prostate cancer.

Hot and spicy sauces

Fiery sauces such as Tabasco and Worcestershire sauce can be helpful in clearing blocked nasal passages. Tabasco is a hot, tangy seasoning made from Mexican chilli peppers, vinegar and salt. Although they are used in such small amounts that they offer few nutritional benefits, they should be avoided by people who suffer from indigestion or who have a peptic ulcer.

Dessert sauces

Sweet sauces, such as hot fudge, elevate the fat and calorie content of an ice cream sundae to dizzying heights. More healthy alternatives include non-fat frozen yoghurt topped with heated frozen berries.

Sausages

See Smoked, cured and pickled meats

Seaweeds

BENEFITS

- An excellent source of iodine
- Provides small quantities of a wide spectrum of minerals, including calcium, copper, iron, magnesium, potassium and zinc
- Some types are rich in the B vitamins, vitamin C and beta carotene
- Some are a source of protein

DRAWBACKS

- Some are very high in sodium

● Myth.......
Kelp tablets, spirulina, chlorella and other seaweed supplements are energy boosters. Some alternative practitioners even claim that they boost the immune system.

.......Reality ●
None of these claims has been proved scientifcally. In fact, some seaweed supplements can cause health problems. High doses of kelp tablets can set off an outbreak of acne. The high iodine content can cause thyroid disorders; and varieties containing iron can provoke iron overload.

There are more than 2,500 varieties of seaweed, which include everything from the algae that forms on ponds to kelp and other marine plants. In general, seaweed is classified according to its colour – brown, red, green and blue-green.

A remarkably versatile and tasty vegetable, seaweed can be used in a broad spectrum of ways. In Japan, for example, seaweed is used to enhance flavours in a variety of dishes, from salads and soups to meat and seafood dishes. Kombu, a type of kelp (a brown plant that is one of the most common seaweeds), is used to flavour soup stocks. Wakame, another type of kelp, is used in Japan in soups and stir-fries.

Seaweeds are found in the diets of other cultures. For example, laver, a red algae called nori by the Japanese, is used by the Irish and Welsh to make flat cakes. The Scots use a seaweed called dulse to make soup. Irish moss, a red algae that is a major source of carrageenan, is used in the industrialised world as a thickening agent in such products as jellies and low-fat salad dressings. It is vital that these seaweeds are recovered from unpolluted waters. An excellent source of many essential nutrients, including protein, seaweeds are a rich source of iodine. The thyroid gland needs iodine to make the hormones that regulate body metabolism.

The mineral content of the various types of seaweed differs, but most provide some calcium, copper, iron, potassium and magnesium. Some, such as nori, supply beta carotene, a precursor of vitamin A.

Seaweed is also low in calories; 2 tablespoons of kelp (10g) contains about 2kcal. The same amount also provides 0.2g of protein, almost 18mcg of folate, 12mg of magnesium and useful amounts of iron and calcium.

The major drawback to seaweed is that many types are high in sodium, so anyone on a low-salt diet should avoid foods containing seaweed.

Seaweed supplements

Kelp tablets are an easy way to include seaweed in the diet. Because of their high iodine content, some herbalists prescribe them for mild thyroid disorders. Freshwater algae such as spirulina and chlorella are increasingly popular. They contain all the nutrients found in green vegetables, including beta carotene, vitamin C, calcium and iron, along with protein and vitamin B_{12}. They may help to detoxify the body and possibly increase immunity, and can also help people with liver disease.

Seaweed as 'medicine'

A lot of research is being done into the use of various types of seaweed in bio-medicine. For example, seaweed is being examined for its curative properties in relation to conditions such as tuberculosis, arthritis and flu and colds, as well as in the treatment of worm infestations. Being so readily available, seaweed could provide sustainable sources of medicines if these qualities are proved.

The truth about aphrodisiacs

- Herbalists recommend saffron as a sexual stimulant, but there is no evidence of its aphrodisiac effect. Some also recommend summer savory as a sexual stimulant and tonic, and winter savory to dampen sexual desire. Neither claim has ever been proved.

- Chinese ginseng may help to correct impotence by improving erectile function through dilating blood vessels. Animal studies indicate that it increases testosterone levels and sperm production.

- Yohimbe, a tropical tree, is valued as an aphrodisiac in some countries. It has no effect on the mind but may dilate blood vessels and help with impotence. There are conflicting studies about its effectiveness.

- Spanish fly, an extract of dried cantharide beetles, causes irritation in the urinary tract and genitals, which some misinterpret as sexual stimulus. In reality, cantharidin, the active component, is a potentially lethal drug.

Sex drive

EAT PLENTY OF

- Fruit and vegetables for vitamin C

- Oils, nuts and seeds, green vegetables and wheatgerm for vitamin E

- Meat, fish, legumes, nuts and seeds, green vegetables and enriched cereals for iron

- Oysters, meat, poultry, eggs, milk, beans, nuts and whole grains for zinc

LIMIT

- Saturated fats and alcohol

AVOID

- Smoking

Some people vouch for the effect of foods on their sex drive, but extravagant claims for aphrodisiacs are not borne out by scientific studies. While sexual function may be our physical response to a cascade of hormones, sexual drive is basically maintained by an active mind in a healthy body.

A healthy sex life depends on good nutrition. Good nerve function, healthy hormone levels and an unobstructed blood flow to the pelvic area are essential to sexual performance. To keep these systems in working order, a diet should be based on legumes, grain products and other complex carbohydrates, with plenty of fruit and vegetables and modest levels of protein; this diet provides plenty of vitamins and minerals. Particularly important is citrus fruit for vitamin C to strengthen blood vessel walls, and low-fat dairy products, enriched cereals, whole grains and green vegetables for riboflavin to maintain the mucous membranes that line the female reproductive tract.

Vitamin E and sexual function. Although there are no confirming clinical studies, many experts believe that without a good supply of this vitamin from wheatgerm, seeds, nuts, oils, unsaturated margarines and green vegetables sexual function is likely to suffer.

Fatigue and depression are common culprits in sexual complaints. These conditions are often linked, and both may be helped by a programme of regular exercise, which stimulates the production of endorphins (mood-elevating brain chemicals). In some cases, iron-deficiency anaemia may be responsible for fatigue. A good diet that includes meat, fish and shellfish, enriched cereals, nuts and seeds, legumes, leafy greens and dried fruit will replenish iron stores.

Consume more zinc. It is known that zinc is tied to sexual function, although its importance to the sex drive has yet to be explained. With zinc deficiency, sexual development in children is delayed, and men, too, need zinc to make sperm. Zinc is found abundantly in foods of animal origin, including seafood (especially oysters), meat, poultry and liver, as well as eggs, milk, beans, nuts and whole grains.

Eat a diet low in saturated fats. People readily accept the link between a high intake of saturated fats, elevated blood cholesterol levels, and a build-up of atherosclerotic fatty plaques on the blood vessels around the heart. It's less well understood, however, that similar plaques develop on the myriad tiny vessels in the penis. Without free-flowing circulation, the penis cannot physically respond to messages from the sex drive.

Curb alcohol consumption. Alcohol's effect on sexual function was neatly stated by William Shakespeare, who noted that wine 'provokes the desire, but takes away the performance'. Excessive alcohol lifts behavioural inhibitions, but this liberating effect may be cancelled by its depressant effect. Alcohol also has an action similar to the female hormone oestrogen. This can have a devastating effect on masculinity, causing impotence and shrinking of the testes in men who drink heavily. The hops in beer may play a part in reducing the libido in beer drinkers.

Stop smoking. Nicotine is an enemy of the arteries. Nicotine not only promotes the formation of atherosclerotic plaque in the penile blood vessels but it also constricts them.

Shellfish

BENEFITS

- A low-fat source of high-quality protein
- A rich source of minerals, including calcium, fluoride, iodine, iron and zinc
- A good source of B-group vitamins

DRAWBACKS

- Susceptible to spoilage and environmental contamination
- Some are high in cholesterol
- Can provoke allergic reactions in some people

Shellfish is the 'catch-all' term that is applied to molluscs and crustaceans – water-dwelling creatures that wear their skeletons on the outside. Molluscs such as oysters and mussels live enclosed within hinged, rigid two-piece shells, which they affix with threadlike excretions to rocks or pilings. But octopus and squid, which are free swimming and have no shells (squid have a transparent internal quill, or beak), are also molluscs. Another exception is snails, which are molluscs that live on dry land or in the water and move about, carrying their shells.

The soft bodies of crustaceans, such as shrimps, lobsters, prawns, crayfish and crab, are covered by hinged plates of chitin, like suits of armour, that allow mobility but shield them from predators. The flesh lies inside the shell and claws of lobsters.

Nutritional value

Shellfish are among our most valuable sources of high-quality protein. In contrast to protein from warm-blooded animals, shellfish protein is very low in actual fat. Some varieties such as squid and prawns contain cholesterol. The warnings about the cholesterol

Talk of toxins

Mussels accumulate toxins more quickly than other types of shellfish. In fact, scientists who monitor waters for poisons use them as an indicator species. Scallops, on the other hand, pose less of a risk than other bivalves because we don't eat the animal itself but the muscle that holds the halves of the shell together.

content of shellfish have been tempered recently as researchers now believe that dietary cholesterol has relatively little effect on blood levels of cholesterol. Shellfish are very low in saturated fat, the type of fat most likely to raise blood cholesterol levels. Shellfish also contain vitamin B_{12} and fewer calories, weight for weight, than other sources of animal protein.

Shellfish are especially rich in minerals, including calcium and phosphorus needed for healthy bones and teeth; copper to help in the production of blood cells, connective tissue and nerve fibres; iodine for thyroid gland function; iron for healthy red blood cells;

C A U T I O N

Some people are allergic to shellfish, and an allergic reaction to one type often means that the others should be avoided too. A severe reaction, with widespread hives, swelling and difficulty breathing, may indicate possible anaphylaxis, which is a life-threatening emergency. People allergic to shellfish may react to the iodine used in many of the dyes administered for contrast X-rays. Tell your doctor if you have ever had an allergic reaction to shellfish.

magnesium for metabolism, bone growth, and production of genetic material; potassium for nerve and muscle function and general metabolism; zinc for the immune system and reproductive health; and selenium, an important antioxidant

Nutrients in different shellfish

Low in saturated fat and high in protein, shellfish are rich in B vitamins and are useful sources of trace minerals. However, they are prone to contamination, so extra care should be taken when buying, preparing and cooking shellfish. All values below are for 100g of edible flesh except where noted.

SHELL-FISH	PROTEIN (g)	FAT (g)	SODIUM (mg)	VITAMINS	MINERALS
COCKLES (boiled)	12	1	490	Excellent source of vitamin B_{12}.	Excellent source of iron and iodine, rich source of selenium.
CLAMS (canned)	16	1	1200	Useful source of niacin.	Excellent source of iron and fair source of potassium and zinc. Contain some calcium.
CRABS (steamed)	20	2	420	Good source of riboflavin and provide some folate, pantothenic acid, vitamin B_6 and niacin.	Good source of zinc. Contain some iron, magnesium and potassium.
LOBSTERS (boiled)	22	1	395	Excellent source of vitamin B_{12} and niacin. Contain some folate and vitamin E.	Good source of zinc. Contain some magnesium and potassium.
MUSSELS (meat only, steamed)	17	2	210	Contain some vitamins E, riboflavin, niacin, B_{12} and B_6.	Good source of iron. Contain calcium, selenium, zinc and magnesium.
OCTOPUS (raw)	18	1	230	Good source of niacin, B_6 and B_{12}.	Source of zinc, iron, iodine and selenium.
OYSTERS (meat only, raw)	15	2	315	Contain some riboflavin, niacin and B_{12}.	Rich in zinc. Excellent source of iron. Contain some calcium and magnesium.
CRAYFISH (raw)	8	1	150	Excellent source of vitamin B_{12}. Contain folate and niacin.	Excellent source of selenium and rich source of iodine.
PRAWNS (cooked)	21	1	350	Source of niacin, vitamin B_6 and folate.	Source of calcium and iron. Contain some zinc and magnesium.
SCALLOPS (steamed)	22	1	145	Good source of vitamin B_{12} and niacin.	Good source of zinc and provide iron.
SQUID (raw)	17	1	285	Contain some niacin.	Source of iron and zinc.

linked to lower heart disease and cancer risk, and protective against mercury and cadmium.

Potential dangers

If grown in polluted waters, shellfish may be contaminated with bacteria and carry a particular risk for hepatitis. Don't gather shellfish near wharf pilings or built-up areas. Instead, buy them from fish markets and food stores that keep shellfish well covered with ice or, in the case of lobsters, in tanks with circulating water aerated with oxygen.

Fresh shellfish may be covered with ice chips and stored for several hours at 0°C. Eat them on the day they are purchased or caught.

Shallow-water shellfish, such as clams and mussels, are the most susceptible to pollution; sea scallops and other deep-water varieties are less likely to be exposed to waste. Molluscs, such as clams and oysters are filter feeders and will each filter as many as 90 litres of water a day. So if there is any pollution in the water, it is likely to be in the shellfish, too – in a concentrated form, for they are 'biomagnifiers', concentrating heavy metals and bacteria, in their tissues as it passes through.

Always try to check where your shellfish have come from: the safest are those that have been farmed in clean waters.

Never take home shellfish such as mussels from the beach, unless you are absolutely sure they are safe.

From time to time, swarming plankton cause the phenomenon known as 'red tide' in coastal waters. Shellfish exposed to the red tide ingest the micro-organisms, which produce a toxin that can survive cooking. The symptoms of red tide poisoning usually appear within 30 minutes of consuming the contaminated fish; they include facial numbness, breathing difficulty

▶ **Seafood platter**
Shellfish are low in saturated fat and rich in heart-healthy omega-3 fatty acids.

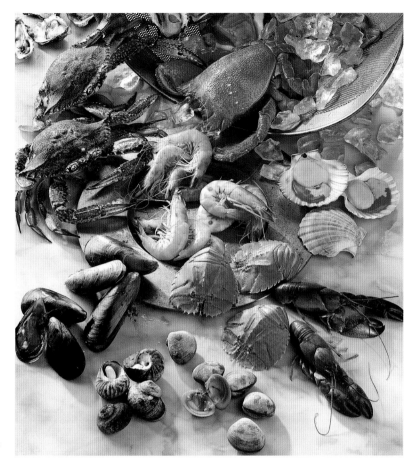

and muscle weakness. Never take shellfish from red-tide areas. ('Red tide' doesn't necessarily mean there is a red tinge to the water.) Mussels tainted with domoic acid, another toxin derived from algae, are undetectable by consumers.

Buying shellfish

Because of their susceptibility to spoilage, shellfish should be kept alive until they are ready to be cooked or served. Buy mussels only if the shells close tightly when tapped. An open shell indicates that the shellfish has died and is therefore not safe to eat. Conversely, when steaming or boiling molluscs in the shell, discard any that have failed to open by the end of the specified cooking time.

Fresh shellfish, whether in the shell or shucked, should smell briny, without any hint of iodine or fishiness. Oysters and clams show their freshness by 'flinching' when you squeeze lemon juice on them.

If possible, buy unopened oysters and shuck them yourself. Do not put these live oysters into the refrigerator or they will die. Instead, store them in a damp hessian bag in an insulated cool box. Once opened, they are best eaten quickly, but they can be stored in a light brine in the refrigerator. Do not store oysters near any strongly flavoured foods, such as canteloupe or blue cheeses, as the oysters will pick up the flavours and become unpalatable.

In Britain it is illegal to harvest oysters during summer when they are spawning – hence the tradition of saying you should only eat oysters when there is an R in the name of the month. However, the Pacific oyster, which is commercially farmed in the UK these days, is unable to spawn in cold British waters. So oysters can be enjoyed here all year round.

Preparing shellfish

Prawns can be bought uncooked as green prawns or cooked to their familiar orange/pink colour. Store them in their shells, in a bowl in the refrigerator, covered with a moist kitchen towel. If fresh, they should keep for up to two days. Green prawns can be cooked in their shells or the shells can be removed before cooking. Make a cut down the back of the prawn and carefully remove the black vein.

Lobsters and crabs should be kept in the coldest section of the refrigerator. Place them on a shallow dish and cover them with plastic wrap or aluminium foil. Like finned fish, shellfish have fragile flesh that should be cooked just to the point where the protein coagulates. The tissues toughen or dry out and fall apart if cooked for too long.

Commercially prepared shellfish are often needlessly high in calories and fat because they are coated with batter or bread crumbs before being deep fried.

The dips and sauces often served with shellfish add calories and saturated fat; cocktail and tartare sauces are highly calorific. Finely chopped shallots blended with lemon juice and herbs complement clams, lobsters and other shellfish. Or simply serve shellfish with lemon or lime.

To make a calcium-rich sauce, you can pound the shells of prawns and lobster smooth, then boil them down with clam juice, lemon juice, white wine and herbs.

S

Shingles

CONSUME PLENTY OF

- Olive and other vegetable oils, nuts, seeds, peanut butter, avocados and wheat germ for vitamin E

- Citrus fruits, apricots, cherries, papaya and tomatoes for antioxidants and bioflavonoids

Herpes zoster the medical term for shingles, is a reactivation of the varicella-zoster virus that causes chickenpox. The cause is unknown, but it often develops when the immune system is suppressed. The virus replicates and migrates along a nerve where it causes localised tingling and burning sensation of the skin. A few days later blisters similar to those of chickenpox develop along the path of the nerve. There can be serious complications if the virus infects an eye or migrates to the brain.

Some doctors believe that good nutrition may help to prevent postherpetic neuralgia, which is a long-term complication marked by nerve pain even after symptoms of shingles disappear.

Beneficial nutrients. Vitamin E, an antioxidant found in wheatgerm, nuts, seeds and vegetable oils, and the bioflavonoids found in fruit and vegetables that are high in vitamin C may also help to prevent the inflammation associated with postherpetic neuralgia.

Vitamin C supports your body's immune system, as do zinc-rich foods like seafood, meat, poultry, milk, yoghurt, beans, nuts and whole grains. If neuralgia does develop, however, the pain may be eased with applications of an ointment that contains capsaicin, the essence of chilli seeds.

Shingles can occur in childhood, but older people are usually more susceptible to the condition.

Sinusitis

CONSUME PLENTY OF

- Fluids such as water, weak teas, herbal teas and juice

- Fresh fruit and vegetables for vitamin C and bioflavonoids

- Garlic, onions and chillies to alleviate sinus congestion

AVOID

- Smoking and dry, overheated rooms

- Milk

Sinusitis is a painful inflammation of the membranes lining the sinus cavities in the skull. It occurs most often in people who suffer from hay fever or other allergies involving the nasal passages, or after a cold. Normally, the mucus produced drains through narrow ducts into the nasal cavity.

Acute sinusitis most often follows a cold – that is, a viral infection. It can be caused by other infections or inflammation, including an allergy such as hayfever. Chronic sinusitis is caused either by allergy or a mixed bacterial infection and is common in asthmatics.

Regardless of the cause, the sinus lining swells and blocks the passages, resulting in a stuffed-up feeling and, possibly, swelling and a deep, dull headache. A clue in diagnosing sinusitis is that pressure on the cheek bones causes pain and bending over increases it. There may also be a thick nasal discharge.

Depending upon the cause, your GP may prescribe antihistamines, decongestants, antibiotics or even steroids to relieve the symptoms.

Dietary and other approaches

Although nutrition does not play a direct role in sinusitis, some dietary measures may help. Studies have suggested that people with chronic

An all-too-common ailment
Many people have at least one episode of sinusitis every year, making it one of the most common ailments. Researchers speculate that the dramatic rise in the incidence of sinusitis in the past ten years may be due to increased pollution and increased resistance to antibiotics.

sinusitis should cut down milk and dairy products in their diets, as milk is mucus-forming.

Fluids can help to dilute secretions and promote drainage. Drink at least 2 litres daily of water, juice, tea or clear soup.

Eat plenty of fresh fruit and vegetables for vitamin C. Citrus fruit (rather than just the juice), grapes and blackberries are useful because they also contain bioflavonoids, plant pigments that have anti-inflammatory properties. Vitamin E, too, has similar benefits. Dietary zinc is also an important immune booster and may have anti-inflammatory properties. Zinc-rich foods include seafood, meat, poultry, milk, yoghurt, beans, nuts and whole grains.

Some foods are natural decongestants. These include garlic, onions, chillies and horseradish. Decongestant herbs and spices include ginger, thyme, cumin, cloves and cinnamon.

If you smoke, make every effort to stop. Smoking causes nasal and sinus inflammation, as can passive smoking. Heat and dry air can cause swollen, dry nasal membranes that are predisposed to sinusitis; a humidifier may be a simple solution.

For fast relief, cover the face with hot, wet towels to promote drainage and increase blood flow to the area. Steam inhalation also promotes drainage. Hot tea may help to reduce congestion; it contains theophylline, a compound believed to ease breathing by relaxing the smooth muscles in the walls of the airways.

S

Sleep and diet

Eating to sleep well

The quality of sleep has an enormous impact on daily life, since poor or interrupted sleep can affect your work, concentration and ability to interact with others. During sleep, both physical and mental restoration take place, allowing you to feel fresh and alert in the morning.

Sleep needs vary from one person to another; the optimal average is 7 to 9 hours. You can judge whether or not you're getting the right amount by how you feel the next day – too much or too little sleep leaves you feeling tired and irritable. Because growth hormones are released during sleep, babies, children and adolescents require more sleep than adults do.

Sleep researchers discount the common myth that older people require less sleep; instead, the amount of sleep that an adult needs remains fairly constant. With age, however, the nature of sleep changes and the incidence of sleep disorders rises. The time spent in the deeper stages of sleep often lessens with age, and an older person is likely to wake more frequently during the night.

WHAT MAKES US SLEEP?
This is still not fully understood, but scientists know that a person's circadian rhythm is set shortly after birth and is then maintained as a 'body clock'. Some natural chemicals in the body enhance sleep, and diet plays a part. Here are some things that are known to affect sleep:

EATING TOO MUCH OR TOO LITTLE CAN DISRUPT SLEEP. A light snack at bedtime can promote sleep, but too much food can cause digestive discomfort that leads to wakefulness.

ALCOHOL IS A DOUBLE-EDGED SWORD. Small amounts of alcohol can help you to fall asleep. But as the body metabolises the alcohol, sleep may become fragmented. Alcohol makes insomnia worse and impairs rapid eye movement (REM) sleep, the time when the body is in its restorative phase. It can also dehydrate you, leaving you tired the next day.

CAFFEINE CAN DISTURB SLEEP. For some people, any food or beverage with caffeine in it can disturb sleep. If you are sensitive to caffeine, avoid it in the afternoon and evening.

CUT THE FAT. If you have a high-fat meal in the evening or eat foods that cause you indigestion and heartburn, your sleep can be disturbed.

DO NOT EAT LATE AT NIGHT. Sufferers from heartburn or acid reflux should avoid late, heavy meals that delay the emptying of the stomach. Lying down with a full stomach encourages acids and gastric juices to flow up into the oesophagus, causing heartburn that disturbs sleep.

DRINKING FLUIDS TOO CLOSE TO BEDTIME CAN CAUSE PROBLEMS. Avoid fluids after dinner to reduce the need to go to the bathroom during the night.

MILK AND HONEY PROMOTE SLEEP. Milk contains tryptophan, an essential amino acid that is a natural dietary sleep inducer. Tryptophan increases the amount of serotonin, a natural sedative, in the brain. This is why so many folk remedies include warm milk with a spoonful of honey, a simple sugar. (Carbohydrates facilitate the entry of tryptophan into the brain.) A turkey sandwich is a sleep-inducing combination of tryptophan and carbohydrates. A banana with milk gives you vitamin B_6, which helps to convert tryptophan to serotonin.

HELPFUL HERBS
Many herbs are said to be useful for inducing sleep; one of the most popular and reliable is valerian. Its use as a sedative has been supported by research demonstrating that active ingredients in the valerian root depress the central nervous

system and relax smooth muscle tissue. Valerian that is brewed into a tea or taken as a capsule or tincture can lessen the time it takes to fall asleep and produce a deep rest. It does not cause dependency or a 'hungover' feeling. It is not recommended for use during pregnancy or breastfeeding, as it has not been studied for these conditions. Other remedies suggested for sleep problems include teas made of chamomile, hops, lemon balm and peppermint, but there is not much evidence that they work.

THE ROLE OF MELATONIN

A hormone produced by the brain, melatonin helps to regulate the body's sleep–wake cycle. Researchers think that it may control the onset of puberty, a woman's menstrual cycle, mood and the release of growth hormones. Melatonin can alleviate insomnia, although It may not help you to stay asleep. When taken correctly, it may prevent jet lag, but the many other claims for melatonin – for example, that it can boost immunity and forestall ageing – are unproven.

Melatonin is not sold over-the-counter in the UK but is available on the internet. It appears to be safe when it's taken in small amounts (doses range from 0.3mg to 5mg), for a temporary bout of insomnia. But experts caution against taking large doses or long-term use because of its potential side effects, which include grogginess, depression and sexual dysfunction. Melatonin should not be taken by women who are attempting to conceive, or who are pregnant or breastfeeding; nor should it be given to children or used by anyone with severe allergies, mental illness, rheumatoid arthritis or other auto-immune diseases and lymphoma and other types of cancers.

SLEEP DISORDERS

Insomnia can be one of the symptoms of anxiety, depression or stress, or it can be caused by a medical problem. Overcoming the cause is essential to improving the quality of sleep. Obesity may interfere with sleep if it affects breathing. Sleep apnoea is a common and potentially serious sleep disorder in which a pattern of loud snoring builds to a crescendo, after which the person stops breathing and awakens briefly. This condition affects an estimated 4 per cent of people in the UK and is common in overweight people, especially middle-aged men. People with obstructive apnoea can stop breathing for 10 seconds or longer a hundred or more times a night. Muscle cramps and restless legs, a vague discomfort relieved only by moving the legs, can also interfere with sleep.

Problem-solver ideas for insomnia sufferers

- Keep a sleep log for several weeks to help to identify activities and behaviour that may interfere with your sleep. Each day, write down the times you wake up and go to bed, and when you drink caffeinated beverages, exercise and take naps.
- Exercise regularly, preferably in the late afternoon. Do not exercise strenuously within 2 or 3 hours of bedtime.
- Don't take a long nap during the day.
- Eat at regular times during the day, and avoid a heavy meal close to bedtime.
- After lunch, stay away from caffeine.
- Don't smoke; if you can't quit, at least try not to smoke for an hour or two before bedtime.
- Avoid excessive mental stimulation before bedtime.
- Establish a schedule to help to regulate your body's inner clock. Go to bed and get up at about the same times every day, and follow the same bedtime preparations each night to create a sleep ritual.
- A warm bath or reading in bed, listening to soothing music or meditating are all useful sleep rituals.
- Keep your bedroom dark and quiet. If you can't block outside noise, mask it with an inside noise, such as the hum of a fan.
- Use your bedroom only for sleeping, not for working or watching TV.
- Wear loose-fitting and comfortable nightclothes.
- If your worries keep you awake at night, deal with them some other time. Devote 30 minutes after dinner to writing down problems and possible solutions, and then try to set them aside.
- If you can't sleep, don't stay in bed fretting for more than 15 minutes or so. Get up, go to another room and read or watch TV until you are sleepy. Be sure to get up at your regular time the next day.

Smoked, cured and potted meats

BENEFITS

- Used sparingly, add flavour without excessive fat or calories

DRAWBACKS

- Nitrites in preserved meats may form cancer-causing nitrosamines

- High sodium content may cause future problems with high blood pressure

- Preserved meats must be carefully handled to prevent food poisoning

- Sausages made with cereal fillers may cause symptoms in people sensitive to these grains

- Cured meats may contain high levels of tyramine, which triggers migraine in susceptible people and causes serious reactions in those taking certain drugs

Before there was refrigeration, people the world over used similar methods for preserving meat: salting, smoking, and air drying. Although curing is no longer essential in industrialised countries, our taste for salty, smoky flavours still persists.

Cancers of the oesophagus and stomach are more common where people eat large quantities of smoked and salt-cured foods, such as in the Far East and Central Asia.

In the UK, however, deaths due to stomach cancer have been decreasing since the 1930s, although consumption of smoked and processed meat has increased. The reason for this may be that cured foods are less heavily treated with preservatives here than in countries where refrigeration is not widely available. Also, most foods sold as 'smoked' are not smoke-cured but are flavoured with a smoke extract that does not have the same carcinogenic potential.

Warning: Tyramine, a metabolic product of the amino acid tyrosine, is found at high concentrations in cured meats. It can trigger migraine attacks in susceptible people. More seriously, it can cause an abrupt rise in blood pressure, headache and even fatal collapse in persons taking monoamine oxidase (MAO) inhibitors to treat depression.

Smoke curing

Smoking preserves meat and fish both by slow cooking at a low temperature and by treatment with chemicals in the smoke. More than 200 components have so far been identified in smoke, including alcohols, acids, phenols and several toxic – and possibly cancer-causing – substances. These chemicals inhibit the growth of micro-organisms that cause meat spoilage, and the phenols slow the oxidation of fat and prevent it from becoming rancid. Smoking is now used primarily for flavour – for example, the distinctive hickory aroma associated with smoked bacon, and mesquite and other aromatic wood chips that are used to enhance the taste of grilled foods.

Air curing

Preserving by drying is another name for air curing, and it has been used for thousands of years. Drying food generally concentrates some nutrients, especially minerals, but the vitamin content of dried meat is much less than that of fresh. Native peoples in North America dried venison, buffalo meat and fish – sometimes mixing them with fat and dried berries – to make a nutritious and long-lasting food. Chipped beef or biltong, as it is called in South Africa, is an air-dried throwback to pioneer preserving methods. Prosciutto is air-cured ham. As with other preservation techniques, air curing has been superseded by refrigeration and is now used mainly to give flavour and texture, although dried meats keep well.

Salt curing

Whether in a brine solution or a dry salt bed, salt curing draws water from the meat and from bacteria and moulds through the process of osmosis. While the meat remains wholesome, the micro-organisms shrivel and die. We no longer need to salt meat to store it over winter, but the method is still used because people like the taste of salty meats, such as ham and bacon.

The more salt used in curing, the better the meat's keeping qualities but the greater the loss of nutrients. When heavily salted meat is soaked to make it palatable, even more vitamins and minerals are lost, but today's curing solutions are much weaker than those formerly used, and salted meat seldom needs to be soaked before cooking.

Sausages

Most sausages are made from pork or beef with cereal fillers, herbs and spices and preservatives. People with coeliac disease should avoid those made with cereal fillers.

Because sausages, like minced meat, go through several stages of handling, they are more susceptible

S

Did you know?

How corned beef got its name

Years ago in England, when ice was the only refrigeration, butchers faced a problem every Friday. They had to close for the weekend, but the ice would melt over two days and meat would spoil. To preserve the meat, butchers soaked it in strong brine or covered it with grains of coarse salt, called 'corns'. The name has stuck ever since.

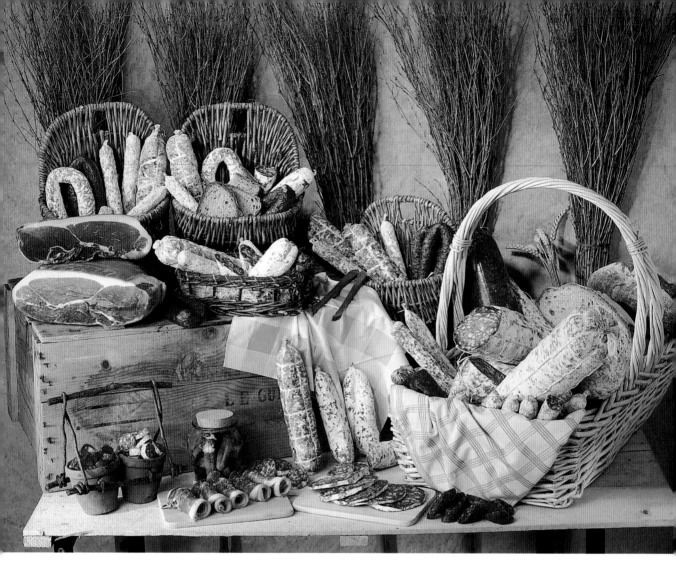

▲ Delicatessen delights
Smoked and cured meats such as salamis and prosciutto are tempting and tasty favourites, but their high saturated fat content means that they should be consumed in moderation.

to contamination than fresh meat and should be cooked thoroughly. Sausages in the wurst family vary in their meat, filler and additive content. Kosher frankfurters and bologna generally contain less filler. In addition, kosher products must be made only with approved cuts of meat; they do not contain scraps and certain organ meats.

All pork and beef sausages are high in salt and saturated fat. Reduced-fat sausages are available, but the benefits of lower fat may be offset by the higher amounts of salt added to boost flavour.

Liverwurst varies in ingredients according to the brand. While high in minerals such as iron, as well as being high in vitamin A and the B vitamins, liverwurst is also high in saturated fat. If flavoured with bacon, the sodium content will be substantially higher.

The famous Italian salami is a particularly unhealthy sausage as it contains dramatically high levels of both sodium and fat, compared with other sausages. Although it is not eaten in such great quantities, as other sausages, only 50g of salami provides a third of the salt that an adult should allow themselves in one day. Salamis, frankfurters and other smoked sausages contain tyramine, a substance which causes headache and even migraine in susceptible people.

Potted meats
Europeans love potted meats. They are made by cooking pork, duck or goose very slowly in order to render, or extract, the fat. The well-cooked meat is then shredded (although small joints of poultry may be left whole), mixed with some of the fat, packed in earthenware or glass jars and then sealed with the remaining fat to keep out air. The shredded meats are usually spread on bread or toast, while the whole joints are used in hearty, long-baked legume dishes, such as cassoulet. Potted meats conserve most of the nutrients of fresh meat, however,

they are quite high in saturated fat and should be eaten only rarely and in very small amounts.

Nitrites and nitrates

The reddish-pink colour of cured meats, including the cold cuts at the deli counter, is due to the presence of nitrites, chemicals that enhance the effect of salt by inhibiting bacterial growth and slowing fat oxidation.

Critics claim that nitrites should be banned because they combine with amino acids during cooking and digestion to form cancer-causing nitrosamines. What's more, nitrite itself can cause tumours in laboratory animals that consume it in very high doses. But the meat industry and the government insist that nitrite should be retained because it is extremely effective against *Clostridium botulinum*, the micro-organism that causes botulin poisoning, or botulism. They also point out that only about a fifth of the nitrites that form nitrosamines comes from meats – the rest are formed in the body from nitrates in vegetables and various plant foods.

C. botulinum thrives in oxygen-free surroundings (such as sealed cans, jars and plastic packaging), and its spores survive long boiling. If vacuum-packed or canned meats are allowed to reach 10°C, any spores present may develop into active bacteria and produce the lethal toxin. Botulin toxin is destroyed at temperatures of about 70°C, but cold cuts are not usually cooked before eating, and even a baked or boiled ham may not be cooked long enough to reach a high enough temperature in the centre.

Not only does nitrite suppress active bacteria, but it also weakens the heat-resistant *C. botulinum* spores. This means that the spores can be destroyed without the need for pressure cooking and reduces

the risk that spores will develop if the meat is carelessly handled. The risk of cancer from nitrites in the doses currently used is much less than the risk of contracting botulism from tainted meat. However, even these risks are smaller than the risk of coronary disease from excessive consumption of the saturated fats that are, in general, plentiful in nitrite-preserved foods. If you enjoy smoked and salted meats, make sure you eat them only occasionally and in moderate amounts.

Smoothies

BENEFITS

- An excellent source of calcium
- Fruit and vegetables add vitamins, minerals and phytochemicals
- A fast, tasty, nutritious breakfast or snack food

Though often high in calories, smoothies are good-quality nutrition in a glass. They are quick to make and a great way to give calcium to children. All you need is a blender or food processor, plus fruit or vegetables and yoghurt or milk and you have a delicious drink rich with vitamins, minerals, antioxidants and fibre. A smoothie can be a breakfast, a beneficial drink before or after a strenuous workout or a meal replacement for people on the go.

> **Super smoothie**
> For a nutrition-packed drink that will appeal to children, try a combination of banana and mango. Bananas are loaded with potassium and mangoes are rich in vitamin C. Dice half a ripe mango and blend it with a small banana, 175ml low-fat milk, 125ml orange juice and 2 tablespoons of vanilla yoghurt. On busy days this can serve as a healthy, quick breakfast.

Ideally it should contain a variety of foods and nutrients: vegetables and fruit, milk and milk products, a protein source and grains.

You can make smoothies out of any combination of things, but typically they include milk and/or yoghurt, fruit, either fresh, canned or frozen, and sometimes juice. The milk provides calcium, riboflavin, potassium, protein and more. A 200ml glass of milk contains 240mg of calcium, over a third of the daily requirement, as well as 7g of protein and 213mg of potassium. If you are allergic to cow's milk or prefer not to drink it, you can use a fortified soya or rice beverage. The fruit provides vitamin C, folate, beta carotene, bioflavonoids and other antioxidants. The healthiness of your smoothie can be boosted even further by adding some wheatgerm, bran cereal, tofu or skimmed milk powder. Making smoothies does not have to be complicated; check your

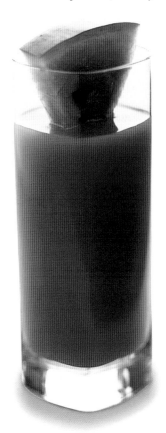

S

refrigerator for any usable leftovers such as last night's fruit salad. Experiment with different flavours – sweet, tart or a combination. Smoothies sold in juice bars are large (often 500ml) and can be very high in calories. Ask for skimmed milk and fruit or share the smoothie.

Snack foods

BENEFITS

- Snacks based on nutritious foods can help to meet nutritional recommendations
- Fruit and vegetables are ideal snacks, high in vitamins and minerals
- Well-timed, low-calorie snacks can take the edge off hunger and help to prevent over-eating at mealtimes

DRAWBACKS

- Snacking on muesli bars and high-fat foods adds empty calories and saturated fats.
- Many commercially prepared snacks and dips are high in sodium.

The human body is programmed to send out hunger signals whenever it needs an energy boost, which may occur between meals. The stores of carbohydrate (glycogen) in the liver and muscles, which help to keep a normal level of blood sugar, are used up in 4 to 6 hours. Healthy snacks replenish them.

Properly handled, snacking can be a healthy response to hunger. The trouble is that many people reach for a snack even when they're not hungry – while watching TV, attending a sporting event or simply out of boredom. And often the snacks they eat are poor nutritional choices – potato crisps, sweets and chocolate – foods often referred to as 'junk' foods. Entire supermarket aisles are devoted to these fat-laden,

Do one simple thing

Try to avoid foods that contain trans fats

Trans fats are even worse than saturated fats as far as health risks are concerned. Try to reduce consumption of foods that list 'hydrogenated' fats or oils as ingredients. The hydrogenation process, used by manufacturers to extend shelf life, leads to the production of trans fats.

high-calorie extravaganzas, and it's easy to fall into the trap of reaching for them. Weight gain can result.

Snacks don't have to be fattening. Eating a low-calorie snack during a long stretch between meals can take the edge off hunger and prevent overeating at the next meal. If snacks are well timed, they won't spoil the appetite for meals and may help to boost flagging energy, especially in children. Some people intentionally blunt their appetites with a low-calorie snack before an event where snack foods are served.

For many people, snacking or having frequent small meals is an alternative to the usual three large ones. This is a good solution for young children whose small stomachs can't consume enough at one sitting to sustain their need for energy. Older adults often can eat only small portions; supplemental

Proof positive

Some studies show that eating frequent small meals is a better strategy for weight management than eating one or two large meals. It's also an effective way to lower cholesterol and regulate blood sugar levels. A UK study showed that middle-aged and older adults who ate frequently throughout the day had lower LDL cholesterol compared with those who tended to eat one or two large meals a day. In fact, many experts think that dividing the day's food into five or six small meals daily is best for overall health.

snacks can help them to maintain a balanced diet. The same is true for people who are convalescing.

Fast-growing adolescents may find snacks useful to fuel their growth and compensate for lapses in their eating patterns. Athletes of all ages typically have an increased demand for energy, especially from carbohydrates, which the body converts to glucose, its major fuel. Pregnant women often suffer bouts of nausea during the early months, and heartburn or a feeling of constant fullness towards the end of pregnancy. Many are happier snacking than eating a large amount at one time.

Smart snacking

If you are among those who snack regularly, it is important to consider snacks in your overall nutrition plan. Choose those that will provide balanced nutrition as well as energy.

Snacks can be the same as small meals, so a sandwich, a bowl of hearty vegetable soup, cheese and biscuits, yoghurt with fruit or a toasted muffin will be good choices, nutritionally. If you are looking for salty, crunchy taste, choose pretzels, bread sticks or air-popped popcorn. Combine them with a low-fat yoghurt-based dip or a bean dip to increase their nutritional value. Other healthy snacks include a bowl of cereal with skimmed milk and fresh fruit, or mini-pizzas made from English muffins topped with pizza sauce and fat-reduced mozzarella cheese.

Snacks can provide several of the recommended daily servings of starchy foods or the two servings of fruit and five of vegetables. An apple, or a pitta pocket filled with chopped raw vegetables, makes a filling, nutritious snack that can be worked into the day's meal plan. Other quick, low-fat foods, such as bags of fresh raw vegetables and dips such as hummous or other bean dips, or a mixture of low-fat yoghurt blended with herbs are good after-school snacks. For a satisfying beverage, make a latte (½ regular or soya milk and ½ decaffeinated coffee) or a smoothie out of yoghurt, fruit and juice.

Snack traps

Everybody knows that a raw carrot is healthier than an iced doughnut, but some snack foods that sound nutritious are not much better than a doughnut. Read labels carefully to find hidden sugar and fats. For example, beware of muesli bars; they are often loaded with sugar and fat. Fruit drinks may contain very little fruit juice but have large amounts of added sugar. Microwave popcorn is often high in fat, as are corn crisps and most crackers. Dried fruits appeal to people with a sweet tooth, and they are easy to take to work or school, but snackers should be careful to brush their teeth after eating them to remove clinging remnants that can promote cavities.

Coping with hunger

When travelling or at work, if you look for a snack once hunger pangs have hit, you're likely to find yourself at the mercy of a vending machine. Instead, anticipate snack attacks with nutritious, low-calorie foods that require little preparation. Take snacks to work or buy them when you buy lunch.

Any number of simple and speedy solutions can fill in the gaps after school, work or play. Canned, juice-packed peach or pear slices, for example, mixed with a sliced banana, chopped apple and a few blueberries or other fruit make an instant fruit salad. For a quick dessert, cut a banana lengthways, add low-fat yoghurt and top with berries. Another great idea is to mash a banana with a sprinkling of cinnamon and spread it on a rice cake. Buy ready-cut carrot sticks and dip them into hummous.

On cold days a cup of soup is a warming snack. Many canned and dried soups contain high levels of sodium, however, and may not be suitable for people on low-salt diets. Homemade soups are preferable. Another hearty cold-weather snack is half a baked potato topped with low-fat cottage cheese and chives.

Add several healthy snacking foods to your weekly shopping list. When you have the right foods on hand, it's easy to prepare snacks to take on trips, to school or to work. Stay away from prepackaged high-fat items, such as potato crisps and tortillas. Dried fruit, nuts and seeds provide valuable nutrients with their calories.

Don't forget dental hygiene. Remind children to brush after snacking or to rinse their mouths vigorously with plain water.

▶ **Healthy snack**
Snacking on healthy foods like vegetables and low-fat dip helps to prevent overeating at mealtime.

Top twenty 100kcal snacks

SNACK	AMOUNT
Almonds	15g
Apple	1 large
Baked tortilla chips	10
Banana	1
Cereal bars	1 small
Cheesestick	1
Chocolate-coated raisins	15 (22g)
Dates	2
Fruit-juice ice lolly	1
Grapes	(150g)
Hard-boiled egg	1 large
Low-fat yoghurt, plain or artificially sweetened	1 carton (200g)
Low-fat custard	135g pot
Oatcakes	2
Orange	1 large
Peanut butter	3 teaspoons
Pistachios (in shells)	1 handful
Pretzels	40 thin sticks
Pumpkin or sunflower seeds	1 small handful (20g)
Rice crackers	10
Sultanas	2 tablespoons (30g)

S

Soft drinks

BENEFITS

- Carbonated drinks provide a quick energy boost from their calories or caffeine

- Sipping ginger ale can help to quell nausea and provide energy for people unable to take solid food

DRAWBACKS

- Many contain large amounts of sugar and acids that can lead to weight gain and dental decay

- High phosphorus content may interfere with calcium absorption

- Caffeine may cause health problems in adults or behaviour and development problems in children

The British first began to bottle lemonade during the 1700s, using sulphur dioxide to preserve it. By 1789 Nicholas Paul of Geneva had developed a method of making carbonated waters in bulk. The taste for carbonated drinks (originally hangover cures) has never faltered.

Soft drinks consist mostly of carbonated water mixed with sugar or an artificial sweetener, plus natural or artificial flavourings and colouring agents. Many of them also contain caffeine. Apart from a quick energy boost from the caffeine or sugar, soft drinks offer little or no nutritional value. A 200ml can of cola contains about 86kcal; a diet soft drink, because it is artificially sweetened, is less than 1kcal, although it may have caffeine in it and its acid can damage teeth.

Health implications

An occasional soft drink may not cause problems, but drinking them regularly contributes empty calories that can add to weight problems. These drinks are also bad for the teeth. Their sugar encourages the growth of cavity-causing bacteria, and they contain acids that can erode tooth enamel. Consumers should read labels carefully to determine what's actually in various soft drinks and mineral waters. Colas, for example, contain large amounts of phosphates, which may impair calcium absorption. A greater concern is that soft drinks cause a decrease in calcium intake by displacing milk from the diet. Children and young people who drink soft drinks instead of milk are missing the calcium critical to the growth of their bones. A 27kg child who drinks a 375ml cola containing 50mg of caffeine is getting the same dose of caffeine that an 80kg man would get from several cups of coffee. A child who is restless or sleepless may be feeling the effects of too many soft drinks. In adults, excessive caffeine may raise blood pressure and cause irregular heart-beats. People who react to caffeine should choose a decaffeinated drink.

When a person can't take other foods and liquids, soft drinks can provide energy during the illness. Some people find that sipping flat ginger ale quells the nausea associated with migraine and morning sickness.

Don't be misled by fruit-flavoured drinks. On close reading, labels will disclose that non-carbonated fruit drinks often contain less than 10 per cent fruit juice while harbouring large amounts of sweeteners and dyes.

Soft drinks need not be harmful if consumed only occasionally. The danger is that if taken regularly in large amounts, they may satisfy hunger and take the place of essential nutrients in the diet. Children who fill up on sugary drinks shortly before and during meals may spoil their appetite for more healthy and nutritious foods.

Medical proof that soft drinks and obesity are linked

A US study published in *The Lancet* medical journal suggests that a soft drink a day gives a child a 60 per cent greater chance of becoming obese. The study, from the Children's Hospital in Boston, Massachusetts, followed 548 children aged 11 and 12 for two school years.

The researchers found that for every can or glass of sugar-sweetened beverage a child drank during that time, their body mass index rose and their chances of becoming obese increased 60 per cent. This held true regardless of initial body mass, diet, television viewing habits and physical activity.

One possible explanation for this link might be that while people tend to eat less at a meal if they have consumed excess calories at a previous one, they don't tend to do that if those extra calories come from beverages. It is not likely that a child would eat less food to compensate for the extra soft drink calories. The overall result would be that more calories are taken in than are burned off - with the inevitable increase in weight.

The soft drink–fast food link

One reason that soft drinks are linked to obesity may be because they are often consumed with fast foods that are loaded with fat. The sugar in the soft drink activates the pancreas to produce insulin, but insulin also tells the body to store fat. So, as the pancreas is feeling the effects of the soft drink, the hamburger and fries arrive, and since the body has more insulin than it needs for the meal, it stores the fat instead of burning it.

Healthy drinks

You can make refreshing and economical drinks at home by mixing sparkling mineral water with fruit juice, a mixture of chopped fresh fruit or any of the wide variety of fruit nectars now sold in food stores and supermarkets.

Sore throat

CONSUME PLENTY OF

- Fruit and vegetables for vitamin C
- Liver (unless you're pregnant), carrots and spinach for vitamin A and beta carotene
- Oily fish for vitamin D
- Olive oil and avocados for vitamin E
- Seafood, lean meat and grains for zinc
- Bio-yoghurt to protect against the side effects of antibiotics
- Non-alcoholic and caffeine-free fluids

AVOID

- Alcohol and tobacco smoke

A raw, stinging throat can often be the first sign of a viral upper respiratory infection, such as a cold or flu, or less commonly, a bacterial infection, such as a 'strep throat'. In children, swollen and infected tonsils can cause a sore throat; among adults, smoking is a common cause of mild, chronic throat pain. Respiratory viruses and streptococcus organisms spread easily from one person to another, but good hygiene and nutrition helps to prevent many episodes.

Dietary factors

Get lots of vitamin C. Although scientific evidence is lacking, many people are convinced that high doses of vitamin C help to reduce the duration and severity of a sore throat and other symptoms of viral respiratory infections. Like other antioxidants, vitamin C is vital in immune function, so adequate amounts can protect against viruses, bacteria and other infectious agents. What constitutes 'adequate', however, remains unresolved. A recent US study indicates that 200mg of vitamin C a day may be a better amount than the present Reference Nutrient Intake (RNI) of 30 to 40mg. The same study found that doses above 200mg are of no added benefit, because body tissues are unable to absorb more than that amount. Indeed, for many people, higher amounts may be detrimental because they can lead to iron overload and other problems.

Eat lots of fruit and vegetables. It is recommended that we eat two servings of fruit and five of vegetables a day, and a diet like this can easily provide 200mg of vitamin C, as well as other essential vitamins and minerals. Especially rich sources of vitamin C include citrus and other fruit, berries, peppers, melons and dark green vegetables. One orange or eight large strawberries contain more than 100 per cent of the RNI for adults. These foods are also high in beta carotene, which the body converts to vitamin A, another antioxidant that is instrumental in building immunity. Vitamin E, found in avocados, is helpful, too.

Try zinc lozenges. Several studies have demonstrated that zinc lozenges can shorten the duration and/or severity of a sore throat. Zinc nasal sprays are also available. A diet that provides adequate zinc strengthens the body's immune defences. Good sources include yoghurt and other dairy products, oysters and other seafood, lean meat, eggs and grains. Taking zinc supplements for a cold or as a preventive measure has been shown to be effective but don't take more than 40mg per day as it can weaken your immune system, making it less able to fight against disease.

Avoid alcohol. Because it reduces immunity and irritates inflamed mucous membranes, alcohol should be avoided until the sore throat clears up. It is also a good idea to cut down on, or completely eliminate, caffeine; possible diuretic effects of large quantities could increase the loss of body fluids and could result in a drying of the membranes and thickening of mucus. Make every effort to stop smoking, and avoid exposure to secondhand smoke.

Easing symptoms

Non-alcoholic fluids, whether hot or cold, can soothe painful swallowing. Some doctors even advise switching to a liquid diet for a while, to keep up levels of nutrition without exacerbating throat pain. Good choices include milkshakes, fruit

S

Do one simple thing

Soothe a sore throat with lemon tea

Lemons are loaded with vitamin C and can make a soothing and beneficial drink for sore throats when made into a hot drink. Squeeze the juice of a lemon into a cup of boiling water and add a teaspoon of honey.

juices, broths and soups and semi-liquid foods such as custards, puddings and jelly.

Many home sore-throat remedies are useful in alleviating symptoms. The most time-honoured favourite is to gargle with salty warm water; you can make an alternative gargle by adding 2 teaspoons of cider vinegar to a half cup of warm water.

Soups

BENEFITS

- Can be highly nourishing
- An ideal food for convalescents
- Easy to make and economical

DRAWBACKS

- Commercial soups are generally high in salt and fat

▶ **The soup solution**
Whether it's an Italian-style minestrone, a creamy carrot, apple and tomato combination or a Thai-inspired soup with prawns, soup is easy to make and nutritious.

Soup is a staple food worldwide. They are comforting, nourishing and usually economical to make. Clear soups could even facilitate weight loss. In one study, the more soup people ate, the fewer calories they took in overall and the more weight they lost. One likely reason is that soup is high in volume, so it helps you to feel full on fewer calories. (That doesn't mean that the fad diet based on cabbage soup is an effective way to lose weight. Like any severely restrictive diet, you'll get tired of it in no time and return to your old eating habits.)

Homemade soups

Even a novice cook can make a delicious soup with a few basic ingredients: diced carrots, potatoes and other vegetables simmered in a stock with herbs. Leftover meat or seafood can be added for more flavour and nutrition. Cooks who care about quality will simmer leftover chicken or beef bones with vegetables to make a soup stock. Some bought stock cubes are high in monosodium glutamate (MSG), sodium and other additives. Always taste soup before adding salt or seasonings. Salt is not needed with good-quality stock.

Some forms of cooking inevitably rob vegetables of many of their natural vitamins, but soups made with fresh ingredients still provide many nutrients, including vitamins, minerals and protein. Vitamin loss can be minimised by adding the vegetables toward the end of the cooking process, bringing the soup to a boil and cooking only until the vegetables are tender. Making your own soup allows you to control the salt content, which is important, especially if you or your family suffer from high blood pressure. Use herbs and natural vegetable flavours to replace salt.

Chilling the stock forces any fat to congeal on the surface and makes it easy to remove. Another way to remove the fat is by pouring the stock through a de-fatting jug. Cream soups and chowders contain higher amounts of saturated fat, but this can be reduced without losing flavour or texture by substituting evaporated skimmed milk for cream and whole milk. 'Cream' soups can also be made with puréed cooked potatoes and skimmed milk.

Commercial soups

Canned and instant soups have varied quality and nutritional value. Choose soups low in fat and sodium. Although canned soups are not as nutritious as homemade, they are still better than instant soups, which are so highly processed that some experts have described them as little more than a mix of MSG, artificial flavours, sodium, dyes and additives.

Soups and gout

If you suffer from gout, choose soups made from vegetable stock, as meat stocks may contain high levels of purines which raise the amount of uric acid in the body. Asparagus soup also contains purines and is best avoided, too.

Popular, healthy soups

Soups can offer various benefits:
- Bouillabaisse, a thick soup from the Mediterranean, is made with any mixture of fish. It provides lycopene from tomatoes, iron and protein from the fish and magnesium from vegetables.
- Chicken soup features large in traditional treatments for convalescents. It is said to clear a blocked nose. It contains protein and most B vitamins.
- French onion soup is warming and nourishing, and has long been regarded as an antidote to fatigue, chills, head colds and even hangovers.
- Gazpacho is a cold soup, from Spain, made with tomatoes and

salad vegetables such as spring onions and cucumber. It is full of vitamins and antioxidants. Both refreshing and filling, it is an ideal light summer meal.
- Lentil soup is particularly good for vegetarians, as lentils provide fibre and iron, as well as high-quality protein.
- Minestrone is a filling, wholesome soup that originated in Italy. It is made with fresh vegetables, dried beans and pasta or rice, and provides healthy amounts of protein, fibre and lycopene.

Soya

BENEFITS

- A vegetarian source of high-quality protein and iron

- A good source of B vitamins, potassium, zinc and other minerals

- Low in calories and saturated fat

DRAWBACKS

- Fermented soya products are high in sodium and may provoke allergies

- Soya protein may hinder iron absorption

For many years, soya foods were enjoyed mainly by vegetarians as an alternative to meat products. But in recent years as more consumers have pursued healthier lifestyles, the consumption of soya foods has risen steadily, bolstered by growing evidence of the many health benefits of these versatile foods. Research continues, however, as some questions about soya and its health effects remain unanswered.

Soya beans are one of the most nutritious and versatile plant foods available. Volume for volume, soya contains more protein than beef, more calcium than milk, more lecithin than eggs and more iron

Do one simple thing

Add foods high in vitamin C to improve iron absorption

Although many soya products are high in iron, it may not be well absorbed. Improve absorption by adding foods high in vitamin C to your meal, such as orange juice, tomatoes, peppers, strawberries or melons.

than beef. And if that were not enough to rate it as a super-food, soya bean protein contains all of the essential amino acids, making it the only plant protein that approaches or equals animal products in providing a complete source of protein. This makes it a good choice for those looking for alternatives to meat products. Soya beans are also good sources of B vitamins and potassium, zinc and other minerals. And to top it off, soya bean oil is low in saturated fat, unlike the fat that comes from animal sources. Soya contains important phyto-chemicals, including isoflavones, saponins, lignans and phytosterols, all of which have a variety of positive effects on health.

Health benefits of soya

The beneficial effect of soya foods on heart disease, some cancers, osteoporosis and menopausal symptoms is the focus of much research. There is a great deal of evidence supporting the health-protective effects of soya. For example, populations that include high amounts of soya in their diet have low rates of breast cancer, prostate cancer and menopausal symptoms. The evidence is stronger for some benefits than for others.

Heart health

This is an area where the research is conclusive. A large body of evidence indicates that replacing some animal

S

products with soya protein can reduce the risk of heart disease. This is because soya lowers levels of the artery-clogging LDL cholesterol without reducing levels of the beneficial HDL cholesterol.

In the UK, it is legal for foods that contain more than 6.25mg of soya protein per portion to claim that, taken as part of a low-saturated-fat diet, they can lower levels of cholesterol in the blood.

The many faces of soya

Tofu. Comes in firm, soft or silken textures. It's made from puréed soya beans and processed into a 'cake'. This versatile food can be stir-fried, grilled, added to soups, lasagna, cheesecake or blended into dips or smoothies.

Soya beverages. Can be bought fresh or in tetra packs. They can be substituted for other beverages or for milk in recipes. Some products are fortified with calcium and vitamin B_{12}, and they come in many flavours such as vanilla, chocolate and coffee.

Soya beans. Convenient to use, canned soya beans can be added to casseroles or soups, or mashed and added to dips or 'veggie burger' recipes.

Green soya beans (*edamame*). Edamame are bought shelled or still in the pod and can be served as a snack or a vegetable dish.

Soya flour. Adds protein to recipes when substituted for plain flour. It can also be found in cereals, pancake mixes, frozen desserts and other common foods.

Textured vegetable protein. It is made from defatted, dehydrated soya flour. Once rehydrated, it can be used as a meat substitute in a variety of dishes, including pasta sauce or lasagna.

Tempeh. Made from fermented soya beans and formed into a chewy cake, this meat substitute can be used in a variety of dishes.

Miso. A delicious fermented soya bean paste, it can be used as a base for soups or as a seasoning.

Soya nuts. These tasty nuts have more fibre and less fat than other nuts. They can be enjoyed as a snack or sprinkled on salads or in stir-fries.

Soya protein powders. Made from isolated soya protein, these powders can be added to shakes or smoothies for a protein-powered breakfast.

Cancer

Throughout Asia, where soya has long been a dietary staple, the rates of breast and prostate cancer are much lower than in Western countries. Studies of Asians show that it is soya intake early in life that is protective. Soya foods contain compounds called isoflavones, which are a subclass of a much larger group of food components called flavonoids. Genistein and daidzein are the two main types of isoflavones in soya. Some researchers attribute the low incidence of these cancers to these isoflavones, which reduce the effects of oestrogen on breast and prostate tissue. Oestrogen is thought to stimulate tumour growth in genetically susceptible people.

However, the evidence regarding soya and its effect on cancer rates is inconclusive, and much more research needs to be done. While there is evidence that soya plays a role in preventing breast cancer, the jury is out on its effect in women who have the disease. The prudent recommendation is that they should consume soya in moderation and not increase their intake in response to a diagnosis of breast cancer.

Osteoporosis

Recent research has indicated that soya isoflavones may delay bone loss and might even build bone density. Not all research is consistent in this finding, however, with some studies showing that soya has no significant effect on bone loss.

Menopausal symptoms

Diets rich in soya foods can reduce menopausal symptoms, particularly the frequency and severity of hot flushes, in some women. The extent of improvement, however, varies from woman to woman.

Some areas of caution

While there is agreement that soya foods offer distinct health benefits, some researchers have cautioned that there may be some health risks as well, particularly for those who eat large amounts of these foods, or who take soya supplements. Concerns have been raised about the effects of soya on the following:

- Cancer. We still have a lot to learn about isoflavones and how they work. Some recent findings have suggested that high isoflavone levels might actually increase the risk of certain cancers, particularly breast cancer. The concerns have been raised with regard to isolated isoflavones in supplement form, not in whole soya foods. However, until further research helps to clarify the role of isoflavones in human health, it is wise to avoid isoflavone supplements in general. People who are being treated, or who have been treated, for breast or prostate cancer should speak to their GP and/or exercise caution before adding soya to their diet.
- Dementia. Results of a recent study suggested that consuming tofu two or more times a week might increase the risk of dementia. At this point, this study raises more questions than it answers, and these results have not been supported by any other studies to date. In addition, this effect has not been seen in

▶ **Asian flavour**
Triangles of tofu stir-fried with thin slices of meat and vegetables is a delicious way to include soya in your diet.

population studies looking at those who consume high amounts of soya foods.
- Thyroid function. Some studies have linked soya consumption to suppressed thyroid function. It appears that the risk is linked only to taking soya supplements or eating huge amounts of soya foods, but more research is needed to clarify this relationship.
- Infant formula. The use of soya-based infant formula has been reviewed and experts concluded that while phyto-oestrogens have the potential to cause adverse effects, there is no evidence that giving infants soya-based formula has been associated with any demonstrated harm. However, FSA recommends that when breastfeeding is not an option, a modified cow's milk formula should be chosen in preference to a soya-based formula.

The bottom line

Overall, soya is regarded as a nutritious, beneficial food, and a welcome addition to a healthy diet. But it should be regarded as a food, not as a medication. It is a good protein substitute and can be used as an alternative to animal proteins.

However, all foods, including soya, are complex mixtures of substances that researchers are only just beginning to understand. Many components are proving beneficial, but there is the risk with any food or component of food that they can

also be harmful in certain amounts and for certain people. Don't overdo it and don't take soya or isoflavone supplements. There's no substitute for a balanced diet that includes a wide variety of wholesome foods in moderate amounts.

Spices

BENEFITS

- Add a variety of flavours to foods
- Can act as an appetite stimulant

Centuries ago, the taste for spices sparked voyages of discovery and kindled international trade. Today, spices are still prized for the variety they lend to the diet.

For thousands of years, spices have been used as flavourings, medicines, perfumes, dyes and even as weapons of war. They can stimulate the appetite and add flavour and interest to humdrum dishes. Characterised by pungent aromas and flavour, spices are the fruit, flowerbuds, roots or bark of plants. While they are rich in minerals, spices are used only in minute amounts, so they provide

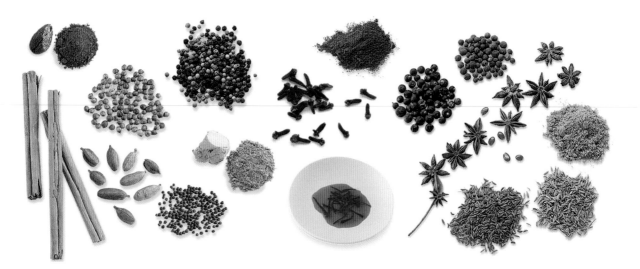

little nutritional value. Because spices lose their pungency on exposure to light, heat and air, store them in a dark, dry cupboard and replace them annually.

Spicy remedies

Through the ages, spices have been used as remedies for almost every ailment. Although most specific health claims have not been borne out by scientific studies, several of the most popular traditional uses do seem to be grounded in fact.

Allspice gets its name from its flavour, which seems to be a blend of the aromas of cinnamon, nutmeg and cloves. It is believed to aid digestion.

Black pepper, like white pepper, is the fruit of a tropical vine; it accounts for 25 per cent of the world's spice trade. It's thought to stimulate digestion, ease flatulence, relieve constipation and improve circulation.

Caraway is a member of the carrot family. Caraway seeds are especially popular as a flavouring for breads, cakes, cheese and red cabbage. Drinking an infusion of caraway may relieve menstrual pain, stimulate milk flow in nursing mothers, and stimulate the appetite. The chemical called limonene in caraway may reduce cancer risk.

Cardamom is used to flavour coffee in Arab countries, sweet breads in Scandinavia, and to enhance the flavour of cooked fruit. Cardamom is also recommended to relieve indigestion. It is sometimes used in the treatment of coughs and colds as well as bronchitis.

Cayenne (also called chilli pepper) and related spices are used to flavour Mexican dishes. They contain capsaicin, a volatile oil, that gives chillies their 'bite' and is used as a topical painkiller. Eating cayenne and other fiery substances is thought to stimulate the production of endorphins, the brain's natural mood enhancers, which may explain the euphoria people feel after eating spicy food. Cayenne may help to clear the airways and so reduce the discomfort from allergies, colds and flu.

Cinnamon, an ancient spice obtained from the dried bark of two Asian evergreens, is a highly versatile flavouring as well as a carminative that relieves bloating and flatulence. Cinnamon may have antibacterial and antimicrobial properties and may also reduce discomfort from heartburn. In an Indian study, the cassia form of cinnamon was found to lower blood glucose, cholesterol and trigycerides in diabetic men and women.

Clove oil, long used as a home remedy for toothaches, is no longer recommended for this purpose because it can burn mucous membranes. However, eugenol, a mild derivative, is used as a flavouring ingredient in some mouthwashes and toothpaste. Eugenol may protect against heart disease by preventing blood clots from forming.

Coriander has been used as a digestive tonic since ancient times. Coriander seed is thought to be helpful in relieving stomach cramps and may have the ability to kill bacteria and fungus. It contains limonene, which is a flavonoid thought to help to fight cancer.

Cumin, a hot spice, blends well in chilli, curries and such Middle Eastern specialties as hummous. It is being investigated for potential antioxidant and anti-cancer effects.

Ginger, popular in Asian dishes as well as in desserts and soft drinks, is a common digestive aid and motion sickness remedy; sipping flat ginger ale may help to ease nausea. Substances in ginger – gingerol, shogaol and zingiberene – have antioxidant capabilities that may help to prevent heart disease and cancer. It has anti-inflammatory properties and may help to protect against arthritis.

S

Taken at the first sign of colds or flu, hot ginger tea is a comforting drink and may help to clear a blocked nose and stimulate the liver to remove toxins from the blood.

Juniper berries Since they have antiseptic properties, juniper berries have been used to treat urinary tract infections such as cystitis. In large doses, juniper acts as a diuretic that may also cause uterine contractions.

Mustard has been used in poultices and smelling salts to relieve pain and congestion since Roman times. Mustard seeds contain allyl isothiocyanates, which some studies suggest inhibit the growth of cancer cells.

Nutmeg and mace come from the same plant; nutmeg is the shelled seed, mace its hull. Both contain myristicin, which can cause hallucinations. Eugenol, a mono-terpene in nutmeg, is thought to help to prevent heart disease by preventing blood cells from forming clots. Nutmeg may also have anti-bacterial properties that may destroy the food-borne bacteria *E. coli*.

Saffron, the most expensive of all spices, is obtained from the stamens of a single variety of crocus. It may ease menstrual and other chronic pain, depression and diarrhoea.

Star anise gets its liquorice flavour from anethole. Anethole-based flavourings have long been used in cough syrups and digestive preparations, as well as in ouzo, arak and anisette liquors. Star anise teas should not be given to children with colic. Doctors have reported a number of adverse reactions to star anise, from nausea to mild convulsions and seizures, all of which were temporary.

Turmeric is essential to Indian curries and gives mustard its yellow colour. Turmeric is a natural anti-biotic used to treat inflammation and digestive disorders and may slow the progress of Alzheimer's.

Spinach

BENEFITS

- A rich source of beta carotene, vitamin K, folate and potassium
- Contains vitamins C and B_6 and riboflavin

DRAWBACKS

- Oxalic acid reduces absorption of the iron and calcium in spinach, and can accelerate the formation of kidney and bladder stones

Contrary to popular belief, spinach is not an especially good source of iron. The myth about its high iron content ignored the fact that its oxalic acid makes its iron unavailable. But the vegetable's dark green leaves do contain many other valuable nutrients, particularly the antioxidants and bioflavonoids that help to block cancer-causing substances and processes. For example, spinach is rich in carotenoids, plant pigments that are responsible for its dark green colour. Among them are lutein and zeaxanthin, which help to prevent macular degeneration, the leading

▼ Versatile vegetable
Young spinach leaves are delicious raw or lightly cooked. Either way, you should wash them thoroughly and discard damaged leaves and tough stalks.

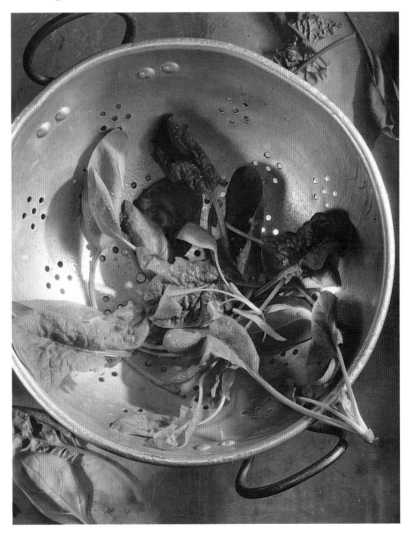

The Popeye myth

The truth behind the myth of Popeye and the strength that eating spinach gave him, dates back to a scientific mistake, made in 1870 by Dr E von Wolf, who misplaced a decimal point and wrongly estimated the iron content of spinach to be ten times greater than it really is.

It wasn't until 1937 that the mistake was discovered, by which time it was too late. The first Popeye cartoons appeared in 1929, and by then the myth about Popeye's phenomenal strength after downing a can of spinach had captured the imagination of children and adults, around the world.

Parents, trying to get their children to eat spinach probably perpetuated Dr von Wolf's mistake.

cause of vision loss in older adults. Cooking spinach helps to convert lutein into more bio-available forms. To enhance the carotenoid absorption, eat spinach with some heart-healthy oil, such as olive oil.

An 80 portion of cooked spinach provides 272mg of potassium, as well as vitamins C and B_{12} and riboflavin, as well as more than 100 per cent of the Reference Nutrient Intake (RNI) for vitamin A and 42mcg of folate, which is 21 per cent of the RNI. Folate is especially important for women who are pregnant or who may be planning a pregnancy, because it helps to prevent congenital neurological defects. Folate deficiency can also cause a severe type of anaemia.

On the negative side, spinach contains iron, calcium and other minerals, but their absorption is hindered by its high concentration

CAUTION

Excess vitamin K can counteract the effects of blood-thinners such as heparin and warfarin. If you are on these medications, keep your intake of vitamin K-rich foods, such as spinach, fairly constant.

of oxalic acid. Absorption can be increased by consuming spinach with other foods that are rich in vitamin C. Oxalic acid is a problem for people susceptible to kidney stones that form from oxalates. Phylloquinone is the most common form of vitamin K found in dark greens such as spinach. Vitamin K is needed for proper blood clotting and it may play a role in preserving bone health. Some research suggests that it may increase bone density and reduce fracture rates. Both the Nurses' Health Study and the Framingham Heart Study found that people who consume the most vitamin K in their diet have a lower risk of hip fractures than those who consume less.

Serving spinach

Spinach can be served either raw or cooked. To avoid overcooking, try steaming or stir-frying it. These cooking methods preserve texture and flavour, and they minimise the loss of many water-soluble vitamins. Although some of these nutrients are lost in cooking, a $\frac{1}{2}$ cup serving of the cooked vegetable actually provides more nutrition than a cup served raw because it takes a full two cups of leaves to cook down into a $\frac{1}{2}$ cup serving. And heating makes the protein in spinach easier to break down, too. The value of raw spinach can be enhanced by serving it with tomato for added vitamin C – which counteracts the effects of oxalic acid.

Before serving spinach, be careful to remove all the sand and dirt. One effective method is to submerge the spinach in a bowl of cold water and let the sand fall to the bottom, then remove and rinse the leaves. Dry them well if making a salad.

If you are cooking the spinach, the water left on the leaves is usually just about the right amount with which to steam it.

Sports nutrition

See Food and fitness

Squash

BENEFITS

- Provide some folate and vitamins A and C

- A good source of potassium and fibre

Squash are members of the same family as courgettes and marrows. There are many types, ranging from the homely pumpkin, through acorn, butternut, gem squashes and the attractively shaped patty pan squash to spaghetti squash with its pale golden strands of flesh.

Some squashes have a soft skin and tender flesh. Because they have a high water content, they are low in calories, with 80g cooked butternut squash having only 26kcal. It also provides about 30 per cent of the Reference Nutrient Intake (RNI) of vitamin C, 25mcg of folate and vitamin B_6, as well as enough beta carotene, which the body converts to vitamin A, to provide 73 per cent of the RNI for vitamin A. Squashes that have an intensely yellow or dark green skin have more beta carotene than paler ones.

Soft-skinned squash can be cooked by stir-frying or steaming to minimise nutrient loss and keep the

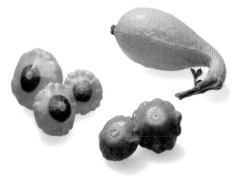

S

vegetable from becoming too mushy. The mild flavour complements stews, soups and mixed vegetables, but using large squash can make some dishes watery. To avoid this problem, lightly salt the slices or pieces of a large squash and place them on absorbent paper towel; rinse and dry the pieces before adding them to the recipe.

Hard-skinned squash

Spaghetti squash has a hard skin and an interesting flesh. The squash is steamed or boiled whole and then cut in half. The flesh can be pulled out with a fork, and resembles strands of spaghetti. It is low in calories, with 80g of the strands having about 18kcal. It provides fibre and small quantities of vitamins and minerals.

Gem squash and butternut can be boiled or steamed, cut open and the flesh scooped out. They will cook more quickly if you stab the hard skins in several places with a sharp knife, before cooking. Butternut is an excellent source of vitamin A; acorn squash provides slightly less.

Strawberries

BENEFITS

- An excellent source of vitamin C
- Contain folate and potassium

Did you know?

Folk remedies feature strawberries

Aside from being delicious, people in many cultures have found strawberries useful for certain conditions. The Chinese, for instance, claim that a handful of the red berries is a good cure for a hangover. Strawberries are also said to whiten teeth and to be useful in getting rid of garlic breath.

- Low in calories and high in fibre
- Provide anti-cancer bioflavonoids

DRAWBACKS

- Provoke allergies in some people

The firm red strawberries that are available for much of the year have been developed from the wild strawberries that have been known for thousands of years and still grow in the wild. The strawberries that predominate in our supermarkets and greengrocers, however, are the much larger, plumper varieties now developed to grow at various times of the year. Those with the best flavour are generally available in late spring and early summer.

Strawberries are delicious, low in calories (about 27kcal in 100g) and very high in vitamin C. In fact, weight for weight, they are almost as good a source of this vitamin as oranges: 80g or eight large strawberries contain about 62mg, or well over 100 per cent of the Reference Nutrient Intake (RNI) for adults. Strawberries also provide useful amounts of folate, potassium, fibre and vitamin B_6.

The seeds in strawberries provide insoluble fibre, which helps to prevent constipation.

Strawberries are also a good source of pectin and other soluble fibres that may help to lower cholesterol. They contain bioflavonoids, including red anthocyanin and ellagic acid, substances that may help to prevent some cancers. Cooking does not destroy ellagic acid, so even strawberry tart and strawberry jam may be beneficial. Remember, though, that these often have a very high sugar content.

Strawberries can be stored whole in the refrigerator for a few days (if sliced, the berries will quickly lose their vitamin C and their flavour). Keep them separate from other foods, as their smell is pervasive.

Better still, wrap their container in cling film to prevent the smell filling your refrigerator. Rinse strawberries gently, just before serving them. Leave the green calyx attached as it prevents water entering the berry and diluting its flavour. Once washed, strawberries need to be consumed soon or they will develop mould.

Because strawberries contain a common allergen as well as a natural salicylate, an aspirin-like compound, some people are allergic to them. However, their salicylate content is responsible for the folklore that they can help those with joint, kidney or liver ailments.

Ways to use strawberries

- Top breakfast cereals such as natural muesli with fresh strawberries.
- For a delicious brunch idea, layer halved strawberries, natural yoghurt and muesli into dessert glasses. Repeat layers until glass is full. Sprinkle top with cinnamon sugar.
- Use fresh or frozen strawberries in smoothies.
- A few strawberries in children's lunchbox make a healthy treat.
- Freeze whole berries for children to eat after school on a hot day – much healthier than ice lollies.
- For a delicious dessert, purée strawberries in a blender with orange juice (or use an orange-flavoured liqueur for adults) and serve over fat-reduced vanilla ice cream or thick Greek-style yoghurt.
- Strawberries can be soaked in liqueur, citrus juice (use a mixture of orange and lemon) or sprinkled with rosewater and dusted with icing sugar just before serving.

S

Stress
Strategies for coping

When people talk about stress, they are usually referring to tension or emotional distress. Medically, however, stress is defined as any condition or situation that places undue strain on the body.

The sources can be a physical illness or injury, as well as numerous psychological factors – including fear, feelings of anger or frustration and even unusual happiness. What constitutes almost unbearable stress to one person may be the spice of life to someone else. In either case, a stressor (a stimulus that causes stress) can trigger the body's automatic stress-response system. This sets the stage for decreased immunity and increased vulnerability to illnesses, ranging from the common cold to heart attacks and cancer.

THE FIGHT-OR-FLIGHT RESPONSE

Stress is not a modern phenomenon. Our early ancestors experienced much more stress than we do – from the constant quest for food to dangers from wild animals and hostile neighbours. Our bodies still respond to any stress much as they would have in prehistoric times. This stress-coping mechanism, called the fight-or-flight response, floods the body with adrenaline and other hormones that raise blood pressure, speed up the heartbeat, tense muscles and put other systems on alert. Metabolism quickens to provide extra energy; and digestion stops as blood is diverted from the intestine to the muscles. While this reaction is appropriate to periodic physical stress, emotional stress is part of daily life and the on-going fight-or-flight reaction has damaging effects.

NUTRITIONAL NEEDS

Good nutrition is especially important during periods of stress. Prolonged stress, whether psychological or physical, plays havoc with digestion and nutritional needs. Food provides energy, vitamins and minerals for dealing with stress and helps to counter the negative

---

Are you stressed?

Because stress can cause many different symptoms, both physical and mental, it's often difficult to determine the true source of many problems. A doctor may order medical tests, even if he suspects that stress is the real cause.
The following are common manifestations of stress:

PHYSICAL SYMPTOMS

- Palpitations, shortness of breath, chest pain and other signs of heart disease (which must be ruled out).
- Unusual rapid breathing, dizziness or light-headedness.
- Tingling sensations in the hands and/or feet.
- Chronic or recurring backache and neck pain.
- Frequent headaches.
- Diarrhoea or constipation.
- Heartburn and other types of digestive problems.

PSYCHOLOGICAL SYMPTOMS

- Difficulty in concentrating and in making decisions.
- Sleep problems.
- Chronic fatigue, even after adequate rest.
- Prolonged anxiety.
- Changes in appetite and an increased reliance on alcohol, nicotine or other drugs.
- Difficulty coping with what normally would be minor setbacks.
- Decreased enjoyment of pleasurable activities and events.

effects on the body's immune system. Citrus fruit, peppers and potatoes are rich in vitamin C, which helps your body to maintain resistance to infection under stress. Also, one study showed that stressed people who took 1,000mg of vitamin C daily had milder increases in blood pressure and lower levels of stress hormones. Foods high in zinc such as seafood, meat, poultry, milk, eggs, whole grains and nuts also help to keep your immune system healthy. The herb valerian can help to lessen anxiety and relaxes the gastro-intestinal tract. Lettuce is known to have a calming effect, too.

When under stress, some people are always hungry and binge on food; others have to force themselves to eat. Because stress interferes with digestion, it may be better to eat four to six small meals spaced throughout the day instead of the traditional three large ones.

Carbohydrate-rich meals can increase the levels of serotonin, a brain chemical that is known to induce a feeling of calm. Studies show that stress-prone people who eat a diet higher in carbohydrates and lower in protein have less stress-induced depression.

TIPS FOR EATING DURING STRESSFUL PERIODS

Here are steps that you can take to help your eating during stressful times:

EAT BREAKFAST. If you are running on empty, stress can be more difficult to handle.

EAT SLOWLY. Eating quickly is often associated with digestive upset and this, coupled with stress, can make your food difficult to digest.

DON'T DIET. Changing eating habits is stressful at the best of times.

Eights ways to relieve stress

1. Make sure you eat regular and healthy meals; several small meals may work best.
2. For a few minutes each day, sit quietly with your eyes closed.
3. Exercise regularly to increase the production of endorphins, brain chemicals that lift mood.
4. Listen to your favourite music; it, too, increases endorphin levels.
5. Learn a relaxation technique, such as yoga, meditation or deep-breathing exercises.
6. Make a things-to-do list for the day; arrange the items by importance. Do one item at a time; move undone items to tomorrow's list.
7. Consider having a pet; stroking an animal can help you to relax.
8. Share your problems with a family member, friend or counsellor.

LIMIT INTAKE OF CAFFEINE AND ALCOHOL. They can affect your mood and sleep patterns. Alcohol can also increase depression and add to stress.

LISTEN TO YOUR BODY and avoid foods that cause you discomfort or digestive upset.

COMFORT FOODS

Almost everyone has a favourite food that provides comfort during stressful times. For some people, it's a food that harks back to childhood, such as milk. Others crave chocolate or sweets, which increase the production of serotonin, a brain chemical that has a calming effect. Soups are also common choices, as are bland nursery favourites like bread pudding, custards, yoghurt and omelettes.

BETTER OFF WITHOUT

Because stress can upset normal digestion, foods that normally are well tolerated may trigger indigestion and heartburn when you are going through a stressful period. Fatty foods, which are digested slowly, should be avoided as much as possible. A few people also find that hot or spicy foods cause them problems during times of stress.

Avoid caffeinated drinks, which can contribute to jittery feelings. Instead, try herbal teas such as chamomile and peppermint, which have a calming effect. Or substitute skimmed milk or fruit juice. If you drink coffee, choose decaffeinated.

Remember you can handle whatever life throws at you much better when you are eating and sleeping well, and by maintaining a positive outlook.

Do one simple thing

Take a multivitamin pill

Studies have shown that chronically stressed people may have depressed levels of nutrients in their body, which can be corrected with a multivitamin and mineral supplement. So although there is no pill that will change the stress you face, if you are not eating well during a difficult period, take a multivitamin and mineral supplement.

S

Stroke

EAT PLENTY OF

- Fresh fruit and vegetables for vitamin C, potassium and important antioxidants
- Nuts, seeds, vegetable oils, wheatgerm for vitamin E
- Oily fish for omega-3 fatty acids
- Oat bran, beans and pulses, linseeds, psyllium and fruit for soluble fibres
- Onions and garlic, which may help to prevent blood clots

LIMIT

- Animal and dairy products that are high in saturated fats and cholesterol
- Salt, which can raise blood pressure
- Alcohol use

AVOID

- Smoking
- Excessive weight gain

More than 100,000 people suffer strokes in England and Wales each year, and almost 60,000 die. Strokes account for 10 per cent of all deaths and are the largest single cause of disability.

Transient ischaemic attacks (TIA), or 'mini-strokes' occur when a clot blocks blood flow to a part of the brain. Most of these clots form in an artery that is already narrowed by athero-sclerosis, either in the brain itself or, more commonly, in the carotid artery in the neck. Ten per cent are haemorrhagic strokes, in which there is bleeding in the brain, such as from a burst blood vessel or severe head injury. Haemorrhagic strokes, which are more likely to be fatal than those caused by clots, are more common in people who already have high blood pressure.

Warning signs of a stroke include sudden weakness or numbness of the face, arm and leg on one side of the body; difficulty in speaking or understanding others; dimness or impaired vision in one eye; and unexplained dizziness, unsteadiness or a sudden fall. Immediate treatment is critical: even if the symptoms disappear, as in the case of a TIA, it is a common prelude to a full-blown stroke. Prompt treatment can be life-saving, and it may also minimise permanent damage, which can include impaired movement, speech, vision and mental function.

Mini-strokes aren't so mini

'Mini-strokes' are transient ischaemic attacks (TIAs), in which a part of the brain is temporarily starved of blood. A recent survey shows that 2.5 per cent of all adults over the age of 18 have had one of these episodes, which are especially common in older adults. Although they usually only last from a few seconds to 24 hours and leave no permanent damage, TIAs are a warning. It is estimated that up to 40 per cent of people who have had these attacks will go on to have a full-blown stroke.

Preventive measures

Despite the fact that we have a better understanding of the underlying causes and key risk factors in strokes and TIAs, such as high blood pressure, heart disease, arteriosclerosis and diabetes, many people persist in a number of unhealthy lifestyle habits that increase the risk of a stroke; these include smoking, excessive use of alcohol, eating too much salt, obesity and a sedentary lifestyle with little or no exercise. Of all these factors, diet is one of the most important.

◀ **Reducing the risks**
The key to avoiding a stroke is a diet low in salt and saturated fat and high in fibre and the omega-3 fatty acids found in some oils and oily fish.

In fact, many of the same nutritional recommendations made for people who have heart disease, high blood pressure and elevated blood cholesterol levels apply to people who are at risk for, or who have had, a stroke.

The Cretan Mediterranean diet, which is high in beneficial oils, whole grains, fruits and vegetables, and low in cholesterol and animal fats is a good place to start; it has been shown to reduce the risk of strokes and heart attacks by 60 per cent over a four year period. The diet is probably so effective because it provides a wide range of antioxidants from vegetables and fruits of all colours.

Eat fruit, lentils, vegetables, legumes and whole grains for their vitamins, minerals and flavonoids. Many of these foods, especially oats, lentils and linseeds, are high in the soluble fibres that help to control cholesterol levels and reduce the risk of atherosclerosis, which narrows the arteries and sets the stage for developing the blood clots that block the flow of blood to the brain. Eating whole grains is important for protection against strokes since data suggests that a wholegrain-based diet may help to reduce the risk for this condition. Preliminary evidence suggests that resveratrol, which is found in grapes, nuts and red wine may inhibit blood clots and also help to relax blood vessels.

Population-based studies suggest that dietary flavonoids, particularly quercetin, which is found in apples, onions and berries, may reduce fat deposits in arteries that can block blood flow to the brain.

Get lots of omega-3s. A number of other foods appear to lower the risk of a stroke. Some fish, for example, are rich in omega-3 fatty acids, which help to prevent blood clots by reducing the stickiness of

Did you know?

Diet alone can reduce the risk of stroke by 43 per cent

A study of more than 43,000 health professionals showed that men who ate about 85g–140g of fish one to three times a month were 43 per cent less likely to have an ischaemic, or clot-related, stroke during 12 years of follow-up. Men who ate fish more often did not reduce their risk any further, suggesting that a small amount works just as well as a larger one.

And, a study of nearly 80,000 women found that eating fish was linked to reductions in the risk of ischaemic strokes, which account for over 80 per cent of all strokes. The study showed that women who ate about 120g of fish two to four times weekly cut their risk by 48 per cent. Slight risk reductions were also found in those who ate fish once a week or less. Another study suggests that both men and women can reduce their ischaemic stroke risk by consuming five to six daily servings of vegetables and fruit.

blood platelets. Doctors recommend eating two fish meals a week, especially salmon, trout, mackerel, sardines or swordfish. Other sources of omega-3 fatty acids include fresh walnuts and walnut oil, rapeseed oil, linseeds, soya beans and leafy green vegetables. Eggs that claim to be omega-3 enriched are available.

Eat plenty of garlic and onions. Garlic and onions appear to decrease the tendency of the blood to clot, and it is thought that they may also boost the body's natural clot-dissolving mechanism.

Consume these foods for the right vitamins, minerals and antioxidants. A growing body of scientific evidence shows that vitamin E, too, reduces the tendency to form blood clots. Foods high in this antioxidant include wheatgerm, nuts, seeds and green leafy vegetables. Other antioxidants include vitamin C, which helps to

strengthen blood vessel walls and thus may protect against brain haemorrhages; most fruit (especially citrus) and vegetables are good sources of vitamin C.

Fruit and vegetables are high in potassium, an electrolyte that is instrumental in maintaining normal blood pressure.

Anyone who has high blood pressure, or a family history of this disease or of strokes, should limit salt intake; the average intake of sodium – a main component of salt – increases the body's fluid volume and is a major cause of raised blood pressure.

Limit alcohol. Numerous studies link excessive alcohol use, defined as more than three drinks a day for men and two for women, to an increased incidence of stroke; the risk is compounded if the person also smokes. The best approach is to abstain completely from smoking and to use alcohol in moderation.

Exercise. Regular exercise is helpful not only in reducing the risk of a stroke and heart attack by helping to control weight and blood cholesterol levels, but also by promoting an enhanced sense of well-being.

Supplements. Grape seed extract may strengthen weak blood vessels, allowing increased blood flow. Dong quai, or Chinese angelica, may prevent the accumulation of platelets in blood vessels. Reports from China indicate that dong quai used after a stroke showed a decrease in the amount of brain damage. Hawthorn is another herb that may help to control high cholesterol and high blood pressure. Turmeric may also be helpful in two ways: first, by lowering 'bad' cholesterol and, second, by preventing platelets from building up at the site of a damaged blood vessel, where they could form clots and cause a blockage.

S

Sugar and other sweeteners

BENEFITS

■ Sugar supplies almost instant energy

DRAWBACKS

■ High amounts may indirectly lead to obesity

■ Sugar fosters the growth of cavity-causing bacteria

Refined sugar is a relatively new food in the human diet, becoming widely available only since the 1500s. However, it didn't take long for this sweetener to become a major commodity.

Sugars have been described as a 'standard currency' for living organisms because all plants and animals store energy chemically as sugar. The sugars adapted for our diet are natural substances produced by photosynthesis in plants.

Nutrition experts distinguish two main types of sugar: intrinsic sugars, which give an appealing taste to such foods as milk, fruit and sweet vegetables, and extrinsic sugars, which are added to our food during its preparation, processing or at the time of consumption.

The main sugar in our diet is sucrose, familiar to us as white sugar. Sucrose comes from sugar cane, sugarbeets or sugars derived from corn, known as corn syrup solids. Food manufacturers in the United States prefer the liquid corn syrup because it is suitable for many processed foods as it provides moistness, extends shelf life and gives a chewy texture.

Food value

At 99.9 per cent sucrose, white sugar is an extremely pure food. Sucrose is a disaccharide (double sugar), which is made up of two monosaccharides (single sugars): glucose (known as blood sugar, dextrose, or grape sugar) and fructose (the sugar in fruit).

The intrinsic sugars in fruit, vegetables and milk are bound up with essential vitamins, minerals, fibre and fats. Extrinsic sugar, however, supplies calories of energy but provides no valuable nutrients, although it satisfies our taste for sweetness and can enhance the flavour of many foods. And while many of the evils blamed on sugar – hyperactivity, acne, high blood pressure, obesity – have been found to be unrelated or only indirectly linked through over-consumption, it is true that sugar is a major cause of tooth decay and that people who turn to sugary fast foods for a quick energy boost may neglect less convenient but much more nutritious foods.

All forms of sugar provide about the same energy value: 4kcal per gram. In everyday terms, a teaspoon of white sugar has 16kcal, and an

A unique sweetener

Artichokes contain cynarin, a unique organic acid that stimulates sweetness receptors in the taste buds. After eating artichokes, some people find that everything – even plain water – tastes sweet for a short time but efforts to convert cynarin into a commercial sugar substitute have not yet been successful.

How much is too much?

There is always dispute about an appropriate quantity of sugar to include in the daily diet. No sugar is actually needed, but since most people like sweet-tasting foods, health authorities try to come up with some recommendation.

An independent report from the World Health Organization (WHO) and the Food and Agriculture Organization of the United Nations (FAO) states that sugar leads to obesity when it displaces other nutrients in the diet. The WHO states that unless people limit their intake of added sugars, including sugar found in soft drinks, to less than 10 per cent of daily calories, they are looking at obesity and dental problems. For most people, that amount of sugar can be found in just a single can of soft drink.

The major problem is that sugar contributes calories but no protein, essential fat, vitamins, minerals or fibre. If you are overweight or obese, you still need essential nutrients, but at the same time you need to reduce calories. It makes good sense to cut back on sugar, especially from foods like soft drinks, sweets, biscuits and many desserts that do not provide essential nutrients with their high sugar (and often fat) content.

individual serving pack has about 24kcal. Although sugar itself is not especially high in calories, many sweet foods, such as chocolates and pastries, are also high in fat, which contains 9kcal per gram.

Icing sugar has about 393kcal in 100g. Although the sugar is pure sucrose, the product is packaged with a small amount of cornflour to prevent clumping. Because of this, people with allergies to corn may suffer adverse reactions from the powdered sugar in icings and desserts. True raw sugar – the first crystals obtained during the refining process – is not sold any more because it is contaminated with soil, plant refuse and insect droppings and parts. What is now sold as raw sugar is highly refined and coloured with a little molasses.

Contrary to the claims of natural food enthusiasts, brown sugar is no more nutritious than white sugar, but consumers who find the taste more appealing can substitute brown for white sugar in any recipe. Brown sugar is made by coating white sugar crystals with molasses. While molasses contains iron and other minerals, the amount in brown sugar is too small to be of nutritional value.

Maple syrup

Both maple sugar and syrup are made by boiling down maple sap – a technique developed by North America's native people long before the arrival of white explorers. Pure maple products are inescapably expensive because production is limited.

A tablespoon of maple syrup (about 15ml) contains about 39kcal. Pure maple products contain traces of potassium, calcium and other minerals, but not in amounts that are sufficient to be of much nutritional value.

Dental problems

All types of sugar – white table sugar, raw sugar, brown sugar, honey, molasses – encourage the growth of the oral bacteria that are responsible for causing cavities. And when starchy foods are broken down by the enzymes in saliva, they also form cavity-causing sugars. More dangerous than the amount of sugar is the length of time the sugar remains in contact with the teeth. Thus, much of the damage can be prevented by brushing soon after eating something sweet.

Sugar alcohols

These sweeteners, such as sorbitol, xylitol, maltitol and lactitol, are used in confectionery, ice cream, chewing gums and some baked goods. They provide fewer calories per gram than sucrose, do not promote tooth decay and do not cause sudden jumps in blood glucose. In some people eating too much of them can cause bloating or diarrhoea. Since sugar alcohols do not cause a sharp rise in insulin levels, they can be used by people with diabetes more readily than table sugar. Less than 10g will cause no significant rise in blood glucose.

Agave nectar

This new liquid sweetener, extracted from the core of the agave cactus, which is native to Mexico, provides a natural, unprocessed sweetener with a low GI. It tastes like a cross between honey and maple syrup, and has caused no known allergic reactions.

▶ **Sugar by any other name**
Molasses, honey and brown sugar provide similar levels of calories per teaspoon.

Supplements

Who needs them?

Each week, nearly a third of all adult Britons take some form of dietary supplement. Some take them because they think they don't eat well enough for their diet to provide optimal levels of nutrients. Others take supplements because of a particular health problem that they want to treat or try to prevent.

Nutritionists have always stressed that our diet is the best source of vitamins, minerals, fatty acids, amino acids and fibre, and that food and nutrients in their natural form are best adapted to the human digestive system. In contrast, supplements usually contain only one isolated form of a nutrient, which lacks the energy, fibre and other dietary components that provide proper nutritional balance.

In recent years, as we have shifted our focus from prevention of deficiency diseases to maximising health and preventing chronic disease, interest in supplements has increased dramatically. However, it is not an easy task for researchers to prove the benefits of supplementation. Their effects depend on the level of nutrients already being absorbed from the diet, as well as factors that influence nutrient absorption and metabolism. Also, supplements may take years to have a significant beneficial effect, making their impact difficult to observe and measure. Despite these challenges, research is beginning to emerge supporting the benefits of certain supplements.

MULTIVITAMINS

The most common supplements are multivitamins. Few studies have addressed at their effects, since most research looks at specific nutrients rather than groups of them. There is some very slight evidence, however, that daily use of a multivitamin is associated with a lower risk of heart disease and stroke, as well as illness from some types of infection. One group of researchers recently concluded that many people could benefit from multivitamins. They may also be important for some women of childbearing years, people who regularly consume more than one or two alcoholic drinks a day, those who do not eat enough fruit and vegetables and the elderly – researchers in the US have concluded that older people should take multivitamins daily as a 'safety net'. But popping a pill can't erase the effects of a poor diet, a sedentary lifestyle, smoking or obesity, and it can't replace healthy food and exercise; foods contain important components, such as fibre, plant chemicals and essential fatty acids.

Remember...

- Supplements won't make up for a bad diet. Eat a varied diet high in fruit and vegetables, whole grains and quality protein foods every day.

- Don't go overboard. While there's no need to worry about the amounts of nutrients in multivitamins, people planning to take therapeutic doses of single nutrients should consult a doctor or an accredited dietitian.

- Beware of the latest cure-all product. Some supplements are heavily marketed without much science to back up their claims. There are no magic bullets.

- Vitamin supplementation should be discussed with your doctor if you are undergoing cancer treatment. In some cases, supplements may be contra-indicated.

FOLIC ACID

There is now good evidence that folic acid can reduce the chances of neural tube birth defects such as spina bifida. This defect occurs when the neural tube of the foetus fails to close, which can result in death, or serious damage to the spinal cord. Folic acid can prevent half of these defects if women take it before conception. So women who could become pregnant are advised to take a supplement of 400mcg of folic acid daily.

There is also some evidence that folic acid may reduce the risk of heart disease. Research shows that people with higher levels of the amino acid homocysteine have a higher risk of heart disease; those who consume more folic acid from a supplement, have lower levels of homocysteine. Again, taking 400mcg a day seems to do the job effectively.

VITAMIN B$_{12}$

Low blood levels of B$_{12}$ are more common in older people because stomach acid, which often decreases with age, is needed for B$_{12}$ absorption. Low levels of this nutrient are associated with higher homocysteine levels, which is a risk factor for heart disease. The type of B$_{12}$ found in supplements does not require gastric acid for absorption, so taking a multivitamin or B-complex containing at least 25mcg of B$_{12}$ will ensure an adequate intake for most. Research suggests many older people would benefit from a B$_{12}$ supplement – but it should always be taken with B-complex, too.

VITAMIN D

Many people don't realise that vitamin D is just as important as calcium for healthy bones. Our main source is sun exposure. But people whose culture or religion does not permit sun exposure, and frail, elderly people who do not get out into the sun may lack vitamin D. Also, as you age, your body becomes less efficient at producing the vitamin from sunlight. There is evidence that a significant number of frail, aged people are vitamin D-deficient, which increases the risk of osteoporosis and fracture. People in these categories would do well to take extra vitamin D. Pregnant women should also take 10mcg of vitamin D a day. It may also help to prevent the onset of multiple sclerosis. Because it is fat soluble, take it with a main meal for best absorption.

CAUTION

Beware of drug/nutrient interactions. Drugs and nutrients share the same route of absorption and metabolism in our body, which creates the potential for interactions. For example, calcium can bind to certain antibiotics, interfering with their absorption. So if you are taking, or planning to take, larger than normal doses of nutrients in supplement form, make sure you find out about the possibility of this type of interaction before you start.

DANGEROUS DOSES

There is growing evidence that more than the recommended daily amount of some nutrients can reduce certain health risks, but excessive quantities of some vitamins and minerals can be extremely dangerous.

Vitamins A and D are fat soluble and cannot be excreted from the body if excess amounts are taken in. High doses of vitamin A can cause liver damage, fatigue, skin problems and other symptoms. Taken before and during pregnancy, it can cause serious birth defects.

High doses of vitamin D can result in calcium deposits in the heart and blood vessels, upset calcium metabolism and bone loss. Taken over an extended period, very large amounts of both vitamins can be fatal. Excessive zinc and some trace minerals have effects ranging from nausea and diarrhoea to death if taken in doses that allow build-up in body tissues.

Make sure all supplements are in child-resistant containers and are kept out of their reach.

Sushi

BENEFITS

■ Contain healthy ingredients, including seaweed, rice, vegetables and fish

■ Low in fat

DRAWBACKS

■ Many varieties are made with raw fish, so should be avoided by pregnant women and those with immune disorders, because of the small risk of exposure to bacteria or parasites

Once considered an esoteric dish, sushi has gone mainstream in restaurants and supermarkets in the UK – and no wonder. This beautiful food is not just delicious and nutritious, it's also an art form that has evolved over centuries.

Technically, the word sushi refers to vinegared rice, but the word is commonly used to describe a variety of bite-sized foods that include raw fish on a bed of rice (nigiri); or rice and seaweed rolls, both thin and larger sizes, filled with fish and/or vegetables (maki). These foods can be eaten as is, or dipped into shoyu (Japanese soy sauce) before eating. Raw fish, chilled and sliced is called sashimi. Much care and attention is put into the creation of these beautiful-looking foods.

Health benefits

Sushi uses rice, seaweed, fish and vegetables – simple, healthy ingredients – and it is low in fat and calories, so it's a great choice for those concerned about their weight or their cholesterol. Those watching their salt intake should go easy on the seaweed (nori) wrapped varieties and especially on the soy sauce.

The bite-sized pieces encourage the diner to eat more slowly and to savour the meal. A typical serving of sushi would consist of a variety of six pieces of nigiri and nori rolls,

all of which would contain about 330kcal. As a general rule, nigiri ranges in calories from 38kcal to 100kcal, with about 28kcal coming from the rice and the remaining calories coming from the various types of fish or topping.

Two pieces of nori roll are about equal to one piece of nigiri, and thick rolls vary considerably depending on their ingredients. One of the most popular items, California roll, which contains fish and avocado, provides about 40kcal per piece.

Caution

Although chefs trained in the art of preparing sushi usually maintain rigorous standards of freshness and cleanliness, eating raw fish carries certain risks. Sushi should always be kept cool, even though the vinegar added to the rice gives some protection against microbial growth. Do not store for more than 8 hours.

Because the fish used in sushi is uncooked, it should not be eaten by pregnant women or those with immune disorders, because of the small risk of exposure to bacteria such as *Listeria monocytogenes*.

For most diners, however, these risks are minimal, as long as the sushi comes from clean premises. For anyone who prefers not to eat raw fish, there are other options, including cooked crab, prawns, egg, tofu or vegetables.

An old art form

Sushi's origins date from the 7th century when South-east Asians first developed a pickling technique. The Japanese adapted this for packing rice and fish. As the fish fermented, the rice produced lactic acid, which pickled the fish. After many improvements throughout the centuries, sushi has developed into a unique, healthy food, and its popularity continues to grow.

Swede

BENEFITS

■ May help to protect against cancer

■ Useful source of vitamin C

DRAWBACK

■ High intakes increase the requirement for iodine

Cruciferous vegetables, which include swedes and turnips, as well as members of the cabbage family, contain chemical compounds that many scientists believe may help to prevent some cancers. The two most widely studied of these chemicals are indoles and isothiocyanates. Experiments indicate that indoles may protect against breast cancer by stimulating enzymes that reduce the effects of the hormone oestrogen, which is thought to encourage this type of cancerous growth. Isothiocyanates are thought to trigger the formation of enzymes that protect DNA against damage by carcinogens.

One disadvantage of these compounds is that they rob the thyroid gland of iodine and can cause an iodine deficiency if you do not get much of this mineral from your diet. Iodine is found in seafood and seaweed, and is needed for the thyroid gland to be able to produce the hormones that control the body's metabolism and therefore its healthy growth and development.

Cooking swedes makes it easier for the body to absorb indoles and isothiocyanates, but as with other vegetables, it reduces the vitamin C content. Nevertheless, a 100g portion of boiled swede provides 12mg (a third of the daily amount needed) as well as useful amounts of folate and vitamin B_1. They are also an excellent food for anyone who is trying to lose weight: a 100g cooked serving contains only 9kcal.

S

Although swedes originated in Bohemia, they came to England via Sweden – hence their name, shortened from Swedish turnips.

Sweetcorn

BENEFITS

■ A good source of folate and thiamin

■ A rich source of lutein

■ Air-popped unbuttered popcorn is low in calories and high in fibre

DRAWBACKS

■ The niacin in corn is not released in the human digestive tract

■ Corn lacks two essential amino acids needed to make a complete protein

Indigenous to the Western world, corn or maize is one of the most abundant grain crops; worldwide, it is exceeded only by wheat and rice as a cereal grain. In many parts of the world, such as the United States, Canada and Africa, corn is allowed to mature on its stalk, and is dried and used as both human food and animal feed, or processed into flour to make cereals and cornmeal.

Sweetcorn, which is harvested while still immature, is the type consumed as a vegetable. It can be cooked in several different ways: on the cob; or with the soft kernels removed and served fresh hot. Baby sweetcorn is boiled and served whole.

Sweetcorn and nutrition

Corn is high in starch and protein, but it lacks two essential amino acids – lysine and tryptophan; as a result, it is not a suitable protein substitute. But when it is eaten with beans and other legumes, however, it provides a complete protein.

One 175g cob contains 116kcal and 18 per cent of the Reference Nutrient Intake (RNI) for folate. Sweetcorn is also a source of potassium, thiamin, fibre and a good source of lutein, a powerful antioxidant that may help to lower the risk of age-related macular degeneration. Most of the niacin in sweetcorn is in the form of niacytin, which is not broken down in the human digestive tract.

Popcorn

A popular snack food, popcorn is a special variety that grows on a cob smaller than those of sweetcorn. As the kernels are heated rapidly, the moisture inside them is converted to steam. When the steam pressure builds to a certain point, it bursts the outer shell and the interior turns into a fluffy mass of starch and fibre many times larger than the original kernel. A 35g portion of air-popped plain popcorn has only 135kcal, making it an ideal, high-fibre snack. Popping the same amount of corn in oil and adding butter increases the calorie content to about 165kcal. Microwavable popcorn may have added fat. Always check the label and try to choose non-fat or low-fat brands.

Sweet potatoes

BENEFITS

■ Orange-fleshed varieties are a rich source of beta carotene

■ A good source of vitamins C and E and potassium

■ Naturally sweet and high in fibre

Sweet potatoes are not related to the common white potato or to yams, with which they are often confused. The sweet tubers, which are highly nutritious, derive their flavour from an enzyme that converts starches to sugar. As the tuber matures and is cooked, it becomes sweeter.

A nutrient-dense vegetable

Like other brightly coloured orange-yellow vegetables, sweet potatoes are an excellent source of beta carotene, a precursor to vitamin A. On average, a 100g medium sweet potato provides more than 200 per cent of the RNI for vitamin A, about 100 per cent of the RNI for vitamin C and excellent amounts of vitamins E and B_1 and potassium. It supplies 87kcal, compared with 74kcal for the same sized white potato.

Sweet potatoes also contain plant sterols, which are cholesterol-lowering compounds, and the soluble fibre pectin which also affects cholesterol. They are an excellent source of insoluble fibre, which may help to prevent constipation and diverticulosis.

There are two types of sweet potato – purple-skinned with soft, orange flesh, or white-skinned with a dry, creamy grey flesh.

They spoil quickly; discard any that have mouldy spots or are shrivelled. Keep them cool but not in the refrigerator. Their skins are delicate, so if peeling is necessary, it is easily done after they are cooked.

S

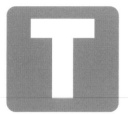

Tacos

See Fast food

Tea

BENEFITS

- A refreshing, calorie-free drink
- Contains antioxidants and bioflavonoids, which may lower the risk of cancer, heart disease and stroke
- Contains tannins, which may provide protection against tooth decay
- Herbal teas are caffeine-free

DRAWBACKS

- Tannins decrease iron absorption if strong tea is consumed with meals
- May have a diuretic effect
- Contains caffeine
- Strong tea may cause insomnia

Tea is the world's most popular non-alcoholic beverage. Most tea is grown in India, Sri Lanka, China, Japan, Taiwan and Indonesia from a shrub in the camellia family. Like coffees, the best-quality teas are grown in the shade at high altitudes, and the finest leaves are plucked from the youngest shoots and unopened leaf buds, which also contain the highest levels of phenols, enzymes and caffeine. Researchers are discovering evidence that drinking tea also provides a number of health benefits.

An antioxidant brew

Tea contains many compounds, including various flavonoids – phytochemicals with powerful antioxidant properties. A subclass of the flavonoids, the catechins, is responsible for the flavour as well as many of the beneficial health effects of tea.

How much of these compounds are present in the final beverage depends on how the leaves are processed. To make black tea, the dried leaves are crushed to liberate enzymes, which react with the catechins over a few hours to produce changes in colour and flavour. This is often referred to as 'fermentation'.

Green tea is not fermented; it is made by first steaming the leaves to halt any enzyme activity. Oolong tea is partially fermented. The highest concentration of catechins is found in green tea, although black tea is also a good source.

Researchers in Boston, USA, did a study comparing the ORAC capacity of tea with 22 vegetables. ORAC is a measurement of the antioxidant power of foods and other chemical substances. The higher the ORAC score, the greater its antioxidant capacity. Although there was variation among the teas, the highest scoring teas were green tea and black tea, brewed for 5 minutes.

A cup of hot brewed tea has virtually no calories and – with the exception of green tea – no appreciable vitamins or minerals, except for fluoride which may come from the soil and air where the tea is grown. Green tea also contains vitamin K, a nutrient needed for the normal clotting of blood.

Tea's health benefits

Tea is as hydrating as water and is a healthier drink. Many studies confirm the health benefits of tea.

Heart disease. The antioxidants in tea may explain the fact that people who drink a lot of tea are much less likely to die from heart disease. Antioxidants prevent the oxidation of cholesterol, making it less likely to stick to artery walls. A recent study showed that black tea taken after a stressful event was able to speed up the rate at which of the level of the stress homone, cortisol, returned to normal. Acute stress has been linked to a greater risk of heart disease. In the same test, black tea also lowered blood platelet activation – linked to blood-clotting and the risk of heart attacks.

Stroke. One study found that the risk of stroke was reduced by about 70 per cent in men who drank five or more cups of black tea a day. Flavonoids may protect against stroke in two ways. They reduce the ability of blood platelets to form clots, the cause of most strokes. They also block some of the damage

Tea may be a powerful infection fighter

Researchers in the USA say that they have found a chemical in tea that boosts the body's defence against disease fivefold.

They say they isolated from ordinary black tea a substance called L-theanine, also found in green and oolong tea. L-theanine is broken down in the liver to ethylamine, a molecule that primes the response of an immune blood cell called the gamma-delta T cell.

Gamma-delta T cells in the blood are the first line of defence against many types of bacterial, viral and parasitic infections. They might even have some anti-tumour activity. The T cells prompt the secretion of interferon, a key part of the body's chemical defence against infection.

caused to arteries by free radicals, unstable molecules that are released when the body consumes oxygen.

Cancer. A number of studies have shown that tea offers protection against a variety of cancers. A type of catechin called EGCG (epigallo-catechin gallate) is thought to be responsible for tea's anti-cancer properties. EGCG protects the DNA in cells from cancer-causing changes. It may also inhibit an enzyme that cancer cells need in order to replicate.

More benefits. The flavonoids in tea may suppress the growth of harmful bacteria, thus helping to prevent infections. Naturally occurring theophyllines in tea dilate the airways in the lungs and have been found to help some people with asthma and other respiratory disorders to breathe more freely. In fact, they have been developed as drugs to treat asthma and other constrictive lung disorders.

Tannins, which are found in wine as well as tea and some herbal teas, such as peppermint, are chemicals that bind surface proteins in the mouth, producing a tightening sensation and giving the impression of a full-bodied liquid. They also bind and incapacitate plaque-forming bacteria in the mouth. The fluoride in green tea may protect against tooth decay, but high levels in some black teas may pose a problem if the local water supply is already fluoridated.

Other effects

Tea leaves contain twice as much caffeine, weight for weight, as coffee beans do. But when made, tea has only half as much caffeine as coffee because tea is drunk weaker. A cup of black or green tea contains 35 to 45mg of caffeine. Tea may trigger a migraine headache in people who are hypersensitive; for others, it may alleviate headaches when taken with aspirin or similar painkillers. Theobromine, which is also found in tea, has effects similar to those of caffeine but milder.

The tannins in strong tea can cut iron absorption by more than 80 per cent when tea is drunk with an iron-rich meal. Vegetarians who drink tea with a meal may be especially susceptible. People with a tendency to anaemia can drink citrus juice at mealtimes to promote iron absorption; squeezing a wedge of lemon or adding milk to tea also binds the tannins and partly blocks their effect on iron.

Tea drinking between meals does not affect iron absorption. Young children should not drink tea, as the relative dose of caffeine is much higher for them. Tannins can stain natural teeth. Some mouthwashes may even intensify the staining.

Did you know?

Green tea may help cholesterol problems

Researchers have found that people who drink five cups of green tea daily may improve their cholesterol levels.

Iced tea

Iced tea becomes cloudy because caffeine and pigment molecules crystallise at low temperatures. Tea, made by steeping several tea bags in lukewarm water for several hours, is less likely to become cloudy than tea brewed with hot water.

Commercial iced teas, flavoured with fruit syrups and sweetened with sugar, contain as many calories as soft drinks.

Tea, like coffee, has a diuretic effect, which increases the kidneys' output of urine. Excessive urination can upset the body's fluid and chemical balance by washing potassium from the body.

Herbal teas

Many plants, especially herbs, can be brewed into teas, also called infusions or tisanes. Because most of them do not contain caffeine, they offer a pleasant alternative for people who prefer to avoid the stimulant. Some herbal teas aid the digestion, and their soothing warmth can promote relaxation at bedtime.

Always choose herbs carefully. Although the herbs and spices that flavour herbal teas have been widely used and are suitable as seasonings, a few herbs and spices are known to be unsafe when used medicinally. Nutmeg, for example, is harmless when used as a flavouring but can cause severe symptoms, including hallucinations, when brewed into a strong tea.

Other herbs, such as oregano, have a stimulating effect and can cause wakefulness. Comfrey, if taken regularly, is toxic to the liver; it is no longer used internally in Britain

Scientific information is unclear regarding the safety of various herbs and herbal products during pregnancy and while breastfeeding. The herbal teas considered safe if used in moderation include citrus peel, ginger, lemon balm, orange

T

Working against cancer

In test tubes, the catechins in tea are powerful inhibitors of cancer growth and animal studies have suggested that tea can inhibit growth of tumour cells in laboratory animals. But it's unclear whether tea works the same way in the human body. Some studies have found that heavy tea-drinking appears to lower the rates of breast, skin, stomach, colorectal and other cancers. Other studies have shown no link between cancer prevention and tea consumption. Ongoing research is exploring the subject. For example, scientists are studying the potential of green tea supplements and topical applications to slow or prevent skin cancer.

Cancer researchers in Arizona, USA, studied heavy smokers who were asked to drink four cups of decaffeinated green tea daily for four months. Test showed that DNA damage (which could lead to cancer) dropped 30 per cent in that group, but not in control groups who drank decaffeinated black tea or water.

Other US researchers, at the University of Rochester, found that two flavonoids in tea, EGCG and EGC, inhibit a molecule called the aryl hydrocarbon (AH) receptor. Tobacco smoke acts on this molecule and causes it to trigger potentially carcinogenic gene activity. By shutting down the AH receptor, green tea may help to prevent smoking-related cancers.

peel and rose hip. Pregnant women should always discuss the use of any herbal infusions with their doctor.

Folk healers have long prescribed herbal teas for medicinal purposes, but few herbal teas have been tested scientifically. Care is needed when self-treating with herbal teas, especially if the herbs have been gathered in the wild. Many plants are poisonous, and these may be picked in error. Among the more popular herbal teas are the following:

Chamomile. A mild sedative, chamomile tea has long been used to ease indigestion, calm the nerves and reduce anxiety. It is said to aid sleep, and used tea bags, once cold, can be applied to soothe inflamed or itching eyes.

Dandelion. Tea made from this common weed is mildly diuretic. Some women use it to reduce premenstrual bloating.

Elderflower. Extracts of elder make a comforting tea if suffering from flu, catarrh or painful sinuses. It is said to have anti-inflammatory, properties and causes perspiration. It is also useful for chesty conditions and may help to ease hay fever.

Fennel. With a flavour similar to liquorice, fennel tea is used to soothe an upset stomach. If taken by a breastfeeding mother, it may increase milk flow and at the same time relieve colic in the baby.

Lavender flower. Tea brewed from dried lavender flowers is said to be mildly sedative.

Lemon balm. This minty tea may help to soothe jittery nerves, without causing drowsiness. It can also aid digestion and alleviate feverish conditions such as flu.

Nettle. Made from the same plant that causes stinging skin irritation, nettle tea is a tonic, providing some vitamin C and several minerals, including iron. It may relieve allergic reactions such as hay fever or nettle rash.

Peppermint. Tea from this mint plant is refreshing and may aid digestion and relieve flatulence. It can be used to control nausea and is useful in the treatment of colds and flu. People with hiatus hernias should avoid it, however, because peppermint may promote reflux of the stomach contents into the oesophagus.

Raspberry leaf. Herbalists recommend raspberry tea to ease menstrual cramps, but it may also stimulate contractions of the uterus, making it unsuitable for use in early pregnancy. It is mildly astringent and can be used as a mouthwash or gargle.

Rooibos. Pronounced 'roy-boss', this totally caffeine-free tea is high in antioxidants. It grows in South Africa's Western Cape region.To get its full flavour, it should be allowed to brew for as long as possible.

Rose hip. Rich in vitamin C, rose hip tea can be taken to ward off colds and infection. Lemon juice or peel enhances its mild flavour.

Rosemary. Tea from this popular garden herb is said to relieve wind and colic; it can ease headaches and is used as a pick-me-up.

Thyme. Herbalists recommend thyme tea for all types of infection, including colds, flu, bronchitis, ear-ache and sinusitus. It is also said to relieve indigestion and lift the spirits.

Instant tea

Powdered or instant tea is made by brewing strong tea, then evaporating the water to leave a powder.

Thyroid disorders

EAT PLENTY OF

■ Seafood, dark green leafy vegetables and dairy products for iodine

LIMIT

■ Alcohol and caffeine, if the thyroid gland is overactive

■ Raw vegetables in the cabbage family, turnips, swedes, peanuts and mustard if the thyroid gland is underactive

The thyroid, a butterfly-shaped gland that lies over the windpipe (trachea) and just below the Adam's apple (larynx), produces T_3 and T_4, iodine-containing hormones that influence almost every function of the body. These hormones regulate metabolism, physical and mental development, nerve and muscle function and circulation. Thyroid hormones also affect the actions of other hormones; for example, they intensify the action of insulin and the body's response to the adrenal hormones (catecholamines) that are instrumental in reacting to stress.

The thyroid needs iodine to produce its hormones, but too much or too little iodine can cause the thyroid to malfunction. Goitre, an overgrown thyroid that is marked by a swelling in the lower neck, usually signals a thyroid disorder. It is common in parts of Africa where crops are raised in iodine-poor soil and people do not receive iodine supplements in the diet. Goitre is also common among the Japanese, who often consume very large amounts of iodine-rich seaweed.

Iodine deficiency, although still a common cause of thyroid disorders in developing nations, can be wiped out by the use of iodised salt. Because seawater contains high levels of iodine, food crops grown on coastal farmlands generally have sufficient levels of the mineral. So saltwater fish and seaweed products are good sources. Eggs, yoghurt, milk and hard cheese are also useful sources of iodine.

Although they affect both sexes, thyroid disorders tend to occur more frequently in women. A type of mental retardation and growth deficiency, cretinism, is a birth defect caused by a lack of iodine in the mother during pregnancy. It is not seen in developed countries, however, where babies are routinely tested for thyroid deficiency. Thyroid problems usually involve either overactivity or underactivity of the gland. Although there is some overlap, the symptoms of one disorder present almost a mirror image of the other. The usual causes of thyroid problems are an infection, auto-immune disorder, hormonal imbalance, tumour, exposure to high levels of ionising radiation or congenital or hereditary problems.

Hyperthyroidism

People with overactive thyroids (hyperthyroidism, or Graves' disease) tend to be nervous and jittery. Their metabolism speeds up, and they experience unusual hunger, weight loss, rapid heartbeat and muscle weakness among other symptoms. They find heat hard to bear and sweat excessively. Whether or not a goitre distorts the neck, a person with an overactive thyroid develops protuberant eyes.

Treatment is aimed at the cause and involves reducing hormone production either by giving radioactive iodine or anti-thyroid drugs or by surgery to remove all or parts of the thyroid.

Hypothyroidism

An underactive thyroid, or hypothyroidism, slows down metabolism, causing weight gain and lethargy. Early symptoms are easily overlooked: sleepiness, muscle weakness and progressive fatigue. People with hypothyroidism often complain of concentration and memory problems. They feel cold, even on hot days, and develop dry skin and thinning hair. Nails grow slowly and become brittle. Because metabolism slows down, weight gain is common, even though the person may be eating less than normal. Women often develop menstrual irregularities; constipation is another common problem. Hypothyroidism is frequently caused by chronic inflammation due to an auto-immune disorder. Treatment usually requires lifelong hormone replacement with thyroxine pills.

Dietary approaches

The Reference Nutrient Intake (RNI) for iodine is 140mcg a day for children over 15 and adult men and women. Boys and girls aged 11 to 14 need only 130mcg. The use of iodised salt in the typical diet, which provides 2g to 6g of salt each day, could easily supply more than these recommended amounts of iodine. However, it is not widely used in the processed foods that supply over 80 per cent of our salt. Even people on low-salt diets can get plenty of iodine from seafood, green leafy vegetables and dairy products. Certain vegetables, mainly cabbage, broccoli and swedes and turnips, contain substances known as goitrogens, which block the effects of thyroid hormones and may lead to goitre. Cooking these foods inactivates the goitrogens; consumption of sufficient iodine also prevents adverse effects.

If you have a thyroid disorder, use small amounts of iodised salt and eat plenty of seafood, dairy products, spinach and other

T

vegetables for iodine. Fish, dairy products, eggs, as well as deep yellow or orange vegetables and fruit, as well as dark green vegetables, provide vitamin A. The conversion of beta carotene to vitamin A is accelerated by thyroxine. People with hypothyroidism may need a higher intake of beta carotene to meet vitamin A needs.

Stay away from caffeine. It may worsen the jittery feeling in someone with an overactive thyroid, so drink decaffeinated coffee and tea or water – they refresh without adding to nervousness. The nicotine in tobacco also adds to feelings of nervousness. Alcohol may aggravate the sleepiness and fatigue in a person with an underactive thyroid gland.

Tofu

See Soya.

Tomatoes

BENEFITS

- A useful source of vitamins C and E, beta carotene, folate and potassium
- A good source of lycopene, an antioxidant that may protect against prostate cancers

DRAWBACKS

- Raw or cooked, may cause indigestion and heartburn
- A possible cause of allergies

Equally delicious raw or cooked, tomatoes are low in calories and rich in vitamins and other healthy substances. Tomatoes, like potatoes, aubergines and peppers, belong to the nightshade family. Brought to Europe from Central America by the Spanish during the 16th century, tomatoes were originally grown as decorative

Did you know?

Tomatoes were once called 'the apple of love'?

The tomato, which is botanically a fruit, used to be called a love apple. This was nothing to do with its voluptuous, shape or passionate colour. In fact, in Italy it was called *pomi dei mori*, 'the apples of the moors'. When said aloud, it sounded to French ears like *pomme d'amour* – in English, 'apple of love'.

plants in northern Europe, where it was feared that the poisons in the leaves might be present in the fruit as well. However, the Spanish and Italians discovered that tomatoes were indeed edible, and began to use them widely in their cuisines. Today, the tomato is one of the world's leading vegetables (although technically the tomato is a fruit).

Special benefits

A Harvard University study showed that men who regularly ate tomato-based foods had lower rates of prostate cancer. Other studies also support this observation. The researchers theorise that lycopene – which is a powerful antioxidant – is the natural cancer-fighting agent in tomatoes. Other studies show that lycopene provides defence against a number of other conditions, such as other cancers and heart disease. It is known to slow down damage to human cells caused by ageing and disease. The best way to get lycopene is through tomatoes in their processed form – tomato sauce, tomato paste, tomato juice and even tomato relish. Lycopene is also found in pink grapefruit and watermelons, but it is most concentrated in tomato paste.

Although no single food can prevent cancer altogether, nutrition experts are unanimous in advising us to eat plenty of fruit and

vegetables, especially tomatoes, that are rich in antioxidant nutrients, which protect against the cancer-causing cell damage that occurs when the body uses oxygen.

Nutritional value

One medium (80g) ripe tomato contains only 15kcal, together with about 14mg of vitamin C and 19mcg of folate. Some of the vitamin C is concentrated in the jelly-like substance that encases the seeds. Some recipes advise removing the seeds in order to prevent the development of a bitter taste during cooking. The jelly-like substance around the seeds is actually high in salicylates, which have an anti-clotting effect on the blood. This may be partially responsible for tomatoes' protection against heart disease.

Commercially prepared tomato sauces for pasta vary in calorie content, depending on added ingredients. Some tomato products may have high levels of added salt; people on low-sodium diets should look for those with no added salt. On average, 200ml of tomato sauce for pasta contains about 95kcal, which may increase substantially with the addition of oil. A 200g portion of canned tomatoes contains only 32kcal. Tomato paste is a concentrated source of nutrients, but as the amount used at any one time is so small, it provides very little extra nutrition. Canned tomato juice, like fresh tomatoes, is a good source of vitamin C. Some vitamin C is lost in the processing, but some

▶ **Tomato varieties**
Tomatoes are actually a type of berry and were called 'love apples' in the 16th century. Their flavour depends more on the variety and how ripe they are than on where they have ripened. Varieties include baby plum, beefsteak, cherry, plum, vine and yellow cherry.

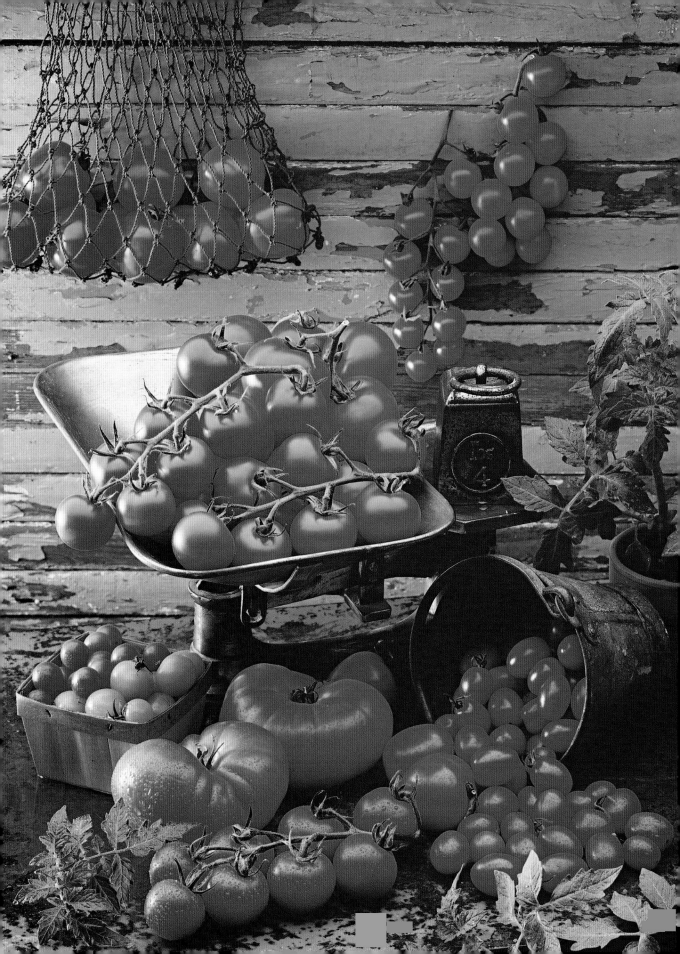

brands are fortified to raise the vitamin C content to the same level as found in fresh tomatoes.

Ripe tomatoes should be stored at room temperature; at 4°C or below, the flesh becomes mealy. The green tomatoes left on the vine at the end of the season should be harvested and cooked or turned into chutney. Sun-dried tomatoes are a delicious addition to dishes, but those packed in oil are high in calories: 100g of sun-dried tomatoes contain about 315kcal and 23g of fat.

Drawbacks

Solanines are toxic substances that are present in minute quantities in all members of the nightshade family; they may trigger headaches in susceptible people. Tomatoes are also a relatively common cause of allergies. An unidentified substance in tomatoes and tomato-based products can cause acid reflux, leading to indigestion and heartburn. People who often have digestive upsets should try eliminating tomatoes for two or three weeks to see if there is any improvement.

Tomato condiments

Many commercially prepared pickles and other condiments are based on tomatoes, including chilli sauce, chutneys and salsa – a sauce that is gaining in popularity. While these preparations certainly add zest

Did you know?

When it comes to tomatoes, redder is better

Tomatoes that have a crimson gene, making them a deep red colour, contain more lycopene than paler tomatoes. A rich, red tomato has up to 50 per cent more lycopene than a paler tomato. Vine-ripened tomatoes have more lycopene than those that are picked early and allowed to ripen off the vine.

Do one simple thing

Leave the skin on and add a little olive oil

Lycopene is in the skin of tomatoes, so if you are making tomato sauce, leave the skin on. Also, lycopene is fat soluble, so cooking tomatoes with a little oil increases absorption.

to food, they contribute little nutrition in the quantities used. In addition, their calorie content is often boosted because of the generous quantities of sugar and oil with which they are made. And because many are high in salt, they should not be eaten by people who need to restrict their sodium intake. The healthiest tomato condiment choice would probably be a homemade salsa.

Trans fats

See Fats

Tuberculosis

CONSUME PLENTY OF

■ Lean meat, poultry, eggs and fish for high-quality protein

■ Fresh fruit and vegetables for vitamin C and beta carotene

■ Fatty fish for vitamin D

■ Lean meat, shellfish, milk, beans and nuts for zinc

AVOID

■ Alcohol, smoking and exposure to second-hand smoke

■ Sharing eating utensils and other personal objects

Poor nutrition and poverty contribute to the incidence of tuberculosis (TB), which is responsible for more deaths globally than any other infectious disease claiming 3 million lives annually. It is estimated that a third of the world's population is infected with one of several strains of *Mycobacterium*, the bacillus that causes TB. Although the disease is inactive in most of these people, at any given time there are probably some 30 million active cases of TB.

Although TB is most prevalent in the developing world, there is fresh cause for concern in Britain. Partly because of improved hygiene and living conditions, the number of TB cases in the UK declined substantially after the 1950s, and vaccination programmes helped to keep the disease in check. However, there was an upswing in 2000, with a 10 per cent increase over the number of cases in 1999. Figures for 2006 show another large increase. Most cases were found in London, mainly among young adults newly arrived from countries where TB is common. There were also several localised outbreaks among schoolchildren. This is especially worrying as there has also been an increase in cases of TB resistant to standard drugs.

The TB bacillus is spread when an infected person coughs or sneezes, releasing the micro-organism into the air. Infection occurs when the bacillus is inhaled and enters the lungs, where it can silently multiply. The immune system usually wipes out the infection at this early stage, but in some people the bacillus remains dormant in the body.

Even so, most infected people never develop symptoms, although they will still have a positive TB skin test, indicating the presence of antibodies against the disease-causing organism.

A latent infection can develop into full-blown TB if the immune system becomes weakened by malnutrition, age, or a serious disease, such as AIDS or cancer. The first symptoms – loss of appetite and weight, night sweats, fever and chills and general malaise – may resemble a lingering bout of flu. But as the disease progresses, more severe manifestations appear: typically, a chronic cough, profuse sputum that may be blood-tinged and smell bad, increasing weakness and eventually, muscle wasting. Although the lungs are TB's most common target organ, it can attack almost any part of the body.

Role of diet

The typical TB treatment calls for long-term daily administration of several powerful antibiotics: usually isoniazid, rifampin, pyrazinamide and ethambutol. While undergoing treatment, patients must abstain from alcohol, which interacts with the drugs and also increases the risk of liver and nerve damage, common side effects of the TB regimen. Both the disease and the medications cause loss of appetite, but it is critical to maintain good nutrition to lessen weight loss, boost immunity and rebuild damaged tissue.

TB diet composition. The diet should provide high-quality protein, from lean meat, poultry, fish, eggs, milk and other animal products. (Some studies show that vegetarians are more vulnerable to TB and its complications than are people whose diets include some animal protein.) Citrus fruit and other fresh fruit and vegetables provide vitamin C and beta carotene, antioxidants that the body needs to boost immunity. Zinc is also important to foster healing and a strong immune system; good sources include oysters and other shellfish, lean meat, milk, beans, nuts and whole grains.

Get lots of vitamin D. Researchers have found out why TB patients who spend time in the sunshine and fresh air often improve faster. White blood cells that are armed with high concentrations of vitamin D appear to be more effective in destroying the bacillus. The body makes vitamin D when the skin is exposed to the sun; dietary sources include margarine, butter, eggs and fatty fish.

Role of vitamin B$_6$. Isoniazid is especially destructive to the nerves. To counter this, some doctors prescribe B$_6$ supplements. Foods that are high in this nutrient include most animal products, grains, spinach and potatoes.

Critical to maintain weight. It is critical to consume more calories than usual to counter the weight loss that is characteristic of TB. The diet should emphasise foods that are dense in calories and easy to digest. Good choices, in addition to the foods already mentioned, include legumes, pasta, grains and other starchy foods; milkshakes or perhaps enriched milk-based drinks; and rich soups, custards, eggs, puddings and ice cream.

Other measures

Because tuberculosis usually damages the lungs, it's important to avoid exposure to tobacco smoke and other pollutants that are harmful to the lungs. It is vital that smokers give up the habit; second-hand smoke should also be avoided as much as possible.

Although tuberculosis is highly contagious, the risk of spreading it can be minimised by practising good hygiene and by not sharing eating utensils and other personal items. When coughing or sneezing, a person with TB should always completely cover his or her mouth and nose with a tissue and then promptly dispose of it.

Because sun and fresh air help to destroy airborne bacilli, the living quarters should be aired frequently and as much sunshine as possible allowed in. Anyone who lives in close contact with a tuberculosis patient should undergo testing for the disease; in some cases, preventive antibiotic treatment may be warranted.

Turnips

BENEFITS

- A useful source of vitamin C, as well as some potassium
- A low-calorie source of fibre
- May protect against certain cancers

DRAWBACKS

- May cause flatulence
- Contain substances that interfere with the production of thyroid hormones

Turnips (including the yellow variety) are economical, healthy and easy to prepare and cultivate (even in soil of poor quality). An 80g serving of boiled turnips yields only 10kcal while providing 8mg of vitamin C (20 per cent of the Reference Nutrient Intake or RNI), 36mg of calcium and 160mg

Did you know?

Turnips can be pink

White turnips are given star billing in the Middle East. In fact, there is even a Lebanese saying that is paid as a compliment: 'Her face is whiter than the inside of a turnip'. In Middle Eastern cuisine, turnips are often pickled with beetroot to give them a pink colour. Small white turnips are sliced or chunked and placed in a glass jar with pieces of beetroot, garlic cloves and celery leaves. Salt (4 to 5 tablespoons) is dissolved in 1 cup of vinegar and 3 cups of water and then poured over the vegetables. The jar is sealed and left in a warm place for about ten days.

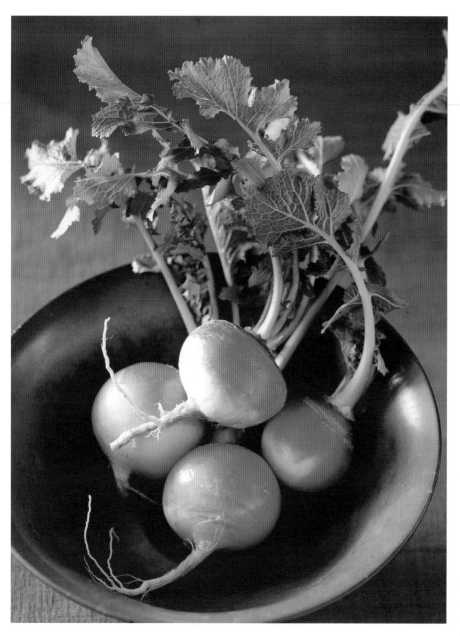

Facts about turnips

- Native to Europe and central Asia, turnips were first cultivated in the Middle East about 4,000 years ago.
- Turnips are used as both table and pig food in eastern Europe.
- The rutabaga evolved from a cross between the turnip and cabbage, and thus it has more vitamin C than turnips do.

Health benefits

The fibre contained in turnips may help to maintain bowel regularity and so may help to prevent colonic or rectal cancer. Also, as members of the cruciferous family, turnips contain sulphurous compounds that may protect against certain forms of cancer. However, like other cruciferous vegetables, turnips can cause bloating and wind.

Warning: Turnips contain two goitrogenic substances, which can interfere with the thyroid gland's ability to make its hormones. These compounds do not pose a risk for healthy people who eat moderate amounts of turnips, but anyone with hypothyroidism should never eat this vegetable raw, since cooking appears to deactivate the goitrogens.

Some herbal practitioners use turnips to treat respiratory ailments, such as asthma and bronchitis, and sore throats, with a few teaspoons a day of homemade turnip syrup, made by boiling chopped turnip in a little water. However, these benefits have not yet been proven scientifically.

▲ **Versatile and tasty complex carbohydrates**
Turnips have been cultivated for 4,000 years and for good reason. They grow in poor soil, are low in calories and high in nutrients, especially the green tops.

of potassium. Turnips provide 1.5g of fibre, including soluble dietary fibres that help to soak up LDL ('bad') cholesterol. The turnip tops, or greens, which many cooks discard, are even more nutritious than the roots themselves: 80g of boiled turnip greens provide only 10kcal, 32mg of vitamin C (more than 75 per cent of the RNI), 78mg of calcium and 62mg of potassium. And unlike the roots, the greens are an excellent source of beta carotene, an important antioxidant nutrient that the body converts to vitamin A.

As well as being boiled, turnips can be baked, braised or steamed, or added to stews, casseroles, soups or vegetable dishes.

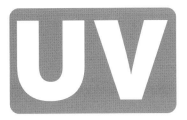

Ulcerative colitis

LIMIT
- Fats, oils and caffeine

AVOID
- Foods that provoke symptoms
- Alcohol in all forms

Ulcerative colitis (once referred to as colitis) is a chronic inflammation of the superficial lining of the colon.

Its causes are not known, although infection, the immune system, diet and heredity have been implicated. It may occur at any age, but is most common between the ages of 15 and 35 and affects 1 in 600 people in the UK. Symptoms include bloody diarrhoea and abdominal cramps. Acute flare-ups of the disease are usually interspersed with periods of remission. When the disease is severe, violent and persistent bloody diarrhoea is accompanied by fever, malaise, loss of appetite and weight, as well as anaemia. When the disease is extensive, there is also a greater risk of colon cancer.

Food and ulcerative colitis
No specific dietary factors have been shown to cause ulcerative colitis. In most cases, it seems to be the presence of any food in contact with the intestine that causes an adverse reaction. It's important to consult a qualified dietitian to ensure good nutrition. Vitamin and mineral supplements are often needed.

Avoid foods high in insoluble fibre. During an acute attack, foods that irritate the bowel often include those high in insoluble fibre: whole grains, unprocessed bran, nuts, seeds and the skins of potatoes and fruit. Less irritating are pectin and other types of soluble fibre, which can be obtained from oats, peeled fruit and leafy green vegetables.

Limit fats and oils. Fatty foods are hard to digest, so keep fats to a minimum. Avoid fried foods and most fast foods.

Avoid caffeine. It is wise to avoid caffeinated drinks, coffee and colas; alcohol; spicy foods and seasonings (such as horseradish and mustard); and beans, cabbage and vegetables that may produce flatulence.

Dairy products. Not all experts think that you should avoid dairy foods. If you are lactose intolerant, then do avoid them, but ensure an adequate intake of calcium and protein from other foods. A calcium supplement with vitamin D aids bone health, particularly if long-term steroid drugs are prescribed.

Omega-3 fats. These fatty acids, which are found in oily fish and all seafood, may be of benefit as they can reduce inflammatory reactions in many parts of the body.

Folic acid. Taking a supplement may reduce the risk of colon cancer and replaces the folic acid depleted by drug treatment.

Chamomile tea. Made from the herb boswellia, chamomile tea may reduce inflammation of the colon. In one study 350mg capsules, three times a day, produced remission in 82 per cent of patients.

Eat plenty of protein and other nutrients. Eggs, fish, poultry and lean meat supply high-grade protein. Red meat is an important source of iron for people who are constantly losing blood from the bowel. Eat vegetables and fruit, without seeds and skins if necessary.

During a severe flare-up, to avoid producing stools, stick to clear broth, weak tea, white bread or toast, eggs or low-fibre cereals. As healing progresses, fish, poultry and lean meats can be added, along with baked or boiled skinless potatoes and, eventually, steamed vegetables and cooked fruit. In severe cases, liquid supplements provide helpful nutrition during a flare-up.

Avoid fast food. People who eat fast food twice a week or more have four times the risk of ulcerative colitis than those who don't.

Drug therapy
Corticosteroids or aminosalicylates are used as suppositories for short periods, mainly during flare-ups of mild cases; they are taken orally when the disease is more extensive. For maintenance treatment, doctors prescribe amino-salicylates, such as sulphasalazine, which is the mainstay of treatment. It is a combination of sulphapyridine and 5ASA. Newer agents include mesalazine, balsalazide and olsalazine. In severe cases, immuno-suppressive drugs may be prescribed and surgery is common.

Ulcers

CONSUME
- A balanced, varied diet
- Lean meat, poultry, wholegrain breads and cereals, legumes and dried fruit for iron lost through bleeding
- Cranberry juice

AVOID
- Coffee, including decaffeinated and other sources of caffeine
- Spices such as pepper, chilli, cloves and garlic, which trigger acid secretion
- Alcohol, smoking and fatty foods
- Late-night snacks or large meals

All sores that erode the mucous membranes or skin and penetrate the underlying muscle are referred to as ulcers. Those that occur in the lower part of the oesophagus, the stomach or the duodenum are known more specifically as 'peptic ulcers', because they form in areas exposed to stomach acids and the digestive enzyme, pepsin. Peptic ulcers affect 1 in 10 men and 1 in 20 women in the UK. When the erosion occurs in the duodenum, the upper part of the small intestine, the term duodenal ulcer is used; an ulcer in the stomach is called a gastric ulcer.

A person with an ulcer may describe the pain as gnawing or burning and can often pinpoint the exact spot. With gastric ulcers, the pain may be made worse by food; with duodenal ulcers the pain occurs when the sufferer is hungry and is eased by food. Some people never have ulcer pain, but may develop intestinal bleeding, heart-burn, bloating and wind, as well as nausea and vomiting.

Causes of ulcers

Over-secretion of stomach acid causes ulcers as well as indigestion and heartburn. Although excess acid secretion plays a role, most ulcers develop when a bacterium, called *Helicobacter pylori*, infects the intestinal tract. Smoking, emotional stress and heavy drinking can also contribute to a person's risk of ulcers. Ulcers frequently occur in people subjected to extreme physical stress, such as serious burns or surgery.

The other major cause of ulcers is the heavy use of drugs like aspirin, ibuprofen, naproxen and other non-steroidal anti-inflammatory drugs (NSAIDs), which erode the mucous membranes. Aspirin is a particular problem, because it inhibits blood clotting and promotes bleeding.

Medical treatment

Better understanding of the causes of ulcers has enabled doctors to devise new treatments. If *H. pylori*, is suspected, the treatment includes antibiotics to eradicate the bacteria and an acid secretion inhibitor to prevent secretion of acids by the cells of the stomach. The bacteria are usually eradicated in a week, but many patients experience side effects such as nausea, diarrhoea or a metallic taste. A daily yoghurt supplement with live lactobacilli and bifidobacteria during treatment may reduce these symptoms.

Stop smoking. It is one factor closely linked to the poor healing of gastric ulcers and the likelihood of relapse and recurrence of duodenal ulcers. Smokers may continue to suffer from ulcers until they quit.

Stop harmful medications. People with ulcers caused by using NSAIDs must discontinue the offending drug. People with a condition such as arthritis should ask their doctor to prescribe a gentler alternative.

Exercising raises your endorphin level. Mindful that 'it's not what you're eating, it's what's eating you', people with ulcers may benefit from relaxation techniques and bio-feedback to cope with stress. Regular exercise promotes the release of endorphins, brain chemicals that dull pain and elevate mood.

Do one simple thing

Eat moderate-sized meals at regular intervals

When and how people eat may be more important than what they eat. Doctors no longer recommend frequent small meals, which can provoke rebound symptoms. Rather, they suggest several moderate-size meals spaced at regular intervals. Late-evening snacks should be avoided, because they stimulate acid secretion during sleep.

Did you know?

The presence of *H. pylori* bacteria increases your risk of stomach cancer

H. pylori, the bacterium that causes peptic ulcers, weakens the mucous coating that protects the stomach lining, allowing acid to do damage. Infection by the bacteria increases stomach cancer risk two to sixfold, whether or not you develop an ulcer.

Home remedies

Many people self-treat ulcer pain with non-prescription drugs or with home remedies concocted from bicarbonate of soda to neutralise stomach acid. But long-term use of antacids containing aluminium hydroxide can prevent the body from absorbing phosphorus and result in the loss of bone minerals. Prolonged ingestion of bicarbonate of soda or antacids containing calcium carbonate may lead to a build-up of calcium and alkali, resulting in nausea, headache and weakness, with a risk of kidney damage. Check with a doctor before using acid-suppressant drugs.

One home remedy that works well is a form of liquorice called DGL which is sold in wafer form at health-food stores. Another is aloe vera juice which should be taken three times a day. Probably best of all is cranberry juice which is thought to reduce the risk of stomach ulcers, because phytochemicals in the juice prevent bacteria from sticking to the stomach walls.

Diet and ulcers

A bland diet was once the basis of treatment, but there is no evidence that it speeds the rate of healing. The main goal of diet is to avoid extreme elevations in gastric acid secretion and irritation of the gastrointestinal lining.

U

Avoid trigger foods. Triggers vary from person to person, but common offenders are coffee (including decaffeinated), caffeine in beverages and chocolate, alcohol, peppermint and tomatoes and tomato-based products. Peppermint and chocolate can also interfere with the closing of the valve that connects the oesophagus to the stomach, allowing acidic juices to 'reflux' up the oesophagus. This can cause heartburn. Fatty foods can slow down stomach emptying and stimulate acid release. Milk and dairy products temporarily relieve pain but can delay healing, possibly by promoting increased gastric secretion. Foods and seasonings that stimulate gastric acid secretion such as black pepper, garlic, cloves and chilli powder should be limited or avoided if they cause problems. Citrus juices may cause discomfort for some people.

Under weight

EAT PLENTY OF

- Larger portions and healthy high-calorie choices

- Nutritious between-meal snack

LIMIT

- Alcohol, caffeine and smoking, which can suppress the appetite

In a society that prizes leanness and spends billions on weight-loss products, people find it hard to accept that excessive thinness (unrelated to anorexia nervosa) is unhealthy. But while obesity is dangerous, surveys show that people who are of average weight at age 50 live longer than those who are markedly underweight.

There's no such thing as a perfect weight; however, for every height and build there is a desirable range in which the rates of disease and death are lowest. Underweight is defined as a Body Mass Index of less than 18.5. (To work out your own BMI see page 275). Mild under-weight is not associated with serious health hazards, but people who are very thin lack energy reserves, are vulnerable to infections and often feel the cold because they lack insulating fat. Patients weighing less than 80 per cent of their desirable weight on admission to a hospital are at high risk of complications. Severely underweight people confined to bed rest can develop pressure sores over bony areas.

When thinness is a problem

Thinness is a problem if it is a result of poor nutrition, such as chronic dieting, which can lead to infertility in women. For those who do conceive, being underweight during pregnancy may cause anaemia, heart and lung complications and a high risk of toxaemia. Their babies are often premature, have a low birth weight and may experience slow growth and development.

Adolescents with erratic schedules may slip below their ideal weight – especially if they exercise a lot. They need to make time to eat.

A corrective diet

Gaining even 1kg a month requires an extra 250kcal a day. The aim should be to build up muscle tissue and increase the level of energy to sustain the weight gain. Unless extremely weak, underweight people should exercise regularly to help to build lean tissue and store some fat.

Ten healthy ways to increase calories

1 Eat at least three well-balanced meals, including a hearty breakfast, and snacks throughout the day. For some people, it might be easier to eat smaller, more frequent meals than three large meals.

2 Eat hearty soups such as lentil, minestrone or split pea soups rather than clear soups. Make your canned soup with regular milk or evaporated milk instead of water and top it with Parmesan cheese and croûtons.

3 Eat cereals with added fruit or nuts instead of the puffed varieties. Make cooked cereal with milk instead of water.

4 Add powdered milk to puddings, baked goods, milkshakes and mashed potatoes.

5 To boost the calories and protein of a glass of milk, add a malted milk powder to your regular milk.

6 Dried fruit such as raisins, dates, prunes or dried apricots can be eaten as a snack or added to cereal or in baking.

7 Salads are low in calories but can be made more substantial by adding avocado, chickpeas, sunflower seeds or raisins.

8 Nuts are high in healthy fat and calories and make a good snack.

9 Choose desserts that have nutritional value but also are high in calories. Puddings and ice creams, breads such as banana bread, carrot cake or carrot muffins and oatmeal cookies are all suitable.

10 Don't take any supplements that are 'guaranteed to put on weight'. Be patient, try to keep a positive attitude about food, eat lots of healthy food, exercise regularly and you will gradually start to see results.

U

It is extremely important to increase dietary calories from healthy fats. A plan for increasing weight focuses, first, on eating more food and, secondly, on consuming foods that provide lots of calories in a compact volume.

Raw vegetables, for example, are nutritious but satisfy hunger long before they have provided any significant calories.

And although a low-fat diet is important, an underweight person may need to relax the rules about eating fat until the desired weight goal has been reached. Increasing dietary fat can rapidly make a difference, because fat contains more than twice as many calories (9kcal per gram) as protein and carbohydrates do (4kcal per gram).

Increase your portions of calorie-dense foods. Nutrition experts advise adhering to your food guide recommendations, but gradually increasing portions and choosing the more nutrient and calorie-dense foods within each group: peanut butter or cheese instead of tofu or cottage cheese, avocados instead of cucumbers, a milkshake instead of skimmed milk. Because caffeine suppresses the urge to eat, replace tea or coffee with juices and milk.

Augment your diet with liquid supplements. People who have lost weight due to illness may benefit from a concentrated liquid formula. Doctors and dietitians may suggest liquid supplements.

Many underweight people feel uncomfortably full when they begin eating larger, more frequent portions to gain weight. This feeling will pass with time. People trying to gain weight occasionally reach a plateau and seem to stay there for a while. Increasing their calorie intake again is necessary in order to restart the weight-gain process and eventually reach their ideal weight.

Urinary tract infections

CONSUME PLENTY OF

- Non-alcoholic and caffeine-free fluids to flush out the urinary system
- Cranberry juice
- Citrus fruit and fresh fruit and vegetables for vitamin C

AVOID

- Bladder irritants, such as coffee, tea and alcoholic beverages

Also known as cystitis, most urinary tract infections (UTIs) affect the bladder, but some may involve the kidneys, the ureters (the tubes that carry urine to the bladder) and the urethra (the tube through which urine exits the body). The most common symptom is an urgent need to urinate, even when the bladder is not full. Urination may cause pain or burning and, in severe cases, small amounts of blood. There may also be a low-grade fever and an ache in the lower back.

Most urinary infections are caused by *E. coli* bacteria, organisms that live in the intestinal tract but that can travel to the bladder. Chlamydia, a sexually transmitted organism, is another cause of UTIs. Women are more vulnerable to urinary infections because the female urethra is shorter than that of males, and its location provides a convenient entryway for bacteria. Many women develop so-called 'honeymoon cystitis', inflammation caused by sexual activity.

Role of diet

Antibiotics are needed to cure bacterial UTIs, but there are some dietary

approaches that may be able to speed healing and help to prevent recurrences of the condition.

- Doctors advise drinking at least eight to ten glasses a day of fluids to increase the flow of urine and to flush out infectious material.
- Avoid coffee, tea, colas and alcoholic drinks, since these increase bladder irritation. Some people find that spicy foods also aggravate the urinary tract.
- Cranberry juice is a favourite home remedy for clearing up UTIs, and one that is supported by research. The phytochemicals in cranberry juice speed the elimination of bacteria by preventing them from sticking to the bladder wall. However, they are only effective for about 10 hours, so to get maximum protection, you should drink 200ml of cranberry juice both morning and evening.

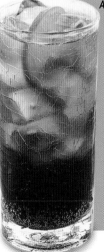

Do one simple thing

Drink berry juice

A Finnish study followed 150 women who had a urinary tract infection but were not taking antibiotics. They found that giving women one glass of cranberry-lingonberry juice daily for 6 months significantly reduced recurrences of UTIs compared to women who received a placebo. Another study, published in the *American Journal of Clinical Nutrition*, showed that berry juices, particularly raspberry, cranberry, strawberry and currant juices, taken one to three times a week were associated with a lower risk of UTI recurrence compared with drinking berry juice less than once a week. This same study showed that women who consumed fermented dairy products, which contained probiotic bacteria (such as yoghurt with *Lactobacillus acidophilus*), also had a decreased risk.

- Vitamin C helps to strengthen the immune system, fight infection and acidify the urine; calcium may reduce bladder irritability.
- Consuming probiotic yoghurts and drinks may be helpful since they are thought to inhibit the growth of micro-organisms that cause UTIs. They are thought to foster the growth of friendly flora in the body, which may be reduced by antibiotic therapy.

Additional preventive tactics

Hygiene measures can help women to avoid recurrent UTIs; many doctors recommend the following.

- Wear loose-fitting underwear made from cotton and pantyhose that have a cotton crotch.
- Avoid douching and using vaginal deodorants, which can cause bladder irritation.
- If you use a diaphragm, ask your doctor to check the size; one that is even slightly too large can irritate the urethra and bladder.
- Urinate and drink a glass of water before sexual intercourse and urinate within an hour afterwards to flush out the urinary tract.
- After a bowel movement, wipe from the front to the back to reduce the risk of carrying intestinal bacteria to the urethra.

Vegetables

BENEFITS

- Many are rich in beta carotene and vitamin C and folate, potassium and other minerals
- High fibre aid regular bowel function
- Rich in bioflavonoids that help to prevent disease

DRAWBACKS

- May contain pesticide residues

Plants combine water, nutrients from the soil and carbon dioxide from the air to synthesise all the compounds necessary for animal life. We live on vegetables whether we eat them directly or through animal intermediaries.

Root vegetables, such as beetroot, carrots, parsnips and turnips, are food storage organs and valuable sources of carbohydrates. Stems, such as celery and fennel, conduct nutrients between roots and leaves, and in some plants, underground stems have evolved into storehouses for starch. Vegetables with dark green leaves, including members of the cabbage family (such as broccoli, cauliflower, bok choy, kale and rocket) and spinach, are rich in antioxidants, bioflavonoids and the B vitamins. The leaves of all vegetables are factories for the production of sugars through photosynthesis. They are the most fragile parts of the plant, which is why they shrink most when cooked. The leaves of plants in the onion family grow into fleshy bulbs that store carbohydrates and water to nourish the plant during its next year of growth. The flowers of some plants are also eaten; broccoli stems with their unopened flower buds are a delicacy.

How much is enough?

It is highly recommended that we eat at least five servings of fruit and vegetables daily. A serving is 80g – about 3-4 heaped tablespoons – of raw or cooked vegetables, a cup of leafy salad vegetables or a 150ml glass of 100 per cent pure vegetable juice. Nutritionists recommend choosing a variety of vegetables, both raw and cooked, including richly coloured orange, red, dark green and yellow ones, vegetables from the cruciferous family and allium vegetables such as onion and garlic. These plants

contain antioxidants, vitamins and minerals and the disease-fighting compounds known as phyto-chemicals.

Nutritional value

Most vegetables are excellent sources of vitamins, fibre, folate and potassium, as well as some other minerals. They are also rich in various phytochemicals that provide protection from disease, and are low in fat and calories.

Green vegetables get their bright colour from chlorophyll, the pigment that traps the energy from sunlight and makes it available for the production of sugars from water and carbon dioxide. Although chlorophyll is soluble only in fats, cooking vegetables in water liberates the enzyme chlorophyllase, which breaks chlorophyll down into water-soluble components. This has no nutritional consequence, but the green colour of the vegetable is diminished. Some vitamins are also water soluble, and are leached out into the cooking water. That's one reason nutritionists recommend using the minimum of water when cooking and, if possible, saving the water for making soup or stock.

Colour is a useful guide to the vitamin content of vegetables. The larger and darker the leaves, the more vitamin C and beta carotene they contain; the pale inner leaves of lettuce and cabbage, for instance, have only about 3 per cent of the carotene found in the dark outer leaves. Unfortunately, outer leaves

V

are often discarded because they are damaged, their texture is too coarse or their flavour too strong.

Deep yellow, orange or dark green vegetables derive their colour from carotenoid pigments; these include beta carotene, an antioxidant that is converted to vitamin A. Because these pigments are stable in cooking and soluble in fat, the nutritional content is well preserved during baking or boiling.

Soluble and insoluble fibre in vegetables keeps bowel function regular and thereby reduces the colon's exposure to potentially toxic by-products of digestion. In some people, however, fibre can cause flatulence and bloating.

Anti-cancer foods

Cancer develops when mutant cells escape the body's immune system. Plants are also susceptible to cellular damage and have developed their own protective mechanisms. Beta carotene, vitamins C and E and phytochemicals are natural antioxidants that hinder cell damage by finding and inactivating free radicals, the unstable molecules that are released when the body uses oxygen. Some phyto-chemicals in vegetables block the growth of blood vessels that feed tumours, others inactivate the enzyme systems that allow cancer cells to spread and still others suppress the hormones that promote cancer growth.

Indoles, found in cruciferous vegetables such as broccoli, cabbage, cauliflower, turnip and rocket, appear to stimulate enzymes that offer some cancer protection. Lutein, the antioxidant found in sweetcorn, dark leafy greens and peppers, may help to prevent the age-related eye disease called macular degeneration, which leads to vision loss. Lycopene, which is found in tomato products, watermelon and pink grapefruit, has been shown to lower the risk of prostate cancer as well as provide protection from heart disease. Onions and garlic contain sulphur compounds, many of which also offer disease protection. Research suggests that rates of stomach cancer are lower in populations who eat large quantities of onions.

In fact, studies have found that people who eat ample vegetables and fruit enjoy a reduced incidence of many cancers and that people who eat few or no vegetables are more likely to develop colon cancer. Vegetables have a protective effect that goes far beyond what vitamin pills can offer. Most vegetables have multiple benefits. Broccoli, for example, contains beta carotene, vitamin C, fibre, folate and the phytochemical sulforaphane. It is this variety of protective nutrients, plant chemicals and as-yet-unidentified compounds in vegetables that helps to keep cancer at bay.

Preserving nutrients

While vegetables provide small quantities of starches, sugars and proteins, their main contributions are vitamins, minerals, fibre and protective phytochemicals. Their nutrient content, colour and texture are affected by the way they are prepared, the length of cooking time and the volume of water used.

The yellow carotene pigments are not water soluble and are well preserved in cooking, but vitamin C and the B vitamins leach into the cooking liquid. Vitamin C is also destroyed on exposure to oxygen. Up to 20 per cent of the vitamin C in a vegetable may be lost for every minute that it takes the water to heat from cold to boiling. This is because an enzyme that destroys vitamin C becomes more active as temperature rises; however, it stops at the boiling point.

For this reason, vegetables

should be added to water that is already boiling. Steaming or cooking vegetables in a small amount of water retains more than twice as much vitamin C as boiling them.

The yellow and orange carotenoid pigments are changed only by the high temperatures reached with pressure cooking. The green of chlorophyll in plant tissues is dulled when heat causes chemical changes, but as chlorophyll cannot affect the human body internally as it is not absorbed, this doesn't matter.

Some cooks blanch vegetables such as beans and broccoli in boiling water for a minute or two, then put them into cold water to hold the colour. This works for vegetables that are served cold, but if they are served hot, they need rapid reheating, with further loss of nutrients.

To preserve the betacyanin in beetroots, avoid boiling them in water – it's best to roast, bake, steam or microwave whole beetroot in their skins. Peeled or cut beetroot leaches its pigments (and thus the betacyanin is lost). Also, boiling in water depletes beetroots of their folate, which is water soluble.

Storing vegetables

Once harvested, most vegetables lose their flavour, sweetness and texture as they use up their own food stores, so the shorter the time stored, the better. Sweetcorn and peas can lose up to 40 per cent of their sugar if they are kept at room temperature for just six hours after picking. Beans and stem vegetables, such as broccoli and asparagus, are known to become tougher the longer they are left out of the refrigerator.

Vegetables that originated in warm climates (including beans, aubergines, courgettes, tomatoes, okra and pumpkins) keep best at 10°C. Most other vegetables keep best in the crisper section of the fridge. Tomatoes should not be stored in the refrigerator: the cold temperature ruins the flavour. They are best kept at room temperature and used within a few days.

Greens should be washed, drained, wrapped in paper or cloth towels and stored in a tightly sealed container in the refrigerator. If bought in airtight packaging, store them as they are. Peppers should be stored in the refrigerator, away from fruit to prevent tainting. Potatoes convert their starch to sugar below 4°C; so keep them cool and out of the light to prevent the formation of toxic alkaloids. Potatoes, pumpkins and sweet potatoes are best stored in a cool place, but not in the fridge.

Possible hazards

Most vegetables are safe to eat either raw or cooked. The exceptions are lima and kidney beans and other legumes, which contain toxic substances that are inactivated through cooking.

Cruciferous vegetables harbour goitrogenic compounds that can interfere with iodine metabolism. Cooking inactivates them, but eating large amounts of these vegetables raw may worsen a pre-existing thyroid condition.

Most vegetables do not provoke allergies, but some people react to members of the nightshade family, which includes aubergines and tomatoes. Sweetcorn and celery are also common allergens.

V

Vegetarian diets

How healthy are they?

Vegetarian diets were once questioned for their nutritional adequacy, but most of these concerns have faded in recent years, as researchers have begun studying their role in both the prevention and treatment of disease.

There has been a growing appreciation for the benefits of vegetarian diets or those that include generous amounts of plant foods and limited amounts of animal foods. Many health organisations now recommend vegetarian diets.

Technically, a vegetarian is defined as a person who does not eat meat, fish or fowl, or products that contain them. However, in reality, the eating patterns of vegetarians can vary considerably. Different degrees of vegetarianism are shown on the right.

HEALTH BENEFITS

Much of what we know about the health benefits of vegetarian diets comes from studies of Seventh-Day Adventists. A high percentage of vegetarians is found among the adherents of this religious group. Many are strict vegans, others merely avoid meat. However, Seventh-Day Adventists, as well as other vegetarians, often have healthier lifestyles in general, so it is difficult to link the health benefits of their lifestyle to any single dietary factor, such as the absence of animal foods. People who give up meat are also likely to drink very little alcohol, be non-smokers, and take plenty of exercise.

OBESITY. In addition to exercise, Plant-based diets have long been associated with decreased obesity, which is a risk factor for many chronic diseases, including heart disease, high blood pressure, diabetes and some cancers.

Some factors that may help to explain lower body weight in vegetarians include lower fat intake, higher fibre consumption and greater consumption of vegetables.

CARDIOVASCULAR DISEASE. Numerous studies have shown a decreased incidence of heart disease among vegetarians compared with non-vegetarians. This may be explained in part by lower blood cholesterol levels in vegetarians. Compared with non-vegetarians, vegans and vegetarians have blood cholesterol levels 35 per cent and 14 per cent lower, respectively.

Although most vegetarians don't eat low-fat diets, their saturated fat intake is considerably lower than that of non-vegetarians. They also consume more fibre, which may be a factor in helping to reduce blood cholesterol levels. In addition, a vegetarian diet has the benefit of the many phytochemicals found in plant foods that have antioxidant properties, and antioxidants make blood cholesterol less likely to stick to artery walls.

However, there are anomalies: a large proportion of the Asians in Britain are vegetarian, but have a higher rate of coronary heart disease than the national average.

HYPERTENSION. In addition to having lower blood pressure in general, vegetarians also have lower rates of high blood pressure (or hypertension) than non-vegetarians. Researchers have looked at possible explanations for this difference, including lower body weight, decreased dietary fat, absence of meat or milk protein, or differences in potassium, magnesium or calcium intakes, but so far they have not been able to draw any conclusions.

CANCER. Vegetarians in general have a lower cancer rate compared with the general population. This difference is most significant for

> **Four rules for healthy vegetarian eating**
>
> 1 Choose a variety of foods, including whole grains, vegetables, fruits, legumes, nuts, seeds and, if desired, dairy products and eggs.
>
> 2 Choose whole, unrefined foods often and limit highly sweetened, fatty, and heavily refined foods.
>
> 3 If dairy products and eggs are included, choose lower-fat dairy products.
>
> 4 Use a regular source of vitamin B_{12} such as yoghurt, milk or eggs, or soya beverage with added B_{12}.

V

prostate cancer and colorectal cancer. A number of factors in vegetarian diets may affect cancer risk, such as eating less fat, lower levels of haem iron (from animal sources) and more fibre, more fruit and vegetables, and a higher intake of phytochemicals like isoflavones, the hormone-like plant compounds found in soya and other plant foods.

DIABETES. There is some evidence that vegetarians have lower rates of diabetes. This protective effect may be the result of lower body weight among vegetarians, as well as a higher fibre intake, which can both improve blood sugar control.

ENSURING ADEQUATE NUTRIENT INTAKE

The nutritional needs of vegetarians are the same as those of non-vegetarians and can mostly be met by following general dietary recommendations. However, adjustments need to be made in a few areas to make up for the lack of animal sources of several nutrients, including protein, vitamin B_{12}, calcium, zinc and iron.

Vegetarian variations

The reasons for being vegetarian are varied, including health concerns, ethics, religion, economics, as well as taste. Here are a few of the varieties:

- **Semi-vegetarians.** Largely practise a vegetarian diet, but may include occasional animal foods in their diet.
- **Lacto-ovo-vegetarians.** Include milk and products made from milk, as well as eggs, but avoid meat, fish and poultry.
- **Lacto-vegetarians.** Include milk and products made from milk.
- **Pescatarians.** Include fish in their diet.
- **Vegans.** Consume no meat, poultry, fish, dairy, eggs or gelatine and may also exclude honey.

INCLUDING ANIMAL FOODS

Lacto-vegetarians, lacto-ovo-vegetarians and pescatarians can adequately meet their nutritional needs by following a balanced diet. A variety of foods should be included, with an emphasis on complex carbohydrates and lower-fat choices, such as grains, legumes, fruit and vegetables and lower-fat dairy products, as well as moderate amounts of eggs, nuts and seeds, to ensure enough energy and protein, and provide good sources of all key nutrients.

VEGAN DIETS

Vegans need to plan their diets more carefully to make sure that their energy and nutrient needs are being met, particularly those of children, adolescents, pregnant and breastfeeding women and older adults whose needs may be greater than normal.

PROTEIN. Vegans can meet their protein needs by combining complementary plant protein sources to make complete proteins. Adults don't need to eat complementary plant proteins at each meal as long as they are eaten in the same day, and as long as a balanced and varied diet provides enough protein on a

V

regular basis. For growing children, whose protein needs are higher, complete protein sources at each meal, such as bread with peanut butter, or beans and rice, are recommended.

CALORIES. Because plant-based diets are high in fibre and lower in calorie-dense foods, care needs to be taken to make sure there is adequate energy in the diet, especially for children. Foods with higher energy density, such as nuts, seeds and dried fruit, should be included in meals and snacks.

VITAMIN B$_{12}$. Because plant foods don't contain B$_{12}$, vegans need to include a reliable source in their daily diet, such as a soya drink with added B$_{12}$, or a B$_{12}$ supplement.

VITAMIN D. Our best source of vitamin D is exposure to the sun. Foods that are fortified with vitamin D, such as margarine and some fortified soya drinks also provide some vitamin D. If sun exposure and intake of fortified foods are not adequate, vitamin D supplements are recommended.

TRACE MINERALS. Iron, zinc, calcium and other trace minerals are not as readily available from plant sources, so vegans need to develop strategies to make sure they're

Do one simple thing

Eat complementary proteins

Although plant foods contain various proteins, they are of an 'incomplete' variety. This means they do not contain all the essential amino acids that the body needs. But combining plant foods to make a complete protein can be as simple as eating a legume (peanut butter) with a grain (wholemeal bread). Alternatively, nuts and seeds can be combined with grains. Examples of complementary plant-protein combinations are:

- Rice and beans.
- Bean-vegetable chilli served with tortillas.
- Baked beans and corn bread.
- Hummous (made with chickpeas and sesame seeds).
- Breadsticks with sesame seeds.
- Multigrain bread made with sunflower seeds.
- Split-pea soup served with a wholegrain roll.

getting adequate amounts, such as: eating iron-enriched cereals, including sources of vitamin C at meals to help absorption of iron from plant foods, and eating tofu, legumes, almonds, sesame seeds and dark green vegetables, to ensure adequate calcium intake.

CHILDREN'S NEEDS

Children have high nutrient requirements, but they have small stomachs, so a strict vegetarian diet, with mainly fruit and vegetables, whole grains and a lot of bulky fibre, may be too low in calories and nutrients to meet a child's needs.

But with some careful planning, a balanced vegan diet with good sources of protein and some concentrated sources of energy can adequately support growth and nutrition. Their daily diet should include: three meals plus plenty of appealing snacks like dried fruit-and-nut mix, muffins and fruit; sources of fat, such as nuts, seeds, avocados and peanut butter; and plenty of protein-rich foods like tofu, soya drinks, soya cheese and yoghurt.

VEGETARIANS MAY NEED MORE IRON AND ZINC

Phytates, compounds found mostly in cereal grains, legumes and nuts, bind with iron and prevent the body from using it.

Vegetarians should increase their intake of plant foods that are rich in iron, or should discuss the use of an iron supplement with their GP. Vitamin C can help to reduce the effects of phytates and cooking vegetables also releases some of the iron that is bound to the phytates. Zinc is found in nuts, seeds (especially pumpkin seeds), lentils, wheat germ, whole grains, peas and spinach.

Vinegar

BENEFITS

- Basis for a low-calorie salad dressing
- Can be used to preserve other foods

DRAWBACKS

- May trigger an allergic reaction in people sensitive to moulds

For centuries, vinegar was a by-product of wine and beer making; in fact, the name comes from the French word *vinaigre*, which means sour wine. Apple cider and wine remain the most popular basic ingredients, but almost any product that produces alcoholic fermentation can be used to make vinegar – there are dozens of varieties available today.

Although various healing powers have been attributed to vinegar over the years, they are difficult to prove. It does, however, provide a low-sodium, low-calorie flavouring.

All vinegars are 4 to 14 per cent acetic acid. They are made in two stages. First, yeasts or other moulds are added to turn the natural sugars in the basic ingredient into alcohol. Then, bacteria are introduced to convert the alcohol into acetic acid.

Varieties of vinegar

Plain white (clear) distilled vinegar is the type used for making pickles and other condiments. It can be transformed into a flavoured or gourmet vinegar simply by adding various herbs, spices or fruit – for example, dill, tarragon, lemon balm, mint, garlic, green peppercorns, chillies, citrus or raspberries. These and many other varieties are widely available, or you can make your own by adding fresh herbs or fruit to distilled, cider or wine vinegars. Cover tightly and store in a dark cupboard. The acetic acid keeps the herbs or fruit from spoiling.

Health benefits

Vinegar is virtually devoid of calories – the only exception is balsamic, with about 18kcal per tablespoon. To reduce its acid bite, most vinegar can be mixed with orange juice or fruit syrup and a little oil.

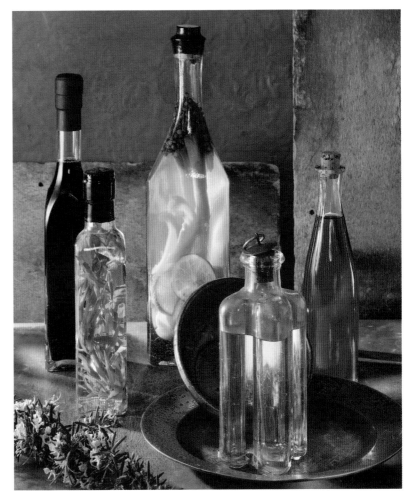

▲ **Sharp flavours**
As a preserving liquid, vinegar has no equal – once sealed, it can last indefinitely. Enliven salads with (from left to right) balsamic, tarragon, citrus, wine and sherry vinegars.

Various vinegars have often been recommended as a treatment for arthritis, indigestion and other ailments. Such claims have never been proved scientifically, but some arthritis sufferers insist that a tonic of cider vinegar and honey does alleviate joint pain.

A note of caution: people who are allergic to moulds may react to vinegar as well as to foods preserved with it. Symptoms to watch for include a tingling or itching sensation around the mouth, and possibly an outbreak of hives.

Did you know?

Why balsamic vinegar is expensive

It's the ageing process. Rich, dark and mild-flavoured balsamic vinegar originated in Modena, Italy. Many consider it to be the best quality vinegar available. Balsamic vinegar is produced from a type of red wine, and the most prized – and expensive – varieties are aged 15 to 50 years.

V

Vitamins
Essential nutrients

For more than 2,000 years, folk healers and physicians have known that eating certain foods prevents or cures diseases. As far back as 400 BC, Hippocrates found that eating liver cured night blindness.

I n 1747, James Lind, a British naval surgeon, discovered the link between diet and scurvy. He advocated eating lemons and limes to prevent the dreadful disease that was common in sailors who lived on biscuits and salt pork on long voyages.

To date, 13 vitamins essential to health have been discovered. Other vitamin-like substances, such as bioflavonoids, have also been identified. Some appear to be essential to health, but Reference Nutrient Intakes (RNIs) for them have not yet been established. Researchers believe there are probably many more substances that may optimise health and may fall into the vitamin category. That is why they recommend eating a variety of foods for complete nutrition.

CLASSIFICATION

Vitamins are classified according to how they are absorbed and stored in the body. Vitamins A, D, E and K are soluble only in fats, whereas vitamin C and the B vitamins are soluble in water. The body can store fat-soluble vitamins in the liver and fatty tissue. Since most excess water-soluble vitamins are excreted in the urine, they need to be eaten more often.

Provitamins are substances that the body can convert into vitamins. Examples include beta carotene, a precursor of vitamin A, as well as a type of steroid in the skin that, after exposure to the sun, is used by the body to make vitamin D.

FAT-SOLUBLE VITAMINS

These vitamins need fat to be absorbed into the bloodstream from the intestinal tract. Thus, people who have fat-malabsorption disorders can develop deficiency symptoms even though their diet supplies adequate amounts of a vitamin. On the other hand, toxic amounts may build up if a person takes high-dose supplements.

VITAMIN A: There are several forms of this vitamin. The preformed, or active, ones are retinol, retinoic acid and retinyl esters. Beta carotene is a precursor form. Vitamin A is essential to normal vision and to prevent night blindness. But it is also necessary for normal cell division and growth, the development of bones and teeth and for the health of skin, mucous membranes and the epithelial tissue that lines the intestine, airways and other organs. Its antioxidant qualities help to prevent the cancer-causing cell damage inflicted by free radicals. The body also needs vitamin A to synthesise amino acids, thyroxine and other hormones.

In general, supplementation with vitamin A is not recommended. Excessive vitamin A can cause toxicity, which can lead to death in extreme cases. A woman considering pregnancy should never take high-dose vitamin A supplements or isotretinoin (Roaccutane), a powerful acne drug derived from vitamin A. Because vitamin A is stored in the body, these should be stopped at least three months before attempting to conceive.

VITAMIN D: There are two forms of this vitamin: D_2, which comes from plants, and D_3, which the body synthesises when the skin is exposed to ultraviolet (UV) rays from the sun. For adequate vitamin D, part of the skin (for example the arms) needs about 10 minutes' sun exposure per day. The body must

Why are they called vitamins?

In 1912 Dr Casimir Funk, a Polish bio-chemist, put forth the theory that foods contained essential chemical substances that were vital to life. He coined the term *vitamines* referring to them as 'vital amines', or nitrogen compounds. His 1922 work was titled *The Vitamines*. It later turned out that some of these substances were not amines and the e was dropped. The term 'vitamin' has been part of our vocabulary ever since.

V

have vitamin D in order to absorb calcium. Vitamin D also promotes absorption of phosphorus and prevents the kidneys from excreting protein in the urine. Because of its role in mineral absorption, vitamin D promotes the growth of strong bones and teeth. A deficiency causes rickets in children and osteomalacia in adults (osteomalacia is the adult form of rickets; it is extremely rare in the industrialised world). Other deficiency symptoms include convulsions and muscle twitching.

VITAMIN E: The tocopherols in vitamin E prevent oxidation, which results in the rancidity of fats and the destruction of vitamins A and D. They also help to maintain healthy red blood cells and muscle tissue, protect the lungs from pollutants and regulate the synthesis of vitamin C and DNA.

The value of vitamin E supplementation for heart disease prevention remains controversial. Although early studies of people with cardiovascular disease have shown 20 to 40 per cent reductions in coronary disease risk, findings in several large, recent randomised trials with similar subjects have shown no benefits. It may be that protection by vitamin E supplementation is afforded mainly to people without known coronary disease or a subset of heart disease patients, but this has yet to be determined.

Unlike other fat-soluble vitamins, tocopherols do not accumulate to toxic levels in the body. Any excess is excreted in the stools. People taking a blood-thinning medication, such as warfarin, or undergoing surgery should not take vitamin E without their doctor's approval, as it has anti-clotting properties.

VITAMIN K: The liver requires vitamin K to manufacture blood proteins that are essential for blood clotting. Intestinal bacteria make half the needed vitamin K; the rest comes from the diet. New research suggests that vitamin K may increase bone density and also reduce fracture rates. Both the Nurses' Health Study and the Framingham Heart Study found that people who consume the most vitamin K have a lower risk of hip fractures than those who consume less. Deficiency is characterised by excessive bleeding from even minor cuts. Some newborn infants are especially vulnerable to vitamin K deficiency, because they lack the intestinal bacteria needed to make it.

WATER-SOLUBLE VITAMINS

As water-soluble vitamins, the B vitamins and vitamin C are more easily absorbed than fat-soluble vitamins because there is always fluid in the intestine. However, deficiencies may develop more quickly because the body stores water-soluble vitamins in only small amounts.

BIOTIN: Closely related to folate, pantothenic acid and vitamin B_{12}, biotin is essential for the proper metabolism of carbohydrates, especially glucose, as well as proteins and fats. Some biotin is made by intestinal bacteria; it is also found in many foods. Deficiency occurs mostly in infants. In adults, it can be induced by eating lots of raw egg whites, which contain avidin, a substance that destroys biotin.

FOLATE: Also referred to as folic acid or folacin, this B vitamin is converted into enzymes that the body needs to make DNA, RNA and red blood cells, and to carry out other important metabolic functions. During pregnancy, folate helps to prevent neurological defects, particularly spina bifida, in the developing foetus. Alcohol and oral contraceptives interfere with absorption, increasing the risk of deficiency.

NIACIN: Also known as vitamin B_3, nicotinic acid and nicotinamide, niacin is important in energy metabolism, normal growth and the synthesis of fatty acids, DNA and protein. Mild niacin deficiency causes mouth sores and diarrhoea. Severe deficiency can lead to pellagra, a disease characterised by diarrhoea, dermatitis, dementia and, if untreated, death.

When consumed in high doses, niacin may lower blood cholesterol levels. But such high doses should be taken only under careful medical supervision, with frequent blood checks for liver damage and high blood sugar. High doses can also cause flushing of the face, neck and arms. It may even cause fainting as a result of blood being 'stolen' from the heart.

(continued on page 382)

All about vitamins

VITAMIN	BEST FOOD SOURCES	ROLE IN HEALTH
FAT-SOLUBLE VITAMINS		
Vitamin A (from retinols in animal products or beta carotene in plant foods)	Retinols: Liver; salmon and other cold-water fish; egg yolks; and full-cream dairy products. Beta carotene: Orange, yellow and green fruit and vegetables, such as carrots, pumpkin and spinach.	Prevents night blindness; needed for growth and cell development; maintains healthy skin, hair and nails, as well as gums, glands, bones and teeth; may help to prevent lung cancer.
Vitamin D (calciferol)	Butter and fortified margarine; egg yolks; fatty fish; fish-liver oils. (Also made by the body when exposed to the sun.)	Necessary for calcium absorption; helps to build and maintain strong bones and teeth.
Vitamin E (tocopherols)	Wheat germ; nuts and seeds; eggs, vegetable oils, margarine and mayonnaise.	Protects fatty acids; maintains muscles and red blood cells; important antioxidant.
Vitamin K	Spinach, cabbage, and other green leafy vegetables; pork, liver; and green tea.	Essential for proper blood clotting.
WATER-SOLUBLE VITAMINS		
Biotin	Egg yolks, soya beans, cereals and yeast.	Essential for energy metabolism.
Folate (folic acid, folacin)	Liver; yeast; broccoli and other cruciferous vegetables; avocados; legumes; many raw vegetables.	Needed to make DNA, RNA and red blood cells, and to synthesise certain amino acids.
Niacin (vitamin B_3, nicotinic acid, nicotinamide)	Lean meats, poultry and seafood; milk; eggs; legumes; fortified breads and cereals.	Essential for energy metabolism; promotes normal growth. Large doses lower cholesterol.
Pantothenic acid (vitamin B_5)	Almost all foods.	Essential for energy metabolism; normalising blood sugar levels; and synthesising antibodies, cholesterol, haemoglobin and some hormones.
Riboflavin (vitamin B_2)	Milk and other dairy products; fortified cereals; lean meat and poultry; raw mushrooms.	Essential for energy metabolism; aids adrenal function.
Thiamin (vitamin B_1)	Pork; legumes; nuts and seeds; fortified cereals; and grains.	Essential for energy metabolism; helps to maintain normal digestion, appetite and proper nerve function.
Vitamin B_6 (pyridoxine, pyridox-amine, pyridoxal)	Meat, fish and poultry; grains and cereals; green leafy vegetables, potatoes and soya beans.	Promotes protein metabolism; metabolism of carbohydrates and release of energy; proper nerve function; synthesis of red blood cells.
Vitamin B_{12} (cobalamins)	All animal products.	Needed to make red blood cells, DNA, RNA and myelin (for nerve fibres).
Vitamin C (ascorbic acid)	Citrus fruit and juices; melons, berries and other fruit; peppers, broccoli, potatoes; and many other fruits and vegetables.	Strengthens blood vessel walls; promotes wound healing; promotes iron absorption; helps to prevent atherosclerosis.

This table presents daily Reference Nutrient Intakes (RNIs). The RNIs are set to meet the known needs of practically all healthy people. Source: Department of Health

V

| DAILY REFERENCE NUTRIENT INTAKES FOR ADULTS OVER 19 | | | |
MALES	FEMALES	SYMPTOMS OF DEFICIENCY	SYMPTOMS OF EXCESS
700mcg	600mcg	Night blindness; stunted growth in children; dry skin and eyes; increased susceptibility to infection.	Headaches and blurred vision; fatigue; bone and joint pain; appetite loss and diarrhoea; dry, cracked skin, rashes and itchiness; hair loss. Can cause birth defects if taken in high doses before and during early pregnancy.
None set; 10mcg for over-65s	None set; 10mcg for over-65s	Weak bones, leading to rickets in children and osteomalacia in adults.	Headaches, loss of appetite, diarrhoea and possible calcium deposits in heart, blood vessels and kidneys.
None set; safe intake 4mg	None set; safe intake 3mg	Unknown in humans.	Excessive bleeding, especially when taken with aspirin and other anti-clotting drugs.
None set; safe intake 1mcg/kg	None set; safe intake 1mcg/kg	Excessive bleeding; easy bruising.	May interfere with anti-clotting drugs; possible jaundice.
None set; safe intake 10-200mcg	None set; safe intake 10-200mcg	Scaly skin; hair loss; depression; elevated blood cholesterol levels.	Apparently none.
200mcg	200mcg	Abnormal red blood cells and impaired cell division; anaemia; weight loss and intestinal upsets; deficiency may cause birth defects.	May inhibit absorption of phenytoin, causing seizures in people with epilepsy taking this drug; large doses may inhibit zinc absorption.
17mg; 16mg for over-50s	13mg; 12mg for over-50s	Diarrhoea and mouth sores; pellagra (in extreme cases).	Hot flushes; liver damage; elevated blood sugar and uric acid.
None set; safe intake 3-7mg	None set; safe intake 3-7mg	Unknown in humans.	Very high doses may cause diarrhoea and oedema.
1.3mg	1.1mg	Vision problems and light sensitivity; mouth and nose sores; swallowing problems.	Generally none, but may interfere with cancer chemotherapy.
1.0mg; 0.9mg for over-50s	0.8mg	Depression and mood swings; loss of appetite and nausea; muscle cramps. In extreme cases, muscle wasting and beriberi.	Deficiency of other B vitamins.
1.4mg	1.2mg	Depression and confusion; itchy, scaling skin; smooth, red tongue; weight loss.	Sensory nerve deterioration.
1.5mcg	1.5mcg	Pernicious anaemia; nerve problems and weakness; smooth or sore tongue.	Apparently none.
40mg	40mg	Loose teeth; bleeding gums; bruises; loss of appetite; dry skin; poor healing. In extreme cases, scurvy and internal haemorrhages.	Diarrhoea; kidney stones; urinary tract irritation; iron build-up; bone loss.

V

(continued from page 379)

PANTOTHENIC ACID: Its name comes from the Greek term for 'widespread' and it is found in almost all plant and animal foods. It is also made by intestinal bacteria. Pantothenic acid is required for the metabolism of carbohydrates, proteins and fats and is used to make hormones, red blood cells and fats. Deficiency of pantothenic acid is unknown.

RIBOFLAVIN: Essential for the release of energy, riboflavin is needed to metabolise proteins, carbohydrates and fats. It is also necessary to utilise niacin and vitamin B_6, and it may play a role in the production of corticosteroid hormones. Riboflavin deficiency does not cause any specific diseases, but it can contribute to other B vitamin deficiency disorders. It is responsible for the bright yellow colour of the urine which is experienced by supplement takers.

THIAMIN: Also known as vitamin B_1, thiamin is instrumental in turning carbohydrates, proteins, and fats into energy. It is also needed to convert glucose into fatty acids. It promotes normal nerve function, muscle tone, appetite and digestion. A mild deficiency causes fatigue, listlessness, irritability, mood swings, numbness in the legs, digestive problems and retarded growth in children. Severe deficiency leads to beriberi, a disease that is rare in developed countries.

VITAMIN B_6: Made up of three interchangeable and related compounds (pyridoxine, pyridoxamine and pyridoxal), vitamin B_6 is a coenzyme that is essential for protein metabolism. It is needed to release energy in forms that the cells can use, and it is instrumental in the functioning of the nervous and immune systems and the manufacture of red blood cells. Deficiency is noted by oily, scaling skin, especially around the eyes, nose and mouth; weight loss; muscle weakness; a smooth, red tongue; irritability; and depression. High-dose supplements can cause nerve damage.

VITAMIN B_{12}: Like other B vitamins, vitamin B_{12} functions as a coenzyme, an organic molecule that helps the enzymes to function. It is essential for the growth and division of cells, as well as for making red blood cells, genetic material and myelin, the fatty sheath that surrounds nerve fibres. Deficiency can cause pernicious anaemia, neurologic symptoms and weakness.

The majority of cases of vitamin B_{12} deficiency are not due to a poor diet; instead, it is almost always caused by an inability to absorb the vitamin from the intestinal tract due to a lack of intrinsic factor, the production of which declines with age. Many intestinal disorders also result in inadequate intrinsic factor. In these cases, B_{12} must be supplemented.

VITAMIN C: Also called ascorbic acid, vitamin C is necessary to make and maintain collagen, the connective tissue that holds body cells together. It is an important antioxidant, associated with lowering risk of heart disease, certain cancers and even some of the health concerns of ageing. Vitamin C promotes healing of wounds and burns, helps to build teeth and bones and strengthens the walls of capillaries and other blood vessels. In addition, it increases iron absorption. A popular treatment for the common cold, most studies suggest that while it probably won't prevent your cold, it may lessen its severity and slightly shorten its duration. Deficiency symptoms are fatigue, joint pain, sore and bleeding gums, easy bruising, weakened bones that fracture easily and the slow healing of wounds. With severe deficiency, these symptoms worsen into scurvy, gum ulcers form, the teeth loosen and haemorrhages can develop.

A WORD ABOUT CHOLINE

Although not strictly speaking a vitamin, choline was classified in 1998 as an essential nutrient by the US National Academy of Sciences. It was once thought that our bodies made adequate amounts of this nutrient, but it is now recognised that we need to obtain choline from our diets. It is available in eggs, legumes, nuts, meats and dairy products. Choline is an important nutrient in fat metabolism, needed to maintain healthy nerve function. It is also a precursor to acetylcholine, a brain neurotransmitter that is involved in memory.

V

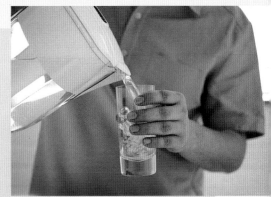

Water
Vital for life

Two parts hydrogen and one part oxygen (H_2O), water is the most abundant substance in the human body, accounting for up to 60 per cent of our body weight.

Even though water has no calories or other nutrients, we can go for only a few days without it. In contrast, a healthy person can survive for six to eight weeks without food. A loss of only 5 to 10 per cent of body water results in serious dehydration, while a 15 to 20 per cent loss is usually fatal.

VITAL FUNCTIONS
Water is essential to virtually every body function, including digestion, absorption and transport of nutrients, elimination of body waste and regulation of body temperature, as well as other chemical processes. It provides a protective cushion for body cells, and in the form of amniotic fluid protects a developing foetus. Water is needed to build all body tissues and is the base of all blood and fluid secretions such as tears, saliva and gastric juices, as well as the fluids that lubricate our organs and joints. It keeps skin soft and smooth.

As the body ages, it becomes drier. The body of a newborn infant is 75 to 80 per cent water, compared with 50 per cent after 65 or 70. This drying out is reflected in the wrinkled skin, reduced saliva flow and stiffened joints that occur naturally with ageing.

HOW MUCH DO WE NEED?
The human body needs enough water to ensure that the urine is pale, not dark or bright yellow. For the average adult this may translate to six to eight glasses of water a day. Most of this comes from drinks – plain water, coffee, tea, juices, soft drinks – but surprisingly there's a substantial amount in foods as well. Fruit and vegetables, for example, are 70 to 95 per cent water, compared with 75 per cent of an egg, 50 to 70 per cent of meat, poultry and fish and 35 per cent of bread.

Our daily needs vary a lot. We need more water in hot weather, during exercise or when we have a fever, cold or other illness. We also need more during pregnancy to provide for the amniotic fluid and the expanded blood volume, as well as to meet the needs of the developing foetus. Breastfeeding mothers need to increase their fluid intake to produce milk, which is 87 per cent water.

As a general rule, the amount of water we take in from fluids and foods should be equal to what is excreted. Many factors can affect this balance. For example, taking diuretics or other drugs that increase urination increases our needs for fluids. Drinking large amounts of strong tea or coffee has a similar diuretic effect, which can offset the fluid intake from these drinks. And eating salty foods also increases our need for extra water to maintain proper fluid balance.

Thirst decreases with age, so elderly people should drink water often even if they don't

---

Six interesting facts about bottled water

1 By law, natural mineral water must specify its mineral composition, but this is not the case for spring waters.

2 Mineral water often has lower levels of minerals than tap water.

3 Unlike some water supplies, bottled water lacks fluoride, which protects against cavities.

4 If you reuse plastic water bottles, wash them thoroughly before refilling.

5 Check the bottling date and 'use by' date to find out how fresh the water is. Bottled water normally contains low numbers of harmless bacteria, but if the water is stored for long periods at room temperatures, these bacteria can multiply rapidly. It's best to store the water in a cool place.

6 Opened containers of bottled water should be refrigerated in case potentially harmful bacteria have been introduced.

W

Home filter systems

Although tap water is safe, to drink, many people use water filters to remove minor traces of chemicals, metals and other substances that may be present. Whatever type of filter system you choose, make sure you replace the filter regularly, according to the manufacturer's instructions. If the filter is used for too long it will start to release pollutants back into the water and bacteria will breed. There are three main types of filter.

- Activated carbon filters sit in the jug and you pour the water over them. They remove chlorine, pesticides and some chemicals, but not fluoride or nitrates.

- Distillation units remove most impurities through vaporising water and then condensing it. They use a lot of electricity and some people don't like the taste.

- Reverse osmosis systems force filtered water through a membrane and remove virtually all chemicals and minerals, including those such as calcium and magnesium, which benefit health and enhance the flavour of drinking water.

feel thirsty; they may even confuse thirst with hunger. Also, during intense exercise or when it's extremely hot and humid, by the time you feel thirsty, you may already have lost enough fluid to affect exercise performance. If you drink more fluid than you need, the kidneys excrete the excess by increasing the volume of urine. If you drink more water than the kidneys can handle, excess is absorbed by your cells.

IS OUR DRINKING WATER SAFE?

The quality of tap water in the UK is generally high and to ensure that it is safe to drink, the British Government has introduced water quality regulations. These impose far more rigorous standards than those applied to many bottled waters, especially over the content of micro-organisms. Water companies add chlorine to water to disinfect it and prevent bacteria from breeding in it. Furthermore, tap water may contain the valuable minerals calcium, magnesium, potassium and iron, but levels can vary greatly, depending on the source and the region.

Although water is regularly tested, certain pollutants may still be present – albeit in minute quantities. These include fertilisers, weedkillers, industrial chemicals and heavy metals. Some substances – such as chlorine, fluoride and aliminium sulphate – which are added to water by the water authorities have provoked alarm among consumers.

Aluminium. Aluminium sulphate is often added to water during treatment to remove suspended matter. Most of it is removed through filtration, although a small amount of aliminium does pass into the water supply. The current European Community (EC) directive sets the maximum permitted concentration of aliminium at 0.2mg per litre.

Sex hormones. Chemicals that mimic the hormone oestrogen, as used in the contraceptive pill, have been detected in some rivers and lakes from which water supplies are drawn. These compounds have been linked with reduced male fertility in certain fish and reptiles, and some scientists are becoming increasingly concerned that these chemicals could have a harmful effect on human fertility.

Lead pipes. These were once common in older houses, and although most have now been replaced, water can still be contaminated by the lead solder used to join copper pipes. The risks are much higher in soft-water areas, as lead dissolves more easily in soft water. It also dissolves more easily in hot water, so never use water from the hot tap for cooking or filling kettles.

To minimise the risk of absorbing lead, run the cold water tap for a few minutes each morning, so that all the water that has been lying in the pipes all night is flushed away. Use water only from the mains supply – normally in the kitchen – for drinking and cooking.

Fluoride. By hardening tooth enamel and making teeth more resistant to decay, fluoride has played a major part in improving dental health in the UK. In some areas, fluoride is added to water supplies (it is not allowed to exceed 1,000mcg per litre). If you want to know if you live in an area where fluoride is added to your water, contact your water supplier.

Fluoride is added to most toothpastes and must be listed among the ingredients.

However, in rare cases, particularly in areas where natural levels of fluoride are high, children can develop a condition known as fluorosis which involves mottling and staining of the teeth due to overdosing on fluoride. It has also been linked with a higher than normal incidence of hip fractures. As fluoride makes tooth enamel harder, it may also make bones denser and less flexible. Research is ongoing on the effects of fluoride and some people object on the grounds that it is 'mass medication'.

Nitrates. Widely used in fertilisers, nitrates leach into rivers and underground sources of water from farmland. Once nitrates are ingested, bacteria in the lower intestine convert them to nitrites which are then absorbed into the bloodstream and excreted through the salivary glands, in saliva. When they enter the stomach, the nitrites may react with the amines present in food to form nitrosamines – carcinogenic substances which may be linked to some types of gastric cancer.

In Britain, the permissable amount of nitrates in tap water is far lower than is commonly found in almost all foods and is not a major risk. Nitrates occur naturally in vegetables, although levels may be boosted by the widespread use of fertilisers.

EU regulations require the level of nitrate to be tested, particularly in spinach and lettuce, by supermarkets and wholesalers before produce reaches the consumer. Nitrates and nitrites are added to cured meat to prevent botulism and improve colour.

WHERE TO GET ADVICE

If you are worried about your water supply, look for your water supplier's phone number on your account. British water companies carry out more than 3 million tests a year to check on levels of pollutants in drinking water, and have to keep a public register of water-quality tests, which they are obliged to let you see. You can also ask your Environmental Health Officer to test your tap water.

BOTTLED WATER

Not all bottled waters are alike. Make sure you read the fine print so you're getting what you're looking for in terms of source, content and taste. Here's a guide:

Spring water. Flows from a natural underground spring source. Once the water is collected and bottled, it should have the same properties as it did under ground. Spring water has no nutritional advantages over tap water.

Mineral water. Defined as 'ground water obtained from subterranean water-bearing strata that, in its natural state, contains soluble matter'. The typical mineral analysis is listed on the label. In some products, the quantities may not be any greater than would be found in tap water. Some mineral waters are naturally carbonated because they contain carbon dioxide, while it is added to other types.

Drinking water. Bottled water can come from a spring or a municipal water supply. It may be treated by distillation, deionisation or reverse osmosis. Other terms for water treated by one of these processes include 'distilled water', 'deionised water' and 'reverse osmosis water'.

Carbonated water. Bottled water that contains natural or added carbonation. Soda water has no calories, but tonic water contains sugar and is considered a soft drink, not a bottled water.

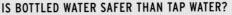

IS BOTTLED WATER SAFER THAN TAP WATER?

Most people think bottled water is purer and healthier than tap water. In fact, bottled waters often contain higher levels of bacteria - albeit harmless - than mains water which is treated with chloride to prevent bacterial growth. Many 'mineral waters' contain levels of minerals that are no higher than mains water.

Some people drink bottled water because they believe it will be low in nitrates, but this is not always true. Levels vary greatly between brands – from under 1mg per litre to 32mg.

Some bottled waters and certain soda waters are high in sodium, which may contribute to high blood pressure. Check the labels, because sodium levels can range from a modest 0.5mg per litre to an unhealthily high 114mg per litre.

Bottled water is definitely safer than tap water when you are travelling in countries notorious for waterborne diseases.

W

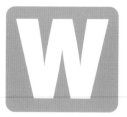

Watercress

BENEFITS

- An excellent source of beta carotene and vitamin C; also provides vitamin E

- A useful source of calcium, iron and potassium

- Rich in antioxidants, which help to prevent cancer and other diseases

DRAWBACKS

- May be contaminated by parasites and bacteria, depending on where it is grown

Whether it is eaten raw, used as a garnish or added to salads, soups and sandwiches, the dark green, peppery leaves of watercress are among the more nutritious greens.

Watercress is a cruciferous vegetable, rich in antioxidants, bioflavonoids and other substances that may protect against certain types of cancer, particularly those of the digestive system. It also has been found to contain a phytochemical called phenylethyl isothiocyanate (PEITC), which may detoxify the carcinogens that are linked to lung cancer. Watercress is also a good source of vitamins A (in the form of beta carotene, its precursor), C and E, antioxidants that protect against cell damage by free radicals, unstable molecules that are produced when the body uses oxygen. A 50g bunch of watercress provides 30 per cent of the Reference Nutrient Intake (RNI) of vitamin A and 70 per cent of the RNI for vitamin C. Yet it contains only 11kcal.

Many alternative practitioners suggest that watercress can alleviate gastrointestinal upsets and help to treat respiratory problems and urinary tract infections. Some claim that it can also be useful as a mild antidepressant, an appetite stimulant and a diuretic. Application of its juice is recommended to clear up acne. However, these health benefits have not been verified.

Buying watercress and using it

Watercress is only available fresh and is usually sold in bunches. Look for crisp leaves and a bright green colour; bypass any with yellow or wilted leaves. Although watercress may be found in small streams, don't pick it in the wild. Streams often contain parasites and bacteria that may cause intestinal infections. Even watercress from a supermarket, which has usually been grown in a controlled environment, should be washed thoroughly before it is served.

The pungency of watercress is complemented by citrus. Use a light citrus dressing on a watercress salad, or toss orange or grapefruit slices with watercress for a refreshing fruit salad. Watercress can also be added to a variety of cooked dishes. However, to preserve its vitamins

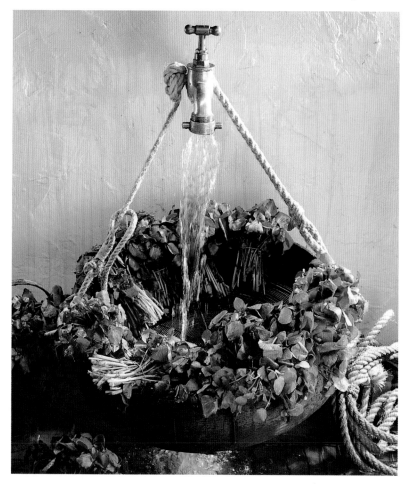

◄ **Cool and fresh**
Watercress, which grows in streams, is at its best in early spring. It should be well washed to remove micro-organisms.

and to prevent the leaves from turning brown, it should be cooked rapidly (microwaving works well) and served at once.

Wheat germ

BENEFITS

- A good source of vitamin E, iron, zinc and thiamin
- Also contains folate, magnesium and fibre

Wheat germ is the nutritional heart of the wheat kernel. The germ is removed during the milling of white flour which, as a result, loses a significant number of important nutrients.

Although it's the smallest part of the grain, the germ is packed with vitamins and minerals, including vitamin E, thiamin, folate, magnesium, iron and zinc.

Two tablespoons of wheat germ _ the amount you might sprinkle over your cereal – contain 36kcal, with good amounts of vitamin E, zinc and vitamin B_6 and useful amounts of other B vitamins, magnesium, copper, potassium, iron and manganese. The same amount of wheat germ has 3g of protein and 1.5g of fibre.

Do one simple thing

Toss a little wheat germ into cakes and puddings

Wheat germ is an exceptionally concentrated source of vitamin E, and this antioxidant may help to prevent cancer, heart disease and vision loss. Take every opportunity to include a little of this delicious whole grain when you're cooking; put it in homemade breads, rice puddings, coffee cakes, apple crumble, pizza dough, pie crusts and homemade biscuits.

Wheat germ may reduce the risk of Type 2 diabetes

It's healthy to eat wheat germ, and it appears to have a positive influence on the risk of diabetes. According to a recent study by Harvard Medical School, eating more wholegrain foods, such as wheat germ, reduces the risk of Type 2 diabetes for women.

Health benefits

Wheat germ offers heart benefits. Its vitamin E is a powerful antioxidant that is linked to heart health as well as a strong immune system. The fat in wheat germ (1g in 2 tablespoons) is predominantly polyunsaturated fat, which can help to lower LDL cholesterol levels when it replaces saturated fat in the diet.

Wheat germ is stabilised to prevent the loss of its vitamins and it is often used to add extra nutrition to foods.

It can be used in baking biscuits, cakes, muffins, breads and pancakes, sprinkled over cereals or salads, added to both meat burgers and veggie burgers, or used as a substitute for breadcrumbs when coating fish, chicken or vegetables.

Once it has been opened, keep the wheat germ tightly sealed and refrigerated to prevent it from going rancid. Wholemeal flour often recombines wheat germ and bran with white flour. Wheat germ oil is particularly rich in vitamin E.

Wine

BENEFITS

- Moderate consumption may decrease the risk of heart disease and certain cancers
- Red wine contains bioflavonoids, phenols and tannins, which have health benefits
- Promotes relaxation

DRAWBACKS

- May trigger allergies and migraine headaches in some people and increase the risk of a rare type of stroke
- Excessive consumption can cause liver disease, cancer and birth defects

Although the art of wine making is some 7,000 years old, the process of fermentation was not understood until the discoveries of Louis Pasteur in the 19th century. Wine tastes good and resists deterioration only after it has undergone fermentation, which is a type of controlled spoilage. Alcohol, a waste product of fermentation, is toxic to all living beings; even the yeasts that excrete it cannot tolerate an environment of more than 15 per cent alcohol, which is why fermentation stops at about this concentration. Most French wines are about 12 per cent alcohol, and Australian and New Zealand wines are about 13 to 14 per cent alcohol. Extra alcohol is added to fortified wines, such as sherry and port.

The components of wine

Red wine is made from purple grapes, but white wine is not necessarily made from white grapes. Many white wines are made from purple grapes, but the skins are removed before they colour the fermenting juice, which is called 'must'. The skins contain most of the bioflavonoids, phenols, tannins and other compounds that give wine its flavour and healthy qualities. The longer the must stays in contact with the skins, the deeper the colour will be. Some dessert wines are made with specially over-ripened grapes to achieve a prized sweetness and a rich consistency.

A small glass (125ml) of red or white wine contains 85kcal. Many varieties have some iron but, more importantly, wine drunk with a meal helps the body to absorb iron from the food.

Wine and the heart

Numerous studies show that a moderate consumption of alcohol – one to two 125ml glasses of wine a day, preferably with a meal – is associated with a lower risk of heart disease. In a research study moderate consumers of red wine were 40 per cent less likely to have a heart attack than those who didn't imbibe. According to a 1991 report, the French had a heart attack rate only a third as high as that of North Americans, despite consuming as much as or more fat than North Americans. Wine consumption may be at least partly responsible for this phenomenon, known as the 'French paradox'. Annual wine consumption in North America is between 8 and 11 litres per person, compared with about 57 litres per person in France.

Researchers have not determined what it is in wine that may prevent heart attacks, but some theorise that compounds such as quercetin and resveratrol in grape skins, as well as other bioflavonoids, may be responsible. These compounds tend to make the blood less sticky and less likely to form clots. It is thought that the French habit of drinking wine with meals may provide the small but regular intake of alcohol needed to reduce clot formation, a cause of most heart attacks.

The bioflavonoids also have anti-oxidant properties and may help to prevent damage to the artery wall and help to keep the arteries dilated. Other research shows that moderate amounts of wine may raise the levels of the protective HDL or 'good', cholesterol.

Other health benefits

Studies are under way, looking at other benefits from the resveratrol found in wine. It is believed that it has a preventive effect on several types of cancer, including colon and prostate cancers. Laboratory studies indicate that the anthocyanin pigments and tannins in wine can fight viruses, but this effect has not been proved in humans. Tannins can inhibit the growth of plaque-forming bacteria on the teeth and may protect against cavity formation.

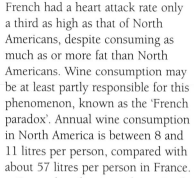

Other studies are exploring the link between the moderate consumption of wine and the lowered risk of dementia.

Some claim that wine makes them sleepier than other alcoholic beverages do; this may be due to ingredients in wine, not the alcohol.

Negative effects

The benefits of moderate wine drinking, which may extend to reducing the risk of some cancers, are lost when daily consumption exceeds two standard drinks for women or four for men. Over-consumption can increase the risk of obesity, stroke, breast cancer, high blood pressure, as well as alcoholism, and cirrhosis and other liver disorders. Even moderate alcohol consumption may raise the risk of haemorrhagic stroke (a burst blood vessel). In addition, heavy use of alcohol in early pregnancy can cause birth defects.

Most wines contain sulphites and preservatives that can trigger allergic reactions in susceptible people. White wine has higher levels of sulphites than red wine. Wine, especially red, is a common trigger of migraines.

W

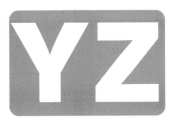

Yams

See also Sweet potatoes
BENEFITS

■ Provides fibre and carbohydrate

■ Useful source of vitamins B$_1$, B$_6$ and C

The staple food crop in much of the tropical world, but particularly in West Africa and New Guinea, the yam grows on a vine and has flesh that is rather like a turnip in texture and ranges in colour from white to bright orange. Some varieties grow to an amazing 2m length and can weigh up to 68kg. The tubers can be stored for up to six months at room temperature.

The yam has almost 50 per cent more protein and more than three times as much complex carbohydrate as the sweet potato (with which it is often confused) and is the better source of energy – 100g of boiled yam provides 133kcal compared with the sweet potato's 84kcal. The yellow-fleshed varieties can be a useful source of beta carotene.

Yeast extracts

BENEFITS

■ An excellent source of most B vitamins

■ Contains potassium and magnesium

■ May be fortified with vitamin B$_{12}$

DRAWBACKS

■ High sodium content

Yeast extract, as well as yeast used in baking and brewing is an excellent source of B vitamins which are needed for maintaining a healthy metabolism. It's also a good source of folate, needed for blood-cell formation, and various minerals, including potassium, magnesium and zinc. However, its high sodium content means that excessive consumption is not advised for people with high blood pressure, or anyone on a low-sodium diet.

Yeast extracts are important source of vitamin B$_{12}$ for vegetarians as it occurs naturally only in foods of animal origin.

Yoghurt

BENEFITS

■ An excellent source of calcium, phosphorus and protein

■ Provides useful amounts of vitamin A, several B vitamins and zinc

■ More digestible than milk for people with lactose intolerance

■ Live yoghurt may help to replace friendly bacteria in the gut after antibiotic treatment

Yoghurt – a protein-rich food that contains valuable immune-enhancing substances – is made by the

Yoghurt goes with everything

■ Fruit smoothie: Combine 125ml natural yoghurt with 150ml diced ripe fruit, add one or two ice cubes and purée in a blender.

■ Yoghurt shake: Blend 125ml fruit-flavoured, frozen nonfat yoghurt with 125ml semi-skimmed milk until creamy.

■ Cucumber dip: Peel, seed and dice a large cucumber and combine with 250ml natural yoghurt, salt, pepper and chopped fresh herbs. Serve as a dip for vegetables, a dressing for salad or a sauce for fish.

■ Mild salsa: Mix 125ml natural yoghurt with 1 mashed ripe avocado, 1 diced tomato and chilli powder to taste. Serve as a dip with tortilla chips or a sauce for enchiladas or hamburgers.

■ Vegetable sauce: Mix natural yoghurt with fresh dill and chopped cashews.

■ Garnish: Top cold cucumber soup or vichyssoise with natural yoghurt and finely sliced chives.

Y

addition of pure cultures of bacteria to pasteurised milk. Fermentation is allowed to proceed until the desired acidity is reached, then it is stopped by cooling the yoghurt. A mixed culture of *Lactobacillus bulgaricus* and *Streptococcus thermophilus* consumes the milk sugar, or lactose, for energy and excretes lactic acid, which curdles the milk. Dried skimmed milk, gelatine or other ingredients may be added for body and taste.

The finished product reflects the fat, mineral and vitamin content of the raw material, whether it be whole or skimmed milk. Fermentation reduces the amount of lactose found in milk, by a third to two-thirds and therefore is more easily digested by people with intolerance to milk.

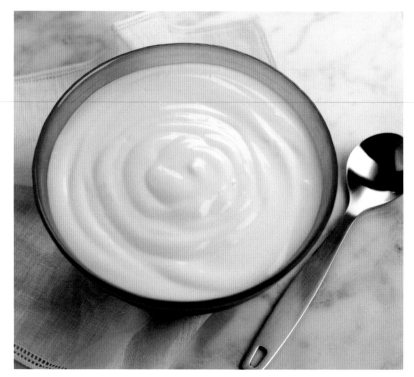

Yoghurt and health

Yoghurt is a healthy food and a useful source of minerals and vitamins. What's more, bio-yoghurts that contain live or 'active' bacteria cultures may help to suppress the growth of harmful micro-organisms in the stomach.

Some scientists question the health benefits of yoghurt, in part because some studies indicate that *L. bulgaricus* does not survive human digestion. But more recent research disputes these findings and backs the age-old observation that yoghurt is useful in restoring normal intestinal flora, the 'friendly' bacteria that inhabit the intestinal tract. Regardless of who is right, eating yoghurt when taking antibiotics (which can upset intestinal flora) does no harm and may be helpful.

It seems to help to relieve gastrointestinal disorders, diarrhoea and constipation. It can also reduce bad breath associated with some digestive disorders.

Yoghurt or any fermented milk product must contain 100 million bacteria per dose to be effective.

It should be absolutely fresh and contain live cultures of acidophilus or bifidobacteria, preferably both. Products that are heavily pasteurised or that have been kept in the refrigerator for too long will have very few active bacteria.

An excellent quick snack and a versatile dessert, yoghurt can be served chilled or frozen, plain or flavoured. Frozen yoghurt contains about 148kcal in a 100ml serving and gives almost the same pleasure as ice cream, with fewer calories and less of the harmful saturated fats.

Because yoghurt contains the same amount of fat as the milk it was made with, low-fat yoghurt is the best choice for people on a low-fat diet. A 200g serving of natural yoghurt made with whole milk contains 166kcal, compared with 132kcal for the same-size glass of whole milk. A 200g serving of natural yoghurt contains 400mg of calcium, about 560mg of potassium and 1.4mg of zinc. Vitamins include 0.4mcg of vitamin B$_{12}$, 36mcg of folate and 0.75mg of riboflavin.

Calorie content rises considerably when sugar and fruit purées are added: 200g of low-fat yoghurt flavoured with fruit and sugar contains about 160kcal.

Low-fat, smooth yoghurts, flavoured with vanilla or toffee, contain 48-50kcal per 120g pot, with only 0.1g of saturated fats, but sugar content is quite high at 6.6g. These virtually fat-free yoghurts have the fewest calories of any of the dessert yoghurts available in supermarkets.

High-fibre yoghurts with added soluble fibre are being promoted for their cholesterol-lowering properties. They are also claimed to promote a feeling of fullness.

Greek-style yoghurts, usually made with ewe's milk, contain about 160kcal per 150g pot.

Yoghurt can be made at home by mixing a few spoons of commercial yoghurt that is made with live cultures into low-fat milk and leaving the covered mixture overnight at lukewarm or room temperature.

Z

Glossary

adipocyte A fat cell.

adrenaline An adrenal hormone that prepares the body to react to stressful situations.

aflatoxin A toxin produced by moulds that grow mainly on peanuts, cottonseed and corn.

ajoenes Phytochemicals, found in garlic, that reduce LDL ('bad') cholesterol and may have anti-clotting, anti-cancer and anti-fungal properties.

albumen A protein, found in most animal and many plant tissues, that coagulates on heating.

allicin A chemical that forms when garlic is crushed or cut and may help to reduce LDL cholesterol levels. Responsible for garlic's pungent smell, allicin produces many sulphur compounds, possibly with antibacterial properties.

allyl sulphides Found in garlic, onions, leeks, shallots and other members of the onion family, these sulphur compounds help to lower the risk of heart disease, stimulate the immune system and are under review for their potential to fight cancer.

alpha carotene Like beta carotene, alpha carotene is an antioxidant carotenoid and a precursor to vitamin A. It is found in apricots, carrots, pumpkins and orange-fleshed sweet potatoes.

alpha linolenic acid An omega-3 essential fatty acid that cannot be made in the body and so must be obtained from foods. ALA is important for the maintenance of cell membranes and for creating substances in the body that protect against inflammatory conditions. ALA may be converted in the human body into two omega-3 fatty acids: EPA (eicosapentaenoic acid) and DHA (docosahexaenoic acid) – but this conversion is not very efficient. It is found in linseeds, rapeseed oil, soya bean oil and walnuts. Smaller amounts are also in dark green leafy vegetables.

amino acids The building blocks of protein. Twenty amino acids are necessary for proper human growth and function. Nine amino acids are termed essential, because they must be provided in the diet; the body produces the remaining 11 as they are needed.

anthocyanins Responsible for the red and blue pigments found in certain fruit and vegetables, anthocyanins are flavonoids with the potential to suppress tumour cell growth, to lower LDL ('bad') cholesterol levels and to prevent blood from forming clots. They are found in apples, berries, cherries, cranberries, blackcurrants, red and black grapes, plums and pomegranates.

antigen A foreign substance that stimulates the body to defend itself with an immune response.

arteriosclerosis The stiffening and hardening of the arterial walls.

bacteria Single-celled micro-organisms that are found in air, food, water, soil and in other living creatures, including humans. 'Friendly' bacteria prevent infection and synthesise certain vitamins; others cause disease.

basal metabolic rate The energy that is required by the human body in order to maintain vital processes during a 24 hour period.

beta carotene One of the most studied of the carotenoids, beta carotene is a potent antioxidant plentiful in red, orange and yellow plant foods (as well as in dark green vegetables where the orange colour is masked by chlorophyll). It is converted by the body into vitamin A. Food sources include: apricots, carrots, Brussels sprouts, dark leafy greens, green peas, pumpkin, spinach and orange-fleshed sweet potatoes.

beta glucan A type of soluble dietary fibre that helps to lower blood cholesterol levels. It is found in oats, oat bran, barley, brown rice bran and shiitake mushrooms.

beta sitosterol A plant sterol similar in structure to cholesterol, beta sitosterol may help to manage benign prostatic hyperplasia (BPH), as well as protect against high cholesterol and cancer. It is found in avocados, corn oil, rice bran, seeds, soya foods and wheat germ.

B-group vitamins Although not chemically related to one another, many of the eight B vitamins occur in the same foods, and most of them perform closely linked tasks within the body, mostly by helping enzymes carry out their work. B vitamins are known by numbers or names, or both: B_1, thiamin; B_2, riboflavin; B_3, niacin; B_5, pantothenic acid; B_6, pyridoxine; B_{12}, cobalamin; biotin; and folate.

boron This bone-nourishing mineral is thought to enhance the body's ability to use calcium, magnesium and vitamin D. It is found in beans and nuts.

bromelain An enzyme derived from pineapples, bromelain is believed to have anti-inflammatory and pain-reducing properties.

calories Basic units for measuring the energy value of food and the energy needs of the body. One calorie is so small that figures are expressed as units of 1,000 calories or kilocalories (kcal), Calories with a capital C or, loosely, calories.

carotenoids Pigments that give certain foods their characteristic orange, yellow and red colours. They may possess potent anti-oxidant properties to fight heart disease, certain types of cancer as well as degenerative eye diseases such as cataracts and macular degeneration. To date, more than 600 carotenoids have been identified, including alpha carotene, beta carotene, beta cryptoxanthin, lutein, lycopene and zeaxanthin.

cellulose One of the main ingredients of plant cell walls, this indigestible carbohydrate is an important source of insoluble fibre.

chlorophyll The green pigment of leaves and plants, chlorophyll helps to freshen breath. Sources include dark leafy greens, kiwi fruit, parsley, peas and peppers.

coenzymes Compounds that work with enzymes to promote biological processes. A coenzyme may be a vitamin, contain a vitamin or be manufactured in the body from a vitamin.

collagen Fibrous protein that helps to hold cells and tissue together.

complementary proteins These are proteins that lack one or more of the essential amino acids but which, when paired, can supply a complete protein. For example, grains are high in the essential amino acid methionine, but they lack lysine. This essential amino acid is plentiful in dried beans, peanuts and other legumes, which are deficient in methionine. By combining a grain food with a legume, a complete range of amino acids is obtained.

complete protein Contains all the essential amino acids. It is found in single animal foods; it can also be constructed by combining two or more complementary plant foods.

complex carbohydrates Starches in legumes, vegetables and grains are complex carbohydrates. A diet rich in complex carbohydrates can help to protect against cardiovascular disease, control blood sugar levels, relieve diarrhoea and ease insomnia. Sources include fruit, grains, legumes, potatoes, pasta and rice.

cruciferous vegetables A family of phytochemical-rich vegetables named for their cross-shaped flowers, cruciferous vegetables are valued for their compounds that exhibit cancer-fighting activity in laboratory studies. Cruciferous vegetables include bok choy, broccoli, Brussels sprouts, cabbage, cauliflower, kale, mustard greens, radishes, rocket, turnips and watercress.

deoxyribonucleic acid (DNA) The basic genetic material of all cells, DNA is the 'genetic blueprint' that causes characteristics to be passed on from one generation to the next.

DHA An omega-3 fatty acid, DHA (docosahexaenoic acid) is important for all phases of the human life cycle. A major building block of human brain tissue and the primary structural fatty acid in the grey matter of the brain and the retina, DHA is vital for brain and eye health. Studies indicate that DHA may have cardiovascular benefits as well as neurological benefits. Although the body has enzymes that convert alpha-linolenic acid to DHA, you get it much more efficiently by eating oil-rich fish, including herring, mackerel, salmon, sardines and trout.

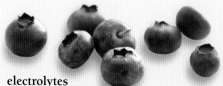

electrolytes Substances that separate into ions that conduct electricity when fused or dissolved in fluids. In the human body, sodium, potassium and chloride are electrolytes essential for nerve and muscle function and for maintaining the fluid balance as well as the acid-alkali balance of cells and tissues.

ellagic acid A phenolic compound with potent antioxidant capabilities, ellagic acid is thought to fight cancer by inducing cancer cell death as well as by neutralising carcinogens such as tobacco smoke or air pollution. Sources include apples, apricots, berries, grapes, pomegranates and walnuts.

endorphins Natural painkillers made by the brain, with effects similar to those of opium-based drugs, such as morphine.

enzymes Protein molecules that are catalysts for many of the chemical reactions that take place in the body.

EPA An omega-3 fatty acid, eicosapentaenoic acid (EPA) is linked to cardiovascular and anti-cancer benefits, and may help to improve inflammatory conditions such as rheumatoid arthritis. Although the body has enzymes that convert alpha linolenic acid to EPA, you get it much more directly and more efficiently by eating oily fish and other seafood.

essential fatty acids (EFAs) The building blocks of necessary fats, EFAs must be obtained through foods. They help to form cell membranes, aid in immune function and produce important hormones. Food sources include vegetables, oils, fish (such as herring, mackerel, salmon, sardines and trout), flax or linseeds, sunflower seeds, walnuts and wheat germ.

fibre, insoluble Made of the indigestible parts of plants, it adds bulk to stools, slowing their transit through the digestive system and easing elimination. Insoluble fibre may promote satiety as well. Sources include wheat bran, whole grains, fruit and vegetables.

fibre, soluble Soluble fibre forms a gel-like mass around food particles, that slows down the rate of digestion and absorption and prevents cholesterol from being absorbed. Pectin and beta glucan are two types of soluble fibre that are particularly good for lowering cholesterol levels. Soluble fibre also helps to manage diarrhoea and may regulate levels of blood glucose as well. Sources include apples, barley, beans and lentils, citrus fruit, peas, oats and psyllium.

flavonoids Powerful antioxidants, flavonoids are phytochemicals linked to a reduced risk of cardio-vascular disease and may impede the development of cancer. The free-radical scavenging properties of flavonoids are thought to inhibit clot formation, act as natural antibiotics, slow age-related decline in memory function, bolster blood vessels and improve the potency of immune cells. Some important flavonoid compounds include anthocyanins, hesperidin, isoflavones, quercetin and resveratrol. They are found in fruit, grains, tea, vegetables and wine.

free radicals Unstable, highly reactive molecules that are the products of metabolism and also form as a result of environmental pollution such as cigarette smoke. Free radicals contribute to 'oxidative stress', which is implicated in premature ageing as well as the onset of many diseases.

fructo-oligosaccharides (FOS) Indigestible carbohydrate compounds, FOS are thought to encourage the growth of friendly bacteria in the body and may reduce the number of toxins produced by unfriendly flora in the colon. They are found in asparagus, bananas, garlic, onions and Jerusalem artichokes.

gamma linolenic acid One of the omega-6 fatty acids found in evening primrose oil.

genistein A potent isoflavone with oestrogen-like activity, genistein may help to balance hormones and might reduce the risk for hormone-related cancer, such as prostate cancer, as well as helping to prevent fibrocystic breasts and premenstrual syndrome. It is found primarily in soya products.

glucose A simple sugar (mono-saccharide) that is the body's prime energy source. Blood levels of glucose are regulated by several hormones, including insulin.

gluten A protein in barley, rye and wheat. Certain people, particularly those with coeliac disease, have an intolerance to it and must avoid foods made with these grains through-out life. Failure to do so can lead to anaemia, osteoporosis and other problems.

glycogen A form of glucose which is stored in the liver and muscles, which is converted back into glucose when needed.

goitrogens When eaten in large quantities, goitrogens in uncooked foods have the potential to interfere with the absorption of iodine and slow thyroid function. Goitrogens are primarily found in cabbage, turnips, mustard greens and radishes, but only in small quantities.

haem iron Found in animal foods such as red meat, pork, fish and poultry; the body absorbs about four times as much haem iron as non-haem iron, which is found in plants and eggs.

haemoglobin The iron-containing pigment in our red blood cells that carries oxygen.

hesperidin A flavonoid found in citrus fruit and juices, hesperidin may improve the integrity of capillary linings.

high-density lipoproteins (HDLs) The smallest and 'heaviest' lipo-proteins, they retrieve cholesterol from the tissues and transport it to the liver to be removed from the body; called 'good cholesterol', because high blood levels of HDLs are considered desirable in lowering heart disease risk.

histamine A chemical in the body's immune defence, it is released during allergic reactions to cause swelling, itching, rash and sneezing.

homocysteine A compound resulting from the breakdown of methionine, an essential amino acid, At high levels in the blood, homo-cysteine increases the risk of atherosclerosis and possibly other serious conditions. An estimated 20 to 40 per cent of people with clogged arteries, or those who have suffered strokes or heart attacks, have abnormally high levels of homocysteine. Researchers have discovered that several B vitamins, folate, vitamin B_6 and B_{12}, can help to lower homocysteine levels.

hormones Chemicals, secreted by the endocrine glands, that trigger body activities, including growth, development and reproduction.

hydrogenation A process used to make liquid oil more solid. This process lengthens shelf life and provides the stability of many baked goods and processed foods. But the process creates trans fatty acids, which raise LDL ('bad' cholesterol) and lower HDL ('good' cholesterol), increasing the risk of heart disease.

incomplete proteins Proteins, usually from plant sources, that lack one or more essential amino acids.

indoles Partially responsible for the strong taste of broccoli and Brussels sprouts, indoles are glucosinolate phytochemicals in cruciferous vegetables and may stimulate cancer-fighting enzymes.

indole-3 carbinol A well-studied compound and a member of the glucosinolate phytochemical family, indole-3-carbinol is abundant in broccoli and other cruciferous vegetables. It may offer protection against hormone-dependent cancers, such as breast cancer.

insulin A hormone that regulates the metabolism of carbohydrates.

isoflavones Found primarily in soya foods, isoflavones are a major class of phyto-oestrogens, plant chemicals with mild oestrogen activity. Genistein and daidzein are the most prominent isoflavones. Soya isoflavones are being studied for their potential to ease the symptoms of menopause and to protect against osteoporosis-related fractures, Alzheimer's disease, high cholesterol and hormone-dependent

cancers, such as breast and prostate cancer.

ketones Potentially toxic waste products produced from the body's partial burning of fatty acids for fuel.

kilojoule Another basic unit of measurement for the energy value of food and the energy needs of the body. Its symbol is kJ. $1kJ = 4.2kcal$.

lecithin A phospholipid constituent of cell membranes and lipoproteins, lecithin is a natural emulsifier that helps to stabilise cholesterol in the bile. Lecithin is not an essential nutrient, because it is synthesised by the liver.

lentinan A polysaccharide (carbohydrate compound) extracted from shiitake mushrooms, lentinan may enhance immunity, as well as protect against cancer, high blood pressure and high cholesterol.

lignans Phyto-oestrogens with mild oestrogen-like activity. They may have anti-tumour effects, antimicrobial benefits and provide relief from PMS and protection against osteoporosis. Food sources include ground linseeds or flaxseeds, linseed oil, and soya foods and grains.

limonene A phytochemical found in lemons, limes and oranges. Its potential to inhibit tumours and protect the lungs is being studied.

linoleic acid One of the omega-6 essential fatty acids.

lipid A fatty compound made of hydrogen, carbon and oxygen, lipids are insoluble in water. The chemical family includes fats, fatty acids, oils, cholesterol and waxes.

lipoprotein A lipid and protein combined, that carries cholesterol in the bloodstream. The main types are high density (HDL), low density (LDL) and very low density (VLDL).

low-density lipoproteins (LDLs) These so-called 'bad' lipoproteins carry most of the circulating cholesterol; high levels are associated with atherosclerosis and heart disease since this form of cholesterol builds up on artery walls.

lutein and zeaxanthin Found in foods that are bright yellow, orange and green, lutein and zeaxanthin are pigments in the carotenoid family that are linked to a reduced risk of cataracts and macular degeneration. Lutein is found in green leafy vegetables such as rocket, kale, spinach and watercress, as well as corn and egg yolks. Zeaxanthin is found in vegetable greens, red peppers and sweetcorn.

lycopene A powerful antioxidant that lends red colour to tomatoes and tomato products, pink grapefruit and watermelon. Studies have shown lycopene to be protective against prostate cancer and possibly lung cancer, and heart disease.

macronutrients Our food provides two types of essential building blocks, or nutrients, known as macronutrients and micronutrients. Most food is primarily water, a macronutrient. The remaining macronutrients – carbohydrate, protein and fat – are vital energy-yielding nutrients that work in harmony with micronutrients to keep the body functioning well.

metabolism The collective term for the body's physical and chemical processes that are needed to maintain life, including the derivation of energy from food.

micronutrients Required in small amounts, vitamins and minerals are non-calorie essential nutrients. Vital for normal growth, development and good health. Micronutrients promote and regulate chemical reactions vital for life and participate in all body processes, such as getting energy from macronutrients, transmitting nerve impulses and battling infections.

monoterpenes A family of phytochemicals that includes limonene, monoterpenes are studied for their ability to detoxify carcinogens, slow cancer cell growth and lower cholesterol levels. Food sources include cherries, citrus fruit, olive oil, caraway, dill and spearmint.

monounsaturated fat Found in olive oil, rapeseed oil, peanut oil, some margarine, avocado, nuts and seeds, heart-healthy mono-unsaturated fat is not easily damaged by oxidation, so is less likely than saturated fat and trans fats to clog arteries. When eaten in place of saturated and trans fats, monounsaturated fats help to lower LDL cholesterol levels.

neurotransmitters Chemicals released from nerve endings that relay messages from cell to cell.

nitrates Nitrogen-containing compounds that occur naturally in certain foods, nitrates are used as preservatives in some meat products, as fertilisers and also in vasodilator drugs.

nitrites These are compounds that are produced in the body by the action of bacteria on nitrates. Nitrites are also used as meat preservatives.

nitrosamines Compounds that are formed in food or in the body through the reaction of nitrites with amines. They are considered carcinogens, although no definite link has been established between nitrosamines and cancer in humans.

oleic acid When consumed in place of saturated fat, this mono-unsaturated fat is linked to healthier cholesterol levels. Food sources include olive oil, rapeseed oil and avocados.

oxalates Found most in green vegetables, oxalates are compounds that can bind the calcium, iron and zinc in vegetables, blocking their absorption in the body. They do not block absorption of minerals from other foods consumed at the same meal. Food sources include beetroot tops, chocolate, nuts, parsley, rhubarb, spinach, tea, cranberries, strawberries, and wheat bran.

oxidation This is a chemical process that burns food with oxygen to release energy.

pasteurisation The process of heating milk or other fluids to destroy micro-organisms that might cause disease.

pectin A soluble fibre that helps to lower artery-damaging LDL cholesterol. Pectin may also be useful for managing diarrhoea and diabetes. Sources include apples, apricots, bananas, carrots, figs, kiwi fruit and sweet potatoes.

peristalsis Muscle contractions that help food and fluids to move along through the digestive tract.

phenylketonuria (PKU) Caused by a genetic defect that prevents the metabolism of the amino acid phenylalanine. People with PKU are identified at birth and must follow a low-phenylalanine diet and avoid aspartame which is most commonly found in artificial sweeteners and desserts that may make low-calorie claims.

phytochemicals Naturally occurring plant chemicals that offer protection against a variety of diseases.

phyto-oestrogens Compounds found in plants that exhibit oestrogen-like activity and may lower the risk of hormone-related cancers, as well as relieve fibrocystic breasts, osteoarthritis and symptoms of the menopause. The two major classes of phyto-oestrogens are isoflavones and lignans. Food sources include beans and soya.

plasma The clear yellow fluid that makes up about 55 per cent of the blood and carries cells, platelets and vital nutrients throughout the body.

platelets Disc-shaped cells, made in the bone marrow, that are needed for blood coagulation.

polyphenols A class of antioxidants, polyphenol phytochemicals are studied for their potential to suppress tumour growth, detoxify carcinogens, interfere with the damaging effects of high oestrogen levels, lower the risk of stroke, and prevent plaque build-up in the arteries. Sources include fruit, vegetables, extra virgin olive oil, tea and red wine.

polyunsaturated fats Fats which contain a high percentage of fatty acids that lack hydrogen atoms and have extra carbon bonds. They are liquid at room temperature (corn and sunflower oils, for instance) unless hydrogen is added. When hydrogen is added, these fats become more like saturated fats and have an adverse effect on blood cholesterol.

prostaglandins Chemicals involved in many body processes, including allergic reaction, inflammation, blood clotting, pain sensitivity and smooth muscle contraction.

purines Compounds that form uric acid when metabolised, purines are found in a number of foods, particularly high-protein foods, such as offal. Caffeine (in coffee and tea), theobromine (in chocolate) and theophylline (in tea) are related compounds. People prone to gout or kidney stones should avoid high levels of purines.

pyridoxine One of the B vitamins, more commonly called B_6, it is essential for protein metabolism and the production of red blood cells. It is important for a healthy nervous and immune system. Food sources include meat, fish, whole grains, avocado, banana and potatoes.

quercetin Red onions, apples, grapes, red wine and berries are rich sources of quercetin, a potent flavonoid linked to a reduced risk of cancer, cardiovascular disease and cataracts.

resveratrol A phytochemical abundant in the skin of red grapes, it is studied for its potential to improve cholesterol levels, prevent atherosclerosis, and reduce the risks for stroke and cancer. Sources include red and black grape juice and red wine.

ribonucleic acid (RNA) It is a substance present in every cell that translates the information contained in DNA into instructions telling the cell which proteins to synthesise.

salicylates Compounds related to salicylic acid, used for making aspirin and other painkillers and as a preservative. Naturally occurring salicylates in fruit or vegetables, honey or tea may produce allergic reactions in people who are sensitive to aspirin.

salmonella Bacteria that are a frequent cause of food poisoning.

saturated fat Fat found in animal products such as meat and full-fat dairy products, as well as oils such as palm and coconut, and also formed during the processing of oils. They are linked to an increased risk of heart disease, certain cancers and other diseases.

serotonin A neurotransmitter that helps to promote sleep and regulates many body processes, including pain perception and the secretion of pituitary hormones.

sucrose Better known as table sugar, sucrose is composed of glucose and fructose. It is obtained from sugar cane; small quantities are also present in honey, fruit and vegetables.

sulphoraphane A notable sulphur compound, sulphoraphane may increase the activity of cancer-fighting enzymes in the body, reduce tumour growth, block carcinogens from initiating cancer and fight hormone-related cancer. Best food sources are broccoli and cabbage.

sulphur compounds These phytochemicals containing sulphur, are abundant in garlic and the onion family, and include allyl sulphide and ajoenes. Certain sulphur compounds are thought to stimulate cancer-fighting enzymes.

tannins Also called proanthocyanidins, tannins may detoxify carcinogens and scavenge harmful free radicals. The tannins in cranberries may protect against urinary tract infections. Tannins reduce the absorption of iron. Sources include blackberries, blueberries, cranberries, grapes, lentils, tea and wine.

toxins Poisons produced by living organisms – plants, animals or bacteria – that, when introduced into the body, are capable of causing an adverse effect.

trans fatty acids Fats that are formed when vegetable oils are hydrogenated to improve their stability and make them more solid. A food that lists 'hydrogenated vegetable oil' on its list of ingredients contains trans fatty acids. Research suggests that high intakes of trans fatty acids may contribute to heart disease by elevating LDL ('bad') cholesterol and reducing HDL ('good') cholesterol.

triglycerides The most common form of dietary and body fat; high blood triglyceride levels have been linked to heart disease.

tryptophan An essential amino acid, tryptophan is converted by the body into the B vitamin niacin. Tryptophan stimulates production of serotonin, a neurotransmitter that supports mental health. Complex carbohydrates enhance the absorption and use of tryptophan in the brain.

uric acid A nitrogen-containing waste product of the metabolism of protein, uric acid causes gout when it builds up.

zeaxanthin See *lutein and zeaxanthin*.

Index

*Headwords in **bold** indicate main entries in the book.

Editor Rachel Warren Chadd

Assistant editor Jill Steed

Art editor Conorde Clarke

Proofreader Barry Gage

Indexer Marie Lorimer

Reader's Digest, London

Editorial director Julian Browne

Art director Anne-Marie Bulat

Head of book development Sarah Bloxham

Managing editor Nina Hathway

Picture resource manager Sarah Stewart-Richardson

Pre-press account manager Dean Russell

Production Editor Rachel Weaver

Product production manager Claudette Bramble

Production controller Katherine Bunn

Origination Colour Systems Limited, London

Printed and bound in China

Adapted from Foods that Harm, Foods that Heal
Second edition published in 2006 by
Reader's Digest (Australia) Pty Limited

Photo Credits

13 Stockbyte. **43** Alan Richardson. **48** Stockbyte. **50** Creatas.
81 Jay Hostetler/Still Life Stock. **87** Tim O'Leary/Taxi/Getty
Images Ltd. **105** Douglas Kirkland/Corbis. **111** H. Amiard.
140 *b* Corbis. **171** Julia Bigg. **238** *b* Charles Gold/Corbis.
299 *b* Annie Griffiths Belt/Corbis. **300** Corbis. **376** Corbis.
384 *b* Corbis. **389** Gerrit Buntrock/The Anthony Blake
Photo Library.

Additional photo acknowledgments:

Digital Stock, Digitalvision, Image100, Index Stock, PhotoDisc,
PictureQuest, and The Reader's Digest Association, Inc./GID

Foods that Harm, Foods that Heal

was published by
The Reader's Digest Association Limited
11 Westferry Circus, Canary Wharf
London E14 4HE

Revised and updated edition copyright © 2007
Reprinted 2008

First edition copyright © 1996

We are committed both to the quality
of our products and the service we
provide to our customers. We value your
comments, so please do contact us on
08705 113366 or via our website at
www.readersdigest.co.uk
If you have any comments or suggestions
about the content of our books, email us at
gbeditorial@readersdigest.co.uk

Book code 400-323 UP0000-3
ISBN 978 0 276 44229 2
Concept code SA 0200/IC
Oracle code 250010600H.00.24